Handbook of Nutraceuticals and Natural Products

Handbook of Nutraceuticals and Natural Products

Biological, Medicinal, and Nutritional Properties and Applications

Volume 2

Edited by

Preetha Balakrishnan

Sreerag Gopi
ADSO Naturals Private Limited
Bangalore, India

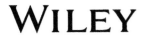

This edition first published 2022
© 2022 John Wiley & Sons, Inc.

The right of Preetha Balakrishnan and Sreerag Gopi to be identified as the authors of the editorial material in this work has been asserted in accordance with law.

Registered Office
John Wiley & Sons, Inc., 111 River Street, Hoboken, NJ 07030, USA

Editorial Office
111 River Street, Hoboken, NJ 07030, USA

For details of our global editorial offices, customer services, and more information about Wiley products visit us at www.wiley.com.

Wiley also publishes its books in a variety of electronic formats and by print-on-demand. Some content that appears in standard print versions of this book may not be available in other formats.

Limit of Liability/Disclaimer of Warranty
In view of ongoing research, equipment modifications, changes in governmental regulations, and the constant flow of information relating to the use of experimental reagents, equipment, and devices, the reader is urged to review and evaluate the information provided in the package insert or instructions for each chemical, piece of equipment, reagent, or device for, among other things, any changes in the instructions or indication of usage and for added warnings and precautions. While the publisher and authors have used their best efforts in preparing this work, they make no representations or warranties with respect to the accuracy or completeness of the contents of this work and specifically disclaim all warranties, including without limitation any implied warranties of merchantability or fitness for a particular purpose. No warranty may be created or extended by sales representatives, written sales materials or promotional statements for this work. The fact that an organization, website, or product is referred to in this work as a citation and/or potential source of further information does not mean that the publisher and authors endorse the information or services the organization, website, or product may provide or recommendations it may make. This work is sold with the understanding that the publisher is not engaged in rendering professional services. The advice and strategies contained herein may not be suitable for your situation. You should consult with a specialist where appropriate. Further, readers should be aware that websites listed in this work may have changed or disappeared between when this work was written and when it is read. Neither the publisher nor authors shall be liable for any loss of profit or any other commercial damages, including but not limited to special, incidental, consequential, or other damages.

Library of Congress Cataloging-in-Publication Data applied for:

9781119746812[hard back]
9781119746799[set]

Cover Design: Wiley
Cover Images: © Kseniya Tatarnikova/Shutterstock; Anna-Ok/Getty Images

Set in 9.5/12.5pt STIXTwoText by Straive, Pondicherry, India

Contents

List of Contributors

Himanshu Agrawal
Molecular Endocrinology Laboratory,
Department of Biotechnology,
Indian Institute of Technology Roorkee,
Roorkee, Uttarakhand, India

Iffath Badsha
Department of Nanotechnology,
Anna University, Chennai, Tamil Nadu, India

Siddhi Bagwe-Parab
Department of Pharmacology, Shobhaben
Pratapbhai Patel School of Pharmacy &
Technology Management, SVKM's NMIMS,
Mumbai, Maharashtra, India

Harpal S. Buttar
Department of Pathology and Laboratory
Medicine, Faculty of Medicine, University of
Ottawa, Ottawa, ON, Canada

Xiao Chen
School of Chemical Sciences, University of
Auckland, Auckland, New Zealand

Ritu Dahiya
Department of Pharmacology, Delhi
Pharmaceutical Science and Research
University, New Delhi, Delhi, India

Neeladrisingha Das
Molecular Endocrinology Laboratory,
Department of Biotechnology,
Indian Institute of Technology Roorkee,
Roorkee, Uttarakhand, India

Emmanuel Duhoranimana
Department of Biotechnologies, Faculty of
Applied Fundamental Sciences, Institutes
of Applied Sciences, INES-Ruhengeri,
Ruhengeri, Republic of Rwanda

Jean Claude Dusabumuremyi
Department of Biotechnologies, Faculty of
Applied Fundamental Sciences, Institutes
of Applied Sciences, INES-Ruhengeri,
Ruhengeri, Republic of Rwanda

Hassan Esmaeili
Department of Horticultural Science, School
of Agriculture, Shiraz University,
Shiraz, Iran
Department of Agriculture,
Medicinal Plants and Drugs Research Institute,
Shahid Beheshti University,
Tehran, Iran

Souvik Ghosh
Molecular Endocrinology Laboratory,
Department of Biotechnology, Indian
Institute of Technology Roorkee, Roorkee,
Uttarakhand, India
Tissue Engineering Laboratory, Centre
of Nanotechnology, Indian Institute of
Technology Roorkee, Roorkee,
Uttarakhand, India

Suresh K. Gupta
Department of Pharmacology, Delhi
Pharmaceutical Science and Research
University, New Delhi, Delhi, India

L. Inbathamizh
Department of Biotechnology, School of Bio
and Chemical Engineering, Sathyabama
Institute of Science and Technology,
Chennai, Tamil Nadu, India

Akbar Karami
Department of Horticultural Science, School
of Agriculture, Shiraz University, Shiraz, Iran

Ginpreet Kaur
Department of Pharmacology, Shobhaben
Pratapbhai Patel School of Pharmacy &
Technology Management, SVKM's NMIMS,
Mumbai, Maharashtra, India

Viney Kumar
Molecular Endocrinology Laboratory,
Department of Biotechnology,
Indian Institute of Technology Roorkee,
Roorkee, Uttarakhand, India

Deo Paranav Milind
Molecular Endocrinology Laboratory,
Department of Biotechnology, Indian
Institute of Technology Roorkee, Roorkee,
Uttarakhand, India

C. Valli Nachiyar
Department of Biotechnology, Sathyabama
Institute of Science and Technology, Chennai,
Tamil Nadu, India

S. Karthick Raja Namasivayam
Department of Biotechnology, Sathyabama
Institute of Science and Technology, Chennai,
Tamil Nadu, India

Sandip Nathani
Molecular Endocrinology Laboratory,
Department of Biotechnology, Indian
Institute of Technology Roorkee, Roorkee,
Uttarakhand, India

Jayshree Nellore
Department of Biotechnology,
Sathyabama Institute of Science and
Technology, Chennai,
Tamil Nadu, India

Harvinder Popli
Department of Pharmacy, Delhi
Pharmaceutical Sciences and Research
University, New Delhi,
Delhi, India

D. Prabavathy
Department of Biotechnology, School of Bio
and Chemical Engineering, Sathyabama
Institute of Science and Technology,
Chennai, Tamil Nadu, India

G. Ranimol
Department of Biotechnology Engineering,
Sahrdaya College of Engineering and
Technology, Thrissur,
Kerala, India

K. Renugadevi
Department of Biotechnology, Sathyabama
Institute of Science and Technology,
Chennai, Tamil Nadu, India

Partha Roy
Molecular Endocrinology Laboratory,
Department of Biotechnology,
Indian Institute of Technology
Roorkee, Roorkee,
Uttarakhand, India

Divya Sachdev
Department of Basic and Applied Sciences,
National Institute of Food Technology,
Entrepreneurship and Management,
Sonipat, Haryana, India

Saakshi Saini
Molecular Endocrinology Laboratory,
Department of Biotechnology,
Indian Institute of Technology
Roorkee, Roorkee,
Uttarakhand, India

D.P. Shivaprasad
Department of Basic and Applied Sciences,
National Institute of Food Technology,
Entrepreneurship and Management, Sonipat,
Haryana, India

Amritpal Singh
Department of Basic and Applied Sciences,
National Institute of Food Technology,
Entrepreneurship and Management, Sonipat,
Haryana, India

Debabrata Sircar
Plant Molecular Biology Laboratory,
Department of Biotechnology, Indian
Institute of Technology Roorkee, Roorkee,
Uttarakhand, India

S. Sudha
Department of Biotechnology, School of Bio
and Chemical Engineering, Sathyabama
Institute of Science and Technology, Chennai,
Tamil Nadu, India

Swetha Sunkar
Department of Bioinformatics, Sathyabama
Institute of Science and Technology,
Chennai, Tamil Nadu, India

Neetu Kumra Taneja
Department of Basic and Applied Sciences,
National Institute of Food Technology,
Entrepreneurship and Management,
Sonipat, Haryana, India

Pankaj Taneja
Department of Biotechnology,
Sharda University, Greater Noida,
Uttar Pradesh, India

Pratik Yadav
Department of Pharmacology,
Shobhaben Pratapbhai Patel School of
Pharmacy & Technology Management,
SVKM's NMIMS, Mumbai,
Maharashtra, India

Preface of Volume 2

Handbook of Nutraceuticals and Natural Products – Biological, Medicinal, and Nutritional Properties and Applications

Nutraceuticals and Natural Product analyzes the nutraceutical and natural product research published over the last decade, paying particular attention to applications and recovery effects. The book emphasizes the great need for both nutritionists and pharmacologists to understand how these drugs can benefit human health. Topics explore innovative sources, bioavailability, pharmacokinetics, translating novel pathways and mechanisms of action into their clinical use, personalized nutrition and natural product medicine, the convergence between nutraceuticals and western medicine, interactions between drugs, nutrients, the microbiome and lifestyles, industrial applications and commercialization, metabolomics, nano-delivery systems and function, and more. Nutraceutical is the hybrid of "nutrition" and "pharmaceutical." Nutraceuticals, in broad, are food or part of food playing a significant role in modifying and maintaining normal physiological function that maintains healthy human beings. The principal reasons for the growth of the nutraceutical market worldwide are the current population and the health trends. The food products used as nutraceuticals can be categorized as dietary fiber, prebiotics, probiotics, polyunsaturated fatty acids, antioxidants, and other different types of herbal/natural foods. These nutraceuticals help in combating some of the major health problems of the century such as obesity, cardiovascular diseases, cancer, osteoporosis, arthritis, diabetes, cholesterol, etc. In whole, "nutraceutical" has led to the new era of medicine and health, in which the food industry has become a research-oriented sector.

This book addresses (14 chapters) nutraceutical/natural product development from a number of perspectives: the process itself, health research that may provide opportunities, idea creation, regulation, and processes and ingredients. It also features case studies that illustrate real product development and commercialization histories. Written for food scientists and technologists, and scientists working in related fields, the book presents practical information for use in functional food product development. It is intended for use by practitioners in functional food companies and food technology centers and will also be of interest to researchers and students of food science.

The first chapter discusses about the nutritional supplements in health care. As the title indicates, the following chapters focus mainly on the preventive and health care aspects of nutraceuticals and functional foods. Topics on regulations and safety were also taken into consideration. The chapter contributors of this book are respected authors and professionals from key institutions around the world. The primary target audience for this book are users of functional foods, food supplements, and nutraceuticals, food technology students, nutritionists, researchers on natural products and phytochemistry, chemistry students, and public and private health practitioners. Additionally, the general public will find this book useful.

1

Nutritional Supplements in Health Care

Iffath Badsha[1], C. Valli Nachiyar[2], S. Karthick Raja Namasivayam[2], K. Renugadevi[2], Swetha Sunkar[3], and Jayshree Nellore[2]

[1] *Department of Nanotechnology, Anna University, Chennai, Tamil Nadu, India*
[2] *Department of Biotechnology, Sathyabama Institute of Science and Technology, Chennai, Tamil Nadu, India*
[3] *Department of Bioinformatics, Sathyabama Institute of Science and Technology, Chennai, Tamil Nadu, India*

1.1 Nutritional Supplements

A nutritional supplement can be defined as any nutrient compound that is added to the diet to benefit human health. These nutritional supplements are used worldwide and represent a broad array of ingestible products that are distinguishable from conventional foods and drugs and are intended to meet essential nutritional requirements. These nutritional supplements include several probiotics, plant-derived, and animal-derived products. The class of nutrient compounds comprises of vitamins, minerals, amino acids, fatty acids, and carbohydrates (Hollenstein 1994; Mason 2011; Watson et al. 2011), which can be either extracted from natural or from synthetic sources either individually or in combination (Cupp and Tracy 2003; Begins and Kreft 2014).

The products sold as nutritional supplements are available in many forms such as tablets, capsules, gelatin capsules, soft gels, liquids, lozenges, chewable preparations and powders, solutions or syrups. (Dietary Supplements: Background Information 2011). The nutritional supplements of essential vitamins and minerals are important when nutritional requirements are not met through diet alone. Nevertheless, the role of dietary supplementation when nutritional sufficiency has already been achieved remains vigorously debated, as potential deleterious effects of excessive intake have been identified for some micronutrients. A huge variety of supplements are currently available on the market, with multiple chronic disease outcomes to be considered before consumption (http://ebrary.ifpri.org/utils/getfile/collection/).

1.2 Historical Overview

Since the beginning of human civilization, human diet was mostly plant-based foods and sea foods that could be easily gathered. Hunter-gatherers later contributed meat and meat products by big game. This was the diet of most humans until 10 000 BCE, when the development of agriculture and animal husbandry provided more meat and grains. People were not aware of vitamins, minerals, proteins, carbohydrates, fats, and their role in human nutrition. Various people in the continents of the Earth developed nutritious local cuisines with mostly local products that sustained their health, whereas by trial and error choose a variety of foods and cooking methods that could lead to physical strength, health, and fertility. The common wisdom of native cultures recognized which foods and herbs had special properties for energy, nutrition and extra additional health benefits for infants, pregnant women, and elders. Everyday diets were "supplemented" to compensate for deficiencies as far back as native cultures. Native Americans, for example, knew to drink a tea made from pine bark and needles containing high concentration of ascorbic acid to treat scurvy, which was later found by science to be a vitamin C deficiency disease. In 1749, Dr. James Lind discovered citrus fruits prevented scurvy (high in vitamin C content) (Brody 1999; Shils et al. 2006; Fraga 2010).

The discovery of the role of micronutrients was a major scientific achievement in understanding the interrelation between nutrition, health, and disease. The first half of the twentieth century witnessed the identification, isolation, and synthesis of essential micronutrients and their role in nutritional deficiency diseases such as scurvy, beriberi, pellagra, rickets, xerophthalmia, and nutritional anemias. Research on the role of nutrition in complex noncommunicable chronic diseases, such as cardiovascular disease, diabetes, obesity, and cancers, is accelerating over the past two or three decades. This created strong paradigm for nutrient-focused approaches on dietary research, guidelines, and policy to address malnutrition (Mozaffarian et al. 2018).

1.3 Timeline of Nutritional Supplements

Casimir Funk in 1913 found that a "vital amine" in food, originating from the observation that the hulk of unprocessed rice protected chickens against a beriberi-like condition (Eijkman 1929). This "vital amine" or vitamin was first isolated in 1926 and named thiamine, and subsequently synthesized in 1936 as vitamin B_1. In 1932, vitamin C was isolated and documented, for the first time, to protect against scurvy (Albert 2002) some 200 years after ship's surgeon James Lind tested lemons for treating scurvy in sailors (Lind 1753).

By the mid-twentieth century (1910s–1950s), all major vitamins had been isolated and synthesized. Their identification in animal and human studies validated the nutritional basis of serious deficiency diseases and led to dietary strategies to tackle beriberi (vitamin B_1), pellagra (vitamin B_3), scurvy (vitamin C), pernicious anemia (vitamin B_{12}), rickets (vitamin D), and other deficiency conditions. Nevertheless, the chemical synthesis of vitamins led to food-based strategies being supplanted by treatment with individual vitamin supplements. This augured the modern-day use and marketing of multivitamins to guard against deficiency, thus launching an entire vitamin supplement industry. This new science of single nutrient deficiency diseases also paved the way for the fortification of selected staple foods with micronutrients, such as iodine in salt and niacin (vitamin B_3) and iron in wheat flour and bread (Backstrand 2002; Bishai and Nalubola 2002; Fletcher et al. 2004). These approaches proved to be effective at reducing the prevalence of many common deficiency diseases, including goiter (iodine), xerophthalmia (vitamin A), rickets (vitamin D), and anemia (iron). Around the world, foods have then been fortified with calcium, phosphorus, iron, and specific vitamins (A, B, C, D), depending on the composition of local staple foods (Tazhibayev et al. 2008; Wirth et al. 2012; Van den Wijngaart et al. 2013).

This new science with focus on single nutrients and their deficiencies coincided with one of the greatest accidents of nutrition history – the Great Depression (1929) and Second World War (1939), during which there was a widespread fear of food shortages. This led to even further emphasis on preventing deficiency diseases. In 1941, the first RDAs (Recommended Dietary Allowance) were announced at the National Nutrition Conference on Defense, providing new guidelines for total calories and selected nutrients including protein, calcium, phosphorus, iron, and specific vitamins (National Nutrition Conference for Defense 1941). These historical events led the nutrition research and policy recommendations to focus on single nutrients linked to specific disease states.

During the next 20–30 years (1950s–1970s), calorie malnutrition and specific vitamin deficiencies declined sharply in high income countries because of economic development and massive increase in staple foods fortified with minerals and vitamins at low cost. At the same time, the rising burdens of diet related noncommunicable diseases began to be recognized, leading to new research directions. Accordingly, agricultural science and technology emphasized production of low cost, shelf stable, and energy dense starchy staples such as wheat, rice, and corn, with corresponding breeding and processing to maximally extract and purify the starch. As in high-income nations, these efforts were accompanied by fortification of staple foods (Fletcher et al. 2004; Tazhibayev et al. 2008; Wirth et al. 2012), as well as food assistance programs, to promote survival and growth of infants and young children in vulnerable populations.

In 1970s to 1990s, accelerating economic development and modernization of agricultural, food processing, and food formulation techniques continued to reduce single nutrient deficiency diseases globally. Coronary mortality also began to fall in high-income countries, but many other diet-related chronic diseases like obesity, diabetes, and cancers were increasing. Accordingly, the 1980 dietary guidelines remained heavily nutrient focused to eat foods with adequate starch and fiber, to avoid fat and cholesterol, and to avoid the intake of too much sodium and sugar (Davis and Saltos 1999). Similarly, the International guidelines were also nutrient focused leading to a proliferation of industrially crafted food products low in fat, saturated fat, and cholesterol and fortified with micronutrients, as well as expansion of other nutrient focused technologies to reduce saturated fat such as partial hydrogenation of vegetable oils. Iron, vitamin A, and iodine were the major micronutrient targets during this period. Evidence was increasing that vitamin A supplements could prevent child mortality from infections such as measles, as well as preventing night blindness and xerophthalmia (Sommer and West 1996). These findings precedented the widespread micronutrient supplementation, especially during pregnancy, with iron and vitamin A, and for fortification of salt with iodine to prevent goiter and developmental abnormalities such as congenital hypothyroidism and hearing loss. Scientific investigations further focused on other environmental factors such as infection and poor sanitation, which may interact with micronutrients and dietary proteins leading to environmental enteric dysfunction (also called tropical enteritis or environmental enteropathy) (Scrimshaw et al. 1968; Harper 1972; Keusch et al. 1972).

In the mid-1990s, scientists were intrigued by the potential health benefits of dietary supplements and carried out numerous research projects (epidemiologic, clinical, in vivo, and in vitro). This interest was fueled in part by studies demonstrating that nutrient antioxidants (such as vitamins C and A, E and β-carotene, selenium) have a role in protecting cells from oxidative free radical damage. Furthermore, these studies demonstrated that a diet rich in fruits and vegetables and abundant in antioxidants, nutrients, and other substances reduced the risk of coronary heart disease and certain cancers. Hence, antioxidant-fortified dietary supplements and a large range of special foods and plants appeared on the market with incredibly superficial health benefits. Another trend in the last decades, which is characteristic of American consumers and people from Western developed countries (Canada, W. Europe, Australia), is that increasingly large numbers of middle-class people became disenchanted with rising health care costs and the perceived impersonal nature of conventional "Western" medicine. In many countries, there is a dramatic rise in the popularity of various complementary and alternative practices, including Chinese herbal medicine, ayurvedic medicine (an Indian holistic medical system incorporating foods and herbs), acupuncture, and homeopathy. During the last decade, the Food and Drug Administration (USFDA) and the European Union attempted to increase regulation of herbal products and other botanicals and dietary supplements, as well as health labeling and creating a platform of basic information among consumers and forcing dietary supplements manufacturers to follow hygiene practices and safety regulations. In the United States, the Dietary Supplement Health and Education Act (DSHEA) of 1994 classifies herbs as dietary supplements and in the EU countries, the European Traditional Herbal Medicinal Products Directive (2004/24/EC) has provided a simplified registration scheme for traditional herbal medicinal products suitable for self-medication (De Smet 2003; Fermer 2005; WHO 2005; Valavanidis 2006; Bent 2008; Walker 2015).

1.4 Global Market of Nutrient Supplements

Dietary supplements are consumed with a prime intention to enhance the intake of essential nutritional components in the human body. Population in the United States, Europe, and Japan is aging, persuading consumers to seek a variety of dietary supplements for maintaining and enhancing the overall health and well-being. The growing importance of health as a lifestyle choice is expected to boost the future growth of dietary supplements globally and has attracted many companies to enter into the vitamin, mineral, and botanical segments of the dietary supplement market, which is preliminarily driven by the paradigm shift toward preventive health management practices, amid rising healthcare costs and increasing burden of lifestyle diseases. Based on the product type, the vitamin segment is steadily growing, whereas the fatty acid segment represents the fastest growing supplement segment due to the popularity of omega-3-based supplements. The herbal supplements are also expected to drive the market growth in the future. Asia-Pacific is the fastest growing region in the dietary supplements market, driven by major investment opportunities especially for herbal and Ayurveda extract-based products. In the recent years, this has witnessed rapid growth in both developed and developing countries with the increasing demand for supplements in countries like India, China, and Japan, owing to the considerable presence of the aging population in such developing countries. Supplements are most in demand, owing to their various health benefits. The dietary supplements market in the region is anticipated to offer major investment opportunities, especially for herbal and ayurveda extract-based products. This is because of the ample availability of raw materials in India and Southeast Asian countries (https://www.researchandmarkets.com).

The prevalence of dietary supplement use ranges from 22 to 53% in studies conducted in the United States (Bailey et al. 2011), Canada (Shakur et al. 2012), Korea (Lee and Kim 2009), United Kingdom (Lentjes et al. 2015), Sweden (Messerer et al. 2001) Germany (Li et al. 2010), and France (Pouchieu et al. 2013). Multivitamins with or without minerals were the most frequently used supplements in the United States (Bailey et al. 2011), whereas in Canada, vitamin C was the most frequently used supplement overall, with vitamin D the most prevalent supplement among women (Shakur et al. 2012).

1.5 Global Need for the Dietary Supplements

Inadequate nutrient intake is widely prevalent at global level and is a main risk factor for noncommunicable diseases (NCDs) (Bruins et al. 2018). Due to the expanding aging global population, related NCDs including musculoskeletal disorders, dementia, loss of vision, and cardiovascular diseases will place an increasing burden on health systems and costs. Dietary and nutritional supplement approaches are of utmost importance in the management of NCDs. Nutrient surveys indicate that the aging population is at particular risk for poor nutrient intake, which may result in increased risk for chronic fatigue, and cardiovascular, cognitive, and neuromuscular disorders in older adults. Noncommunicable diseases such as cancer, CVD, chronic respiratory disease, and diabetes mellitus are the major causes of death globally and have become a major global burden in both developed and developing nations. An estimated 36 million deaths were caused by noncommunicable diseases, including CVD (48.0%), cancer (21.0%), chronic respiratory disease (12.0%), and diabetes mellitus (3.5%) (WHO, World Health Statistics 2015). The annual number of deaths from CVD is expected to rise from 17 million to 25 million between 2008 and 2030 owing to population growth and increased longevity (WHO, World Health Statistics 2015). A similar increase is expected for cancer-related deaths in the same time frame (from 7.6 million to 13.0 million). Furthermore, in 2008, 80% of all deaths from noncommunicable diseases occurred in low-income and middle-income countries, with a higher proportion of premature ($\leq$70 years) deaths recorded in middle-income countries than in high-income countries (48% versus 26%) (WHO, World Health Statistics 2015). Therefore, an urgent need exists for simple and effective preventive strategies and treatments that can be applied on a global scale.

On the other hand, various nutrients have been reported to play a role in reducing the risk for ischemic heart disease, stroke, myocardial infarction, heart failure, hypertension, and diabetes with varying levels of effect size and evidence. B-vitamins reduced the risk for stroke by reducing homocysteine levels. Vitamin C and D may reduce hypertension, omega-3 long chain polyunsaturated fatty acids (LCPUFAs) may have positive effect on blood lipid profiles, and omega-3-LCPUFAs, vitamin D, and chromium may reduce diabetes risk factors.

Inadequate vitamin D, calcium, and vitamin K intake are generally reported in the aging population and have been associated with musculoskeletal disorders, such as increased bone fracture risks. Increased vitamin D in combination with increased calcium and possibly also vitamin K may reduce the risk for hip fractures, thus beneficially impacting musculoskeletal health. Inadequate B vitamins intake, in particular folic acid, vitamins B_6 and B_{12}, has been associated with age-related cognitive decline, while supplementation has been reported to improve cognitive performance. Similarly, evidence has been reported for vitamin C, D, E, and omega-3-LCPUFAs to slow down dementia progression. Increased intake of lutein and zeaxanthin has been demonstrated to improve macular pigment optical density measures, a marker of age-related macular degeneration (Bruins et al. 2019).

Therefore, adequate nutrient intake may help to improve health and well-being in older populations and slow the progression of NCDs. Implementing a long-term preventative strategy to promote healthy aging and break down the barriers to adequate nutrition for older adults could result in significant healthcare cost savings. Nutrition is increasingly acknowledged and integrated into public health policies and programs to manage healthy aging (Bruins et al. 2019). Promoting nutrient-rich diets and adequate nutrient intakes for healthy aging should be considered part of an integral approach to address NCDs in health policies. Accordingly, there is a need for public and/or private partnerships where governments, health authorities, academics, and the food sector jointly promote the benefits of healthy nutrient-rich diets and lifestyle to manage NCDs.

1.6   Malnutrition

Every single country in the world is affected by one or more forms of malnutrition. Poverty amplifies the risk of malnutrition, and combating malnutrition in all its forms is one of the greatest global health challenges. People of developing countries especially women, infants, children, and adolescents are at particular risk of malnutrition. Malnutrition is a group of conditions in children and adults generally related to poor quality or insufficient quantity of specific nutrient intake, absorption, or utilization, which may increase the health care costs, reduce productivity, and slow economic growth, that can perpetuate a cycle of poverty and ill-health (http://www.who.int/features/qa/malnutrition/en). Optimizing nutrition early in life ensures long-term benefits (https://www.who.int/news-room/fact-sheets/detail/malnutrition).

Malnutrition is also defined by simple anthropometry, which captures a broad range of exposures and risk factors for serious infection in addition to inadequate nutritional intake. There is a bi-directional relationship between malnutrition and infection as the malnourished children are at increased risk of infection, and chronic, repeat, or recurrent infections often contribute to malnutrition. Dysbiosis and pathogen colonization resulting in mucosal dysfunction and inflammatory activation also affect nutritional status, as well as risks of life-threatening infection. While malnutrition leads to increased incidence, severity, and case fatality of common infections, risks continue beyond acute episodes leading to significant post-discharge mortality. A well-established concept of a "vicious-cycle" between nutrition and infection has evolved to encompass dysbiosis and pathogen colonization as precursors to infection, enteric dysfunction constituting malabsorption, dysregulation of nutrients and metabolism, inflammation, and bacterial translocation. All of those interact with a child's diet and environment. Thus, additionally to a diet low in specific nutrients, a good range of antenatal and postnatal environmental exposures, acute infection, chronic illness, or psychosocial neglect may result in malnutrition (Walsona and Berkley 2018).

The various types of malnutritions can be broadly divided into two major categories:

- Protein malnutrition – resulting from the lack of dietary protein in varying proportions.
- Micronutrient malnutrition – resulting from a deficiency of specific micronutrients

1.6.1 Protein Malnutrition

Protein malnutrition is a form of malnutrition that is defined as a range of pathological conditions emerging due to the lack of dietary protein in varying proportions. The condition has mild, moderate, and severe degrees. It is common worldwide in both children and adults and accounts for 6 million deaths annually (https://www.nap.edu/read/11537/chapter/14). Protein malnutrition affects children the most because they have less protein intake. The few rare cases found in the developed world are almost entirely found in small children as a result of fad diets, or ignorance of the nutritional needs of children, particularly in cases of milk allergy (Liu et al. 2001). It can also be secondary to other conditions such as chronic renal disease (Muscaritoli et al. 2009) or cancer cachexia (Bosaeus 2008). Protein malnutrition is detrimental at any point in life, but protein malnutrition prenatally has been shown to have significant lifelong effects. During pregnancy, diet should contain at least 20% protein for the health of the fetus. Diets that consist of less than 6% protein in utero have been linked with many deficits (https://en.wikipedia.org).

The prenatal protein nutrition is vital to the development of the fetus, especially the brain, the susceptibility to diseases in adulthood, and even gene expression. When pregnant females of various species were given low-protein diets, the offspring were shown to have many deficits. This highlights the great significance of adequate protein in the prenatal diet.

The consequences of prenatal protein malnutrition are decreased brain size (Portman et al. 1987), impaired neocortical long-term potentiation (Hernandez et al. 2008), altered fat distribution (Bellinger et al. 2006), increased obesity (Sutton et al. 2010), increased stress sensitivity (Augustyniak et al. 2010), decreased sperm quality (Toledo et al. 2011), altered cardiac energy metabolism

(Slater-Jefferies et al. 2011), increased passive stiffness (Toscano et al. 2010), decreased birth weight, and gestation duration (Rasmussen and Habicht 2010).

Although protein malnutrition is more common in low-income countries, children from higher-income countries are also affected, including children from large urban areas in low socioeconomic neighborhoods. This may also occur in children with chronic diseases and children who are institutionalized or hospitalized for a different diagnosis. Risk factors include a primary diagnosis of intellectual disability, cystic fibrosis, malignancy, cardiovascular disease, end stage renal disease, oncologic disease, genetic disease, neurological disease, multiple diagnoses, or prolonged hospitalization. In these conditions, the challenging nutritional management may get overlooked and underestimated, resulting in an impairment of the chances for recovery and the worsening of the situation ("Marasmus and Kwashiorkor." Medscape Reference. May 2009).

A large percentage of children that suffer from protein malnutrition also have other comorbid conditions such as diarrhea, malaria, sepsis, severe anemia, bronchopneumonia, HIV, tuberculosis, scabies, chronic suppurative otitis media, rickets, and keratomalacia. These comorbidities affect already malnourished children and may increase the likelihood of death (Ubesie et al. 2012). The general explanation of increased infectious comorbidity in malnourished people is that malnutrition tends to cause mild or moderate immunodeficiency, eroding the barriers that normally keep infectious diseases at bay (https://en.wikipedia.org).

There are three stages of protein malnutrition in children:

Protein malnutrition	Manifestation	Rationale
Acute malnutrition	Wasting/thinness (low weight-for-height)	Inadequate nutrition leading to rapid weight loss or failure to gain weight normally
Chronic malnutrition	Stunting/shortness (low height-for-age)	Inadequate nutrition over long period of time leading to failure of linear growth
Acute and chronic malnutrition	Combination of underweight and stunting	A combination measure of acute and chronic malnutrition, occurring as a result of wasting, stunting, or both

Source: Reference: http://conflict.lshtm.ac.uk/page_115.htm.

1.6.2 Micronutrient-Related Malnutrition

Micronutrients are essential elements required in varying optimal quantities throughout life to orchestrate a range of physiological functions to maintain health. These micronutrients enable the body to produce enzymes, hormones, and other substances that are essential for proper growth and development. Inadequacies in intake of micronutrients such as vitamins and minerals lead to micronutrient-related malnutrition. Micronutrient deficiencies affect more than two billion people of all ages in both developing and industrialized countries (https://en.wikipedia.org).

1.7 Importance of Dietary Supplements in Healthcare

1.7.1 Amino Acids as Dietary Supplement

Amino acids are defined as organic substances containing both amino group and acid group. Apart from being the building blocks of proteins, many amino acids have specific functions of their own and are indispensable for certain vital biological processes. They function as neurotransmitters, as precursors for neurotransmitters, and many important metabolites, including crucial oligo- and polypeptides, as a stimulus for hormonal release, and in inter-organ nitrogen transport and nitrogen excretion (MCG Van de Poll et al. 2013). Consequently, maintaining optimum amino acid levels by dietary or topical supplementation may support and modulate these specific functions.

On the basis of needs from the diet for nitrogen balance or growth, amino acids were traditionally classified as nutritionally essential (indispensable) or nonessential (dispensable) for humans and animals. **Essential amino acids** are defined as either those amino acids whose carbon skeletons cannot be synthesized or those that are inadequately synthesized de novo by the body in response to the needs and which must be provided from the diet to meet optimal requirements. **Conditionally essential amino acids** are those that can be normally synthesized in adequate amounts by the body, but which must be provided through the diet to meet optimal needs under conditions where rates of utilization are greater than rates of synthesis. However, functional needs (e.g. reproduction and disease prevention) should also be a criterion for classification of essential or conditionally essential amino acids. **Nonessential amino acids** are those amino acids that can be synthesized de novo in adequate amounts by the body to meet optimal requirements. It should be recognized that all of the 20 protein amino acids and their metabolites are required for normal cell physiology and function (El Idrissi 2008; Lupi et al. 2008; Novelli and Tasker 2008; Phang et al. 2008). **Semi-essentials** are those amino acids that are not essential under normal circumstances but may be in certain situations (https://www.healthline.com). Abnormal metabolism of an amino acid disturbs whole body homeostasis, impairs growth and development, and may even cause death (Wu et al. 2004; Orlando et al.2008; Willis et al. 2008). Growing evidence shows that besides their role as building blocks of proteins and polypeptides, certain amino acids are important regulators of key metabolic pathways that are necessary for the growth, reproduction, and immunity in organisms, therefore maximizing efficiency of food utilization, enhancing protein accretion, reducing adiposity, and improving health. They are called **functional amino acids** (Wu 2009).

Essential amino acids	Nonessential amino acids	Semi essential amino acids	Conditional amino acids	Functional amino acids
Methionine	Alanine	Arginine	Arginine	Arginine
Arginine	Asparagine	Histidine	Cysteine	Cysteine
Threonine	Aspartate		Glutamine	Glutamine
Valine	Glutamine		Tyrosine	Leucine
Isoleucine	Glutamate		Glycine	Proline
Leucine	Cysteine		Proline	Tryptophan
Lysine	Serine		Serine	
Phenylalanine	Glycine			
Histidine	Proline			
Tryptophan	Tyrosine			

Amino acids display remarkable metabolic and regulatory versatility. They serve as essential precursors for the synthesis of a variety of molecules with enormous importance and also regulate key metabolic pathways and processes that are vital to the health, growth, development, reproduction, and homeostasis of organisms.

Dietary supplementation with one or a mixture of amino acids may be beneficial for:

1) Ameliorating health problems at various stages of the life cycle (e.g. fetal growth restriction, neonatal morbidity and mortality, weaning-associated intestinal dysfunction and wasting syndrome, obesity, diabetes, cardiovascular disease, the metabolic syndrome, infertility, and infection)
2) Optimizing efficiency of metabolic transformations to enhance protein synthesis, muscle growth, milk production, egg and meat quality, and athletic performance, while preventing excess fat deposition and favoring reduction of adiposity in humans and animals (Wu 2009).

1.7.1.1 Importance of Amino Acids in Biological Pathways

- Nutrient absorption and metabolism (e.g. nutrient transport, protein turnover, fat synthesis and oxidation, glucose synthesis and oxidation, amino acid synthesis and oxidation, urea and uric synthesis for ammonia detoxification, and efficiency of food utilization) (Amino Acids: Biochemistry and Nutrition, Wu 2009).
- Cellular signaling via mTOR, cAMP, and cGMP activation pathways, as well as the generation of NO, CO, and H_2S.
- Hormone synthesis and secretion (e.g. insulin, glucagon, growth hormone, glucocorticoids, prolactin, placental lactogen, and epinephrine).
- Endothelial function, blood blow, and lymph circulation.
- Reproduction and lactation (e.g. spermatogenesis, male fertility, ovulation, ovarian steroidogenesis, embryo implantation, placental angiogenesis and growth, fetal growth and development, and lactogenesis).
- Immune function and health (e.g. T-cell proliferation and B-cell maturation, antibody production by B-cells, killing of pathogens, obesity, diabetes, and metabolic syndrome).

Protein deficiency has long been known to impair immune function and increases the susceptibility of animals to disease. However, only in the past 20 years, the underlying cellular and molecular mechanisms began to unfold. A dietary deficiency of protein reduces the availability of most amino acids in plasma, particularly glutamine, arginine, tryptophan, methionine, and cysteine (Li et al. 2007). The roles of glutamine, arginine, methionine, and cysteine in enhancing the immune function have been well established (Li et al. 2007; Van Brummelen and Du Toit 2007; Tan et al. 2008). Because the availability of cysteine is a major factor that limits the synthesis of glutathione (Wu et al. 2004), dietary supplementation with N-acetyl-cysteine (a stable precursor of cysteine) is highly effective in enhancing immunity under various disease states (Grimble 2006). It is noteworthy that a large amount of NO synthesized from arginine by inducible NO synthase is cytotoxic to pathogenic microorganisms and viruses (Bronte and Zanovello 2005). Accordingly, dietary supplementation with arginine improves the immune status of humans and animals (Li et al. 2007; Tan et al. 2008). There has been growing interest in recent years in the role of tryptophan and proline in immune functions (Melchior et al. 2003). A major mediator derived from proline oxidation is H_2O_2, which is cytotoxic to pathogenic bacteria and is also a signaling molecule (Shi et al. 2004). A high activity of proline oxidase in placentae (Wu et al. 2005, 2008) and the small intestine of mammals (Wu 1997) may play a crucial role in protecting these organs from infections during the critical periods of fetal and neonatal development. Further, proline oxidase is present in milk and may play a role in protecting the neonatal intestine from infectious agents (Sun et al. 2002). This may explain, in part, why neonates fed a non-milk diet have a high risk of intestinal dysfunction in comparison with those nursed by their mothers (Wu et al. 1996).

Studies of amino acid nutrition have been largely based on traditional approaches (e.g. digestibility trials, nitrogen balance, assessments of growth and reproductive performance, isotope tracer techniques, as well as northern and western blots) (Dekaney et al. 2008; Mateo et al. 2007, 2008; Wang et al. 2008). However, recent advances of high-throughput functional genomics, microarray, metabolomics, and proteomics (Ptolemy et al. 2007; He et al. 2008; Hu et al. 2008; John et al. 2008; Yan and He 2008; Wang et al. 2009) have provided powerful discovery tools to study regulatory roles for AA in gene expression and protein function.

1.7.1.2 Amino Acid Deficiencies and Supplementation

During undernutrition and disease condition, diminished turnover of amino acids can occur. These deficiencies may concern specific amino acids in certain diseases or a more generalized amino acid deficiency. The resulting functional deficits can contribute to the symptoms, severity, and progress of the disease. These deficits can be counteracted by simple supplementation of the deficient amino acids. Amino acid supplementation is also applied to enhance turnover and improve amino acid function in nondeficient patients (Poll et al. 2005).

S. no.	Essential amino acids	Functions	Dietary source
1.	Arginine $C_6H_{14}N_4O_2$ (https://en.wikipedia.org)	Arginine is involved in many biological pathways • Krebs cycle • Urea cycle – Ammonia detoxification • Acid/base homeostasis • T-cell proliferation • Host immune response and defenses • Collagen synthesis and helps heal injuries • Cardiovascular function • Vasodilation, immunomodulation, neurotransmission, and cell signaling	Turkey, chicken, red meat, pork, seafood, pumpkin seeds, nuts, algae, rice, soybeans, peanuts, spirulina, dairy, chickpeas, lentils. Watermelon also contains high amounts of citrulline and an arginine biosynthetic precursor (https://www.sciencedirect.com/)
2.	Methionine $C_5H_{11}NO_2S$ (https://en.wikipedia.org)	Methionine plays an important role in metabolism and detoxification It is also necessary for tissue growth and flexibility of skin and hair and strong nails. It aids the proper absorption of selenium, zinc, and minerals that are vital to health. It also aids in the removal of heavy metals, such as lead and mercury	Turkey, beef, fish, pork, tofu, milk, cheese, nuts, beans, and whole grains like quinoa (https://www.myfooddata.com)

S. no.	Essential amino acids	Functions	Dietary source
3.	Threonine $C_4H_9NO_3$ (https://en.wikipedia.org)	Threonine is a principal part of structural proteins such as collagen and elastin, which are important components of the skin and connective tissue. It is necessary for healthy skin and teeth, as it is a component in tooth enamel. It also plays a role in fat metabolism and immune function. It may be beneficial for people with indigestion, anxiety, and mild depression Its intermediate glycine is involved in brain development	Cottage cheese, poultry, fish, meat, lentils, black turtle bean and sesame seeds (nutritiondata.self. com)
4.	Lysine $C_6H_{14}N_2O_2$ (https://en.wikipedia.org)	Lysine plays major roles in synthesis and regulation of proteins, hormone, enzyme and antibodies and also regulates the absorption of calcium. It is also important for energy production, immune function It has a vital role in building muscle, maintaining bone strength, aiding recovery from injury or surgery. It may also have antiviral effects Its intermediate carnitine is involved in mitochondrial oxidation of long-chain fatty acids There is not a lot of research available on lysine deficiency, but a study on rats indicates that lysine deficiency can lead to stress-induced anxiety	Meat, specifically red meat, pork, and poultry Cheese, particularly parmesan Certain fish, such as cod and sardines, Eggs Soybeans, particularly tofu, isolated soy protein, and defatted soybean flour, Spirulina, Fenugreek seed, Brewer's yeast, beans and other legumes, and dairy products also contain lysine (http://pennstatehershey.adam. com).
5.	Leucine $C_6H_{13}NO_2$ (https://en.wikipedia.org)	Leucine helps regulate blood sugar levels and aids the growth and repair of muscle and bone Leucine deficiency can lead to skin rashes, hair loss, and fatigue Like valine, leucine is a branched-chain amino acid that is critical for protein synthesis and muscle repair. It also helps regulate blood sugar levels, stimulates wound healing and produces growth hormones Its intermediate ketoisocaproic acid is involved in regulation of energy and protein metabolism, Substrate for glutamine synthesis	High leucine foods include chicken, beef, pork, fish (tuna), tofu, canned beans, milk, cheese, squash seeds, and eggs (https://www.myfooddata.com)

(Continued)

S. no.	Essential amino acids	Functions	Dietary source
6.	Isoleucine $C_6H_{13}NO_2$ (https://en.wikipedia.org)	Isoleucine helps with wound healing, immunity, blood sugar regulation, and hormone production. It is heavily concentrated in muscle tissue and responsible for muscle metabolism It is also important for immune function, hemoglobin production and energy regulation Older adults may be more prone to isoleucine deficiency than younger people. This deficiency may cause muscle wasting and shaking	Beef, chicken, pork, fish, tofu, dairy, beans, lentils, whole grains, nuts, seeds, and vegetables like peas (https://www.myfooddata. com)
7.	Valine $C_5H_{11}NO_2$ (https://en.wikipedia.org)	Valine is essential for mental focus, muscle coordination, and emotional calm. It helps stimulate muscle growth, tissue repair and regeneration and is involved in energy production Deficiency may cause insomnia and reduced mental function	Beef, chicken, pork, fish, tofu, yogurt, beans, podded peas, seeds, nuts, and whole grains like oatmeal (https://www. myfooddata.com)
8.	Phenylalanine $C_9H_{11}NO_2$ (https://en.wikipedia.org)	Phenylalanine helps the body use other amino acids, as well as proteins and enzymes. The body converts phenylalanine to tyrosine, which is necessary for specific brain functions Phenylalanine is often in the artificial sweetener aspartame, which manufacturers use to make diet sodas. Large doses of aspartame can increase the levels of phenylalanine in the brain and may cause anxiety and jitteriness and affect sleep People with a rare genetic disorder called phenylketonuria (PKU) are unable to metabolize phenylalanine. As a result, they should avoid consuming foods that contain high levels of this amino acid Phenylalanine is a precursor for the neurotransmitters like tyrosine, dopamine, epinephrine and norepinephrine. It plays an integral role in the structure and function of proteins and enzymes and the production of other amino acids Phenylalanine deficiency, though rare, can lead to poor weight gain in infants. It may also cause eczema, fatigue, and memory problems in adults	Beef, chicken, pork, tofu, fish, beans, milk, nuts, seeds, pasta, whole grains, and vegetables like sweet potatoes (https://www. myfooddata.com)

S. no.	Essential amino acids	Functions	Dietary source
9.	Tryptophan $C_{11}H_{12}N_2O_2$ (https://en.wikipedia.org)	Tryptophan is necessary for proper growth in infants and maintenance of proper nitrogen balance. It is a precursor of serotonin and melatonin. Serotonin is a neurotransmitter that regulates appetite, sleep, mood, and pain. Melatonin also regulates sleep Tryptophan is a sedative, and it is an ingredient in some sleep aids. One study indicates that tryptophan supplementation can improve mental energy and emotional processing in healthy women Tryptophan deficiency can cause a condition called pellagra, which can lead to dementia, skin rashes, and digestive issues Its intermediates are • Kynureninic acid – CNS inhibition • Quinolinic acid – CNS excitation • Serotonin – Mood regulation, sleep regulation, intestinal motility • Melatonin – Regulation of circadian rhythms	Chicken, eggs, cheese, fish, peanuts, pumpkin and sesame seeds, milk, turkey, tofu and soy, chocolate (https://www.myfooddata.com)
10.	Histidine $C_6H_9N_3O_2$ (https://en.wikipedia.org)	Histidine facilitates growth, the creation of blood cells, and tissue repair. It also helps maintain the special protective covering over nerve cells, which is called the myelin sheath The body metabolizes histidine into histamine, which is crucial for immunity, reproductive health, and digestion. The results of a study that recruited women with obesity and metabolic syndrome suggest that histidine supplements may lower BMI and insulin resistance Deficiency can cause anemia, and low blood levels appear to be more common among people with arthritis and kidney disease	Meat, eggs, tofu, soy, buckwheat, quinoa, and dairy (https://www.medicalnewstoday.com)

Source: Reference (https://www.medicalnewstoday.com/)

Recommended Dietary Allowance (RDA) Reference: (https://globalrph.com)

There is no standard dose of arginine. The safety of long-term arginine supplement use is not clear (https://www.webmd.com).

Different stages of life	Histidine (mg/kg/day)	Isoleucine (mg/kg/day)	Leucine (mg/kg/day)	Lysine (mg/kg/day)	Methionine + cysteine (mg/kg/day)	Phenylalanine + tyrosine (mg/ kg/ day)	Threonine (mg/kg/day)	Tryptophan (mg/kg/day)	Valine (mg/kg/day)
Infant age: 0–6 months	36	88	156	107	59	135	73	28	87
Infant age: 7–12 months	32	43	93	89	43	84	49	13	58
Children age: 1–3 years	21	28	63	58	28	54	32	8	37
Children age: 4–8 years	16	22	49	46	22	41	24	6	28
Boy's age: 9–13 years	17	22	49	46	22	41	24	6	28
Girl's age: 9–13 years	15	21	47	43	21	38	22	6	27
Boy's age: 14–18 years	15	21	47	43	21	38	22	6	27
Girl's age: 14–18 years	14	19	44	40	19	35	21	5	24
Adult's age: 19 years and older	14	19	42	38	19	33	20	5	24
Pregnancy	18	25	56	51	25	44	26	7	31
Lactation	19	30	62	52	26	51	30	9	36

1.7.2 Essential Fatty Acids as Dietary Supplement

Essential fatty acids are fatty acids that humans and other animals must ingest because the body cannot synthesize them but are required for healthy functioning of organism (Robert and Maurice 1980). The term "essential fatty acid" refers only to the fatty acids required for biological processes and does not include the fats that only act as fuel. Only two fatty acids are known to be essential for humans: alpha-linolenic acid (an omega-3 fatty acid) and linoleic acid (an omega-6 fatty acid) (Whitney and Rolfes 2008). Some other fatty acids are sometimes classified as "conditionally essential,", meaning that they can become essential under some developmental or disease conditions; examples include docosahexaenoic acid (an omega-3 fatty acid) and gamma-linolenic acid (an omega-6 fatty acid) (Burr et al. 2007).

Over the past few years, there has been a dramatic increase in the public interest and scientific scrutiny of omega fatty acids and their impact on personal health. Omega-3 fatty acids possess anti-inflammatory, antiarrhythmic, and antithrombotic properties, whereas omega-6 fatty acids are proinflammatory and prothrombotic. Omega-3 and omega-6 fatty acids are essential because they are not synthesized by the body and should be obtained through diet or supplementation. Omega-3 fatty acids are important components of the cell membranes and also provide calories to perform many functions in the heart, blood vessels, lungs, immune system, and endocrine system. Omega-3 fatty acids are found in foods, such as fish (especially cold-water fatty fish, such as salmon, mackerel, tuna, herring, and sardine) and flaxseed, and in dietary supplements, such as fish oil (Cod liver oil), standard fish body oil (e.g. herring, salmon), omega-3 fatty acid concentrate.
Dietary source of predominant essential fatty acids (Covington 2004).

Food sources rich in omega-3 fatty acids	Food sources rich in omega-6 fatty acid
Canola oil	Borage oil
Fish oil	Corn oil
Flaxseed oil	Cottonseed oil
Soybean oil	Grapeseed oil
Walnut oil	Peanut oil
Chia seeds	Safflower oil
Cold water fatty fish such as salmon, mackerel, tuna, herring, and sardines	Sesame oil
	Soybean oil
	Sunflower oil
	Meat, poultry, fish, and eggs

Source: Reference: Covington (2004).

The three important omega-3 fatty acids are alpha-linolenic acid (ALA), eicosapentaenoic acid (EPA), and docosahexaenoic acid (DHA). The retina (eye), brain, and sperm cells contain high levels of omega-3 fatty acids especially DHA. DHA and EPA are found in fatty fish, algae, and other seafood. ALA is found mainly in plant seeds and oils, green leafy vegetables, flaxseeds, beans (soyabean), and nuts (walnuts). Linoleic acid is an omega-6 fatty acid, which is present in grains, meats, and the seeds of most plants (Kris-Etherton et al. 2003). Increased consumption of vegetable oils high in omega-6 fatty acids (such as corn, safflower, sunflower, and cottonseed oils) and meats from animals that were fed with grains high in omega-6 fatty acids has drastically shifted the dietary ratio of omega-6 to omega-3 fatty acids from an estimated 1 : 1 in the early human diet to approximately 10 : 1 in the modern diet (Kris-Etherton et al. 2003).

The dietary intake of omega fatty acids is essential because through an inefficient enzymatic process of desaturation (the rate of conversion is less than 1 percent), ALA produces EPA (20 carbons) and DHA (22 carbons), precursors to a group of eicosanoids (prostaglandins, thromboxanes, and leukotrienes) that are anti-inflammatory, antithrombotic, antiarrhythmic, and vasodilatory. The longer chain fatty acid derivative of linoleic acid (omega-6 fatty acid) is arachidonic acid (20 carbons), and it is a precursor to a different group of eicosanoids that are proinflammatory and prothrombic. ALA and linoleic acid utilize and compete for the same enzymes in the production of their longer chain fatty acids, EPA, and arachidonic acid. The ingestion of fish and fish oil either through natural food or supplement provides EPA and DHA directly, therefore avoiding the competition for enzymes to convert ALA to EPA (Covington 2004)

1.7.2.1 Dosage

The American Heart Association's recommendations for intake of omega-3 fatty acids state that patients without documented CHD should eat at least two servings of fatty fish per week along with other foods rich in omega-3 fatty acids. Persons with CHD are encouraged to eat at least one daily meal that includes a fatty fish or take a daily fish oil supplement to achieve a recommended level of 0.9 g/day of EPA. Most commercial fish oil capsules (1 g) contain 180 mg of EPA and 120 mg of DHA. Therefore, three 1-g capsules per day in divided doses provides the recommended dosage of 0.9 g of omega-3 fatty acids. Fish oil is also available in a more highly concentrated liquid form that provides 1–3 g of omega-3 fatty acids per teaspoon, depending on the product and manufacturer. The effective dosage for treating hypertriglyceridemia is 2–4 g/day, which is significantly higher than the dosage recommended for cardiovascular protection. The FDA has concluded that dietary dosages of up to 3 g/day of omega-3 fatty acids from marine sources are "Generally Recognized as Safe." For persons who are vegetarians or non-fish eaters, a total daily intake of 1.5–3 g/day of ALA seems to be beneficial.

Recommended amount of essential fatty acids through diet.

Life stage	Recommended amount of ALA (g)
Birth to 12 months	0.5 (total omega-3-fatty acids)
Children 1–3 years	0.7 (ALA)
Children 4–8 years	0.9 (ALA)
Boys 9–13 years	1.2 (ALA)
Girls 9–13 years	1.0 (ALA)
Teen boys 14–18 years	1.6 (ALA)
Teen girls 14–18 years	1.1 (ALA)
Men	1.6 (ALA)
Women	1.1 (ALA)
Pregnant teens and women	1.4 (ALA)
Breastfeeding teens and women	1.3 (ALA)

Source: Reference: Covington (2004).

1.7.2.2 Importance of Omega Fatty Acids in Health Care

Omega-3 fatty acids could play an important role in mental health as approximately 50–60% of the adult brain is composed of lipids (dry weight), of which roughly 35% are phospholipids comprised of unsaturated fatty acids (Haag 2003). Of these, the polyunsaturated fatty acids such as docosahexaenoic acid (an omega-3 fatty acid) and arachidonic acid (an omega-6 fatty acid) are found in the highest concentrations. These components of phospholipids have important functions in maintaining nerve cell membrane integrity and fluidity, as well as contributing to neuronal signal transduction.

DHA is important in prenatal brain development, where it appears to play a key role in synaptogenesis (Martin and Bazan 1992; Green et al. 1999). DHA deficiency has been linked to a number of neurophysiological deficits including cognitive impairment (Birch et al. 2000), decreased visual acuity (Birch et al. 1998), and decreased cerebellar function (Jamieson et al. 1999). In the adult biosystem, an optimal balance between omega-3 and omega-6 fatty acids is essential for normal neuronal function, an imbalance in the omega-6 to omega-3 fatty acid ratio may lead to increase in disorders of all kinds (Simopoulos 1999; Sugano and Hirahara 2000; Simopoulos 2003; Kang 2003; Yehuda 2003; de Lorgeril and Salen 2003; Dubnov and Berry 2003; Zampelas et al. 2003; Hamazaki and Okuyama 2003; Chajes and Bournoux 2003; Cleland et al. 2003; Kris-Etherton et al. 2003). This imbalance suggested an etiologic mechanism by which psychiatric disorders may develop (i.e. abnormalities in PUFA metabolism), and in turn, a rationale for ways to treat them (e.g. PUFA supplementation). In both of these regards, depression and schizophrenia have been the two most investigated and speculated on psychiatric disorders. The strong variability in the annual prevalence rates for major depressive disorder, expressed as an almost 60-fold variation across countries (Weissman et al. 1996), parallels the wide cross-national differences in mortality rates from coronary artery disease, suggesting that similar risk factors could be involved in both scenarios (Hibbeln 1998).

In the twentieth century, the increasing lifetime risk of depression has coemerged with a shift in diet involving an increase in omega-6 fatty acid intake and a decrease in the intake of omega-3 fatty acids (Edwards et al. 1998), and this change in the dietary omega-6/omega-3 fatty acid intake ratio has been proposed as being responsible for the increased risk of depression (Smith 1991). At the same time, it has been suggested that these recent changes in the diet are responsible for the increase in cardiovascular and inflammatory disorders (Smith 1991). It is suggested that major depression is strongly predictive of both coronary heart disease and myocardial infarction (Booth-Kewley and Friedman 1987; Pratt et al. 1996) and, some physical illnesses, such as coronary heart disease or diabetes, appear to occur with increased frequency in patients with major depression and schizophrenia (Peet and Horrobin 2002). The mechanism by which diet may affect health, including depression or cardiovascular disease, is thought to involve low levels of omega-3 fatty acid content in biomarkers (e.g. red blood cells [RBCs]) (Edwards et al. 1998; Peet and Horrobin 2002). An omega-3 fatty acid deficiency hypothesis of depression has helped justify treatment with omega-3 fatty acid supplementation (Horrobin and Bennett 1999).

The Diet and Reinfarction Trial (DART) (Burr et al. 1989) was one of the first studies to investigate a relationship between dietary intake of omega-3 fatty acids and secondary prevention of myocardial infarction. Studies conducted in patients with heart disease suggest that dietary and nondietary fatty acids decreased progression of coronary lesions, reduced mortality caused by myocardial infarction, and sudden death caused by cardiac arrhythmias and all-cause mortality in patients with known coronary heart disease. It was reported that men who consumed fish at least once per week had a 50% reduction in the risk for sudden death and a significant reduction in all-cause mortality (Albert et al. 1998). It was also found that higher consumption levels of fish and ALA were associated with a decreased risk of CHD and CHD-related deaths (Hu et al. 2002).

Several studies (Cleland et al. 1988; Kremer et al. 1990; Lau et al. 1993; Volker et al. 2000) have found that fish oil significantly reduced morning stiffness, swollen joints in patients with rheumatoid arthritis. It has been reported that reducing dietary intake of omega-6 fatty acids while increasing consumption of omega-3 fatty acids reduces the inflammatory mediators of rheumatoid arthritis (James and Cleland 1997; Vargova et al. 1998).

Studies also suggest that omega-3 fatty acids could lower plasma triglyceride levels, particularly in persons with hypertriglyceridemia (Harris et al. 1997) by inhibiting the synthesis of very-low-density lipoprotein (VLDL) cholesterol and triglycerides in the liver. Omega-3 fatty acids also appear to have a dose-response hypotensive effect in patients with hypertension (Howe 1997).

But high dosages of fish oil may increase LDL cholesterol levels, but the clinical relevance of this finding remains unclear (Harris et al. 1997). Other potential side effects of omega-3 fatty acids include a fishy after taste and gastrointestinal disturbances, all of which appear to be dose-dependent (Kris-Etherton et al. 2003). Omega-3 fatty acids exert a dose-related effect on bleeding time; however, there are no documented cases of abnormal bleeding as a result of fish oil supplementation, even at high dosages and in combination with other anticoagulant medications (Eritsland et al. 1996). Significant amounts of methylmercury, polychlorinated biphenyls, dioxins, and other environmental contaminants may be concentrated in certain species of fish, such as shark, swordfish, king mackerel, and tilefish (also known as golden bass or golden snapper), however high-quality fish oil supplements usually do not contain these contaminants.

1.7.3 Vitamins and Minerals as Dietary Supplements

In the twentieth century, research has dramatically increased our understanding of the biochemical processes of cellular energy generation and demonstrated the fundamental role of a large number of vitamins and minerals as coenzymes and cofactors in these processes (Huskisson et al. 2007).

The role of vitamins in energy metabolism continues to attract researchers. Studies have emphasized that the B complex vitamins are essential for mitochondrial function and a lack of just one of these vitamins may compromise an entire sequence of biochemical reactions necessary for transforming food into physiological energy (Depeint et al. 2006). As with the B vitamins, the role of certain minerals in energy metabolism is the topic of increasing research interest. It was found that several minerals and trace elements are essential for energy generation, although more research is needed to elucidate their precise role. Inadequate intake of micronutrients, or increased needs, impairs health and increases susceptibility to infection but may also result in tiredness, lack of energy, and poor concentration (Huskisson et al. 2007). For example, an adequate amount of magnesium, zinc, and chromium is required to ensure the capacity for increased energy expenditure and work performance, and that supplemental magnesium and zinc apparently improve strength and muscle metabolism (Lukaski 2000). It was also found that magnesium depletion resulted in increased energy needs and an adverse effect on cardiovascular function during submaximal work (Lukaski and Nielsen 2002). Lukaski has also shown that low dietary zinc also impairs cardiorespiratory function during exercise (Lukaski 2005).

The transformation of dietary energy sources (carbohydrates, fats, and proteins) into cellular energy in the form of ATP requires several micronutrients as coenzymes and cofactors of enzymatic reactions: (i) thiamine pyrophosphate (TPP; vitamin B_1), CoA (containing pantothenic acid [Vit B_5]), flavin mononucleotide (FMN; derived from vitamin B_2), flavin adenine dinucleotide (FAD; derived from vitamin B_2), and nicotinamide adenine dinucleotide (NAD; derived from nicotinamide) are involved in the Krebs cycle and complexes I and II of the respiratory chain; (ii) biotin (Vit B_7), CoA, and FAD are involved in heme biosynthesis, which is an essential part of the cytochromes and important for the latter part of the mitochondrial respiratory chain; (iii) succinyl-CoA can feed into either the respiratory chain or the Krebs cycle depending on the needs of the cell (Huskisson et al. 2007).

1.7.3.1 Inadequate Micronutrient Intake

The serious consequences of profound vitamin deficiencies have been recognized for more than a century. In developed countries, the deficiency diseases such as rickets, pellagra, scurvy, and beriberi are now relatively uncommon as a result of better general nutrition and micronutrient supplementation. But, within the past two decades, a number of investigators (Brubacher 1988; Bassler 1995) have re-introduced the concept of marginal micronutrient deficiency, first proposed by Pietrzik in 1985 (Pietrzik 1985). This showed that long before the clinical symptoms of deficiency appear, micronutrient deficiencies develop progressively through several sub-clinical stages.

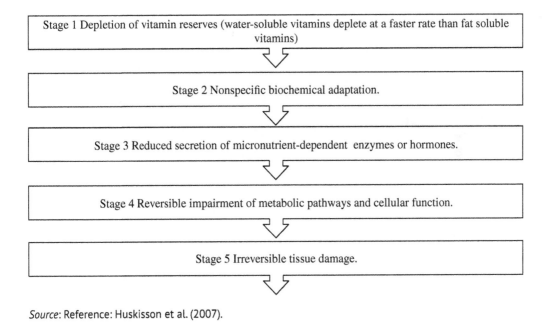

Source: Reference: Huskisson et al. (2007).

Marginal deficiencies may occur as a result of inadequate micronutrient intake, caused by poor diet, malabsorption, or abnormal metabolism. Whether in the developed or the less developed world, the overwhelming majority of cases fall into stages 1–3 and are further referred to as an inadequate micronutrient status. Ideally, a sufficient and balanced diet should cover the overall micronutrient requirements. Unfortunately, even in developed countries, many sections of the population do not receive the essential vitamins and minerals needed from their diet. Several groups in the population are at increased risk for inadequate micronutrient status, usually due to insufficient intake caused by weight-reducing diets, insufficient and/or imbalanced nutrition, eating disorders, or demanding periods such as extensive exercise or emotional and/or physiological stress. Increased requirements may also cause an inadequate vitamin and mineral status; for example, as may occur in pregnancy and lactation, during growth, in the elderly, smokers and chronic alcohol abusers, and in patients with certain underlying diseases (Shankar 2001; Meydani and Han 2001; Rucker et al. 2001; Baessler et al. 2002). Even healthy individuals can be at risk due to lifestyle-related factors such as rushed meals, unhealthy food choices, chronic or periodical dieting, and stress-related behavior, such as smoking, excessive alcohol, and coffee consumption (Huskisson et al. 2007).

Even mild micronutrient deficiencies can result in a lack of well-being and general fatigue, reduced resistance to infections or impaired mental processes (e.g. memory, concentration, attention, and mood) (https://www.ncbi.nlm.nih.gov/books/NBK114310; https://www.ncbi.nlm.nih.gov/books/NBK225483).

There are 13 types of vitamins divided into two broad categories – Fat soluble and water soluble.

There are four fat soluble vitamins (A, D, E, K) and nine water soluble vitamins (B_1, B_2, B_3, B_5, B_6, B_7, B_9, B_{12}, C).

S. no	Water-soluble vitamins	Functions	Deficiency condition	Food sources
1.	Thiamine (vitamin B_1) $C_{12}H_{17}N_4OS^+$ (https://en.wikipedia.org)	• Essential cofactor in the conversion of carbohydrates to energy • Needed for normal muscle function, including the heart muscle. • Involved in oxidative carboxylation reactions, which also require manganese ions. • Needed for healthy skin, hair, muscles, and brain and is critical for nerve function Huskisson et al. (2007)	Beriberi There are 4 types of beriberi 1) Dry beriberi – affects the peripheral nervous system. It also includes Wernicke–Korsakoff syndrome (Brain disorder) 2) Wet beriberi – affects the cardiovascular system and other bodily systems 3) Infantile beriberi – affects the babies of malnourished mothers 4) Gastrointestinal beriberi – affects the digestive system and other bodily systems. (https://en.wikipedia.org)	Milk, nuts, oats, oranges, legumes, brown rice, ham, soymilk, cereals, watermelon, peas and yeast, pork chops, beef, liver, pork, eggs (https://www.livescience.com)
2.	Riboflavin (vitamin B_2) $C_{17}H_{20}N_4O_6$ (https://en.wikipedia.org)	• As a cofactor in the mitochondrial respiratory chain, helps in the release of energy from foods • Component of the main coenzymes FAD and FMN. • Needed for healthy skin, hair, blood, and nervous system Huskisson et al. (2007)	Ariboflavinosis, angular stomatitis (https://en.wikipedia.org)	Milk, eggs, yogurt, cheese, organ meats (such as kidneys and liver), lean meats, green vegetables (such as asparagus, broccoli, and spinach), fortified cereals, bread, and enriched grains (https://ods.od.nih.gov)

(Continued)

S. no	Water-soluble vitamins	Functions	Deficiency condition	Food sources
3.	Niacin (vitamin B_3, nicotinic acid) $C_6H_5NO_2$ (https://en.wikipedia.org)	• As a cofactor in the mitochondrial respiratory chain, helps in the release of energy from foods • Transformed into NAD and NADP, which play a key role in oxidation–reduction reactions in all cells • Needed for healthy skin, hair, blood, and nervous system Huskisson et al. (2007)	Pellagra (https://en.wikipedia.org)	Meat (such as beef and pork), poultry (such as chicken and turkey), fish, fortified and whole grains, mushrooms, avocados, green peas, brown rice, potatoes, peanut butter (https://www.myfooddata.com)
4.	Choline (vitamin B_4) $C_5H_{14}NO^+$ (https://en.wikipedia.org)	• Choline (Vit B_4) also known as adenine or carnitine is neither a vitamin nor a mineral; however, it is often grouped with the vitamin B complex due to its similarities • It is a distant member of the B-complex family and is known as one of the "lipotropic" factors. Lipotropic means that choline possesses properties that prevent the excessive accumulation of fat in the liver. • It poses an antioxidant activity. • It helps with protein synthesis. • When combined with ribose, it forms adenosine which is highly important for normal heart function. • Helps make and release the neurotransmitter acetylcholine, which aids in many nerve and brain activities. Plays a role in metabolizing and transporting fats Huskisson et al. (2007)	Alzheimer's, Parkinson's, schizophrenia, epilepsy, multiple sclerosis, poor memory, cardiovascular disease, atherosclerosis, anxiety, attention-deficit hyperactivity disorder (ADHD), alcoholism, cirrhosis, NAFLD, NASH, hypertriglyceridemia, hyperhomocysteinemia, hypertension, failure to thrive in newborns, infertility, and birth defects (https://www.onlineholistichealth.com)	Brewer's yeast is the best food source of vitamin B_4 Other sources include milk, eggs, liver, salmon, raw honey, whole grains, green leafy vegetables, aloe vera, spirulina, and peanuts Smaller amounts can be found in herbs and spices such as hops, sage, spearmint, caraway, cinnamon, sumac, and ginger (https://www.caasn.com)

| 5. | Pantothenic acid (vitamin B$_5$) C$_9$H$_{17}$NO$_5$

(https://en.wikipedia.org) | • Plays an essential role in the Krebs cycle
• Component of coenzyme A
• Helps convert food into energy and helps make lipids (fats), neurotransmitters, steroid hormones, and hemoglobin
Huskisson et al. (2007) | Burning feet syndrome (https://en.wikipedia.org) | Beef, poultry, seafood, organ meats, eggs (egg yolk), milk, vegetables (such as mushrooms (especially shiitakes), avocados, potatoes, broccoli, tomato), whole grains (such as whole wheat, brown rice, and oats), peanuts, sunflower seeds, and chickpeas (https://ods.od.nih.gov) |
| 7. | Biotin (vitamin B$_7$ or vitamin H) C$_{10}$H$_{16}$N$_2$O$_3$S

(https://en.wikipedia.org) | • As a cofactor, involved in metabolism of fatty acids, amino acids and utilization of B vitamins
• Helps convert food into energy and synthesize glucose. Helps make and break down some fatty acids. Needed for healthy bones and hair
Huskisson et al. (2007) | Alopecia (https://en.wikipedia.org) | Walnuts, peanuts, cereals, milk, and egg yolks, whole meal bread, salmon, pork, sardines, mushroom and cauliflower. Fruits that contain biotin include avocados, bananas and raspberries (https://www.news-medical.net) |

(Continued)

S. no	Water-soluble vitamins	Functions	Deficiency condition	Food sources
8.	Folic acid (vitamin B_9, folate, folacin) $C_{19}H_{19}N_7O_6$ (https://en.wikipedia.org)	• Folates function as a family of cofactors that carry one-carbon (C1) units required for the synthesis of thymidylate, purines, and methionine, and required for other methylation reactions • Folate is essential for metabolic pathways involving cell growth, replication, survival of cells in culture • Around 30–50% of cellular folates are located in the mitochondria • Vital for new cell creation. Helps prevent brain and spine birth defects when taken early in pregnancy; should be taken regularly by all women of child-bearing age since women may not know they are pregnant in the first weeks of pregnancy. Can lower levels of homocysteine and may reduce heart disease risk. May reduce risk for colon cancer. Offsets breast cancer risk among women who consume alcohol Huskisson et al. (2007)	Macrocytic anemia (https://en.wikipedia.org)	Green leafy vegetables (turnip greens, spinach, romaine lettuce, asparagus, okra, Brussels sprouts, broccoli), legumes like black-eyed peas and chickpeas, orange juice, tomato juice, beans, peanuts, sunflower seeds, fresh fruits, fruit juices, whole grains, meat, liver, seafood, eggs, fortified grains, and cereals (https://www.hsph.harvard.edu)

9. Cobalamin (vitamin B_{12})

$C_{63}H_{88}CoN_{14}O_{14}P$

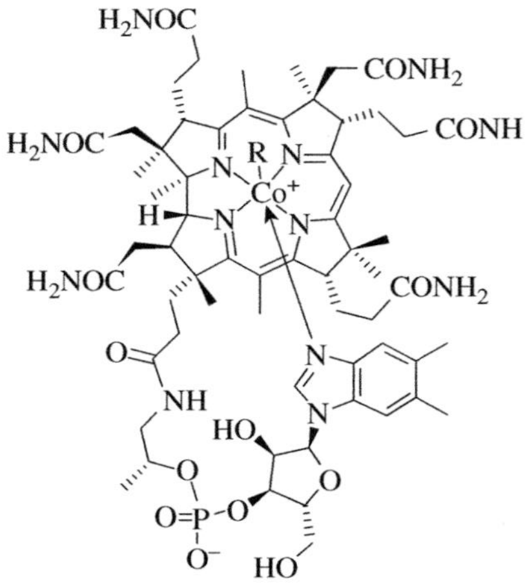

(https://en.wikipedia.org)(https://en.wikipedia.org)

- Aids in lowering homocysteine levels and may lower the risk of heart disease
- Assists in making new cells and breaking down some fatty acids and amino acids
- Protects nerve cells and encourages their normal growth
- Helps make red blood cells and DNA

Huskisson et al. (2007)

Pernicious anemia
(https://en.wikipedia.org)

Meat, poultry, fish, milk, cheese, eggs, fortified cereals, fortified soymilk
(https://ods.od.nih.gov)

(Continued)

S. no	Water-soluble vitamins	Functions	Deficiency condition	Food sources
10.	Ascorbic acid (vitamin C) $C_6H_8O_6$	• Essential for synthesis of carnitine (transports long-chain fatty acids into (ascorbic acid) mitochondria) and the catecholamines, adrenaline and noradrenaline • Ascorbic acid facilitates transport and uptake of nonheme iron at the mucosa, the reduction of folic acid intermediates, and the synthesis of cortisol • Potent antioxidant • Foods rich in vitamin C may lower the risk for some cancers, including those of the mouth, esophagus, stomach, and breast. Long-term use of supplemental vitamin C may protect against cataracts. Helps make collagen, a connective tissue that knits together wounds and supports blood vessel walls. Helps make the neurotransmitters serotonin and norepinephrine. Acts as an antioxidant, neutralizing unstable molecules that can damage cells. Bolsters the immune system Huskisson et al. (2007)	Scurvy (https://en.wikipedia.org)	Fruits with the highest sources of vitamin C include: cantaloupe, citrus fruits and juices, such as orange and grapefruit, kiwi fruit, mango, papaya, pineapple, strawberries, raspberries, blueberries, cranberries and watermelon Vegetables with the highest sources of vitamin C include: broccoli, brussels sprouts, cauliflower, green and red peppers, spinach, cabbage, turnip greens, and other leafy greens, sweet and white potatoes, and tomatoes (https://medlineplus.gov)

Recommended dietary allowances (RDA) for vitamins.

Life stages	Vit A (µg/day)	Vit D (µg/day)	Vit E (mg/day)	Vit K (µg/day)	Vit C (mg/day)	Vit B_1 (mg/day)	Vit B_2 (mg/day)	Vit B_3 (mg/day)	Vit B_4 (mg/day)	Vit B_5 (mg/day)	Vit B_6 (mg/day)	Vit B_7 (µg/day)	Vit B_9 (µg/day)	Vit B_{12} (µg/day)
Infants														
0–6 months	400	10	4	2.0	40	0.2	0.3	2	125	1.7	0.1	5	65	0.4
6–12 months	500	10	5	2.5	50	0.3	0.4	4	150	1.8	0.3	6	80	0.5
Children														
1–3 years	300	15	6	30	15	0.5	0.5	6	200	2	0.5	8	150	0.9
4–8 years	400	15	7	55	25	0.6	0.6	8	250	3	0.6	12	200	1.2
Males														
9–13 years	600	15	11	60	45	0.9	0.9	12	375	4	1.0	20	300	1.8
14–18 years	900	15	15	75	75	1.2	1.3	16	550	5	1.3	25	400	2.4
19–30 years	900	15	15	120	90	1.2	1.3	16	550	5	1.3	30	400	2.4
31–50 years	900	15	15	120	90	1.2	1.3	16	550	5	1.3	30	400	2.4
51–70 years	900	15	15	120	90	1.2	1.3	16	550	5	1.7	30	400	2.4
>70 years	900	20	15	120	90	1.2	1.3	16	550	5	1.7	30	400	2.4
Females														
9–13 years	600	15	11	60	45	0.9	0.9	12	375	4	1.0	20	300	1.8
14–18 years	700	15	15	75	65	1.0	1.0	14	400	5	1.2	25	400	2.4
19–30 years	700	15	15	90	75	1.1	1.1	14	425	5	1.3	30	400	2.4
31–50 years	700	15	15	90	75	1.1	1.1	14	425	5	1.3	30	400	2.4
51–70 years	700	15	15	90	75	1.1	1.1	14	425	5	1.5	30	400	2.4
>70 years	700	20	15	90	75	1.1	1.1	14	425	5	1.5	30	400	2.4
Pregnancy														
14–18 years	750	15	15	75	80	1.4	1.4	18	450	6	1.9	30	600	2.6
19–30 years	770	15	15	90	85	1.4	1.4	18	450	6	1.9	30	600	2.6
31–50 years	770	15	15	90	85	1.4	1.4	18	450	6	1.9	30	600	2.6
Lactation														
14–18 years	1200	15	19	75	115	1.4	1.6	17	550	7	2.0	35	500	2.8
19–30 years	1300	15	19	90	120	1.4	1.6	17	550	7	2.0	35	500	2.8
31–50 years	1300	15	19	90	120	1.4	1.6	17	550	7	2.0	35	500	2.8

Source: Reference (https://www.ncbi.nlm.nih.gov/books).

Tolerable upper intake levels for vitamins reference (https://www.ncbi.nlm.nih.gov/books). Food and Nutrition Board, Institute of Medicine, National Academies.

Life stage group	Vit A (µg/day)	Vit D (µg/day)	Vit E (mg/day)	Vit K (mg/day)	Vit C (mg/day)	Vit B_1 (mg/day)	Vit B_2 (mg/day)	Vit B_3 (mg/day)	Vit B_4 (g/day)	Vit B_5 (mg/day)	Vit B_6 (mg/day)	Vit B_7 (mg/day)	Vit B_9 (µg/day)	Vit B_{12} (mg/day)
Infants														
0–6 months	600	25	ND	ND	ND	ND	ND	ND	ND	ND	ND	ND	ND	ND
6–12 months	600	38	ND	ND	ND	ND	ND	ND	ND	ND	ND	ND	ND	ND
Children														
1–3 years	600	63	200	ND	400	ND	ND	10	1.0	ND	30	ND	300	ND
4–8 years	900	75	300	ND	650	ND	ND	15	1.0	ND	40	ND	400	ND
Males														
9–13 years	1700	100	600	ND	1200	ND	ND	20	2.0	ND	60	ND	600	ND
14–18 years	2800	100	800	ND	1800	ND	ND	30	3.0	ND	80	ND	800	ND
19–30 years	3000	100	1000	ND	2000	ND	ND	35	3.5	ND	100	ND	1000	ND
31–50 years	3000	100	1000	ND	2000	ND	ND	35	3.5	ND	100	ND	1000	ND
51–70 years	3000	100	1000	ND	2000	ND	ND	35	3.5	ND	100	ND	1000	ND
>70 years	3000	100	1000	ND	2000	ND	ND	35	3.5	ND	100	ND	1000	ND
Females														
9–13 years	1700	100	600	ND	1200	ND	ND	20	2.0	ND	60	ND	600	ND
14–18 years	2800	100	800	ND	1800	ND	ND	30	3.0	ND	80	ND	800	ND
19–30 years	3000	100	1000	ND	2000	ND	ND	35	3.5	ND	100	ND	1000	ND
31–50 years	3000	100	1000	ND	2000	ND	ND	35	3.5	ND	100	ND	1000	ND
51–70 years	3000	100	1000	ND	2000	ND	ND	35	3.5	ND	100	ND	1000	ND
>70 years	3000	100	1000	ND	2000	ND	ND	35	3.5	ND	100	ND	1000	ND

(Continued)

Life stage group	Vit A (μg/day)	Vit D (μg/day)	Vit E (mg/day)	Vit K (mg/day)	Vit C (mg/day)	Vit B$_1$ (mg/day)	Vit B$_2$ (mg/day)	Vit B$_3$ (mg/day)	Vit B$_4$ (g/day)	Vit B$_5$ (mg/day)	Vit B$_6$ (mg/day)	Vit B$_7$ (mg/day)	Vit B$_9$ (μg/day)	Vit B$_{12}$ (mg/day)
Pregnancy														
14–18 years	2800	100	800	ND	1800	ND	ND	30	3.0	ND	80	ND	800	ND
19–30 years	3000	100	1000	ND	2000	ND	ND	35	3.5	ND	100	ND	1000	ND
31–50 years	3000	100	1000	ND	2000	ND	ND	35	3.5	ND	100	ND	1000	ND
Lactation														
14–18 years	2800	100	800	ND	1800	ND	ND	30	3.0	ND	80	ND	800	ND
19–30 years	3000	100	1000	ND	2000	ND	ND	35	3.5	ND	100	ND	1000	ND
31–50 years	3000	100	1000	ND	2000	ND	ND	35	3.5	ND	100	ND	1000	ND

ND, not determinable.

Source: Reference (https://www.ncbi.nlm.nih.gov/books).

Minerals.

S. no.	Minerals	Benefits	Deficiency condition	Sources
1.	Calcium	Builds and protects bones and teeth. Helps with muscle contractions and relaxation, blood clotting, and nerve impulse transmission. Plays a role in hormone secretion and enzyme activation. Helps maintain healthy blood pressure (https://www.health.harvard.edu)	Hypocalcemia	Yogurt, cheese, milk, tofu, sardines, salmon, fortified juices, soya beans, nuts, leafy green vegetables, such as broccoli, okra, and kale (but not spinach or Swiss chard, which have binders that lessen absorption) (https://www.nhs.uk; https://www.health.harvard.edu)
2.	Chloride	Balances fluids in the body. A component of stomach acid, essential for digestion (https://www.health.harvard.edu)	Hypochloremia	Chloride is found in table salt or sea salt as sodium chloride. It is also found in many vegetables. Foods with higher amounts of chloride include seaweed, soy sauce, rye, tomatoes, lettuce, celery, olives, and processed foods (https://medlineplus.gov)
3.	Chromium	Enhances the activity of insulin, helps maintain normal blood glucose levels, and is needed to free energy from glucose (https://www.health.harvard.edu)	Impaired insulin function, inhibition of protein synthesis and energy production, type 2 diabetes and heart disease	Whole grain products, some cereals, nuts, certain fruits and vegetables like broccoli, potatoes, grape juice, and oranges are sources of chromium, fat-free or low-fat milk and milk products, fish and fish oils, seafood, lean meat, poultry (turkey), eggs, lean beef, oysters, cheese, legumes (beans and peas), nuts, seeds, and soy products (https://ods.od.nih.gov)
4.	Copper	Plays an important role in iron metabolism and immune system. Helps make red blood cells (https://www.health.harvard.edu)	Problems with connective tissue, muscle weakness, anemia, low white blood cell count, neurological problems, and paleness	Liver, oysters, shellfish, spirulina, shiitake mushrooms, lobsters, whole-grain products, leafy greens, beans, prunes, cocoa, black pepper, nuts, and seeds (https://www.healthline.com)
5.	Fluoride	Encourages strong bone formation. Keeps dental cavities from starting or worsening (https://www.health.harvard.edu)	Dental caries and possibly osteoporosis	Marine fish, blue crab, shrimp, table wine, raisins, coffee, and teas (https://www.myfooddata.com)

(Continued)

S. no.	Minerals	Benefits	Deficiency condition	Sources
6.	Iodine	Part of thyroid hormone, which helps set body temperature and influences nerve and muscle function, reproduction, and growth. Prevents goiter and a congenital thyroid disorder (https://www.health.harvard.edu)	Endemic goiter, hypothyroidism, cretinism, decreased fertility rate, increased infant mortality, and mental retardation or intellectual disability	Iodized salt, processed foods, seafood, fish (such as cod and tuna), seaweed, shrimp, and other seafood, dairy products (such as milk, yogurt, and cheese) and products made from grains (like breads and cereals), fruits, and vegetables (https://ods.od.nih.gov)
7.	Iron	Helps hemoglobin in red blood cells and myoglobin in muscle cells ferry oxygen throughout the body. Needed for chemical reactions in the body and for making amino acids, collagen, neurotransmitters, and hormones (https://www.health.harvard.edu)	Anemia and fatigue	Red meat, liver (chicken, lamb), poultry (chicken and duck), sardines, salmon, lamb, eggs, fruits, green vegetables (kale, broccoli, spinach and green peas), legumes (such as lentils, beans, and chickpeas), firm tofu, tempeh, pumpkin seeds (pepitas) and sunflower seeds, nuts (cashews and almonds), wholegrain cereals (oats or muesli), wholemeal bread, brown rice, dried apricots, amaranth, and quinoa (https://www.healthdirect.gov.au)
8.	Magnesium	Needed for many chemical reactions in the body. Works with calcium in muscle contraction, blood clotting, and regulation of blood pressure. Helps build bones and teeth (https://www.health.harvard.edu)	Diabetes, hypertension, coronary heart disease, osteoporosis, hypocalcemia, hypokalemia, cardiac and neurological manifestations	Green vegetables such as spinach and broccoli, legumes, cashews, sunflower seeds and other seeds, halibut, whole-wheat bread, milk (https://ods.od.nih.gov)
9.	Manganese	Helps form bones. Helps metabolize amino acids, cholesterol, and carbohydrates (https://www.health.harvard.edu)	Impaired growth, impaired reproductive function, skeletal abnormalities, impaired glucose tolerance, and altered carbohydrate and lipid metabolism	Fish, whole grains, oysters, mussels, nuts, soybeans and other legumes, rice, leafy vegetables, coffee, tea, and many spices such as black pepper (https://ods.od.nih.gov)
10.	Molybdenum	Part of several enzymes, one of which helps ward off a form of severe neurological damage in infants that can lead to early death (https://www.health.harvard.edu)	Encephalopathy and intractable seizures	Legumes, nuts, grain products, cereal grains, leafy vegetables, beef liver, and milk (https://ods.od.nih.gov)

#	Mineral	Function	Deficiency	Food Sources
11	Phosphorus	Helps build and protect bones and teeth. Part of DNA and RNA. Helps convert food into energy. Part of phospholipids, which carry lipids in blood and help shuttle nutrients into and out of cells (https://www.health.harvard.edu)	Hypophosphatemia which includes bone diseases such as rickets in children and osteomalacia in adults. An improper balance of phosphorus and calcium may cause osteoporosis	Milk and dairy products, meat, fish, poultry, eggs, liver, green peas, broccoli, potatoes, almonds (https://ods.od.nih.gov)
12	Potassium	Balances fluids in the body. Helps maintain steady heartbeat and send nerve impulses. Needed for muscle contractions. A diet rich in potassium seems to lower blood pressure. Getting enough potassium from your diet may benefit bones (https://www.health.harvard.edu)	Hypokalemia that includes kidney disease	Brown and wild rice, meat, poultry, fish, milk, fruits and vegetables, grains, beans and legumes (https://www.webmd.com)
13	Selenium	Acts as an antioxidant, neutralizing unstable molecules that can damage cells. Helps regulate thyroid hormone activity (https://www.health.harvard.edu)	Keshan disease leading to poor heart function, Kashin–Beck disease leading to osteoarthritis in children and myxedematous endemic cretinism, which results in mental retardation	whole grains and dairy products, including milk and yogurt, pork, beef, turkey, chicken, fish, shellfish, and eggs (https://ods.od.nih.gov)
14	Sodium	Balances fluids in the body. Helps send nerve impulses. Needed for muscle contractions. Impacts blood pressure; even modest reductions in salt consumption can lower blood pressure (https://www.health.harvard.edu)	Hyponatremia	Salt, soy sauce, processed foods, vegetables (https://www.myfooddata.com)
15	Sulfur	Helps form bridges that shape and stabilize some protein structures. Needed for healthy hair, skin, and nails (https://www.health.harvard.edu)	Obesity, heart disease, Alzheimer's and chronic fatigue	Meat, fish, poultry, nuts, legumes, eggs, grains, diary, fruits and vegetables (https://www.healthline.com)
16	Zinc	Helps form many enzymes and proteins and create new cells. Frees vitamin A from storage in the liver. Needed for immune system, taste, smell, and wound healing. When taken with certain antioxidants, zinc may delay the progression of age-related macular degeneration (https://www.health.harvard.edu)	Growth retardation, loss of appetite, impaired immune function, hair loss, diarrhea, delayed sexual maturation, impotence, hypogonadism in males, and eye and skin lesions	Red meat, poultry, oysters, and some other seafood, fortified cereals, beans, nuts (https://ods.od.nih.gov)

Recommended dietary allowances for minerals.

Life-stage group	Ca (mg/day)	Cr (µg/day)	Cu (µg/day)	F (mg/day)	I (µg/day)	Fe (mg/day)	Mg (mg/day)	Mn (mg/day)	Mo (µg/day)	P (mg/day)	Se (µg/day)	Zn (mg/day)	K (mg/day)	Na (mg/day)	Cl (g/day)
Infants															
0–6 months	200	0.2	200	0.01	110	0.27	30	0.003	2	100	15	2	400	110	0.18
7–12 months	260	5.5	220	0.5	130	11	75	0.6	3	275	20	3	860	370	0.57
Children															
1–3 years	700	11	340	0.7	90	7	80	1.2	17	460	20	3	2000	800	1.5
4–8 years	1000	15	440	1	90	10	130	1.5	22	500	30	5	2300	1000	1.9
Males															
9–13 years	1300	25	700	2	120	8	240	1.9	34	1250	40	8	2500	1200	2.3
14–18 years	1300	35	890	3	150	11	410	2.2	43	1250	55	11	3000	1500	2.3
19–30 years	1000	35	900	4	150	8	400	2.3	45	700	55	11	3400	1500	2.3
31–50 years	1000	35	900	4	150	8	420	2.3	45	700	55	11	3400	1500	2.3
51–70 years	1000	30	900	4	150	8	420	2.3	45	700	55	11	3400	1500	2.0
>70 years	1200	30	900	4	150	8	420	2.3	45	700	55	11	3400	1500	1.8
Females															
9–13 years	1300	21	700	2	120	8	240	1.6	34	1250	40	8	2300	1200	2.3
14–18 years	1300	24	890	3	150	15	360	1.6	43	1250	55	9	2300	1500	2.3
19–30 years	1000	25	900	3	150	18	310	1.8	45	700	55	8	2600	1500	2.3
31–50 years	1000	25	900	3	150	18	320	1.8	45	700	55	8	2600	1500	2.3
51–70 years	1200	20	900	3	150	8	320	1.8	45	700	55	8	2600	1500	2.0
>70 years	1200	20	900	3	150	8	320	1.8	45	700	55	8	2600	1500	1.8
Pregnancy															
14–18 years	1300	29	1000	3	220	27	400	2.0	50	1250	60	12	2600	1500	2.3
19–30 years	1000	30	1000	3	220	27	350	2.0	50	700	60	11	2900	1500	2.3
31–50 years	1000	30	1000	3	220	27	360	2.0	50	700	60	11	2900	1500	2.3
Lactation															
14–18 years	1300	44	1300	3	290	10	360	2.6	50	1250	70	13	2500	1500	2.3
19–30 years	1000	45	1300	3	290	9	310	2.6	50	700	70	12	2800	1500	2.3
31–50 years	1000	45	1300	3	290	9	320	2.6	50	700	70	12	2800	1500	2.3

Source: Reference (https://www.ncbi.nlm.nih.gov/books).

Tolerable upper intake levels for minerals.

Life-stage group	Ca (mg/day)	Cr (mg/day)	Cu (µg/day)	F (mg/day)	I (µg/day)	Fe (mg/day)	Mg (mg/day)	Mn (mg/day)	Mo (µg/day)	P (g/day)	K (µg/day)	Se (µg/day)	Zn (mg/day)	Na (g/day)	Cl⁻ (g/day)
Infants															
0–6 months	1000	ND	ND	0.7	ND	40	ND	ND	ND	ND	ND	45	4	ND	ND
7–12 months	1500	ND	ND	0.9	ND	40	ND	ND	ND	ND	ND	60	5	ND	ND
Children															
1–3 years	2500	ND	1000	1.3	200	40	65	2	300	3	ND	90	7	ND	2.3
4–8 years	2500	ND	3000	2.2	300	40	110	3	600	3	ND	150	12	ND	2.9
Males															
9–13 years	3000	ND	5000	10	600	40	350	6	1100	4	ND	280	23	ND	3.4
14–18 years	3000	ND	8000	10	900	45	350	9	1700	4	ND	400	34	ND	3.6
19–30 years	2500	ND	10000	10	1100	45	350	11	2000	4	ND	400	40	ND	3.6
31–50 years	2500	ND	10000	10	1100	45	350	11	2000	4	ND	400	40	ND	3.6
51–70 years	2000	ND	10000	10	1100	45	350	11	2000	4	ND	400	40	ND	3.6
>70 years	2,000	ND	10000	10	1,100	45	350	11	2000	3	ND	400	40	ND	3.6
Females															
9–13 years	3000	ND	5000	10	600	40	350	6	1100	4	ND	280	23	ND	3.4
14–18 years	3000	ND	8000	10	900	45	350	9	1700	4	ND	400	34	ND	3.6
19–30 years	2500	ND	10000	10	1100	45	350	11	2000	4	ND	400	40	ND	3.6
31–50 years	2500	ND	10000	10	1100	45	350	11	2000	4	ND	400	40	ND	3.6
51–70 years	2000	ND	10000	10	1100	45	350	11	2000	4	ND	400	40	ND	3.6
>70 years	2000	ND	10000	10	1100	45	350	11	2000	3	ND	400	40	ND	3.6
Pregnancy															
14–18 years	3000	ND	8000	10	900	45	350	9	1700	3.5	ND	400	34	ND	3.6
19–30 years	2500	ND	10000	10	1100	45	350	11	2000	3.5	ND	400	40	ND	3.6
31–50 years	2500	ND	10000	10	1100	45	350	11	2000	3.5	ND	400	40	ND	3.6
Lactation															
14–18 years	3000	ND	8000	10	900	45	350	9	1700	4	ND	400	34	ND	3.6
19–30 years	2500	ND	10000	10	1100	45	350	11	2000	4	ND	400	40	ND	3.6
31–50 years	2500	ND	10000	10	1100	45	350	11	2000	4	ND	400	40	ND	3.6

Source: Reference (https://www.ncbi.nlm.nih.gov/books).

Recommended dietary allowances for macronutrients.

Life stage group	Total water (l/day)	Carbohydrate (g/day)	Total fiber (g/day)	Fat (g/day)	Linoleic acid (g/day)	α-Linolenic acid (g/day)	Protein (g/day)
Infants							
0–6 months	0.7	60	ND	31	4.4	0.5	9.1
6–12 months	0.8	95	ND	30	4.6	0.5	11
Children							
1–3 years	1.3	130	19	ND	7	0.7	13
4–8 years	1.7	130	25	ND	10	0.9	19
Males							
9–13 years	2.4	130	31	ND	12	1.2	34
14–18 years	3.3	130	38	ND	16	1.6	52
19–30 years	3.7	130	38	ND	17	1.6	56
31–50 years	3.7	130	38	ND	17	1.6	56
51–70 years	3.7	130	30	ND	14	1.6	56
>70 years	3.7	130	30	ND	14	1.6	56
Females							
9–13 years	2.1	130	26	ND	10	1.0	34
14–18 years	2.3	130	26	ND	11	1.1	46
19–30 years	2.7	130	25	ND	12	1.1	46
31–50 years	2.7	130	25	ND	12	1.1	46
51–70 years	2.7	130	21	ND	11	1.1	46
>70 years	2.7	130	21	ND	11	1.1	46
Pregnancy							
14–18 years	3.0	175	28	ND	13	1.4	71
19–30 years	3.0	175	28	ND	13	1.4	71
31–50 years	3.0	175	28	ND	13	1.4	71
Lactation							
14–18 years	3.8	210	29	ND	13	1.3	71
19–30 years	3.8	210	29	ND	13	1.3	71
31–50 years	3.8	210	29	ND	13	1.3	71

Source: Reference (https://www.ncbi.nlm.nih.gov/books).

Acceptable macronutrient distribution ranges.

Macronutrient	Range (percent of energy)		
	Children, 1–3 years	Children, 4–18 years	Adults
Fat	30–40	25–35	20–35
n-6 Polyunsaturated fatty acids (linoleic acid)	5–10	5–10	5–10
n-3 Polyunsaturated fatty acids (α-linolenic acid)	0.6–1.2	0.6–1.2	0.6–1.2
Carbohydrate	45–65	45–65	45–65
Protein	5–20	10–30	10–35

Source: Reference (https://www.ncbi.nlm.nih.gov/books).

1.8 Conclusion

This review provides a comprehensive information about various nutrient requirement and their prescribed daily intake for leading healthy life. Every government has the responsibility to provide the basic nutrient requirement in the form of nutrient supplement either at an affordable price or free of cost for each and every individual to make the nation healthy.

Authors' Contributions

All the authors have contributed equally for this work.

References

Albert, S.G. (2002). *The Discovery of Vitamin C*. American Chemical Society National Historic Chemical Landmarks https://www.acs.org/content/acs/en/education/whatischemistry/landmarks/szentgyorgyi.html.

Albert, C.M., Hennekens, C.H., O'Donnell, C.J. et al. (1998). Fish consumption and risk of sudden cardiac death. *JAMA* 279: 23–28.

Augustyniak, R.A., Singh, K., Zeldes, D. et al. (2010). Maternal protein restriction leads to hyperresponsiveness to stress and salt-sensitive hypertension in male offspring. *American Journal of Physiology. Regulatory, Integrative and Comparative Physiology* 298: R1375–R1382.

Backstrand, J.R. (2002) The history and future of food fortification in the United States: a public health perspective. *Nutrition Reviews* 60: 15–26. doi:https://doi.org/10.1301/002966402760240390

Baessler, K.H., Golly, I., Loew, D. et al. (2002). Vitamin-Lexikon fuer Aerzte. In: *Apotheker und Ernaehrungswissenschaftler*, 3e. Urban & Fischer: Muenchen-Jena.

Bailey, R.L., Gahche, J.J., Lentino, C.V. et al. (2011). Dietary supplement use in the United States, 2003–2006. *Journal of Nutrition* 141: 261–266.

Bassler, K.H. (1995). Definition und Relevanz subklinischer Vitaminmangelzustände. *VitaMinSpur* 10: 112–118.

Begins, K. and Kreft, S. (2014). *Dietary Supplements. Safety, Efficacy and Quality*. Amsterdam: Woodhead Publishing (inprint of Elsevier).

Bellinger, L., Sculley, D.V., and Langley-Evans, S.C. (2006). Exposure to undernutrition in fetal life determines fat distribution, locomotor activity and food intake in ageing rats. *International Journal of Obesity* 3: 729–738. https://doi.org/10.1038/sj.ijo.0803205. PMC 1865484. PMID 16404403.

Bent, S. (2008). Herbal medicine in the united states: review of efficacy, safety, and regulation. *Journal of General Internal Medicine* 23: 854–859.

Birch, E.E., Hoffman, D.R., Uauy, R. et al. (1998). Visual acuity and the essentiality of docosahexaenoic acid and arachidonic acid in the diet of term infants. *Pediatric Research* 44: 201–209.

Birch, E.E., Garfield, S., Hoffman, D.R. et al. (2000). A randomized controlled trial of early dietary supply of long-chain polyunsaturated fatty acids and mental development in term infants. *Developmental Medicine and Child Neurolology* 42: 174–181.

Bishai, D. and Nalubola, R. (2002). The history of food fortification in the United States: its relevance for current fortification efforts in developing countries. *Economic Development and Cultural Change* 51: 37. 5310.1086/345361.

Booth-Kewley, S. and Friedman, H.S. (1987). Psychological predictors of heart disease: a quantitative review. *Psychological Bulletin* 101: 343–362.

Bosaeus, I. (2008). Nutritional support in multimodal therapy for cancer cachexia. *Supportive Care in Cancer* 16: 447–451. https://doi.org/10.1007/s00520-007-0388-7. PMID 1819628.

Brody, T. (1999). *Nutritional Biochemistry*, 2e. Amsterdam, Boston: Academic Press (imprint of Elsevier).

Bronte, V. and Zanovello, P. (2005). Regulation of immune responses by l-arginine metabolism. *Natural Reviews Immunology* 5: 641–654.

Brubacher, G.B. (1988). Assessment of vitamin status in pregnant women. In: *Vitamins and Minerals in Pregnancy and Lactation*, Nestle Nutrition Workshop Series, vol. 16 (ed. H. Berger), 51–57. Vevey: Nestec/New York: Raven Press.

Bruins, M.J., Bird, J.K., Aebischer, C.P., and Eggersdorfer, M. (2018). Considerations for secondary prevention of nutritional deficiencies in high-risk groups in high-income countries. *Nutrients* 10: 47.

Bruins, M.J. Peter Van Dael; Manfred Eggersdorfer (2019) The role of nutrients in reducing the risk for noncommunicable diseases during aging. *Nutrients*, 11: 85. doi:https://doi.org/10.3390/nu11010085.

Burr, M.L., Fehily, A.M., Gilbert, J.F. et al. (1989). Effects of changes in fat, fish, and fibre intakes on death and myocardial reinfarction: diet and reinfarction trial (DART). *Lancet* 2: 757–761.

Burr, G.O., Burr, M.M., and Miller, E. (2007). On the nature and role of the fatty acids essential in nutrition. *Journal of Biological Chemistry* 86: 587–621.

Chajès, V. and Bournoux, P. (2003). Omega-6/Omega-3 polyunsaturated fatty acid ratio and cancer. Omega-6/Omega-3 essential fatty acid ratio: the scientific evidence. *World Review Nutrition and Dietetics* 92: 133–151.

Cleland, L.G., French, J.K., Betts, W.H. et al. (1988). Clinical and biochemical effects of dietary fish oil supplements in rheumatoid arthritis. *Journal of Rheumatology* 15: 1471–1475.

Cleland, L.G., James, M.J., and Proudman, S.M. (2003). Omega-6/omega-3 fatty acids and arthritis. omega-6/omega-3 essential fatty acid ratio: the scientific evidence. *World Review Nutrition and Dietetics* 92: 152–168.

Covington, M.B. (2004). Omega-3 fatty acids. *American Family Physician* 70: 133–140.

Cupp, M.J. and Tracy, T.S. (ed.) (2003). *Dietary Supplements. Toxicology and Clinical Pharmacology*. New York: Humana Press.

Davis, C. and Saltos, E. (1999). Dietary recommendations and how they have changed over time. In: *America's Eating Habits: Changes and Consequences*, Agriculture Information Bulletin No 750 (ed.

E. Frazao). USDA, ERS https://www.ers.usda.gov/webdocs/publications/42215/5831_aib750b_1_.pdf.

De Lorgeril, M. and Salen, P. (2003). Dietary prevention of coronary heart disease: focus on omega-6/omega-3 essential fatty acid balance. Omega-6/omega-3 essential fatty acid ratio: the scientific evidence. *World Review Nutrition and Dietetics* 92: 57–73.

De Smet, P.A.G.M. (2003). Herbal medicine in Europe. Relaxing regulatory standards. *New England Journal of Medicine* 352: 1176–1178.

Dekaney, C.M., Wu, G., Yin, Y.L., and Jaeger, L.A. (2008). Regulation of ornithine aminotransferase gene expression and activity by all trans retinoic acid in Caco-2 intestinal epithelial cells. *Journal of Nutritional Biochemistry* 19: 674–681.

Depeint, F., Bruce, W.R., Shangari, N. et al. (2006). Mitochondrial function and toxicity: role of B vitamins on the one-carbon transfer pathways. *Chemico-Biological Interactions* 163: 113–132.

Dietary Supplements (2011). *Background Information*. Office of Dietary Supplements, US National Institutes of Health (24 June 2011). Retrieved 2 February 2018.

Dubnov, G. and Berry, E.M. (2003). Omega-6/omega-3 fatty acid ratio: the Israeli paradox. Omega-6/omega-3 essential fatty acid ratio: the scientific evidence. *World Review Nutrition and Dietetics* 92: 81–91.

Edwards, R., Peet, M., Shay, J. et al. (1998). Omega-3 polyunsaturated fatty acid levels in the diet and in red blood cell membranes of depressed patients. *Journal of Affective Disorders* 48: 149–155.

Eijkman, C. (1929). Nobel Lecture: the Nobel Prize in Physiology or Medicine. https://www.nobelprize.org/nobel_prizes/medicine/laureates/1929/eijkman-lecture.html.

El Idrissi, A. (2008). Taurine increases mitochondrial buffering of calcium: role in neuroprotection. *Amino Acids* 34: 321–328.

Eritsland, J., Arnesen, H., Gronseth, K. et al. (1996). Effect of dietary supplementation with *n*-3 fatty acids on coronary artery bypass graft patency. *American Journal of Cardiology* 77: 31–36.

Fermer, R.E. (2005). Regulating herbal medicine in the UK. *British Journal of Medicine* 333: 62–63.

Fletcher, R.J., Bell, I.P., Lambert, J.P. (2004) Public health aspects of food fortification: a question of balance. *Proceedings of Nutrition Society* 63: 605–614. doi:https://doi.org/10.1079/PNS2004391

Fraga, C.G. (ed.) (2010). *Plant Phenols and Human Health. Biochemistry, Nutrition, and Pharmacology*. Hoboken, NJ: Wiley.

Green, P., Glozman, S., Kamensky, B. et al. (1999). Developmental changes in rat brain membrane lipids and fatty acids. The preferential prenatal accumulation of docosahexaenoic acid. *Journal of Lipid Research* 40: 960–966.

Grimble, R.F. (2006). The effects of sulfur amino acids intake on immune function in humans. *Journal of Nutrition* 136: 1660S–1665S.

Haag, M. (2003). Essential fatty acids and the brain. *Canadian Journal of Psychiatry* 48: 195–203.

Hamazaki, T. and Okuyama, H. (2003). The Japan Society for Lipid Nutrition recommends to reduce the intake of linoleic acid: a review and critique of the scientific evidence. Omega-6/Omega-3 essential fatty acid ratio: the scientific evidence. *World Review Nutrition and Dietetics* 92: 109–132.

Harper, G.P. (1972) Xylose malabsorption and growth retardation in East Pakistani children. *American Journal of Clinical Nutrition* 25: 1227–1229. doi:https://doi.org/10.1093/ajcn/25.11.1227

Harris, W.S., Ginsberg, H.N., Arunakul, N. et al. (1997). Safety and efficacy of Omacor in severe hypertriglyceridemia. *Journal of Cardiovascular Risk* 4: 385–391.

He, Q.H., Kong, X.F., Wu, G. et al. (2008) Metabolomic analysis of the response of growing pigs to dietary l-arginine supplementation. *Amino Acids* 37: 199–208 doi:https://doi.org/10.1007/s00726-008-0192-9.

Hernandez, A., Burgos, H., Mondaca, M. et al. (2008). Effect of prenatal protein malnutrition on long-term potentiation and BDNF protein expression in the rat entorhinal cortex after neocortical and hippocampal tetanization. *Neural Plasticity* 2008: 1–9. https://doi.org/10.1155/2008/646919. PMC 2442167. PMID 18604298.

Hibbeln, J.R. (1998). Fish consumption and major depression. *Lancet* 351: 1213.

Hollenstein, J. (1994). *Understanding Dietary Supplements*. Boston, MA: Pri-Med Institute.

Horrobin, D.F. and Bennett, C.N. (1999). Depression and bipolar disorder: relationships to impaired fatty acid and phospholipid metabolism and to diabetes, cardiovascular disease, immunological abnormalities, cancer, ageing and osteoporosis. Possible candidate genes. *Prostaglandins Leukotrienes and Essential Fatty Acids* 60: 217–234.

Howe, P.R. (1997). Dietary fats and hypertension. Focus on fish oil. *Annals of New York Academy of Sciences* 827: 339–352.

Hu, F.B., Bronner, L., Willett, W.C. et al. (2002). Fish and omega-3 fatty acid intake and risk of coronary heart disease in women. *JAMA* 287: 1815–1821.

Hu, C.A., Williams, D.B., Zhaorigetu, S. et al. (2008). Functional genomics and SNP analysis of human genes encoding proline metabolic enzymes. *Amino Acids* 35: 655–664.

Huskisson, E., Maggini, S., and Ruf, M. (2007). The influence of micronutrients on cognitive function and performance. *Journal of International Medical Research* 35: 1–19.

James, M.J. and Cleland, L.G. (1997). Dietary *n*-3 fatty acids and therapy for rheumatoid arthritis. *Seminars in Arthritis and Rheumatism* 27: 85–97.

Jamieson, E.C., Farquharson, J., Logan, R.W. et al. (1999). Infant cerebellar gray and white matter fatty acids in relation to age and diet. *Lipids* 34: 1065–1071.

John, J.P.P., Oh, J.E., Pollak, A., and Lubec, G. (2008). Identification and characterization of arsenite (+3 oxidation state) methyltransferase (AS3MT) in mouse neuroblastoma cell line N1E-115. *Amino Acids* 35: 355–358.

Kang, J.X. (2003). The importance of omega-6/omega-3 fatty acid ratio in cell function: the gene transfer of omega-3 fatty acid desaturase. Omega-6/omega-3 essential fatty acid ratio: the scientific evidence. *World Review Nutrition and Dietetics* 92: 23–36.

Keusch, G.T., Plaut, A.G., Troncale, F.J. (1972) Subclinical malabsorption in Thailand. II. Intestinal absorption in American military and Peace Corps personnel. *American Journal of Clinical Nutrition* 25: 1067–1079. doi:https://doi.org/10.1093/ajcn/25.10.1067.

Kremer, J.M., Lawrence, D.A., Jubiz, W. et al. (1990). Dietary fish oil and olive oil supplementation in patients with rheumatoid arthritis. Clinical and immunologic effects. *Arthritis and Rheumatology* 33: 810–820.

Kris-Etherton, P.M., Harris, W.S., and Appel, L.J. (2003). American Heart Association. Nutrition Committee. Fish consumption, fish oil, omega-3 fatty acids, and cardiovascular disease [published correction appears in Circulation 2003;107:512]. *Circulation* 106: 2747–2757.

Lau, C.S., Morley, K.D., and Belch, J.J. (1993). Effects of fish oil supplementation on non-steroidal anti-inflammatory drug requirement in patients with mild rheumatoid arthritis—a double-blind placebo controlled study. *British Journal of Rheumatology* 32: 982–989.

Lee, J.S. and Kim, J. (2009). Factors affecting the use of dietary supplements by Korean adults: data from the Korean National Health and Nutrition Examination Survey III. *Journal of American Dietetic Association* 109: 1599–1605.

Lentjes, M.A., Welch, A.A., and Keogh, R.H. (2015). Opposites don't attract: high spouse concordance for dietary supplement use in the European Prospective Investigation into Cancer in Norfolk (EPIC-Norfolk) cohort study. *Public Health Nutrition* 18: 1060–1066.

Li, P., Yin, Y.L., Li, D.F. et al. (2007). Amino acids and immune function. *British Journal of Nutrition* 98: 237–252.

Li, K., Kaaks, R., Linseisen, J. et al. (2010). Consistency of vitamin and/or mineral supplement use and demographic, lifestyle and health-status predictors: findings from the European Prospective Investigation into Cancer and Nutrition (EPIC)-Heidelberg cohort. *British Journal of Nutrition* 104: 1058–1064.

Lind, J.A. (1753). *Treatise of the Scurvy*. The James Lind Library.

Liu, T., Howard, R.M., Mancini, A.J. et al. (2001). Kwashiorkor in the United States: Fad diets, perceived and true milk allergy, and nutritional ignorance. *Archives of Dermatology* 137: 630–636. PMID 11346341.

Lukaski, H.C. (2000). Magnesium, zinc, and chromium nutriture and physical activity. *American Journal of Clinical Nutrition* 72: 585S–593S.

Lukaski, H.C. (2005). Low dietary zinc decreases erythrocyte carbonic anhydrase activities and impairs cardiorespiratory function in men during exercise. *American Journal of Clinical Nutrition* 81: 1045–1051.

Lukaski, H.C. and Nielsen, F.H. (2002). Dietary magnesium depletion affects metabolic response during submaximal exercise in postmenopausal women. *Journal of Nutrition* 132: 930–935.

Lupi, A., Tenni, R., Rossi, A. et al. (2008). Human prolidase and prolidase deficiency. *Amino Acids* 35: 739–752.

Martin, R.E. and Bazan, N.G. (1992). Changing fatty acid content of growth cone lipids prior to synaptogenesis. *Journal of Neurochemistry* 59: 318–325.

Mason, P. (2011). *Dietary Supplements*, 4e. London: Pharmaceutical Press.

Mateo, R.D., Wu, G., Bazer, F.W. et al. (2007). Dietary l-arginine supplementation enhances the reproductive performance of gilts. *Journal of Nutrition* 137: 652–656.

Mateo, R.D., Wu, G., Moon, H.K. et al. (2008). Effects of dietary arginine supplementation during gestation and lactation on the performance of lactating primiparous sows and nursing piglets. *Journal of Animal Science* 86: 827–835.

Melchior, D., Le Floc'h, N., and Seve, B. (2003). Effect of chronic lung inflammation on tryptophan metabolism in piglets. *Advances in Experimental Medicine and Biology* 527: 359–362.

Messerer, M., Johansson, S.E., and Wolk, A. (2001). Sociodemographic and health behaviour factors among dietary supplement and natural remedy users. *European Journal of Clinical Nutrition* 55: 1104–1110.

Meydani, S.N. and Han, S.N. (2001). Nutrition regulation of the immune response: the case of vitamin E, chapter 41. In: *Present Knowledge in Nutrition*, 8e (ed. B.A. Bowman and R.M. Russel), 449–462. Washington DC: ILSI Press.

Mozaffarian, D. Irwin Rosenberg; Ricardo Uauy (2018) History of modern nutrition science— implications for current research, dietary guidelines, and food policy. *BMJ*, 361:k2392. doi:https://doi.org/10.1136/bmj.k2392.

Muscaritoli, M., Molfino, A., Bollea, M.R., and Fanelli, F.R. (2009). Malnutrition and wasting in renal disease. *Current Opinion in Clinical Nutrition and Metabolic Care* 12: 378–383.

Novelli, A. and Tasker, R.A.R. (2008). Excitatory amino acids in epilepsy: from the clinics to the laboratory. *Amino Acids* 32: 295–297.

Orlando, G.F., Wolf, G., and Engelmann, M. (2008). Role of neuronal nitric oxide synthase in the regulation of the neuroendocrine stress response in rodents: insights from mutant mice. *Amino Acids* 35: 17–27.

Peet, M. and Horrobin, D.F. (2002). A dose-ranging study of the effects of ethyl-eicosapentaenoate in patients with ongoing depression despite apparently adequate treatment with standard drugs. *Archives of General Psychiatry* 59: 913–919.

Phang, J.M., Donald, S.P., Pandhare, J., and Liu, Y. (2008). The metabolism of proline, as a stress substrate, modulates carcinogenic pathways. *Amino Acids* 35: 681–690.

Pietrzik, K. (1985). Concept of borderline vitamin deficiencies. *International Journal of Vitamin and Nutrition Research* 27: 61–73.

Poll, M. C. G. V, Luiking, Y. C., Dejong, C. H. C. et al. (2005). Amino acids: Specific functions. In: *Encyclopedia of human nutrition*, 2e (Caballero, B, Allen, L. and Prentice A), 92–100. Netherland: Elsevier.

Portman, O.W., Neuringer, M., and Alexander, M. (1987). Effects of maternal and long-term postnatal protein malnutrition on brain size and composition in rhesus monkeys. *Journal of Nutrition* 117: 1844–1851. https://doi.org/10.1093/jn/117.11.1844. PMID 3681475.

Pouchieu, C., Andreeva, V.A., Peneau, S. et al. (2013). Sociodemographic, lifestyle and dietary correlates of dietary supplement use in a large sample of French adults: results from the NutriNet-Sante cohort study. *British Journal of Nutrition* 110: 1480–1491.

Pratt, L.A., Ford, D.E., Crum, R.M. et al. (1996). Depression, psychotropic medication, and risk of myocardial infarction. Prospective data from the Baltimore ECA follow-up. *Circulation* 94: 3123–3129.

Ptolemy, A.S., Lee, R., and Britz-McKibbin, P. (2007). Strategies for comprehensive analysis of amino acid biomarkers of oxidative stress. *Amino Acids* 33: 3–18.

Rasmussen, K.M. and Habicht, J.P. (2010). Maternal supplementation differentially affects the mother and newborn. *Journal of Nutrition* 140: 402–406. https://doi.org/10.3945/jn.109.114488. PMID 20032480.

Robert, S.G. and Maurice, E.S. (1980). *Modern Nutrition in Health and Disease*, 6e, 134–138. Philadelphia: Lea and Febinger. ISBN: 978-0-8121-0645-9.

Rucker, R.B., Suttie, J.W., McCormick, D.B. et al. (2001). *Handbook of Vitamins*, 3e. New York: Marcel Dekker.

Scrimshaw, N.S., Taylor, C.E., Gordon, J.E. et al. (1968). *Interactions of Nutrition and Infection*. World Health Organization.

Shakur, Y.A., Tarasuk, V., Corey, P. et al. (2012). Comparison of micronutrient inadequacy and risk of high micronutrient intakes among vitamin and mineral supplement users and nonusers in Canada. *Journal of Nutrition* 142: 534–540.

Shankar, A.H. (2001). Nutritional modulation of immune function and infectious disease, chapter 9. In: *Present Knowledge in Nutrition*, 8e (ed. B.A. Bowman and R.M. Russel), 686–700. Washington DC: ILSI Press.

Shi, W., Meininger, C.J., Haynes, T.E. et al. (2004). Regulation of tetrahydrobiopterin synthesis and bioavailability in endothelial cells. *Cell Biochemistry Biophysics* 41: 415–433.

Shils, M.E., Shike, M., Ross, A.C. et al. (2006). *Modern Nutrition in Health and Disease*, 10e. Philadelphia: Lippincott Williams & Wilkins, Wolters Kluwer.

Simopoulos, A.P. (1999). Essential fatty acids in health and chronic disease. *American Journal of Clinical Nutrition* 70: 560S–569S.

Simopoulos, A.P. (2003). Importance of the ratio of omega-6/omega-3 essential fatty acids: evolutionary aspects. Omega-6/Omega-3 essential fatty acid ratio: the scientific evidence. *World Review Nutrition and Dietetics* 92: 1–22.

Slater-Jefferies, J.L., Lillycrop, K.A., Townsend, P.A. et al. (2011). Feeding a protein-restricted diet during pregnancy induces altered epigenetic regulation of peroxisomal proliferator-activated receptor-α in the heart of the offspring. *Journal of Developmental Origins of Health and Disease* 2: 250–255. https://doi.org/10.1017/S2040174410000425. PMC 3191520. PMID 22003431.

Smith, R.S. (1991). The macrophage theory of depression [erratum appears in Med Hypotheses 36: 178]. *Medical Hypotheses* 35: 298–306.

Sommer, A. and West, K.P.J. (1996). *Vitamin A Deficiency: Health, Survival, and Vision*. Oxford University Press.

Sugano, M. and Hirahara, F. (2000). Polyunsaturated fatty acids in the food chain in Japan. *American Journal of Clinical Nutrition* 71: 189S–196S.

Sun, Y.P., Nonobe, E., Kobayashi, Y. et al. (2002). Characterization and expression of L-amino acid oxidase of mouse milk. *Journal of Biological Chemistry* 277: 19080–19086.

Sutton, G.M., Centanni, A.V., and Butler, A.A. (2010). Protein malnutrition during pregnancy in C57BL/6J mice results in offspring with altered circadian physiology before obesity. *Endocrinology* 151: 1570–1580. https://doi.org/10.1210/en.2009-1133. PMC 2850243. PMID 20160133.

Tan, B.E., Li, X.G., Kong, X.F. et al. (2008) Dietary l-arginine supplementation enhances the immune status in early-weaned piglets. *Amino Acids* 37: 323–331. doi:https://doi.org/10.1007/s00726-008-0155-1

Tazhibayev, S., Dolmatova, O., Ganiyeva, G., et al. (2008) Evaluation of the potential effectiveness of wheat flour and salt fortification programs in five Central Asian countries and Mongolia, 2002–2007. *Food and Nutrition Bulletin* 29: 255–265. doi:https://doi.org/10.1177/156482650802900402

Toledo, F.C., Perobelli, J.E., Pedrosa, F.P. et al. (2011). In utero protein restriction causes growth delay and alters sperm parameters in adult male rats. *Reproductive Biology and Endocrinology* 9: 94. https://doi.org/10.1186/1477-7827-9-94. PMC 3141647. PMID 21702915.

Toscano, A.E., Ferraz, K.M., Castro, R.M. et al. (2010). Passive stiffness of rat skeletal muscle undernourished during fetal development. *Clinics (São Paulo, Brazil)* 65: 1363–1369. https://doi.org/10.1590/s1807-59322010001200022. PMC 3020350. PMID 21340228.

Ubesie, A.C., Ibeziako, N.S., Ndiokwelu, C.I. et al. (2012). Under-five protein energy malnutrition admitted at the University of In Nigeria Teaching Hospital, Enugu: a 10 year retrospective review. *Nutrition Journal* 11: 43. https://doi.org/10.1186/1475-2891-11-43. ISSN 1475-2891. PMC 3487930. PMID 22704641.

Valavanidis, A. (2006). Herbs and traditional therapeutic plants. *Scientific American (Greek Edition)* 92–95. (in Greek).

Van Brummelen, R. and Du Toit, D. (2007). l-Methionine as immune supportive supplement: a clinical evaluation. *Amino Acids* 33: 157–163.

Vargova, V., Vesely, R., Sasinka, M. et al. (1998). Will administration of omega-3 unsaturated fatty acids reduce the use of nonsteroidal antirheumatic agents in children with chronic juvenile arthritis? [Slovak]. *Casopis Lékaru Ceských* 137: 651–653.

Volker, D., Fitzgerald, P., Major, G. et al. (2000). Efficacy of fish oil concentrate in the treatment of rheumatoid arthritis. *Journal of Rheumatology* 27: 2343–2346.

Walker, D.R. (2015). Report on the Regulation of Herbal Medicine and Practitioners. Dpt of Health and the Medicines (UK), Healthcare Products Regulatory Agency. http://www.dcscience.net/Report_on_Regulation_of_Herbal_Medicines_and_Practitioners.pdf.

Walson, J.L. and Berkley, J.A. (2018). The impact of malnutrition on childhood infections. In: *Current Opinion in Infectious Diseases*. Lippincott Williams & Wilkins http://www.ncbi.nlm.nih.gov/pmc/articles/PMC6037284/.

Wang, W.W., Qiao, S.Y., Li, D.F. (2008) Amino acids and gut function. *Amino Acids* 37: 105–110. doi:https://doi.org/10.1007/s00726-008-0152-4

Wang, X., Ou, D., Yin, J., et al. (2009) Proteomic analysis reveals altered expression of proteins related to glutathione metabolism and apoptosis in the small intestine of zinc oxide-supplemented piglets. *Amino Acids* 37: 209–218. doi:https://doi.org/10.1007/s00726-009-0242-y.

Watson, R.R., Gerald, J.K., and Prredy, V.R. (ed.) (2011). *Nutrients, Dietary Supplements, and Nutriceuticals. Cost Analysis versus Clinical Benefits*. Berlin: Springer Science & Business Media.

Weissman, M.M., Bland, R.C., Canino, G.J. et al. (1996). Cross-national epidemiology of major depression and bipolar disorder. *JAMA* 276: 293–299.

Whitney, E. and Rolfes, S.R. (2008). *Understanding Nutrition*, 11e, 154. California: Thomson Wadsworth.

WHO National Policy on Traditional Medicine and Regulation of Herbal Medicines (2005). Report WHO Global Survey, 168 pp. http://apps.who.int/medicinedocs/pdf/s7916e/s7916e.pdf.

Van de Poll, M.C.G., Luiking, Y.C., Dejong, C.H.C. et al. (2013). Amino acids: specific functions. In: *Encyclopedia of Human Nutrition*, 3e (ed. A. Prentice, L. Allen and B. Caballero). Reference module in biomedical sciences, 79–87. Netherland: Elsevier.

Van den Wijngaart, A., Begin, F., Codling, K., et al. (2013) Regulatory monitoring systems of fortified salt and wheat flour in selected ASEAN countries. *Food and Nutrition Bulletin* 34: S102–11. doi:https://doi.org/10.1177/15648265130342S112.

Willis, A., Beander, H.U., Steel, G., and Valle, D. (2008). PRODH variants and risk for schizophrenia. *Amino Acids* 35: 673–679.

Wirth, J.P., Laillou, A., Rohner, F., et al. (2012) Lessons learned from national food fortification projects: experiences from Morocco, Uzbekistan, and Vietnam. *Food and Nutrition Bulletin* 33: S281–92. doi:https://doi.org/10.1177/15648265120334S304

World Health Organization (2015). World health statistics. http://www.who.int/gho/publications/world_health_statistics/2012/en/.

Wu, G. (1997). Synthesis of citrulline and arginine from proline in enterocytes of postnatal pigs. *American Journal of Physiology* 272: G1382–G1390.

Wu, G. (2009) Amino acids: metabolism, functions, and nutrition. *Amino Acids* 37: 1–17. doi:https://doi.org/10.1007/s00726-009-0269-0.

Wu, G., Knabe, D.A., Flynn, N.E. et al. (1996). Arginine degradation in developing porcine enterocytes. *American Journal of Physiology, Gastrointestinal and Liver Physiology* 271: G913–G919.

Wu, G., Knabe, D.A., and Kim, S.W. (2004). Arginine nutrition in neonatal pigs. *Journal of Nutrition* 134: 2783S–2790S.

Wu, G., Bazer, F.W., Hu, J. et al. (2005). Polyamine synthesis from proline in the developing porcine placenta. *Biology of Reproduction* 72: 842–850.

Wu, G., Bazer, F.W., Datta, S. et al. (2008). Proline metabolism in the conceptus: implications for fetal growth and development. *Amino Acids* 35: 691–702.

Yan, G.R. and He, Q.Y. (2008). Functional proteomics to identify critical proteins in signal transduction pathways. *Amino Acids* 35: 267–274.

Yehuda, S. (2003). Omega-6/omega-3 ratio and brain related functions. Omega-6/omega-3 essential fatty acid ratio: the scientific evidence. *World Review Nutrition and Dietetics* 92: 37–56.

Zampelas, A., Paschos, G., Rallidis, L. et al. (2003). Linoleic acid to alpha-linolenic acid ratio: from clinical trials to inflammatory markers of coronary artery disease. Omega-6/omega-3 essential fatty acid ratio: the scientific evidence. *World Review Nutrition and Dietetics* 92: 92–108.

2

Nutraceuticals for Prevention and Treatment of Cancer

Neeladrisingha Das[1], Sandip Nathani[1], Viney Kumar[1], Himanshu Agrawal[1], Debabrata Sircar[2], and Partha Roy[1]

[1] *Molecular Endocrinology Laboratory, Department of Biotechnology, Indian Institute of Technology Roorkee, Roorkee, Uttarakhand, India*
[2] *Plant Molecular Biology Laboratory, Department of Biotechnology, Indian Institute of Technology Roorkee, Roorkee, Uttarakhand, India*

2.1   Introduction

The term "cancer" represents a large group of diseases that may affect different parts of the body under specified conditions. At present, cancer is one of the significant health concerns and the second major reason for death across the world. According to World Health Organization (WHO), cancer is accountable for the 9.6 million deaths or one in six deaths in the year 2018 (WHO 2020). A myriad of experimental, epidemiological, and clinical researches focus on identifying the mechanism of various cancer forms, their prevention as well as management. The transformation of the cancerous cells from normal cells undergoes multistage processes starting from a simple lesion to a malignant tumor. One of the key reasons behind this unsought transmutation is the interactions between the genetic factor and several external carcinogens, including biological (bacteria, viruses, and parasites), physical (ionizing and UV radiation), and chemical (arsenic, asbestos, tobacco, etc.). Besides, aging and nutrition are two more ancillary factors that may brace the cancer progression. Moreover, lifestyle and diets are recently considered the most substantial environmental component linked to cancer. As per the statistics of the world cancer research fund, cancer deaths due to diet and related conditions can range from 10 to 70% (World Cancer Research Fund 2007). Based on the epidemiological evidence, the same report also explored the cancer risks and the impact of dietary factors like body weight gain, physical activity, dietary patterns, nutrients, phytochemicals, and more. Albeit, there is no direct scientific conclusion on the link between cancer risk and diets, but there are a considerable number of evidence acknowledging certain dietary factors and their role in cancer risk, as well as management.

As far as cancer management is concerned, the major treatments implied for cancer are surgery, radiotherapy, and chemotherapy. The most commonly used chemotherapy drugs are DNA interactive, antitubulin, antimetabolite, or specific molecular targeting agents (Hosseini and Ghorbani 2015; Nussbaumer et al. 2011). However, various side effects are associated with the clinical application of these drugs that includes bone marrow suppression, dysfunction of the neurological system, resistance to drugs and cardiac complication, and impairment in the gastrointestinal tract (Dropcho 2011; Monsuez et al. 2010). These complications drive interest toward the anticancer agent derived from natural products due to their broader impact on various cellular signaling pathways along with negligible toxic effects against normal cells.

Complementary and alternative medicines (CAM) are the most reliable form of medicine practiced across the globe. These are very well accepted across various communities due to their link in the traditional practices, folklore forms, and clinical safety. Various forms of CAM include phytotherapy, homeopathy, ayurveda, yoga, and naturopathy, including use of phytochemicals and nutraceuticals. Epidemiological investigations and clinical trials clearly indicate that different chronic diseases such as cancer, diabetes, and neurodegenerative disorders can be avoided by adopting the appropriate lifestyle, environment, and dietary pattern. Consumption of nutritional food that is rich in fruits, vegetables, fish oil can lessen the occurrence and prevalence of these diseases (Mecocci et al. 2014). Nutraceuticals are the products that are obtained from a food source (part of food) and provide promising therapeutic benefits against chronic disease apart from their essential nutritional values (Nasri et al. 2014). Based on food sources, nutraceuticals can be categorized into phytochemicals and non-phytochemicals. Phytochemicals are obtained purely from plants while non-phytochemicals might be obtained from sources other than plants including livestock, marine, and microbes. Phytochemicals are distributed into various subcategories depending on their chemical structure. Phytochemicals that are considered as nutraceuticals are alkaloids, carotenoids, flavonoids, diterpenes, and phenolic acids and some others. Major non-phytochemicals that come into nutraceutical categories are prebiotics, probiotics, marine-based nutraceuticals, and melatonin (Chauhan et al. 2013). The usage of natural dietary products for the prevention of cancer is termed as chemoprevention. This term is different from chemotherapy, where mostly synthetic chemicals are used for the treatment of cancer (Salami et al. 2013). Among different nutraceuticals, phytochemicals with high antioxidant and polyphenol content have shown substantial chemoprotective activities. A large number of evidences suggested a protective effect of organosulfur compounds, flavonoids, carotenoids, and phenolic acids against oxidative stress and cellular pathways that initiate or promote the tumorigenesis (Kapinova et al. 2018; Saldanha and Tollefsbol 2012). Data obtained from various in vitro and in vivo studies postulated that cancer risk could be decreased by a precise consumption of antioxidant-rich phytochemicals, fruits, vegetables, beverages, grains, and vitamins without any remarkable adverse effects (Soerjomataram et al. 2010; Turati et al. 2015). Dietary natural products can exert their anticancer effects by various mechanisms that include protection of normal cells against oxidative damage, inhibition of tumor cell growth and metastasis, and supportive effects toward chemotherapeutic drugs (Lee et al. 2013).

These antioxidants showed chemopreventive properties due to their protective effect against oxidative DNA damage that is mainly associated with tumor initiation. Phytochemicals, after their entry into the cells, can protect them from oxidative stress in different ways. Phytochemicals can either scavenge the free radicles independently or activate the cellular signaling pathways. Activation of NF-E2-related factor 2-Kelch-like ECH-associated protein 1 (Nrf2-Keap1) pathway is the major antioxidant mechanism by phytochemicals to protect cells against oxidative stress (Finley et al. 2011). Nrf-2 pathway activation results in the initiation of cellular defense mechanism that includes synthesis of antioxidant and stress-defense proteins and detoxifying enzymes and transporters. All these molecules participate in the protection of normal cells against reactive oxygen species (ROS), reactive nitrogen species (RNS), and reactive metabolites of carcinogenic species (Lee et al. 2013; Qin and Hou 2016).

In tumor cells, cell growth, survival, and proliferative machinery are dysregulated compared to normal cells. Interestingly, certain dietary phytochemicals also target multiple growth inhibitory mechanisms to prevent tumor progression that includes induction of apoptotic cell death, cell cycle arrest, and angiogenesis inhibition (Hosseini and Ghorbani 2015; Khan et al. 2010). Apart from this, natural products are now being used in combination with anticancer drugs. This combination can improve the efficacy and decrease the dose and weaken the toxic effect of anticancer drugs. Many cancer cells exhibit resistance to apoptosis; however, a combination of certain phytochemicals like grape proanthocyanidin and epigallocatechin gallate (EGCG) with anticancer drugs like doxorubicin has been reported to remarkably inhibit this drug resistance in liver tumor cells and in turn promotes apoptosis (Liang et al. 2010).

On the contrary, certain studies reported against the beneficial effect of few antioxidant phenolics and vitamin supplementation for the prevention of cancer (Calvani et al. 2020). Excess intake of certain dietary component is also positively associated with increased risk of certain types of cancer including ovary, pancreas, prostate, liver, and endometrium. These components include food and beverages containing a high amount of calorie, sugar, alcohol, saturated and trans-unsaturated fatty acids, and red meat (Stepien et al. 2016; Williams et al. 2010). Altogether, human and epidemiological studies imply that an overall antioxidant-rich diet have greater influence compared to individual dietary antioxidants. Therefore, a healthy diet pattern that is rich in anticarcinogenic compounds and deficient for carcinogenic compounds could be an efficient chemopreventive approach for the cure and management of cancer. In this chapter, we will discuss the current progress in context of nutraceuticals and their impact on cancer prevention and treatment. Emphasis has been made on specific cellular and molecular targets of various nutraceuticals for combating cancer.

2.2 Classification of Nutraceuticals

The term *"nutraceutical"* was first coined by Stephen DeFlice (1989), which was derived from the combination of both "nutrition" and "pharmaceutical." A wide range of terms is being used to define the nutraceuticals, including- bioactive compounds, phytochemicals, dietary supplements, medicinal foods, nutritional supplements, and many more. The nutraceuticals research has gained momentum recently due to its potential therapeutic and nutritional benefits and presumed efficacy in terms of toxicity. Although there are not any standard classification systems for nutraceuticals but the wide range of products that come under the canopy of nutraceuticals can be mainly classified into commercial, traditional, and nontraditional nutraceuticals. Figure 2.1 depicts a complete classification of nutraceuticals and their sub-types. The traditional nutraceuticals primarily include- prebiotics, probiotics, nutraceutical enzymes (hemicellulase from mushroom, pancreolipase), and all kinds of chemicals, including nutrients (vitamins, amino acids, etc.), and phytochemicals (flavonoids, polyphenolics, phenolics, etc.). From this segment, the phytochemicals are vividly

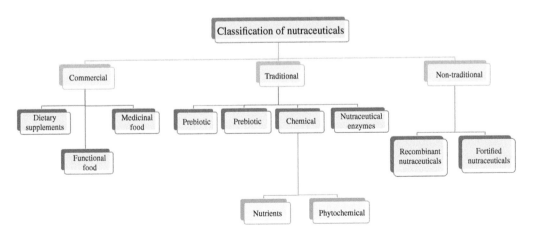

Figure 2.1 Basic classification of nutraceuticals.

studied for their therapeutic potential in various chronic illnesses, including cancer. The nontraditional segment of the nutraceuticals comprises of fortified and recombinant nutraceuticals.

The fortified nutraceuticals include the fortified foods either obtained through the agricultural breeding or added nutritional ingredients. However, certain foods have nutritional value, which are developed either with the help of genetic engineering or using the latest biotechnology approaches. These categories of nontraditional nutraceuticals are placed in recombinant nutraceuticals (e.g. bread, vinegar). The commercial segment of the nutraceuticals is mainly divided into commercially available dietary supplements or nutritional supplements, functional foods, and medicinal foods. In 1994, Dietary Supplement Health and Education Act (DSHEA) of United States defined the term "dietary supplement" as dietary ingredients intended to compensate the nutritional needs and supplement the diet (Food Report 2007). These are mainly available in the form of pills or capsules (e.g. vitamin B capsules) and concentrated liquids. Medicinal foods comprise of specialized diets prescribed under medical supervision and having health benefits. These kinds of foods are mainly prescribed to manage complications like impaired digestion, coeliac disease, and various chronic conditions like cardiac diseases, diabetes, and cancer. Similarly, functional foods are known for their health benefits beyond their traditional nutritional contributions. In some cases, the functional foods undergo a process called nitrification to perpetuate the nutrient content in the food even after its processing. Discussing all types of nutraceuticals and their role in the management of cancer is beyond the scope of this chapter. Hence, the roles of selected nutraceuticals having a key role in cancer management are vividly discussed.

2.3 Cancer and Nutrition

Although role of nutrition in cancer pathogenesis is a vast field, nevertheless, its importance is gradually becoming evident. According to World Cancer Research Fund and American Institute for Cancer Research, with proper diet intake and physical activity, cancer could be prevented about 30–40%. The role of nutrition in cancer has been investigated with a reductionist approach in which a nutrient or a particular food has been explored for its effect on regression or tumor formation (Donaldson 2004).

It is consistently evident from ample epidemiological studies that dietary habits influence the outcomes of several chronic diseases, like gallstone, cataract, type-II diabetes, cardiovascular disease, neurodegenerative diseases (e.g. Parkinson disease), and different kinds of cancer (e.g. colorectal cancer). Dietary habits, responsible for the nutritional profile of an individual, are closely associated with disease prognoses because nutrition modulates several fundamental cellular process, like inflammation, ROS, apoptosis, hormone regulation, and many others (Figure 2.2). Vegetarian diet is generally believed to reduce risks of chronic illnesses and facilitate defined health goals (Angel Nivya et al. 2012). Between naturally occurring and synthetic drugs, although, latter ones have relatively instantaneous onset of action and are associated with more side effects. Thus, prophylactic approaches to achieve targeted health goals and manage disease occurrences through dietary modulations and intake of drugs from natural sources are becoming increasingly popular (Angel Nivya et al. 2012). Besides providing nutrition, plants are rich sources of nonnutritive substances (very low in calories or contain no calories), called phytochemicals. The phytochemicals originally evolved as components of defense mechanisms of plants. However, their inherent defensive properties, like antioxidative, anti-inflammatory, and immune modulatory, to name a few, have proven to be equally beneficial to humans against various disease pathogeneses. Consequently, the past few years have witnessed an increasing demand for food products, dietetics,

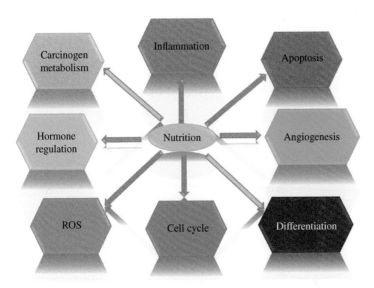

Figure 2.2 Nutrition that can influence cancer development by affecting fundamental cellular processes.

and pharmaceuticals enriched in such phytochemicals (Angel Nivya et al. 2012). Therefore, pharmaceutical industries have focused on developing products containing bioactive compounds in the form of capsules, gels, solutions, liquors, pills, etc. These products enriched in phytochemicals having health-boosting effects can be classified neither as food nor as conventional drugs. Thus, a new term, nutraceutical has been derived from nutrient and pharmaceutical to refer to these products. So, nutraceuticals can be defined as any substance with nutritive, as well as medicinal properties and thus can be used for maintenance of health and treatment and prevention of diseases (Andlauer and Fürst 2002).

The chemotherapeutic value of nutraceuticals in cancer is becoming evident, primarily from animal studies involving certain phytochemicals, like phytoesterogens, flavones, curcumin isoflavonones, capsaicin, genestein, gingerol, epigallocatechin-3-gallate, lycopene, antioxidants, vitamins, and minerals (Tripathi et al. 2005). Self-described testimonies of nutraceutical medicine in favor of liquorice (for peptic ulcer), phosphatidylcholine (for hepatitis), kambocha tea (for arthritis), ginger (for, dizziness, emetic disorder, carminative), glucosamine (for chondroitin), lutein (for antipain), vitamins C, D, E, minerals like Se, Zn, Cu, fenugreek (for osteoarthritis), leupeptin, urokinase inhibitor (for prostate cancer), green tea (for cancer), lycopene, carotenoids, glucans (for cardiovascular disease), *Morinda citrifolia* (for relief from muscle pain and high blood pressure), *Trigonella foenum-graceum* (as anticancer, antidiabetic), *Rhus coriaria* (for antibacterial activity), *Thymus vulgaris, Geranium sanguineum* (as antiviral), and sorrel (for immune system) have accrued success for these compounds over years. Likewise, silbinin, lycopene, vitamin D, shark cartilage (to decrease bone pain and osteoporosis), vitamin E and selenium, green tea, soy, seed extract of grape, pectin, and modified citrus are accepted as preventive food supplements for prostate cancer (Sharma 2009). Nutraceuticals may act as essential nutrient, phytohormone, and biochemical metabolite regulator in the body. There are prominent evidences showing that nutraceuticals, such as vitamin E, lycopene (carotenoids), vitamin C, carotene, glutathione (thiols), lipoic acid, can prevent and inhibit cancer (Figure 2.3). Presence of vitamin E in the lipid domain of plasma lipoprotein and biological membranes prevents polyunsaturated fatty acid (PUFA) lipid peroxidation and effectively reverses the inhibitory effect of lipid peroxidation on cell

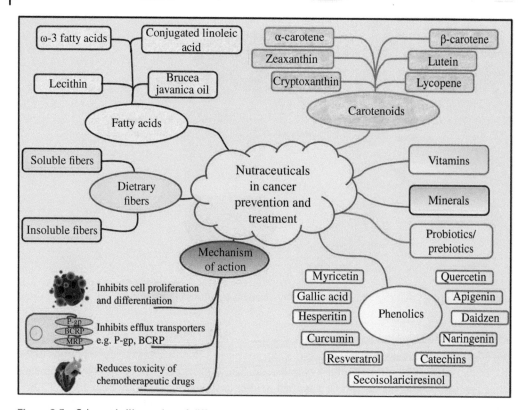

Figure 2.3 Schematic illustration of different nutraceuticals used in cancer prevention and treatment. *Source:* Arora and Jaglan (2016). Reproduced with permission from Elsevier.

proliferation (Conklin 2000). Along with antioxidant activity, vitamin E induces apoptosis by enhancing antineoplastic activity. Apoptosis-inducing property of vitamin E is due to its inhibitory effect on protein tyrosine kinases (PTKs) (Yu et al. 1999). Bleomycin-induced chromosomal breakage was also reduced by vitamin E (Anderson et al. 1995), indicating that antioxidants are potent chemopreventive agents for chemotherapy-induced secondary tumors. Water-soluble antioxidant vitamin C provides protection from lipid peroxidation through ROS scavenging, reducing chromosomal damage and risk of chemotherapy-induced carcinogenesis (Conklin 2000). Likewise, superoxide dismutase (enzyme), co-enzyme Q-10, selenium, zinc (minerals), manganese, and copper are reported to induce apoptosis in isolated cancer cells (Hennekens 1994). In electron transport chain of mitochondria, an indispensable cofactor, i.e. coenzyme Q10 (CoQ10), acts as electron carrier between the enzyme complexes of the respiratory chain. CoQ10 is a lipid-soluble antioxidant that scavenges free radicals within the biological membranes and prevents lipid peroxidative damage of mitochondrial membranes (Solaini et al. 1987). Vegetables like carrot, cabbage, onion, lettuce, tomato with 9–12% fiber content have been reported to show antioxidant property and can inhibit cell proliferation. Fruits like apple, orange, apricot, plum, and pine are also rich in fibers. Apple has higher fiber content (18–30%) compared to many other fruits. The water soluble dietary fibers are also present in dried beans, oats, legumes, and chicory (Sharma 2009). β-Carotene, a lipid-soluble antioxidant, is one of >600 carotenoids that are produced by plants and microorganisms and occurs naturally as a mixture of *cis* and *trans* isomers. *Trans*-isomer form of β-carotene is a less effective antioxidant than *cis*-isomer β-carotene. Chronic low doses of cyclophosphamide also reduced the rate of tumor induction in animals (Alpha-Tocopherol, Beta Carotene Cancer Prevention Study Group 1994). The oligosaccharides, like inulins, fructo-oligosaccharides, lactilol, lactulose, soybean oligosaccharides, xylo-oligosaccharides, galacto-oligosaccharides, lacto-sucrose, gluco-oligosaccharides, isomalto-oligosaccharides, when tested in animals showed reduction in proliferation of cancer cells (Sharma 2009). Similarly, soy isoflavones, curcumin, genistein, epigallocatechin-3-gallate (EGCG), capsaicin lycopene, and gingerol have been established as cancer-protective nutraceuticals (Lambert et al. 2003). The major nutraceuticals are either vitamins, minerals, or phytochemicals. The vitamins A, B6, B12, D, E, and folate are potent anticancer and immunoprotective agents and can significantly reduce cancer risk (Sood and Sood 2007; Slatore et al. 2008; Zhang et al. 2008). Meta-analyses, epidemiological evidences, and randomized trials for biochemical and metabolic activities have revealed that vitamin-containing diets act as anitioxidants in primary and secondary cancers (Bairati et al. 2005, 2008; Hercberg et al. 2006; Park et al. 2009). Among the minerals, Mg, Zn, Se, and Ca have been associated with cancer prevention (Gromadzińska et al. 2008; Huang et al. 2006; Johnson 2004; Lin et al. 2006). Fatty acids, like soy phytoestrogens, and polyphenols, like isoflavones, are potent chemopreventive agents against cancer that can effectively reduce cell proliferation, free radicals, and necrosis and induce apoptosis (Colomer et al. 2007; Ganry 2005; Holzbeierlein et al. 2005; Messina and Wood 2008; Russo 2007; Thomasset et al. 2007; Walle et al. 2007). There are different sources to consume omega-3 PUFA including flax seed oil, flax seed, and cold water fish. While fish oil contains two types of omega-3 PUFA, namely, docosahexaenoic acid (DHA) and icosapentaenoic acid (EPA), flax seed oil mainly contain alpha-linolenic acid (ALA). ALA is also present in walnuts, hemp, and pumpkin seeds. The best sources of omega-3 PUFA are herring, lake trout, salmon, mackerel, canned sardines, albacore tuna, anchovies, lake white fish, and bluefish. PUFAs are effective in preventing primary tumors growth. FOLFOX chemotherapy (a combination of chemotherapy drugs used to treat bowel cancer and made up of (i) folinic acid, (ii) fluorouracil (5FU), (iii) oxaliplatin) showed that PUFAs could increase their efficacy on repetitive chemotherapy-resistant cancers. Combination of FOLFOX and PUFA actually targeted different aspects of chemotherapy-resistant cancers, which resulted in PARP cleavage with increased apoptosis and decreased PI3K/ phosphatase and tensin homolog (PTEN)/Akt/mTORC1 signaling (Vasudevan et al. 2014).

Nutritional modulation is therefore beneficial in cancer patient's treatment. For cancer patients, foods with low carbohydrates, having omega-3 fatty acid, protein, and fibers rich constituents are beneficial (Tuomisto et al. 2004). Besides, nutraceuticals can reduce chemo- and radiotherapy-associated toxicity and cancer cachexia (Grimble 2003). The phytochemicals act at different cellular levels through discrete mechanisms. Although many of them comprise a multifaceted antioxidant sources affecting signaling pathways and modulating transcription factors through redox mechanism, there are others that directly modulate the immunological cascade, enzymes related to inflammation and endocrine system. Besides, few phytochemicals directly affect DNA repair and cleavage processes.

Several known phytochemicals have been analyzed from various nutraceuticals and dietary sources. Majority of them have profound effects in limiting the growth of various types of cancers. These phytochemicals act by targeting particular signaling pathways involved in cancer progression and tumor development/invasion, and their mechanism of action in cellular systems are well validated. Discussing the role of every phytochemicals/nutraceutical is beyond the scope of this review. Hence, in the current section, the focus of our discussion mainly involves the effect of some major nutraceuticals mostly used as a daily dietary ingredient or as folklore medicine and the phytochemicals involved in them. The Table 2.1 in the following section elaborates on the role of various dietary nutraceuticals/phytochemicals for the regulation of cancer progression. Most of the

Table 2.1 List of major nutraceuticals/phytochemicals and their role in cancer research.

SI No	Nutraceuticals/ dietary supplements	Major phytoconstituents	Mechanism of action	References
1.	Apples	Phloretin	• Inhibits tumor cell proliferation, migration, invasion by inhibiting ERKs, Akt, and CDKs	Yang et al. (2015)
			• Induces apoptosis by inducing Bax, PARP, and Bcl2	Delphi and Sepehri (2016)
2.	Berries	Pectin	• Inhibit cell growth by arresting cell cycle at sub G1 phase in 4T1 breast cancer cells	
		Proanthocyanidins	• Reduces cell viability in SKOV-3 ovarian cancer cells by blocking expression of Akt and VEGF	Kim et al. (2012), Kim et al. (2005)
			• Induces apoptosis in human colorectal cancer cell line, SNU-C4 by upregulation of BAX and Caspase-3, and downregulation of Bcl2	
		Quercetin-3-glucuronide	• Inhibits doxorubicin resistance by reducing endoplasmic reticulum stress in hepatocellular carcinoma cells	Wu et al. (2019)
3.	Cruciferous vegetables	Indole-3-carbinol	• Inhibits cell adhesion, spreading, and invasion via upregulation of PTEN and E-cadherin in T47-D breast cancer cells	Meng et al. (2000)
		Diindolylmethane	• Acts syngergystically with capsaicin in human colon cancer cells by modulating NF-κB and p53 genes	Clark et al. (2015)
4.	Carrots	β-carotene	• Induces apoptosis and cell cycle arrest in breast cancer cell line	Gloria et al. (2014)
		Lutein	• Restricts proliferation of human small cell lung cancer cells by inducing apoptosis through PI3k/mTOR/AKT pathway	Zhang et al. (2018), Chew et al. (2003)
			• Inhibits mouse mammary tumor growth by upregulating proapoptotic genes, p53, and Bax and also regulates angiogenic activity	
5.	Coffee	Caffeine	• Synergistic anticancer effect with cisplatin via inhibiting Fanconi anemia group D2 protein mono-ubiquitination in hepatocellular carcinoma cells	Bessler et al. (2012), Oda et al. (2017)
			• Inhibition of TNF-α and IFNγ secretion by peripheral blood mononuclear cells and suppress growth of colon cancer cells	

			References
	Trigonelline	• Activation of apoptosis by inhibition of Nrf2 transcription factor in pancreatic cancer cells • Anti-invasive activity in rat ascites hepatoma cell line AH109A by inhibition of ROS production	Arlt et al. (2013), Hirakawa et al. (2005)
6.	Peanuts		
	Taxifolin	• Enhances andrographolide-induced mitotic arrest and apoptosis in human prostate cancer cells via spindle assembly checkpoint activation • Inhibition of human cervical cancer Hela cell proliferation by upregulation of p53 and p21	Zhang et al. (2013), Zhai et al. (2011)
7.	Garlic		
	S-allylmercaptocysteine	• E-cadherin upregulation, antimetastatic activity in androgen-independent prostate cancer in vivo • Inhibits proliferation of colorectal cancer cells via upregulating cleaved caspase-3 and cleaved PARP1 under in vitro and in vivo conditions	Howard et al. (2007), Liang et al. (2011)
8.	Grapes		
	Chlorogenic acid	• Induces apoptosis in HCT116 cells by inducing DNA fragmentation, caspase-9 activation, and PARP-1 cleavage • Induces cell death in MCF-7 and MDA MB 231 cells by arresting cell cycle in G1 phase	Deka et al. (2017), Gouthamchandra et al. (2017)
	Gallic acid	• Induces apoptosis in DU145 and 22Rv1 cells and also reduces the tumor in DU145 and 22Rv1 xenograft nude mice models • Reduces tumor in transgenic adenocarcinoma of the mouse prostate (TRAMP) model by decreasing expression of Cdk4, Cdk2, and Cdk6 • Inhibits the prostate cancer (DU145) cell growth by iROS generation, arresting cell cycle in G2/M phase, and inhibiting Cdc25C and Cdc2 activities	Chen et al. (2014), Kaur et al. (2009), Raina et al. (2008)
	Resveratrol	• Inhibits the growth of HT29 (colon cancer) cells by suppressing oncogenic miRNA (miR-27a) • Reduces the growth of prostate cancer cells by downregulating AR and its coactivator GRIP-1 and SRC-1 • Inhibits the tumorigenesis in follicular thyroid cancer by inhibiting ST6GAL2-Hippo signaling pathway	Del Follo-Martinez et al. (2013), Nikhil et al. (2014a), Xu et al. (2020)

(Continued)

Table 2.1 (Continued)

Sl No	Nutraceuticals/ dietary supplements	Major phytoconstituents	Mechanism of action	References
9.	Green Tea	Catechin	• Inhibits the cancer cell proliferation by acting on the phosphorylation of VEGF • Promotes in sensitizing chemoresistant hepatocellular carcinoma cells to doxorubicin in murine model by reducing the expression of HIF-1α and MDR1 mRNA	Lamy et al. (2002), Liang et al. (2010)
		Epicatechin	• Limits the cancer cell progression of PC3, SKOV3, U373MG cells • Restricts HCT116 cell growth by inducing the expression of NAG-1 • Enhances ROS generation in MCF-7 and MDA-MB-231 cells and upregulates proapoptotic proteins, namely, BAD and BAX	Baek et al. (2004), Park et al. (2004), Pereyra-Vergara et al. (2020)
		Quercetin-3-o-runtinoside	• Induces apoptosis in MOLT3 (lymphoblastic leukemia) cells by activating mitochondria-dependent caspase cascades • Restricts proliferation of thyroid cancer cells (K1 and BCPAP) in combination with sorafenib and increases the expression of epithelial markers	Celano et al. (2020), Samanta et al. (2010)
10.	Soy	Genistein	• Inhibits the growth of kidney cancer cells by CDKN2a hypomethylation • Inhibits proliferation, invasion, and migration of squamous cell carcinoma by inhibition of ERK/MEK and JNK signaling • Induces apoptosis in tumors implanted from human cells in nude mice	Ji et al. (2020), Li et al. (2020), Zhou et al. (2008)
		Diadzein	• Induces apoptosis in ovarian cancer cell line (SKOV3) by inhibition of MEF/ERK/Raf cascade and inducing cell cycle arrest • Induces apoptosis in MCF-7 cells by mitochondrial pathway • Induces cell cycle arrest and autophagy-related cell death in melanoma cell lines (A-375 cells) by deactivating PI3K/Akt signaling pathway	Chu et al. (2020), Hua et al. (2018), Jin et al. (2010)
		Glycitein	• Inhibits glioma cell (U87MG cell) invasion by downregulating MMP3 and MMP9 expressions • Induces ROS-dependent apoptosis and G0/G1 cell cycle arrest through NF-κB/MAPK/STAT3 pathway	Feng et al. (2019), Lee et al. (2010)

11.	Tomatoes	Lycopene	• Inhibits the growth of MCF-7 cells by arresting cell cycle and inhibiting IGF1 signaling • Restricts the proliferation of prostate cancer cells (PC3 cell) by enhancing miR let-7f1 and decreased expression of AKT2	Karas et al. (2000), Li et al. (2016)
		Rutin	• Attenuates cisplatin-induced renal inflammation and induces apoptosis by caspase-3 activation in Wistar rats • Exerts anticancer activity on renal carcinoma cells • Restores chemosensitivity in mammary carcinoma cell lines (MCF-7 and MDA-MB 231 cells) by inducing cell cycle arrest in G2/M phase	Arjumand et al. (2011), Caparica et al. (2020), Iriti et al. (2017)
12.	Honey	Chrysin	• Induction of apoptosis in MCF7 cells • Induces apoptosis in MDA-MB-231 cells by acting on histone deacetylase inhibitor (HDAC8) enzyme • Induces apoptosis in lungs carcinoma cell lines (A549 cells) by involving p53, caspases, BAX, and Bcl	Mag et al. (2016), Samarghandian et al. (2014), Sun et al. (2012)
		Pinobanksin	• Induction of apoptosis in B-cell lymphoma cancer cell line (M12. C3.F6) • Exerts antiproliferative effect in colon cancer cells (SW480) by inhibiting Wnt cascades	Afrin et al. (2020), Alday et al. (2015)

data indicate the experimental evidences in favor of anticancer properties of these phytochemicals and warrants their health beneficial effects.

2.4 Molecular Targets of Nutraceuticals in Combating Cancer

As mentioned earlier, dietary habits decide our overall health and proneness and reaction to disease contraction, including cancer, which is believed to be modulated mainly at genetic and epigenetic levels. Nutraceuticals, functional foods, and supplemental micronutrients can reduce cancer development through inhibited cell proliferation and induced apoptosis as evident from a collection of natural dietary products showing preventive potentials against cancer by targeting different signaling pathways (Figure 2.4) (Calvani et al. 2020; Zheng et al. 2016).

Natural and dietary nutraceuticals have been reported to function at molecular level, for example, enhancing gap-junctional communication through carotenoids, in vitro, "connexin 43" amplification (Calvani et al. 2020), flavonoids modulate xenobiotic detoxification at phase I and II level, and inhibition of protein kinase C through vitamin E (important enzyme in tumor progression) (Aggarwal et al. 2010). Through clinical trials berberine, resveratrol, and curcumin have been shown to be involved in glucose metabolism/metabolic syndrome, cardiovascular diseases, diabetes, defective

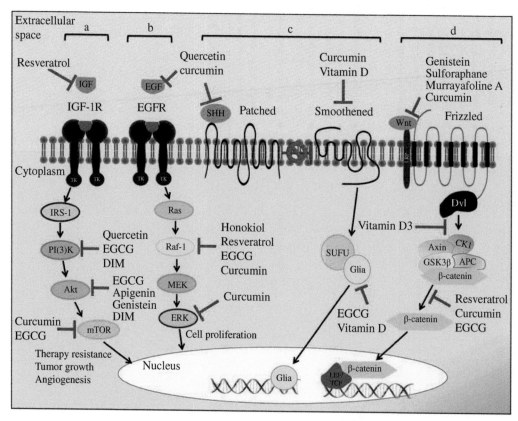

Figure 2.4 Schematic representation of nutraceuticals targeting different signaling pathways involved in cancer. *Source:* Arora and Jaglan (2016). Reproduced with permission from Elsevier.

endothelial function, colorectal adenoma reoccurrence, Alzheimer's disease, age-related macular degeneration, and various kind of cancers (McCubrey et al. 2017). Phytochemicals present in cumin, red pepper, and ginger are potential anticancer agents that can suppress nuclear transcription factor-κB (NF-κB)-mediated signaling pathway involved in cancer pathogenesis. In fact, NF-κB is an appealing therapeutic target for polyphenols and nutraceutics extracted from plants (Kunnumakkara et al. 2018). NF-κB activates genes responsible for both early and late stage progressions of cancer, for example, the early stage targets are apoptosis suppressor proteins (Bcl-XL and Bcl-2) and cyclin D1 that enable cancer cells to override the restrictions on cell proliferation. Among late stage, the targets are vascular endothelial growth factor (VEGF) and matrix-metalloproteases (MMPs) required for angiogenesis and metastasis (Dorai and Aggarwal 2004). NF-κB activity has also been reported to be modulated by resveratrol. Resveratrol is reported to inhibit cyclooxygenase (COX) activity and isoenzyme cytochrome P450 (CYPA1) drug metabolism. It also influences mitochondrial biogenesis, fatty acids oxidation, gluconeogenesis, and respiration (Diaz-Gerevini et al. 2016). Resveratrol can suppress interleukin 17 (IL-17), proinflammatory cytokines, tumor necrosis factor-alpha (TNF-α), and induce activated T-cell apoptosis implicating its potential against autoimmune diseases (Han et al. 2015). Similarly, curcumin and its analogs have been shown to possess superior potentials as anticancer agents due to their antiproliferative, anti-invasive, and antiangiogenic properties proven in vitro (Cen et al. 2009). Curcumin was also found to promote tumor suppressor p53, activate Nrf2 enzymes, and inhibit COX-2 and TGF-β to prevent mouse liver lymphoma (Das and Vinayak 2015).

Dietary natural products like pomegranate, mangosteen, apple, soy, citrus fruits, mango, grape, ginger, cruciferous vegetables, edible macro-fungi, garlic, cereals, and black cumin are effective against progression and development of breast cancer. These natural products can prevent breast cancer by inhibiting proliferation, migration, metastasis, angiogenesis, downregulating the expression and activity of ER-α, inducing arrest of cell cycle and apoptosis, and finally making them sensitive to radiotherapy and chemotherapy (Li et al. 2017).

In the following section, we discuss the cross-talk between various molecular targets in cancer and nutraceuticals involved in their regulations.

2.4.1 Apoptosis

Apoptosis or programmed cell death is employed by the body in self-defense against cancer growth during diseased condition. Vitamin E and selenium in combination can activate molecular targets to trigger apoptosis (Zu and Ip 2003). To prevent cancer, phytochemicals upregulate proapoptotic genes, like Bak and Bax, and/or downregulate antiapoptotic factors, like Bcl-xL and Bcl-2, by triggering the mitochondria-mediated pathway (Davis 2007).

Intake of cruciferous vegetables such as Brussels sprouts, broccoli, cauliflower, and cabbage reduces the chance of occurrence of prostate cancer in humans. Glucosinolates in cruciferous vegetables metabolize mainly into indole-3-carbinol, which under acidic pH converts into polymeric 3,3′-diindolylmethane (DIM). Both indole-3-carbinol and 3,3′-diindolylmethane induce apoptosis in PC3 cells by triggering translocation of cytochrome c to cytosol from mitochondria and activation of initiator caspase-9 and effector caspases-3 and -6 and consequential cleavage of poly ADP-ribose. Thus, indole-3-carbinol and 3,3′-diindolylmethane are potentially inhibitive toward prostate cancer (Nachshon-Kedmi et al. 2004). Besides, hormone-associated cancers like breast and prostate are prevented by indole-3-carbinol through induction of apoptosis via tumor-necrosis-factor-related apoptosis-inducing ligand (TRAIL). TRAIL is already known to be the regulatory pathway of choice for inducing apoptosis in a variety of tumor cell types (Jeon et al. 2003) as it does not affect normal cells. Curcumin has been reported to facilitate TRAIL-mediated apoptosis in several cancer cell lines. TRAIL, the TNF family member, induces apoptosis selectively in cancer cells through four membrane-bound receptors, namely, decoy receptor 1 (DcR1), decoy receptor 2 (DcR2), death receptor 4 (DR4), and death receptor 5 (DR5). Out of these four receptors, DR4 and DR5 have the conserved "death domain" required for TRAIL signaling. However, DcR1 and DcR2 lack this death domain and act as decoy receptors for TRAIL to protect normal cells. Interestingly, curcumin upregulates DR5 in cancer cells and make them more susceptible to TRAIL-mediated apoptosis. Additionally, curcumin downregulates various factors like angiopoitein-1, NF-κ B, inducible nitric oxide to block the activity of Jun N-terminal kinase (Jung et al. 2005). Berberin modulates the expressions of proteins like Bcl-2, BCL-XL, poly (ADP ribose) polymerase 1 (PARP1), Beclin-1, TP53, p21Cip1, MMP9 involved in cell cycle progression, apoptosis, autophagy, and invasion (Dulak 2005). Apigenin (4′,5,7-trihydroxy flavone) available in cabbage, chamomile tea, garlic, guava, and French peas inhibits MAPK activity and stimulates the p53–p21/waf response pathway. Apigenin is known to repress transcription of inducible nitric oxide synthetase (iNOS) and COX-2 by inhibiting IκB kinase activity. Allicin [S-(2-propenyl) 2-propene-1-sufinothioate], found in garlic, induces nuclear condensation, formation of apoptotic bodies, and DNA fragmentation (laddering) in cancerous cells. It activates extrinsic and intrinsic pathways (caspase-3, 8, and 9) and induces cleavage of PARP (Tripathi et al. 2005). Cruciferous vegetables, because of their antioxidative property, can prevent DNA damage from electrophiles and ROS. They can prevent carcinogenesis by restricting their metabolic activation of cytochrome P450 (Talalay and Fahey 2001). Thus, phytochemicals and nutraceuticals are potential prophylactic and therapeutic agents capable of significantly reducing the risks of carcinogenesis by inducing apoptosis (Hecht 1999).

2.4.2 DNA Methylation

Many phytochemicals are engaged in histone modifications, post-transcriptional gene regulation and DNA methylation through affecting especially Micro RNAs (miRNAs), non-coding RNAs (ncRNAs) and long ncRNAs (Krakowsky and Tollefsbol 2015). Epigenetic dietary components are present in human foods, such as sulforaphane, genistein, and EGCG, which protect humans from developing many common cancers through modulation of DNA methylation (Li et al. 2014). These dietary compounds regulate gene expression through histone modification with histone acetyl transferases (HATs) and DNA methylation with histone deacetylases (HDACs) via epigenetic mechanisms. The long-term consumption of bioactive compounds is likely to induce epigenomic modifications pertaining to prevention and cure of metabolic diseases (Nosrati et al. 2017). These are stable, heritable modifications that represent an important memory mechanism witnessed during embryogenesis (Strogantsev and Ferguson-Smith 2012). An appropriate exposure to epigenetic modulators from the diet that target DNA methylation may lead to the fruitful intervention of early epigenetic reprogramming and disease prevention in later life. Three independent DNA methyltransferases (DNMTs), DNMT1, DNMT3A, and DNMT3B, for DNA methylation patterns are required at early embryonic stage for cellular differentiation (Krakowsky and Tollefsbol 2015). In general, kinase inhibitors, chemo-radiotherapeutic agents, immune-stimulatory compounds, personalized antibodies are involved in cancer treatments. Aberrant epigenetic alterations acquired during tumorigenesis can be reversed using HDAC inhibitors and demethylating drugs (Łuczak and Jagodziński 2006). Recent studies support that phytochemicals, natural compounds, and dietary supplements are actually the alternative approach to restore the normal epigenetic marks, which generally changes during carcinogenesis and potential therapy for cancer treatment (Hardy and Tollefsbol 2011). EGCG, quercetin, resveratrol, curcumin, and sulforane are the most studied phytochemicals with respect to epigenetic modulation in cancer (Shankar et al. 2016). Through computational study, EGCG has been shown to inhibit enzymatic activities of DNMT3b and HDAC1 by substrate sequestration, suggesting reactivation of tumor suppressor genes such as cadherin1, retinoic acid receptor β (RAR β), and death-associated protein kinase-1 (Khan et al. 2015). EGCG is shown to repress the hormone responsiveness of androgen receptor through hypoacetylation of the same, thus resulting in increased cell death and decreased cell proliferation in lymph node carcinoma of the prostate (LNCaP) cancer cells. Similar epigenetic modulations of DMNTs and HDACs by EGCG to restore expression of silenced genes like p16INK4a and Cip1/p21 are also evident in cervical and skin cancers (Lee et al. 2012). Likewise, curcumin has been identified for breast cancer therapy because of the presence of an excellent nontoxic hypomethylating agent (Kumar et al. 2017). In estrogen-positive Michigan cancer foundation-7 (MCF-7) breast cancer cell line, curcumin can restore the function of Ras association domain family 1 isoform A (RASSF1A) and inhibit DNMT1 expression by promoter hypomethylation, thus resulting in decreased cell proliferation and breast tumor growth in vivo (Du et al. 2012). Besides, curcumin proved to be an efficient epigenetic downregulator of DNMT3A, thus affecting the expression of RARβ in A549 cell-induced lung cancer in nude mice (Jiang et al. 2015). In brain cancer also, curcumin effectively induced histone hypoacetylation of H3 and H4 proteins to promote neural differentiation. In parallel, it prevented differentiation of astrocytes and induced apoptosis associated with PARP activity (Wu et al. 2013). Similarly, in in vitro cell-based models of acute myeloid leukemia, curcumin downregulated DNMT1 to restore p15INK4b expression and promotion of G1 cell cycle arrest by hypomethylation of its promoter (Yu et al. 2013). In prostate cancer LNCaP cells, curcumin was found to inhibit JNK signaling and repress H3K4me3 epigenetic mark to promote apoptosis in vivo (Zhao et al. 2018). Resveratrol has been shown to regulate many biological functions like cell division, angiogenesis, apoptosis, cell proliferation, and metastasis in different types of cancer and thus confirms its therapeutic effects (Borriello 2017). Resveratrol is reported to reactivate PTEN and promote acetylation by inhibition of the MTA1/HDAC complex and Akt pathway in vivo, consequently resulting in tumor cell death and regression of prostate cancer (Dhar et al. 2015). However, the role of phytochemicals in preventing the occurrence/recurrence of cancer and their potential in nutritional intervention for modulating the functions of epigenetic mechanisms are still under debate.

2.4.3 miRNA

miRNA or miRs have been reported to show both negative and positive regulation of gene expressions. Among these miRs, miR-21 affects many signaling pathways like NF-κB, PI3K/PTEN/AKT, programmed cell death protein 4 (PDCD4). Recent report showed that curcumin regulates miR-21 in different types of cancer. Curcumin binds to the promoter region of miR-21 gene and decreases its expression and simultaneously increasing miR-21exosomes, respectively (Chen et al. 2015). Anticancer effect of curcumin on bladder cancer is attributed to induction of tumor suppressive miR-203 by it. miR-203 is repressed via promoter hypermethylation in bladder cancer. Curcumin demethylates miR-203 promoter region as evident from decrease in miR-203 targets, SRC and AKT2, following its treatment (Saini et al. 2011). In some cancers, curcumin induces DNA hypomethylation and downregulates the expression of DNA methyltransferase 1 (DNMT1) (Yu et al. 2013). Maternally Expressed Gene 3 (MEG3) lncRNA is a tumor suppressor, whose expression in hepatocellular carcinoma is decreased due to promoter methylation. Curcumin reversed the promoter methylation status by upregulating miR-185 and miR-29a. miR-185 inhibited DNMT1, while miR-29a targeted DNMT3A and DNMT3B (Zamani et al. 2015; Zhuo et al. 2016). in vitro, curcumin has been shown to demethylate *Nrf2* promoter to induce its expression that consequently generated stress response to restore the oxidative equilibrium through quinine-1(NQO-1) and NAD(P)H dehydrogenase (Khor et al. 2011).

Genistein can prevent prostate adenocarcinoma by upregulating tumor suppressor genes like ephrin B2 and glutathione S-transferase P1 (GSTP1) and downregulating proliferating factors like Akt, mouse double minute 2 homolog (MDM2), and NF-κB through demethylation of their promoter regions (Vardi et al. 2010). Genistein modulates expressions of various miRNAs like miR-222, miR-1260b, miR-221, miR-574-3p, miR-1296 and miRNA-15. It inhibits cell proliferation and invasion in prostate cancer tissues by reducing the level of overexpressed oncomiR like miR-1260b (Phuah and Nagoor 2014). Similar to genistein, resveratrol reduces promoter methylation of miRNA genes. OncomiRs, miR-17, miR-20a, and miR-106b, target 3'UTR of PTEN to reduce its expression in prostrate cancer. Resveratrol and its derivative, pterostilbene, negatively modulate these oncomiRs to restore PTEN expression in prostrate cancer cells (Dhar et al. 2011, 2015). In breast cancer cell line, MDA-MB-231, and breast cancer stem cells in vivo, tumor-suppressive miR-NAs (like miR-143, miR-141, miR-16 and many others) are shown to be upregulated by resveratrol (Hagiwara et al. 2012). However, there is lack of sufficient in vivo data in support of natural compounds influencing the levels of miRNAs in the context of cancer invoking the need for more preclinical studies to establish the influence of natural compounds in carcinogenesis through miRNA modulation (Kapinova et al. 2018).

2.4.4 Inflammation

Inflammation is responsible for development of several cancers, and it is mainly linked to deregulated expression and activation of nitric oxide synthase (responsible for inflammatory response) and cyclooxygenase (COX-2) (Coussens and Werb 2002). Antioxidative and anti-inflammatory properties of edible and medicinal plants potentially contributes in chemopreventive activities. Resveratrol, EGCG, and curcumin inhibit NOS and COX-2 expression by blocking activation of NF-κB (Surh et al. 2001). Normally, patients at the late stage of cancer has compromised immunity because of less cytokine production and decreased natural killer (NK) cell activity. Therefore, increasing NK activity and the production of cytokines would be necessary for late-stage cancer patients.

Capsaicin helps in decreasing oxidative stress and has great antioxidant potential, and so helps in reducing the ROS generation as was reported in lungs of benzopyrenein-induced mice (Anandakumar et al. 2008). Carnosol reduces the DNA binding activity of NF-κB in activated macrophages by blocking its nuclear translocation through inactivation of IKK (Lo et al. 2002). Quercetin results in attenuation of phorbol-12-acetate-13-myristate (PMA)-induced expression and activation of p38 MAPK and NF-κB in human mast cells in vitro (Min et al. 2007). In response to lipopolysaccharide (LPS) stimulation, ajoene was reported to inhibit production of TNF-α in mice melanoma cells in vivo (Shishodia et al. 2003). Zingerone, allyl isothiocyanate (AITC), and curcumin have been reported to inhibit the release of monocyte chemoattractant protein-1 (MCP-1) from adipocytes and stops the production of nitric oxide and TNF-α significantly (Woo et al. 2007).

2.4.5 Cytokine

Cytokine, mainly interleukin-6 (IL-6), plays important role in immune physiology; however, over-production of IL-6 could be a cause of cancer in various tissues/organs like prostate, breast, lung, ovary, and colon. Hormonal feedback mechanism using sex steroids (testosterone and estrogen) controls the over production of IL-6. The loss of sex steroids after menopause results in large-scale production of IL-6, thus predisposing them to cancer. A large number of therapeutic approaches using soy isoflavones and phytoestrogens were aimed to prevent cancer progression, which might (in)directly target the IL-6 levels as well (daidzein, genistein, biochanin) (Dijsselbloem et al. 2004).

Kaempferol and apigenin inhibited LPS-induced TNF-α production in macrophages and resulted in IL-1β inhibition and diminished MCP-1 production in vitro. Apigenin inhibits the production of prostaglandin E(2), NOS p38, c-JunN-terminal kinase (JNK), and MAPK phosphorylation. It also inhibited the expression of IL-1β and TNF-α genes in macrophages, thus confirming its protective role against inflammation-related cancer (Kowalski et al. 2005).

2.4.6 Growth Factors

In cancer development, angiogenesis process occurs by formation of new blood vessels from endothelial cells with sustained nutrient and oxygen supply to the proliferating cells. During angiogenesis, the endothelial cells are stimulated by various growth factors such as fibroblast growth factor (FGF), VEGF, hepatocyte growth factor (HGF), platelet-derived growth factor (PGDF), angiopoietins, and receptors belonging to the family of epithelial growth factors. FGF and VEGF are considered to be the two important factors in angiogenesis (Fayette et al. 2005). Angio-prevention employs antiangiogenic strategies to control tumor growth. In this regard, both natural and semi-synthetic agents are being explored with encouraging results obtained from various natural resources (Tosetti et al. 2002). Catechins like EGCG present in green tea has the potential to inhibit VEGF, crucial for tumor angiogenesis, at low dose (concentrations achievable through diet) (Béliveau and Gingras 2004). In a similar way, natural polyphenol and the anthocyanidin, ellagic acid, found in several fruits and nuts, can inhibit PDGF and VEGF receptors together as is evident from both in vitro and in vivo assays (Labrecque et al. 2005; Lamy et al. 2006). These evidences clearly suggests the antiangiogenic potentials of phytochemicals in preventing formation of new blood vessels is necessary for cancer management.

2.4.7 Sirtuin

Sirtuins are a class of nicotinamide adenine dinucleotide-consuming enzymes that are implicated in numerous biological pathways and are considered promising target for treating human diseases. There are seven sirtuins in mammals, SIRT1–7. Most of the sirtuins are histone deacetylases, but some have ADP-ribosyl transferases activity also. Phytoalexin production in plants like resveratrol and pterostilbene are linked to the inherent defense mechanisms in them (McCubrey et al. 2017). These compounds affect methylation of genes; however, required concentrations are higher than normal casual consumption of food and beverage products to elicit these changes. Experimental evidences confirmed the effects of these compounds on triple-negative breast cancer (MDA-MB-157) and hepatocellular carcinoma (HCC1806) cell lines. Combination of resveratrol and pterostilbene showed synergistic inhibition of cell proliferation at physiologically relevant concentrations. The combinatorial treatment of resveratrol and pterostilbene induced expressions of gamma-H2A histone family member X (gamma-H2AX), SIRT1, and telomerase in MDA-MB-157 and HCC1806 cells. Upregulated SIRT1 prevented DNMT1-mediated suppression of tumor suppressor genes (Kala et al. 2015).

2.4.8 Topoisomerase

Topoisomerases hold a pivotal role as enzymatic DNA-processing machinery. Therefore, DNA topoisomerases are essential for cell survival. However, specific strand breaks due to topoisomerase activities trigger cell death (Baranello et al. 2013). Modulation of this dual functionality of topoisomerases is being explored for cancer treatments (Baechler et al. 2014; Khadka and Cho 2013; Pommier 2006). Topoisomerases, being crucial for life sustenance, its modulation as anticancer tool is considered a challenging task and relies more on phytochemicals and nutraceuticals. Through slow and prolonged dietary exposure to naturally occurring topoisomerase modulators, the adverse effects associated with pharmaceuticals can be avoided.

Isoflavones, also known as phytoestrogens, mainly present in the *Leguminosae* family, belong to the class of polyphenols. Among several legumes, soybeans, alfalfa, clover, and chickpeas are quite rich in isoflavones. Major isoflavones present in soy are genistein, daidzein, and glycitein and occur in four chemical forms (glycosides, aglycons, malonylglucosides, and acetylglucoside) (Fritz et al. 2013; Jian 2009). In addition to biochanin A and formononetin as dominant ones, isoflavones daidzein and genistein are also present in red clover (Booth et al. 2006; De Rijke et al. 2005). A specific topoisomerase type 2 (Topo-2) inhibitor and the observed cytotoxicity of genistein are associated with its poisoning activity even at micromolar levels, which generates permanent double-strand breaks in DNA at DNA-enzyme binding sites. Topo-2 poisoning mechanism of genistein is similar to the classical topo-2 poison, etoposide (Bandele and Osheroff 2007; López-Lázaro et al. 2007; Mizushina et al. 2013; Salti et al. 2000). However, both biochanin A and daidzein do not have Topo-2 poisoning properties in cell-free DNA cleavage assays and in cells (Bandele and Osheroff 2007). The cytotoxic and DNA-damaging potencies of etoposide and genistein differ considerably, with former exerting stronger cytotoxic and genotoxic effects in human CEM leukemia cells. Etoposide generates more stable covalent Topo-2α- and 2β-DNA intermediates compared to genistein. The intensity of drug interaction with the cleavable complex is believed to be positively correlated to the levels of DNA strand breaks and subsequent toxicity (Bandele and Osheroff 2008; Kalfalah et al. 2011). Genistein forms both stable Topo-2α and 2β/DNA intermediates at nonphysiological concentrations above 100 μm but is thought to exert its genotoxicity mainly through its interaction with Topo-2β isoform (Bandele and Osheroff 2007; Kalfalah et al. 2011; López-Lázaro et al. 2007).

The major polyphenols in green tea are EGCG, epicatechin-3-gallate (ECG), epigallocatechin (EGC), and epicatechin (EC) (Niemeyer and Brodbelt 2007). The tea, produced from the leaves of *Camellia sinensis*, is one of the most widely consumed beverages in the world (Sang et al. 2005). Green tea polyphenols, in particular EGCG, have been assumed to modulate cell signaling transduction pathways associated with several disease preventions including diabetes mellitus, cancer, and cardiovascular disorders (Yang et al. 2009a; Yang and Wang 2011). Over past years, EGCG has gained remarkable attention as a possible cancer chemopreventive compound. DNA integrity is now believed to be modulated by interactions of topoisomerase isoenzymes with catechins. The catechins present in tea can efficiently inhibit Topo-2 activity (Suzuki et al. 2001). Through a redox-dependent mechanism, EGCG has been reported to effectively poison both Topo-2α and 2β in K562 cells incubated with 100 μm EGCG (López-Lázaro et al. 2011).

The most prevalent plant flavonoids are flavonoles including quercetin, fisetin, myricetin, and kaempferol, and they are common in a large number of fruits and vegetables. In grains, leafy plants, and herbs, there are fairly low amounts of flavons such as luteolin, apigenin, and baicalein. Myricetin serves as a Topo-1 inhibitor in K562 leukemia cells (López-Lázaro et al. 2010). Myricitin, quercetin, and fisetin act as a covalent Topo-1 inhibitor, stabilizing enzyme/DNA cleavage complex, and intercalation with DNA, and thus inhibiting both type I and II topoisomerase activities (Austin et al. 1992; Constantinou et al. 1995). Biochemical studies revealed that quercetin has tremendous potential to inhibit Topo-2. IC50 values for quercetin, kaempferol, fisetin, and myricetin, determined biochemically through cell-free drug response assays, are 6.9, 8.1, 8.2, and 11.9 μg/mL, respectively (Constantinou et al. 1995). In a recent study by Shiomi et al., myricetin was found to inhibit Topo-2 activity of human DNA at an IC50 value of 27.5 μM (8.8 μg/mL) (Shiomi et al. 2013). The Topo-2 inhibitory properties of some common flavonoids were found to be as quercetin > kaempferol > fisetin > myricetin (Esselen and Barth 2014; Shiomi et al. 2013).

Curcumin is yet another Topo-2 poison as postulated from its DNA intercalating property and sensitivity of its clastogenicity to topo-2 inhibitors (Martín-Cordero et al. 2003; Snyder and Arnone 2002). Curcumin enhances Topo-2α and 2β activities only in the presence of potassium ferricyanide [$K_3Fe(CN)_6$] as oxidizing agent, suggesting that oxidized metabolites of curcumin, like bicyclopentadione, and several reactive quinine methide intermediates are responsible for the increase of Topo-2-mediated DNA cleavage (Griesser et al. 2011; Ketron et al. 2013; Metzler et al. 2012).

Resveratrol is reported to arrest cell cycle at S-phase with an associated increase in phosphorylated γH2AX, thus implicating DNA double-strand breaks responsible for this process, which is expected since there are reports of resveratrol inhibiting catalytic activity of recombinant human Topo-2 (Baechler et al. 2014; Hwangbo et al. 2012; Leone et al. 2010). Reports have shown that polyphenolic fractions from grape cell culture, crude grape, and grape vine shoot extracts can inhibit human Topo-2, and all these establish the topoisomerase modulating potential of resveratrol (Baechler et al. 2014; Jo et al. 2005, 2006). In addition, the resveratrol oligomers r2-viniferin, hopeaphenol, and the dimer ε-viniferin have also been reported for their Topo2-inhibiting bioactivity (Baechler et al. 2014).

2.4.9 Antioxidant Activity

Fundamental basis of life is an appropriate equilibrium between antioxidants and oxidation. "Oxidative stress" is a result of disruption in the prooxidant–antioxidant balance and induces tissue injury (Rahal et al. 2014). Oxidative stress is a physiological process that occurs in the body when oxidation processes are increased due to lack of an antioxidant-dependent protection. This imbalance can cause activation of various signaling pathways that may even lead to the progression of cancer (Liguori et al. 2018) and also can damage major biochemical constituents of the body (lipids, proteins, DNA, fatty acids, etc.) (Cornelli 2009). Redox imbalance and deregulated redox signals are involved in cancer initiation, malignancy, and resistivity to treatment (Panieri and Santoro 2016). The excellence of antioxidant abilities and the beneficial effects on human health by phytochemicals and many natural food compounds are of particular interest (Na and Surh 2008). Nutritional plant-based chemicals, derived from different vegetables, fruits, herbal products, and spices, were reported to activate Nrf2 and trigger expression of antioxidant or phase II detoxifying enzymes in vitro (Saw et al. 2012; Zhang et al. 2015). Curcumin, resveratrol, and anthocyanins may also reduce inflammation, as they were found to inhibit the production of prostaglandin, activity of NF-κB, and increase the production of cytokine (Calvani et al. 2020).

2.4.10 Glutathione and Glutathione Esters

Glutathione (GSH) is the major water-soluble antioxidant, a tripeptide of glutamic acid, cysteine, and glycine (GluCysGly), present in the nuclei, cytoplasm, and mitochondria of cells. GSH requires GSH peroxidase for performing antioxidant functions. Normal cells (especially kidney cells) take up more GSH than the cancer cells, because an enzyme γ-glutamyl transpeptidase presents only in normal cells that is required for hydrolysis of GSH to Glu and Cys to Gly and transports these products into the cell. This distinction between normal cells and cancer cells provides selective GSH-related protection for normal cells (Zunino et al. 1989). Lycopene is a powerful antioxidant and provides protection against cell damage due to free radicals. Administration of lycopene in rats was found to increase the expressions of heme oxygenase 1 (HO-1), Nrf2, and antioxidant enzymes like glutathione peroxidase (GSH-Px), catalase (CAT), and superoxide dismutase (SOD). As a result, an increase in the intracellular GSH levels and decrease in ROS generation were observed (Calvani et al. 2020).

2.5 Hallmarks of Cancer and the Role of Nutrition and Nutraceuticals

While the characteristics and metabolic alternations in cancer progression were first discovered a century ago, the regular changes in the cancer metabolomics and involvement of diverse pathways in the tumorigenesis have become a topic of renewed interest in the past decade. With the invention of recently developed molecular biology aids, several emerging studies have expanded our knowledge on tumor-associated metabolic alternations in the cells and the hallmarks associated with this. The present perspective in hallmarks and possible targets of cancer progression are expanded rationally with increased innovations in understanding the cancer biology. During 2000, **Hanahan and Weinberg** defined six basic hallmarks of cancer: (i) infinite replicative potential, (ii) sustained angiogenesis, (iii) evading apoptosis, (iv) evading growth repressors, (v) sustained proliferative signaling, and (vi) tissue invasion and metastasis (Hanahan and Weinberg 2000). Almost after a decade, a revised list of hallmarks was prepared by them in which two major emerging mechanisms were included. These mechanisms are reprogrammed energy metabolism and evading immune response and two enabling traits like gene mutations and tumor-associated inflammation (Hanahan and Weinberg 2011). Hence, combinedly, all the aforesaid factors form the next-generation hall marks of the cancer (Figure 2.5). Although each hallmark for cancer has its own significance, the hallmark related to energy metabolism is in the vicinity of cellular nutrition. Since the early twentieth century, after the postulation of Warburg hypothesis, cancer cells were reported to use several abnormal metabolic pathways to compensate for the energy requirements (Alfarouk et al. 2014; Warburg 1925). Notably, cancer cells acquire necessary nutrients from the tumor microenvironment and utilize the same to build new biomass and sustained cell proliferation. Hence, the relationship between nutrients consumption and cancer progression has become one of the essential research topics from nutraceutical aspects. Factors like overeating, obesity, and irregularities in glucose metabolism are responsible for the carcinogenesis and is in line with the energy metabolism hall mark of the cancer progression (Calle et al. 2003). Describing each hallmark and its impact due to nutrition is beyond the scope of this review. Hence, some relevant hallmarks of cancer and their correlation to nutrition are described under.

2.5.1 Sustained Proliferative Signaling

Sustained proliferative signaling is the most significant hallmark of all cancer cells. Abnormality in cell physiology and increased sensitivity to allied growth factors are the key regulators in the sustained proliferation of these cells. Diet is either directly or indirectly involved in the regulation of various growth factors required for the cell growth. Among various growth factors, insulin-like growth factor 1 (IGF-1) plays a vital role in cell proliferation in normal and healthy conditions. But

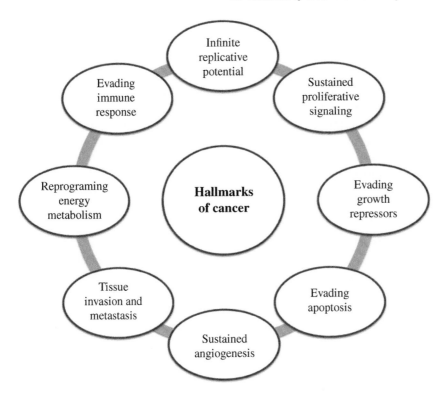

Figure 2.5 Various hallmarks of cancer.

the same plays a key role in cancer cells by encouraging tumorigenic pathways and inhibiting the pathways associated with apoptosis and cell cycle arrest (Mawson et al. 2005; Párrizas et al. 1997). As per a report by Levine et al., low protein intake reduced the expression of IGF-1 and resulted in decreased cancer mortality (Levine et al. 2014). Similarly, insulin, a key regulator of IGF-1 axis, also plays a pivotal role in the regulation of cancer. Accumulating evidences suggest that insulin have potent growth-promoting and anabolic responses, and this may help in the progression of cancer (Clayton et al. 2011; Fisher et al. 1996). As per a study by Fenton et al., curcumin (a prime component of turmeric) and docosahexaenoic acid (derived from omega 3 rich foods) are effective in reducing cell proliferation in insulin-induced colon carcinoma cells (Fenton and McCaskey 2013). The report shows the inhibition of MEK, which is an upstream segment of ERK signaling and responsible for enhanced transcription of the proteins responsible for proliferation.

Now, if we consider the growth factors in cancer cell progression and the dietary inputs, several hypotheses come into account. Dietary inputs and cancer management has been a conspiracy theory and an ever-debating topic. Although there is no consensus on the dietary factor and cancer risk, the high consumption of fruits and vegetables are consistently associated with reduced cancer rates (Wiseman 2008). Folate is one such dietary supplement whose deficiency may result in the epithelial malignancies, including ovary, breast, lungs, cervix, and pancreas (Kim 2007; Yang et al. 2009b). Green leafy vegetables are generally highly rich in folates. As mammals cannot synthesize folate de novo, these are either taken directly through diets or produced in body by various enzymatic processes. Series of evidences from case–control, retrospective, and perspective human studies reveals that people having regular high folate diet inclusions and high folate concentration in blood plasma have relatively low risk of developing colon cancer (Sanjoaquin et al. 2005). Since the correlation between obesity and cancer is identified, recent studies are carried out on the role of dietary fats in regulating cancer. As per an earlier report by Vechhia (1992), a higher dietary saturated fat level is responsible for increased cancer cell proliferation in various cancer types (La 1992). Most of the recent studies are mainly focused on understanding the molecular mechanisms responsible for fat-induced cell proliferation in different cancers like breast, ovary, endometrium, osteosarcoma, to name a few (Henderson and Feigelson 2000). However, trans-fatty acids (TFA), monosaturated fatty acids (MUFA), and saturated fatty acids (SFA) are found to be involved in breast tumorigenesis (MacLennan and Ma 2010). As per another study by Kwon et al. 2016, high fat is responsible for prostatic interstitial neoplasia with the downregulation of PTEN, which is a potent tumor-suppressor protein (Kwon et al. 2016).

2.5.2 Evading Growth Repressors

Evading growth repressors is one of the critical hall marks of cancer and is mainly associated with tumor-suppressor genes. There are various tumor suppressors identified, which limit cancer cell proliferation. These genes control cell proliferation by their involvement in a myriad of signaling pathway and arresting the cell cycle machinery. For example, retinoblastoma (Rb) protein is associated with E2F (transcription factor) and controls the cell proliferation and cell cycle mechanism in normal conditions. In the case of cancer, Rb is inactivated by phosphorylated cyclin/cdk complex, which in turn releases free E2F resulting in enhanced cell proliferation. Now, if we consider the dietary nutrients and tumor suppressor genes, several experimental evidences showed the role of bioactivities in the activation of these tumor-suppressor genes. As per a study by Yao et al. 2012, blueberry extracts reduced prostate cancer by activation of the tumor-suppressor genes. The same report showed that the extract was found to increase the percentage of cells in G0/G1 phase, whereas it reduced the S and G2/M population. As per the report, the cell cycle arrest was supported by the reduced expression of cyclinE/Cdk2 and CyclinD1/Cdk4 and an increased expression of p27, an inhibitor of cyclin/cdk complex (Yao et al. 2012). As per another report by Nikhil et al. (2014b), a conjugate of ptersostilbene (a stilbenoid common in berries) along with isothiocyanate (commonly found in cruciferous vegetables) was effective in reducing the breast cancer cells by acting on PPARγ. The report claims the agonistic effect of the conjugate that activates PPARγ, which in turn triggers the upregulation of tumor-suppressor gene, i.e. PTEN and caspases-3, -7, and -9, thus resulting in apoptosis (Nikhil et al. 2014b). Another study by Butelli et al. (2008) showed the anticancer effect of pterostilbene on the gastric carcinoma cells. In this study, pterostilbene induced the cell cycle arrest by attenuating the protein expression of cyclin/cdk complex and phosphorylated Rb. Hence, this is another example of how bioactive components reactivates the tumor-suppressor system, thus leading to the cell death (Butelli et al. 2008). Undoubtedly, single bioactive components from the dietary supplements have beneficial role in reactivating the tumor-suppressor genes. In contrast to this, another study focused on evaluating the mixed anthocyanidines from mixed berries. As per the report, the mixed anthocynanidines synergistically reduced the non-small-cell lung carcinoma cell proliferation by reducing cyclinB1 and cyclinD1 levels (Kausar et al. 2012). Curcumin, a major component of turmeric, is another well-studied bioactive having potential in reactivating the tumor-suppressor system as well regulating the cell cycle machinery. As per a report by Shishodia et al. 2005, curcumin alleviated the proliferation of human mantle cell lymphoma (MCL) cell lines. The report claimed that curcumin induced a cell cycle arrest in G0/G1 phase, and there was an involvement of NF-κB pathway (Shishodia et al. 2005). To support the above finding, another recent study by Zhang et al. 2020 showed the effect of curcumin on gastric cancer cell lines through Gli1-β-catenin pathway. As per the study, curcumin induced cytoskeletal remodeling and cell cycle arrest in S-phase.

In addition to this, authors also claimed the effect of curcumin in reducing the epithelial to mesenchymal transitions (EMT) and inhibition of *shh* and *wnt* signaling pathways (Zhang et al. 2020).

2.5.3 Reprogramming of Energy Metabolism

Abnormality in cellular energetics is a cancer hallmark in which tumors undergo various changes and altered pathways. The cancer cells synthesize different macromolecules to compensate the energy requirement for rapid cell proliferation. Hence, in order to develop therapeutic candidates, recently, research targeting metabolic pathways has gained momentum. De novo lipogenesis is one of the most vital factors for cancer cell survival, especially in a stressed environment (Rysman et al. 2010; Schug et al. 2015). In normal conditions, acetyl Co A originated from tricarboxylic acid (TCA) cycle is responsible for fatty acid biosynthesis. However, in cancer conditions, when the carbon source is low, acetyl-Co A is synthesized by the action of acetyl-CoA synthetase 2. This phenomenon helps the cancer cells for their sustained proliferation in the lipid-depleted stressed microenvironment (Alderton 2015; Schug et al. 2015). Similarly, acetyl-CoA synthetase 1 is also involved in the synthesis of acetyl-Co A. Unlike acetyl-CoA synthetase 2, the synthesis of acetyl-Co A by acetyl-CoA synthetase 1 takes place in mitochondria. These facts suggest that both acetyl-CoA synthetase 1 and 2 can be potential targets for inhibiting the cancer cell proliferation. As per a study by Focke et al. 1990, allicin (a major bioactive constituent of ginger) is responsible for inhibiting the acetyl-Co A synthetase (Focke et al. 1990). Another report by Chu et al. 2012 showed the antiproliferative effect of allicin in the hepatocarcinoma cells by targeting p53. These studies altogether provides insights about the involvement of bioactive constituents from ginger in the energy metabolism of carcinoma cells (Chu et al. 2012).

In cancer cell energetics, anaerobic glycolysis is an important hallmark of all cancer tissues. Therefore, targeting the pathways involved in the glycolysis mechanism is also considered an alternative approach to combat the disease. Accumulating evidences shows the involvement of various phytochemicals in the energy metabolism of cancer cells (Focke et al. 1990; Tosetti et al. 2009). Hypoxia inducible factor-1 (HIF-1) plays a vital role in the anaerobic glycolysis. This helps in promoting energy production by an alternative approach other than oxidative phosphorylation. HIF-1 activates phosphoinositide-dependent kinase (PDK)1, which in turn deregulates the pyruvate dehydrogenase and thus hindering pyruvate to enter TCA cycle (Kim et al. 2007; Semenza 2010). Apart from this, HIF-1 is also involved in the induction of hexokinase II, which is responsible for higher rate of aerobic glycolysis in cancer cells (Gwak et al. 2005; Riddle et al. 2000). Tocotrienols, a form of vitamin E, is vividly studied phytochemical from dietary source for their role in suppressing HIF-1 and VEGF (Kannappan et al. 2012). Trocotienols are naturally present in various vegetable oils, palms, rice barns, and oats (Siles et al. 2013). As per a report by Kannapan et al. (2012), tocotrienols inhibit cancer cell growth by their involvement in multiple pathways including HIF-1 (Kannappan et al. 2012). Another report by Bi et al. 2010 showed that γ- tocotrienols were responsible for the reduced expression of HIF-1 and VEGF in both normal and hypoxic conditions (Bi et al. 2010).

As far as cancer cell energetics is concerned, adenosine triphosphate (ATP) synthesis is quite inefficient in carcinoma condition (Kaelin and Thompson 2010). Hence, more glucose is required to compensate the energy need in tumor microenvironment. Tumors, therefore, overexpress certain transporters to enhance glucose influx inside the cells. Glucose transporter 1 (GLUT-1) is among such transporters, which are highly expressed in different types of tumors (Haber et al. 1998; Krzeslak et al. 2012). Flavone apigenin, which is widely distributed in many fruits and vegetables, is found to have profound effect on the reduction of the GLUT-1 in the pancreatic cancer cells via inhibition of PI3K/Akt pathway (Melstrom et al. 2008). As per another report by Liao et al. 2015, curcumin reduced the lungs cancer invasion and metastasis by acting on the GLUT1/MT1-MMP/ MMP2 pathway (Liao et al. 2015). However, the nature of cancer cells to adapt as per the requirement predisposes them to myriad of molecular mechanisms, and involvement of various metabolites is often observed. Apparently, the correlation between nutrition and cellular energetics is being studied vividly to find mechanisms responsible for cellular adaptations.

2.5.4 Activating Invasion and Metastasis

"Invasion and metastasis" is the deadliest cancer hallmark among all. Different factors like heterogeneity in tumor cell population and stemness limit various cancer therapeutic options. The whole process of EMT occurs through a series of well-orchestrated event. The cell adhesion proteins like E-cadherin, N-cadherin, and vimentin have been reported to play vital role in the whole process (BenAyed-Guerfali et al. 2019; Loh et al. 2019). Apart from this, proteins associated with cell polarity, extracellular matrix, and motility, i.e. RHO family proteins and MMPs, also play crucial role in EMT (Lee et al. 2008; Loh et al. 2019; Vega and Ridley 2008). Recent studies revealed the role of various phytochemicals from the dietary source in combating this advanced form of cancer. Sulforaphane is a sulfur-rich compound found in cruciferous vegetables (Sita et al. 2018; Wiczk et al. 2012). Series of evidences suggest the role of sulfarophane in inhibiting the invasion and metastasis in various cancer cell lines and animal models (Singh et al. 2009; Wang et al. 2009; Wiczk et al. 2012). Similarly, curcumin also exerts antimetastatic potential in various carcinoma conditions. According to a report by Shao et al. (2002), curcumin restricts the ER-negative breast cancer cell proliferation by downregulating MMP2 and upregulating TIMP-1 and 2 (Shao et al. 2002). The same report also showed the role of curcumin in inhibiting FGF and VEGF in ER-negative breast carcinoma cells. Another study by Farhangi et al. 2015 showed the antimetastatic potential of curcumin in 4T1 mouse breast carcinoma cell line. The study reported that curcumin exerted the antimetastatic potential by inhibiting NF-κB, which in turn downregulated VEGF, MMP9, and COX2 (Farhangi et al. 2015). Resveratrol, another major component from berries, has a profound effect against metastasis and invasion. As per a recent study by Yin et al. 2020, resveratrol suppressed the inhibition of gastric cancer cell metastasis by acting on β-catenin/Wnt signaling pathway (Yin et al. 2020). Recent evidences showed a direct correlation between EMT and cancer stem cell populations (Fritz et al. 2020; Singh and Settleman 2010; Wilson et al. 2020; Yang et al. 2020). EMT can activate stemness in the cancer cell population either by activating the signaling pathways responsible for stem cell regulators or by the epigenetic modifications (Wilson et al. 2020). According to another recent study by Sun et al., it showed that resveratrol inhibited renal cancer stem cell populations by modulating the sonic hedgehog pathway (Sun et al. 2020).

All the dietary components discussed here for their role against metastasis and advanced form of cancer are quite well explained with mechanisms of actions. Nevertheless, it is quite unclear that consuming the dietary components directly can induce any translational effect or not. Hence, it can be deduced that consuming foods containing these kinds of phytochemicals may provide a balanced diet and provide prophylactic benefits to humans.

2.6 Limitations of Nutraceuticals

The potential bio-efficacy of any nutraceutical or any food bioactive component depends upon its bioavailability, which defines the fraction of ingested food actively available to the circulatory system of the body. Bioavailability is an extremely complicated process that includes different phases

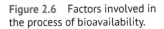

Figure 2.6 Factors involved in the process of bioavailability.

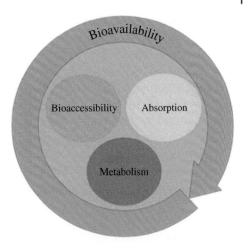

like digestion, absorption, metabolism, and excretion (Parada and Aguilera 2007) (Figure 2.6). In order to pursue a beneficial effect on health, any bioactive components from food need to be bioavailable. However, the productive benefits of many nutraceuticals are not observed because of their relatively low and variable bioavailability (Fernández-García et al. 2012; Rein et al. 2013). Some barriers are responsible for the poor bioavailability of nutraceuticals like chemical modification during the digestion process, hindrance in solubility with gastrointestinal fluids, low absorption in intestinal epithelium cells, and first-pass metabolism in the liver to name a few (Actis-Goretta et al. 2013; Moelants et al. 2012).

2.6.1 Factors Limiting the Bioavailability of Nutraceuticals

In the following section, we discuss some of the factors that are linked to the bioavailability of nutraceuticals.

2.6.1.1 Bioaccessibility
This factor is the first step in the bioavailability of any food components or drugs. It defines the amount of bioactive components that leach out from the food matrix and are available for absorption in the gastrointestinal tract. Digestion process and break down of food initiates from the mouth by mastication and continues throughout the gastrointestinal tract by a mixture of various digestive enzymes. The physiological parameters like pH, temperature, and composition of food matrix have an impact on the bioaccessibility of any nutraceutical (Fernández-García et al. 2009). The primary factor that limits the bioaccessibility of any nutraceutical is its ability to be released from the food matrix. Carotenoid is an example of such a nutraceutical, which is trapped within the cellular structure of vegetables, and due to this, its accessibility in the gastrointestinal tract is limited (Failla et al. 2008). Another factor that limits bioaccessibility is the solubility of nutraceuticals in digestive fluid. This factor mostly affects hydrophobic nutraceuticals, which need to be engulfed into micelles due to their low solubility in water (Porter et al. 2008). Some physiological changes imposed by the volume of food matrix and its caloric content may affect the bioaccessibility of bioactive molecules from digested food. It has been reported that bioavailability of isoflavonoids from high fat and protein-containing food is better than supplementary isoflavonoids taken without food (Walsh et al. 2003). Other studies also showed higher absorption of carotenoids from full-fat salad dressing in comparison to fat-free salad dressing (Brown et al. 2004). Interaction of nutraceuticals with other

components of digested food or digestive fluids also plays a significant role in determining their bioaccessibility. A recent study showed that ferulic acid of whole-grain wheat has a high binding affinity to the polysaccharides, which limits its bioaccessibility to less than 1% (Mateo Anson et al. 2009).

On the other hand, about 60% of bioavailability has been observed when free ferulic acid is added to wheat flour (Mateo Anson et al. 2009). The bioaccessibility of specific nutraceuticals may also be limited by the presence of particular components within ingested food matrices, such as ionic biopolymers or chelating agents. Phytic acid is the primary storage form of phosphorus in cereals, legumes, and nuts, which is known to limit the bioaccessibility of micronutrients like zinc, iron, calcium. The digestive tract of a human lacks enzyme phytase, which is responsible for the chelating effect of phytic acid on micronutrients (Gupta et al. 2013).

2.6.1.2 Absorption

It is an essential factor that plays a very crucial role in the bioavailability of nutraceuticals. It defines uptake of bioactive components from digested food into intestinal epithelial cells and, ultimately, in the circulatory system of the body. Intestinal epithelial cells are known to form mucus layer, which limits the passing of substances of more than 400 nm size (Cone 2009). The flavonoids have sugar moiety β-glucosides, which limits their absorption in the small intestine (Bravo 2009). However, according to an earlier report, improved absorption of flavonoids is due to additional rhamnose moiety, which is cleaved off by microbiota of large intestine (Erlund et al. 2000). Apart from size and structure, the absorption of nutraceuticals also depends on their stereoisomer configuration. Catechin and lycopene have been shown to exhibit different bioavailability with their distinct stereoisomers (Ottaviani et al. 2011). Absorption of nutraceuticals also depends on their ability to cross nonpolar phospholipid bilayer. The value of the oil–water partition coefficient decides this ability of a molecule to cross the hydrophobic bilayer. Any molecule having a value of greater than 10, for this coefficient is considered to have higher permeability through epithelial cells (Dahan and Miller 2012). Although some bioactive molecules have low bilayer membrane permeability, they can still cross this bilayer by passing through paracellular space available between adjacent cells. The tight junctions are responsible for this narrow space, which allows the passing of less than 0.7 nm size molecules, especially amino acids and sugars (Seki et al. 2008; Tsutsumi et al. 2008). The bilayer membrane also consists of some active transporters made up of single or multiple proteins. Some vitamins and phytochemicals are transported inside epithelial cells through these active transporters (Dudhatra et al. 2012; Tso et al. 2004). This type of transport mechanism depends on the concentration of nutraceuticals and other molecules that compete for the binding with a transporter. On the other hand, some efflux transporters present on epithelial cells have a role in transporting nutraceuticals and some flavonoids back into the lumen and thus reducing their bioavailability (Misaka et al. 2013).

2.6.1.3 Metabolism

Metabolism and chemical transformation in the gastrointestinal tract is another major factor that limits the bioavailability of many nutraceuticals. This metabolic process involves different types of enzymes, such as reductases, esterases, cytochrome P450, and dehydrogenases. Nutraceuticals or any other drug pass through phase I metabolism, which takes place in enterocytes and the product of this metabolic reactions pass through phase II, which occurs in liver or spleen (Chen et al. 2014). Some collective metabolic transformation includes oxidation of carotenoids, hydrolysis of some polyphenols, breakdown of curcumin in an alkaline environment (Tsao 2010). Resveratrol, quercetin, and epicatechin have been shown to be metabolized by specific enzymes present in the gastrointestinal tract (Petri et al. 2003; Planas et al. 2012). The metabolism of lipophilic nutraceuticals increases their polarity due to the addition of hydrophilic groups, which ultimately promotes reabsorption in the kidney and excretion from the body. Some nutraceuticals are not absorbed in the small intestine, but they undergo a fermentation process by the colonic bacteria of large intestine and enters into the circulatory system (Monagas et al. 2010). For example, highly hydrophilic anthocyanins are not readily absorbed within the small intestine, but they may be metabolized by enzymes in the colon and converted to forms suitable for absorption, such as protocatechuic, syringic, vanillic, and 4-hydroxybenzoic acids (Stevenson et al. 2011).

2.7 Safety Aspects of the Nutraceuticals

Generally dietary supplements are commonly considered safe; however, it is not applicable to all categories of nutraceuticals. Some reports demonstrate that excess consumption of fat-soluble vitamins could be toxic. For example, high dose of α-tocopherol (800–1200 mg/day) could lead to bleeding due to its antiplatelet function, whereas if dose exceed than 1200 mg/day may cause severe complication such as gonadal dysfunction, diarrhea, and blurred vision (Selhub and Rosenberg 1996). The result of randomized trials indicate an increased chances of cancer recurrence in head and neck cancer patient that had undergone radiation therapy and were prescribed vitamin E supplementation (Bairati et al. 2005). A higher incidence of lung cancer and mortality was observed in the male alcohol users receiving the vitamin A supplements (Omenn et al. 1996). Recently, another large clinical trial demonstrated a higher risk of lung cancer in smokers that are recipient of β-carotene supplements (Middha et al. 2019). Excess consumption of vitamin A supplements is also closely associated with contrasting effect on bone health that includes reduced density of bone minerals and increased chances of bone fracture (Jackson and Sheehan 2005). Most nutraceuticals possess antioxidant and anti-inflammatory effects and are rarely toxic. However, very little information is available about their toxic effects. A report stated that EGCG can lead to the liver injury by promoting the liver cell dysfunctions (Mazzanti et al. 2009). It has also been reported that soy-derived isoflavones in purified form have potent estrogenic properties both in vitro and in vivo model systems (Badger et al. 2009; Ronis et al. 2018). But the biggest challenge is deciding the exact dosages for them since its consumption has been reported to be associated with adverse impacts on male hormonal and reproductive system that includes reduction in testes size, suppression of androgen level, and fertility (Chen and Rogan 2004; Ronis et al. 2016). Additionally, its consumption also promotes the estrogen-dependent tumor growth (Ronis et al. 2018). In women, endometriosis cases have also been reported following the excess consumption of isoflavone supplements (Mahady et al. 2003).

2.8 Conclusion

The implications of our broadening knowledge of cancer biology and the influence of nutrient and phytochemical intake and metabolism may potentially be used to prevent and/or slow the progression of tumor development and metastasis. Nutraceuticals not only destroy cancer cells but also protect healthy tissues, help maintain a strong immune system, and above all make cancer therapies more conducive compared to conventional therapeutic systems. Researches on natural products, phytochemicals, and nutraceuticals are currently gaining momentum due to their less toxicity and assertive efficacy in various cancer conditions. This adds an advantage over the modern drugs, which exacerbates the patients' health condition under regular chemotherapy. The complex interactions among genotype, diet, and environment are deciphering new knowledge, which will facilitate personalized nutritional recommendations. Although the individual phytochemicals present in the dietary supplements are very well studied, their translational features in terms of clinical outcomes are often questioned. However, it can be suggested that a healthy food intake regularly can ease the possible complications of various disorders including cancer. Therefore, all these facts warrants more comprehensive clinical studies involving a large population size in order to decipher the potential of these nutraceuticals and their future use as an alternative and complementary medicine.

References

Actis-Goretta, L., Lévèques, A., Rein, M. et al. (2013). Intestinal absorption, metabolism, and excretion of (-)-epicatechin in healthy humans assessed by using an intestinal perfusion technique. *American Journal of Clinical Nutrition 98* (4): 924–933. https://doi.org/10.3945/ajcn.113.065789.

Afrin, S., Haneefa, S.M., Fernandez-Cabezudo, M.J. et al. (2020). Therapeutic and preventive properties of honey and its bioactive compounds in cancer: an evidence-based review. *Nutrition Research Reviews 33* (1): 50–76. https://doi.org/10.1017/S0954422419000192.

Aggarwal, B.B., Sundaram, C., Prasad, S., and Kannappan, R. (2010). Tocotrienols, the vitamin E of the 21st century: its potential against cancer and other chronic diseases. *Biochemical Pharmacology 80* (11): 1613–1631. https://doi.org/10.1016/j.bcp.2010.07.043.

Alday, E., Valencia, D., Carreño, A.L. et al. (2015). Apoptotic induction by pinobanksin and some of its ester derivatives from Sonoran propolis in a B-cell lymphoma cell line. *Chemico-Biological Interactions 242*: 35–44. https://doi.org/10.1016/j.cbi.2015.09.013.

Alderton, G.K. (2015). Metabolism: acetate nourishes stressed tumour cells. *Nature Reviews Cancer 15* (2): 67. https://doi.org/10.1038/nrc3899.

Alfarouk, K.O., Verduzco, D., Rauch, C. et al. (2014). Glycolysis, tumor metabolism, cancer growth and dissemination. A new pH-based etiopathogenic perspective and therapeutic approach to an old cancer question. *Oncoscience 1* (12): 777.

Alpha-Tocopherol Beta Carotene Cancer Prevention Study Group (1994). The effect of vitamin E and beta carotene on the incidence of lung cancer and other cancers in male smokers. *New England Journal of Medicine 330* (15): 1029–1035. https://doi.org/10.1016/S0002-9149(99)00324-0.

Anandakumar, P., Kamaraj, S., Jagan, S. et al. (2008). Capsaicin modulates pulmonary antioxidant defense system during Benzo(a)pyrene-induced lung cancer in swiss albino mice. *Phytotherapy Research 22*: 529–533. https://doi.org/10.1002/ptr.

Anderson, D., Basaran, N., Blowers, S.D., and Edwards, A.J. (1995). The effect of antioxidants on bleomycin treatment in in vitro and in vivo genotoxicity assays. *Mutation Research, Fundamental and Molecular Mechanisms of Mutagenesis 329* (1): 37–47. https://doi.org/10.1016/0027-5107(95)00017-D.

Andlauer, W. and Fürst, P. (2002). Nutraceuticals: a piece of history, present status and outlook. *Food Research International 35* (2–3): 171–176. https://doi.org/10.1016/S0963-9969(01)00179-X.

Angel Nivya, M., Raja, K., Kumaravel, M. et al. (2012). Role of nutraceuticals in cancer. *International Journal of Pharmacy and Pharmaceutical Sciences 4* (SUPPL. 4): 415–420. https://doi.org/10.4018/978-1-5225-7039-4.ch017.

Arjumand, W., Seth, A., and Sultana, S. (2011). Rutin attenuates cisplatin induced renal inflammation and apoptosis by reducing NFκB, TNF-α and caspase-3 expression in wistar rats. *Food and Chemical Toxicology 49* (9): 2013–2021. https://doi.org/10.1016/j.fct.2011.05.012.

Arlt, A., Sebens, S., Krebs, S. et al. (2013). Inhibition of the Nrf2 transcription factor by the alkaloid trigonelline renders pancreatic cancer cells more susceptible to apoptosis through decreased proteasomal gene expression and proteasome activity. *Oncogene 32* (40): 4825–4835. https://doi.org/10.1038/onc.2012.493.

Arora, D., Jaglan, S., (2016). Nanocarriers based delivery of nutraceuticals for cancer prevention and treatment: a review of recent research developments. *Trends in Food Science & Technology*, 54, 114–126. doi: https://doi.org/10.1016/j.tifs.2016.06.003.

Austin, C.A., Patel, S., Ono, K. et al. (1992). Site-specific DNA cleavage by mammalian DNA topoisomerase II induced by novel flavone and catechin derivatives. *Biochemical Journal 282* (3): 883–889. https://doi.org/10.1042/bj2820883.

Badger, T.M., Gilchrist, J.M., Pivik, R.T. et al. (2009). The health implications of soy infant formula. *American Journal of Clinical Nutrition 89* (5): 1668–1672. https://doi.org/10.3945/ajcn.2009.26736U.

Baechler, S.A., Schroeter, A., Dicker, M. et al. (2014). Topoisomerase II-targeting properties of a grapevine-shoot extract and resveratrol oligomers. *Journal of Agricultural and Food Chemistry 62* (3): 780–788. https://doi.org/10.1021/jf4046182.

Baek, S.J., Kim, J.S., Jackson, F.R. et al. (2004). Epicatechin gallate-induced expression of NAG-1 is associated with growth inhibition and apoptosis in colon cancer cells. *Carcinogenesis 25* (12): 2425–2432. https://doi.org/10.1093/carcin/bgh255.

Bairati, I., Meyer, F., Gélinas, M. et al. (2005). A randomized trial of antioxidant vitamins to prevent second primary cancers in head and neck cancer patients. *Journal of the National Cancer Institute 97* (7): 481–488. https://doi.org/10.1093/jnci/dji095.

Bandele, O.J. and Osheroff, N. (2007). Bioflavonoids as poisons of human topoisomerase IIα and IIβ. *Biochemistry 46* (20): 6097–6108. https://doi.org/10.1021/bi7000664.

Bandele, O.J. and Osheroff, N. (2008). The efficacy of topoisomerase II-targeted anticancer agents reflects the persistence of drug-induced cleavage complexes in cells. *Biochemistry 47* (45): 11900–11908. https://doi.org/10.1021/bi800981j.

Baranello, L., Kouzine, F., and Levens, D. (2013). DNA topoisomerases: beyond the standard role. *Transcription 4* (5): 37–41. https://doi.org/10.4161/trns.26598.

Bardia, A., Tleyjeh, I.M., Cerhan, J.R. et al. (2008). Efficacy of antioxidant supplementation in reducing primary cancer incidence and mortality: systematic review and meta-analysis. *Mayo Clinic Proceedings 83* (1): 23–34. https://doi.org/10.4065/83.1.23.

Béliveau, R. and Gingras, D. (2004). Green tea: prevention and treatment of cancer by nutraceuticals. *The Lancet 364* (9439): 1021–1022.

BenAyed-Guerfali, D., Dabbèche-Bouricha, E., Ayadi, W. et al. (2019). Association of FOXA1 and EMT markers (Twist1 and E-cadherin) in breast cancer. *Molecular Biology Reports 46* (3): 3247–3255. https://doi.org/10.1007/s11033-019-04784-w.

Bessler, H., Salman, H., Bergman, M., and Djaldetti, M. (2012). Caffeine alters cytokine secretion by PBMC induced by colon cancer cells. *Cancer Investigation 30* (2): 87–91. https://doi.org/10.3109/07357907.2011.636113.

Bi, S., Liu, J.R., Li, Y. et al. (2010). γ-Tocotrienol modulates the paracrine secretion of VEGF induced by cobalt(II) chloride via ERK signaling pathway in gastric adenocarcinoma SGC-7901 cell line. *Toxicology 274* (1–3): 27–33. https://doi.org/10.1016/j.tox.2010.05.002.

Booth, N.L., Overk, C.R., Yao, P. et al. (2006). Seasonal variation of red clover (Trifolium pratense L., Fabaceae) isoflavones and estrogenic activity. *Journal of Agricultural and Food Chemistry 54* (4): 1277–1282. https://doi.org/10.1021/jf052927u.

Borriello, A. (2017). Resveratrol in cancer prevention and treatment: focusing on molecular targets and mechanism of action. *Proceedings 1* (10): 976. https://doi.org/10.3390/proceedings1100976.

Bravo, L. (2009). Polyphenols: chemistry, dietary sources, metabolism, and nutritional significance. *Nutrition Reviews 56* (11): 317–333. https://doi.org/10.1111/j.1753-4887.1998.tb01670.x.

Brown, M.J., Ferruzzi, M.G., Nguyen, M.L. et al. (2004). Carotenoid bioavailability is higher from salads ingested with full-fat than with fat-reduced salad dressings as measured with electrochemical detection. *American Journal of Clinical Nutrition 80* (2): 396–403. https://doi.org/10.1093/ajcn/80.2.396.

Butelli, E., Titta, L., Giorgio, M. et al. (2008). Enrichment of tomato fruit with health-promoting anthocyanins by expression of select transcription factors. *Nature Biotechnology 26* (11): 1301–1308. https://doi.org/10.1038/nbt.1506.

Calle, E.E., Rodriguez, C., Walker-Thurmond, K., and Thun, M.J. (2003). Overweight, obesity, and mortality from cancer in a prospectively studied cohort of US adults. *New England Journal of Medicine 348* (17): 1625–1638.

Calvani, M., Pasha, A., and Favre, C. (2020). Nutraceutical boom in cancer: inside the labyrinth of reactive oxygen species. *International Journal of Molecular Sciences 21* (6): 1–25. https://doi.org/10.3390/ijms21061936.

Caparica, R., Júlio, A., Araújo, M.E.M. et al. (2020). Anticancer activity of rutin and its combination with ionic liquids on renal cells. *Biomolecules 10* (2): https://doi.org/10.3390/biom10020233.

Celano, M., Maggisano, V., Bulotta, S. et al. (2020). Quercetin improves the effects of sorafenib on growth and migration of thyroid cancer cells. *Endocrine 67* (2): 496–498. https://doi.org/10.1007/s12020-019-02140-3.

Cen, L., Hutzen, B., Ball, S. et al. (2009). New structural analogues of curcumin exhibit potent growth suppressive activity in human colorectal carcinoma cells. *BMC Cancer 9*: 1–8. https://doi.org/10.1186/1471-2407-9-99.

Chauhan, B., Kumar, G., Kalam, N., and Ansari, S.H. (2013). Current concepts and prospects of herbal nutraceutical: a review. *Journal of Advanced Pharmaceutical Technology & Research 4* (1): 4–8. https://doi.org/10.4103/2231-4040.107494.

Chen, A. and Rogan, W.J. (2004). Isoflavones in soy infant formula: a review of evidence for endocrine and other activity in infants. *Annual Review of Nutrition 24*: 33–54. https://doi.org/10.1146/annurev.nutr.24.101603.064950.

Chen, Z., Zheng, S., Li, L., and Jiang, H. (2014). Metabolism of flavonoids in human: a comprehensive review. *Current Drug Metabolism 15* (1): 48–61. https://doi.org/10.2174/138920021501140218125020.

Chen, J., Xu, T., and Chen, C. (2015). The critical roles of miR-21 in anti-cancer effects of curcumin. *Annals of Translational Medicine 3* (21): 1–7. https://doi.org/10.3978/j.issn.2305-5839.2015.09.20.

Chew, B.P., Brown, C.M., Park, J.S., and Mixter, P.F. (2003). Dietary lutein inhibits mouse mammary tumor growth by regulating angiogenesis and apoptosis. *Anticancer Research 23* (4): 3333–3339.

Chu, Y.L., Ho, C.T., Chung, J.G. et al. (2012). Allicin induces p53-mediated autophagy in Hep G2 human liver cancer cells. *Journal of Agricultural and Food Chemistry 60* (34): 8363–8371. https://doi.org/10.1021/jf301298y.

Chu, H., Li, J., Liu, T. et al. (2020). Anticancer effects of Daidzein against the human melanoma cell lines involves cell cycle arrest, autophagy and deactivation of PI3K/AKT signalling pathways. *Journal of B.U.ON. 25* (1): 485–490.

Clark, R., Lee, J., and Lee, S.H. (2015). Synergistic anticancer activity of capsaicin and 3,3′-diindolylmethane in human colorectal cancer. *Journal of Agricultural and Food Chemistry 63* (17): 4297–4304. https://doi.org/10.1021/jf506098s.

Clayton, P.E., Banerjee, I., Murray, P.G., and Renehan, A.G. (2011). Growth hormone, the insulin-like growth factor axis, insulin and cancer risk. *Nature Reviews Endocrinology 7* (1): 11–24. https://doi.org/10.1038/nrendo.2010.171.

Colomer, R., Moreno-Nogueira, J.M., García-Luna, P.P. et al. (2007). n-3 fatty acids, cancer and cachexia: a systematic review of the literature. *British Journal of Nutrition 97* (5): 823–831. https://doi.org/10.1017/S000711450765795X.

Cone, R.A. (2009). Barrier properties of mucus. *Advanced Drug Delivery Reviews 61* (2): 75–85. https://doi.org/10.1016/j.addr.2008.09.008.

Conklin, K.A. (2000). Dietary antioxidants during cancer chemotherapy: impact on chemotherapeutic effectiveness and development of side effects. *Nutrition and Cancer 37* (1): 1–18. https://doi.org/10.1207/S15327914NC3701_1.

Constantinou, A., Mehta, R., and Runyan, C. (1995). Flavonoids as dna topoisomerase antagonists. *Journal of Natural Products 58* (2): 217–225.

Cornelli, U. (2009). Antioxidant use in nutraceuticals. *Clinics in Dermatology 27* (2): 175–194. https://doi.org/10.1016/j.clindermatol.2008.01.010.

Coussens, L.M. and Werb, Z. (2002). Inflammation and cancer. *Nature 420* (6917): 860–867. https://doi.org/10.1038/nature01322.

Dahan, A. and Miller, J.M. (2012). The solubility-permeability interplay and its implications in formulation design and development for poorly soluble drugs. *The AAPS Journal 14* (2): 244–251. https://doi.org/10.1208/s12248-012-9337-6.

Das, L. and Vinayak, M. (2015). Long term effect of curcumin in restoration of tumour suppressor p53 and phase-II antioxidant enzymes via activation of Nrf2 signalling and modulation of inflammation in prevention of cancer. *PLoS One 10* (4): 1–22. https://doi.org/10.1371/journal.pone.0124000.

Davis, C.D. (2007). Nutritional interactions: credentialing of molecular targets for cancer prevention. *Experimental Biology and Medicine 232* (2): 176–183. https://doi.org/10.3181/00379727-207-2320176.

De Rijke, E., Aardenburg, L., Van Dijk, J. et al. (2005). Changed isoflavone levels in red clover (Trifolium pratense L.) leaves with disturbed root nodulation in response to waterlogging. *Journal of Chemical Ecology 31* (6): 1285–1298. https://doi.org/10.1007/s10886-005-5286-1.

Deka, S., Gorai, S., Manna, D., and Trivedi, V. (2017). Evidence of PKC binding and translocation to explain the anticancer mechanism of chlorogenic acid in breast cancer cells. *Current Molecular Medicine 17* (1): 79–89. https://doi.org/10.2174/1566524017666170209160619.

Del Follo-Martinez, A., Banerjee, N., Li, X. et al. (2013). Resveratrol and quercetin in combination have anticancer activity in colon cancer cells and repress oncogenic microRNA-27a. *Nutrition and Cancer 65* (3): 494–504. https://doi.org/10.1080/01635581.2012.725194.

Delphi, L. and Sepehri, H. (2016). Apple pectin: a natural source for cancer suppression in 4T1 breast cancer cells in vitro and express p53 in mouse bearing 4T1 cancer tumors, in vivo. *Biomedicine and Pharmacotherapy 84*: 637–644. https://doi.org/10.1016/j.biopha.2016.09.080.

Dhar, S., Hicks, C., and Levenson, A.S. (2011). Resveratrol and prostate cancer: promising role for microRNAs. *Molecular Nutrition & Food Research 55* (8): 1219–1229. https://doi.org/10.1002/mnfr.201100141.

Dhar, S., Kumar, A., Li, K. et al. (2015). Resveratrol regulates PTEN/Akt pathway through inhibition of MTA1/HDAC unit of the NuRD complex in prostate cancer. *Biochimica et Biophysica Acta-Molecular Cell Research 1853* (2): 265–275. https://doi.org/10.1016/j.bbamcr.2014.11.004.

Diaz-Gerevini, G.T., Repossi, G., Dain, A. et al. (2016). Beneficial action of resveratrol: how and why? *Nutrition 32* (2): 174–178. https://doi.org/10.1016/j.nut.2015.08.017.

Dijsselbloem, N., Vanden Berghe, W., De Naeyer, A., and Haegeman, G. (2004). Soy isoflavone phyto-pharmaceuticals in interleukin-6 affections: multi-purpose nutraceuticals at the crossroad of hormone replacement, anti-cancer and anti-inflammatory therapy. *Biochemical Pharmacology 68* (6): 1171–1185. https://doi.org/10.1016/j.bcp.2004.05.036.

Donaldson, M.S. (2004). Nutrition and cancer: a review of the evidence for an anti-cancer diet. *Nutrition Journal 3*: 1–21. https://doi.org/10.1186/1475-2891-3-19.

Dorai, T. and Aggarwal, B.B. (2004). Role of chemopreventive agents in cancer therapy. *Cancer Letters 215* (2): 129–140. https://doi.org/10.1016/j.canlet.2004.07.013.

Dropcho, E.J. (2011). The neurologic side effects of chemotherapeutic agents. *CONTINUUM Lifelong Learning in Neurology 17* (1): 95–112. https://doi.org/10.1212/01.CON.0000394676.67372.87.

Du, L., Xie, Z., Wu, L.C. et al. (2012). Reactivation of RASSF1A in breast cancer cells by curcumin. *Nutrition and Cancer 64* (8): 1228–1235. https://doi.org/10.1080/01635581.2012.717682.

Dudhatra, G.B., Mody, S.K., Awale, M.M. et al. (2012). A comprehensive review on pharmacotherapeutics of herbal bioenhancers. *The Scientific World Journal 2012*: https://doi.org/10.1100/2012/637953.

Dulak, J. (2005). Nutraceuticals as anti-angiogenic agents: hopes and reality. *Journal of Physiology and Pharmacology 56* (SUPPL. 1): 51–67.

Erlund, I., Kosonen, T., Alfthan, G. et al. (2000). Pharmacokinetics of quercetin from quercetin aglycone and rutin in healthy volunteers. *European Journal of Clinical Pharmacology 56* (8): 545–553. https://doi.org/10.1007/s002280000197.

Esselen, M. and Barth, S.W. (2014). Food-borne topoisomerase inhibitors: risk or benefit. In: *Advances in Molecular Toxicology*, 1e, vol. 8. Elsevier B.V. https://doi.org/10.1016/B978-0-444-63406-1.00004-0.

Failla, M.L., Huo, T., and Thakkar, S.K. (2008). in vitro screening of relative bioaccessibility of carotenoids from foods. *Asia Pacific Journal of Clinical Nutrition 17* (SUPPL. 1): 200–203. https://doi.org/10.6133/apjcn.2008.17.s1.48.

Farhangi, B., Alizadeh, A.M., Khodayari, H. et al. (2015). Protective effects of dendrosomal curcumin on an animal metastatic breast tumor. *European Journal of Pharmacology 758*: 188–196. https://doi.org/10.1016/j.ejphar.2015.03.076.

Fayette, J., Soria, J.C., and Armand, J.P. (2005). Use of angiogenesis inhibitors in tumour treatment. *European Journal of Cancer 41* (8): 1109–1116. https://doi.org/10.1016/j.ejca.2005.02.017.

Feng, Y.Z.Y., Zhai, Y.L.Y., Wang, Y.F.J., and Jin, C.Y.C. (2019). Glycitein induces reactive oxygen species-dependent apoptosis and G0/G1 cell cycle arrest through the MAPK/STAT3/NF-κB pathway in human gastric cancer cells. *Drug Development Research 80* (5): 573–584. https://doi.org/10.1002/ddr.21534.

Fenton, J.I. and McCaskey, S.J. (2013). Curcumin and docosahexaenoic acid block insulin-induced colon carcinoma cell proliferation. *Prostaglandins, Leukotrienes, and Essential Fatty Acids 88* (3): 219–226. https://doi.org/10.1016/j.plefa.2012.11.010.

Fernández-García, E., Carvajal-Lérida, I., and Pérez-Gálvez, A. (2009). in vitro bioaccessibility assessment as a prediction tool of nutritional efficiency. *Nutrition Research 29* (11): 751–760. https://doi.org/10.1016/j.nutres.2009.09.016.

Fernández-García, E., Carvajal-Lérida, I., Jarén-Galán, M. et al. (2012). Carotenoids bioavailability from foods: from plant pigments to efficient biological activities. *Food Research International 46* (2): 438–450. https://doi.org/10.1016/j.foodres.2011.06.007.

Finley, J.W., Kong, A.N., Hintze, K.J. et al. (2011). Antioxidants in foods: state of the science important to the food industry. *Journal of Agricultural and Food Chemistry 59* (13): 6837–6846. https://doi.org/10.1021/jf2013875.

Fisher, W.E., Boros, L.G., and Schirmer, W.J. (1996). Insulin promotes pancreatic cancer: evidence for endocrine influence on exocrine pancreatic tumors. *Journal of Surgical Research 63* (1): 310–313. https://doi.org/10.1006/jsre.1996.0266.

Focke, M., Feld, A., and Lichtenthaler, H.K. (1990). Allicin, a naturally occurring antibiotic from garlic, specifically inhibits acetyl-CoA synthetase. *FEBS Letters 261* (1): 106–108. https://doi.org/10.1016/0014-5793(90)80647-2.

Fritz, H., Seely, D., Flower, G. et al. (2013). Soy, red clover, and isoflavones and breast cancer: a systematic review. *PLoS One 8* (11): 1–18. https://doi.org/10.1371/journal.pone.0081968.

Fritz, A.J., Hong, D., Boyd, J. et al. (2020). RUNX1 and RUNX2 transcription factors function in opposing roles to regulate breast cancer stem cells. *Journal of Cellular Physiology, December 2019*: 1–12. https://doi.org/10.1002/jcp.29625.

Ganry, O. (2005). Phytoestrogens and prostate cancer risk. *Preventive Medicine 41* (1): 1–6. https://doi.org/10.1016/j.ypmed.2004.10.022.

Gloria, N.F., Soares, N., Brand, C. et al. (2014). Liposomes as delivery systems for carotenoids. *Food & Function 5* (6): 1232–1240.

Gouthamchandra, K., Sudeep, H.V., Venkatesh, B.J., and Shyam Prasad, K. (2017). Chlorogenic acid complex (CGA7), standardized extract from green coffee beans exerts anticancer effects against cultured human colon cancer HCT-116 cells. *Food Science and Human Wellness 6* (3): 147–153. https://doi.org/10.1016/j.fshw.2017.06.001.

Griesser, M., Pistis, V., Suzuki, T. et al. (2011). Autoxidative and cyclooxygenase-2 catalyzed transformation of the dietary chemopreventive agent curcumin. *Journal of Biological Chemistry 286* (2): 1114–1124. https://doi.org/10.1074/jbc.M110.178806.

Grimble, R.F. (2003). Nutritional therapy for cancer cachexia. *Gut 52* (10): 1391–1392. https://doi.org/10.1136/gut.52.10.1391.

Gromadzińska, J., Reszka, E., Bruzelius, K. et al. (2008). Selenium and cancer: biomarkers of selenium status and molecular action of selenium supplements. *European Journal of Nutrition 47* (SUPPL. 2): 29–50. https://doi.org/10.1007/s00394-008-2005-z.

Gupta, R.K., Gangoliya, S.S., and Singh, N.K. (2013). Reduction of phytic acid and enhancement of bioavailable micronutrients in food grains. *Journal of Food Science and Technology 52* (2): 676–684. https://doi.org/10.1007/s13197-013-0978-y.

Gwak, G.Y., Yoon, J.H., Kim, K.M. et al. (2005). Hypoxia stimulates proliferation of human hepatoma cells through the induction of hexokinase II expression. *Journal of Hepatology 42* (3): 358–364. https://doi.org/10.1016/j.jhep.2004.11.020.

Haber, R.S., Rathan, A., Weiser, K.R. et al. (1998). GLUT1 glucose transporter expression in colorectal carcinoma: a marker for poor prognosis. *Cancer 83* (1): 34–40.

Hagiwara, K., Kosaka, N., Yoshioka, Y. et al. (2012). Stilbene derivatives promote Ago2-dependent tumour-suppressive microRNA activity. *Scientific Reports 2*: 1–9. https://doi.org/10.1038/srep00314.

Han, G., Xia, J., Gao, J. et al. (2015). Anti-tumor effects and cellular mechanisms of resveratrol. *Drug Discoveries & Therapeutics 9* (1): 1–12. https://doi.org/10.5582/ddt.2015.01007.

Hanahan, D. and Weinberg, R.A. (2000). The hallmarks of cancer review douglas. *Cell 100* (7): 57–70. https://doi.org/10.1007/s00262-010-0968-0.

Hanahan, D. and Weinberg, R.A. (2011). Hallmarks of cancer: the next generation. *Cell 144* (5): 646–674. https://doi.org/10.1016/j.cell.2011.02.013.

Hardy, T.M. and Tollefsbol, T.O. (2011). Epigenetic diet: impact on the epigenome and cancer. *Epigenomics 3* (4): 503–518. https://doi.org/10.2217/epi.11.71.

Hecht, S.S. (1999). Biochemistry and physiology chemoprevention of cancer by isothiocyanates, modifiers of carcinogen metabolism. *Journal of Nutrition 129* (March): 768–774.

Henderson, B.E. and Feigelson, H.S. (2000). Hormonal carcinogenesis. *Carcinogenesis 21* (3): 427–433. https://doi.org/10.1093/carcin/21.3.427.

Hennekens, C. (1994). Antioxidant, Vitamins and Cancer. *The American Journal of Medicine 97* (C): 305–352. https://doi.org/10.1016/S0083-6729(08)60288-5.

Hercberg, S., Czernichow, S., and Galan, P. (2006). Antioxidant vitamins and minerals in prevention of cancers: lessons from the SU.VI.MAX study. *British Journal of Nutrition 96* (S1): S28–S30. https://doi.org/10.1079/bjn20061695.

Hirakawa, N., Okauchi, R., Miura, Y., and Yagasaki, K. (2005). Anti-invasive activity of niacin and trigonelline against cancer cells. *Bioscience, Biotechnology, and Biochemistry 69* (3): 653–658. https://doi.org/10.1271/bbb.69.653.

Holzbeierlein, J.M., McIntosh, J., and Thrasher, J.B. (2005). The role of soy phytoestrogens in prostate cancer. *Current Opinion in Urology 15* (1): 17–22. https://doi.org/10.1097/00042307-200501000-00005.

Hosseini, A. and Ghorbani, A. (2015). Cancer therapy with phytochemicals: evidence from clinical studies. *Avicenna Journal of Phytomedicine 5* (2): 84–97. https://doi.org/10.22038/ajp.2015.3872.

Howard, E.W., Ling, M.T., Chee, W.C. et al. (2007). Garlic-derived S-allylmercaptocysteine is a novel in vivo antimetastatic agent for androgen-independent prostate cancer. *Clinical Cancer Research 13* (6): 1847–1856. https://doi.org/10.1158/1078-0432.CCR-06-2074.

Hua, F., Li, C.H., Chen, X.G., and Liu, X.P. (2018). Daidzein exerts anticancer activity towards SKOV3 human ovarian cancer cells by inducing apoptosis and cell cycle arrest, and inhibiting the Raf/MEK/ERK cascade. *International Journal of Molecular Medicine 41* (6): 3485–3492. https://doi.org/10.3892/ijmm.2018.3531.

Huang, H.Y., Caballero, B., Chang, S. et al. (2006). The efficacy and safety of multivitamin and mineral supplement use to prevent cancer and chronic disease in adults: a systematic review for a National Institutes of Health state-of-the-science conference. *Annals of Internal Medicine 145* (5): 372–385. https://doi.org/10.7326/0003-4819-145-5-200609050-00135.

Hwangbo, K., Zheng, M.S., Kim, Y.J. et al. (2012). Inhibition of DNA topoisomerases I and II of compounds from Reynoutria japonica. *Archives of Pharmacal Research 35* (9): 1583–1589. https://doi.org/10.1007/s12272-012-0909-x.

Iriti, M., Kubina, R., Cochis, A. et al. (2017). Rutin, a Quercetin Glycoside, restores chemosensitivity in human breast cancer cells. *Phytotherapy Research 31* (10): 1529–1538. https://doi.org/10.1002/ptr.5878.

Jackson, H.A. and Sheehan, A.H. (2005). Effect of vitamin A on fracture risk. *Annals of Pharmacotherapy 39* (12): 2086–2090. https://doi.org/10.1345/aph.1G028.

Jeon, K.I., Rih, J.K., Kim, H.J. et al. (2003). Pretreatment of indole-3-carbinol augments TRAIL-induced apoptosis in a prostate cancer cell line, LNCaP. *FEBS Letters 544* (1–3): 246–251. https://doi.org/10.1016/S0014-5793(03)00473-3.

Ji, Z., Huo, C., and Yang, P. (2020). Genistein inhibited the proliferation of kidney cancer cells via CDKN2a hypomethylation: role of abnormal apoptosis. *International Urology and Nephrology 52* (6): 1049–1055. https://doi.org/10.1007/s11255-019-02372-2.

Jian, L. (2009). Soy, isoflavones, and prostate cancer. *Molecular Nutrition & Food Research 53* (2): 217–226. https://doi.org/10.1002/mnfr.200800167.

Jiang, A., Wang, X., Shan, X. et al. (2015). Curcumin reactivates silenced tumor suppressor Gene RARβ by reducing DNA Methylation. *Phytotherapy Research 1245* (March): 1237–1245.

Jin, S., Zhang, Q.Y., Kang, X.M. et al. (2010). Daidzein induces MCF-7 breast cancer cell apoptosis via the mitochondrial pathway. *Annals of Oncology 21* (2): 263–268. https://doi.org/10.1093/annonc/mdp499.

Jo, J.Y., De Mejia, E.G., and Lila, M.A. (2005). Effects of grape cell culture extracts on human topoisomerase II catalytic activity and characterization of active fractions. *Journal of Agricultural and Food Chemistry 53* (7): 2489–2498. https://doi.org/10.1021/jf048524w.

Jo, J.Y., Gonzalez De Mejia, E., and Lila, M.A. (2006). Catalytic inhibition of human DNA topoisomerase II by interactions of grape cell culture polyphenols. *Journal of Agricultural and Food Chemistry 54* (6): 2083–2087. https://doi.org/10.1021/jf052700z.

Johnson, I.T. (2004). Micronutrients and cancer. *Proceedings of the Nutrition Society 63* (4): 587–595. https://doi.org/10.1079/pns2004389.

Jung, E.M., Lee, T.J., Park, J.W. et al. (2005). Curcumin sensitizes tumor necrosis factor-related apoptosis-inducing ligand (TRAIL)-induced apoptosis through reactive oxygen species-mediated upregulation of death receptor 5 (DR5). *Carcinogenesis 26* (11): 1905–1913. https://doi.org/10.1093/carcin/bgi167.

Kaelin, W.G. and Thompson, C.B. (2010). Q and A: cancer: clues from cell metabolism. *Nature 465* (7298): 562–564. https://doi.org/10.1038/465562a.

Kala, R., Shah, H.N., Martin, S.L., and Tollefsbol, T.O. (2015). Epigenetic-based combinatorial resveratrol and pterostilbene alters DNA damage response by affecting SIRT1 and DNMT enzyme expression, including SIRT1-dependent γ-H2AX and telomerase regulation in triple-negative breast cancer. *BMC Cancer 15* (1): 1–18. https://doi.org/10.1186/s12885-015-1693-z.

Kalfalah, F.M., Mielke, C., Christensen, M.O. et al. (2011). Genotoxicity of dietary, environmental and therapeutic topoisomerase II poisons is uniformly correlated to prolongation of enzyme DNA residence. *Molecular Nutrition & Food Research 55* (SUPPL. 1): 127–142. https://doi.org/10.1002/mnfr.201000509.

Kannappan, R., Gupta, S.C., Kim, J.H., and Aggarwal, B.B. (2012). Tocotrienols fight cancer by targeting multiple cell signaling pathways. *Genes & Nutrition 7* (1): 43–52. https://doi.org/10.1007/s12263-011-0220-3.

Kapinova, A., Kubatka, P., Golubnitschaja, O. et al. (2018). Dietary phytochemicals in breast cancer research: anticancer effects and potential utility for effective chemoprevention. *Environmental Health and Preventive Medicine 23* (1): 1–18. https://doi.org/10.1186/s12199-018-0724-1.

Karas, M., Amir, H., Fishman, D. et al. (2000). Lycopene interferes with cell cycle progression and insulin-like growth factor I signaling in mammary cancer cells. *Nutrition and Cancer 36* (1): 101–111. https://doi.org/10.1207/S15327914NC3601_14.

Kaur, M., Velmurugan, B., Rajamanickam, S. et al. (2009). Gallic acid, an active constituent of grape seed extract, exhibits anti-proliferative, pro-apoptotic and anti-tumorigenic effects against prostate carcinoma xenograft growth in nude mice. *Pharmaceutical Research 26* (9): 2133–2140. https://doi.org/10.1007/s11095-009-9926-y.

Kausar, H., Jeyabalan, J., Aqil, F. et al. (2012). Berry anthocyanidins synergistically suppress growth and invasive potential of human non-small-cell lung cancer cells. *Cancer Letters 325* (1): 54–62. https://doi.org/10.1016/j.canlet.2012.05.029.

Ketron, A.C., Gordon, O.N., Schneider, C., and Osheroff, N. (2013). Oxidative metabolites of curcumin poison human type II topoisomerases. *Biochemistry 52* (1): 221–227. https://doi.org/10.1021/bi3014455.

Khadka, D.B. and Cho, W.J. (2013). Topoisomerase inhibitors as anticancer agents: a patent update. *Expert Opinion on Therapeutic Patents 23* (8): 1033–1056. https://doi.org/10.1517/13543776.2013.790958.

Khan, N., Adhami, V.M., and Mukhtar, H. (2010). Apoptosis by dietary agents for prevention and treatment of prostate cancer. *Endocrine-Related Cancer 17* (1): 39–52. https://doi.org/10.1677/ERC-09-0262.

Khan, M.A., Hussain, A., Sundaram, M.K. et al. (2015). Epigallocatechin-3-gallate reverses the expression of various tumor-suppressor genes by inhibiting DNA methyltransferases and histone deacetylases in human cervical cancer cells. *Oncology Reports 33* (4): 1976–1984. https://doi.org/10.3892/or.2015.3802.

Khor, T.O., Huang, Y., Wu, T.Y. et al. (2011). Pharmacodynamics of curcumin as DNA hypomethylation agent in restoring the expression of Nrf2 via promoter CpGs demethylation. *Biochemical Pharmacology 82* (9): 1073–1078. https://doi.org/10.1016/j.bcp.2011.07.065.

Kim, Y.I. (2007). Folate and colorectal cancer: an evidence-based critical review. *Molecular Nutrition & Food Research 51* (3): 267–292. https://doi.org/10.1002/mnfr.200600191.

Kim, Y.J., Park, H.J., Yoon, S.H. et al. (2005). Anticancer effects of oligomeric proanthocyanidins on human colorectal cancer cell line, SNU-C4. *World journal of gastroenterology: WJG 11* (30): 4674.

Kim, J. W., Gao, P., Liu, Y. C., Semenza, G. L., & Dang, C. V. (2007). Hypoxia-inducible factor 1 and dysregulated c-Myc cooperatively induce vascular endothelial growth factor and metabolic switches hexokinase 2 and pyruvate dehydrogenase kinase 1. *Molecular and Cellular Biology*, *27*(21), 7381–7393. doi:https://doi.org/10.1128/MCB.00440-07

Kim, K.K., Singh, A.P., Singh, R.K. et al. (2012). Anti-angiogenic activity of cranberry proanthocyanidins and cytotoxic properties in ovarian cancer cells. *International Journal of Oncology 40* (1): 227–235. https://doi.org/10.3892/ijo.2011.1198.

Kowalski, J., Samojedny, A., Paul, M. et al. (2005). Effect of apigenin, kaempferol and resveratrol on the expression of interleukin-1β and tumor necrosis factor-α genes in J774.2 macrophages. *Pharmacological Reports 57* (3): 390–394.

Krakowsky, R.H.E. and Tollefsbol, T.O. (2015). Impact of nutrition on non-coding rna epigenetics in breast and gynecological cancer. *Frontiers in Nutrition 2* (May): 1–25. https://doi.org/10.3389/fnut.2015.00016.

Krzeslak, A., Wojcik-Krowiranda, K., Forma, E. et al. (2012). Expression of GLUT1 and GLUT3 glucose transporters in endometrial and breast cancers. *Pathology and Oncology Research 18* (3): 721–728. https://doi.org/10.1007/s12253-012-9500-5.

Kumar, U., Sharma, U., and Rathi, G. (2017). Reversal of hypermethylation and reactivation of glutathione S-transferase pi 1 gene by curcumin in breast cancer cell line. *Tumor Biology 39* (2): 1–8. https://doi.org/10.1177/1010428317692258.

Kunnumakkara, A.B., Sailo, B.L., Banik, K. et al. (2018). Chronic diseases, inflammation, and spices: how are they linked? *Journal of Translational Medicine 16* (1): 1–25. https://doi.org/10.1186/s12967-018-1381-2.

Kwon, O.J., Zhang, B., Zhang, L., and Xin, L. (2016). High fat diet promotes prostatic basal-to-luminal differentiation and accelerates initiation of prostate epithelial hyperplasia originated from basal cells. *Stem Cell Research 16* (3): 682–691. https://doi.org/10.1016/j.scr.2016.04.009.

La, C.V. (1992). Cancers associated with high-fat diets. *Journal of the National Cancer Institute. Monographs* 1992 (12): 79–85.

Labrecque, L., Lamy, S., Chapus, A. et al. (2005). Combined inhibition of PDGF and VEGF receptors by ellagic acid, a dietary-derived phenolic compound. *Carcinogenesis 26* (4): 821–826. https://doi.org/10.1093/carcin/bgi024.

Lambert, J.D., Lee, M.J., Lu, H. et al. (2003). Epigallocatechin-3-gallate is absorbed but extensively glucuronidated following oral administration to mice. *Journal of Nutrition 133* (12): 4172–4177. https://doi.org/10.1093/jn/133.12.4172.

Lamy, S., Gingras, D., and Béliveau, R. (2002). Green tea catechins inhibit vascular endothelial growth factor receptor phosphorylation. *Cancer Research 62* (2): 381–385.

Lamy, S., Blanchette, M., Michaud-Levesque, J. et al. (2006). Delphinidin, a dietary anthocyanidin, inhibits vascular endothelial growth factor receptor-2 phosphorylation. *Carcinogenesis 27* (5): 989–996. https://doi.org/10.1093/carcin/bgi279.

Lee, Y.H., Albig, A.R., Regner, M. et al. (2008). Fibulin-5 initiates epithelial-mesenchymal transition (EMT) and enhances EMT induced by TGF-β in mammary epithelial cells via a MMP-dependent mechanism. *Carcinogenesis 29* (12): 2243–2251. https://doi.org/10.1093/carcin/bgn199.

Lee, E.J., Kim, S.Y., Hyun, J.W. et al. (2010). Glycitein inhibits glioma cell invasion through down-regulation of MMP-3 and MMP-9 gene expression. *Chemico-Biological Interactions 185* (1): 18–24. https://doi.org/10.1016/j.cbi.2010.02.037.

Lee, Y.H., Kwak, J., Choi, H.K. et al. (2012). EGCG suppresses prostate cancer cell growth modulating acetylation of androgen receptor by anti-histone acetyltransferase activity. *International Journal of Molecular Medicine 30* (1): 69–74. https://doi.org/10.3892/ijmm.2012.966.

Lee, J.H., Khor, T.O., Shu, L. et al. (2013). Dietary phytochemicals and cancer prevention: Nrf2 signaling, epigenetics, and cell death mechanisms in blocking cancer initiation and progression. *Pharmacology and Therapeutics 137* (2): 153–171. https://doi.org/10.1016/j.pharmthera.2012.09.008.

Leone, S., Cornetta, T., Basso, E., and Cozzi, R. (2010). Resveratrol induces DNA double-strand breaks through human topoisomerase II interaction. *Cancer Letters 295* (2): 167–172. https://doi.org/10.1016/j.canlet.2010.02.022.

Levine, M.E., Suarez, J.A., Brandhorst, S. et al. (2014). Low protein intake is associated with a major reduction in IGF-1, cancer, and overall mortality in the 65 and younger but not older population. *Cell Metabolism 19* (3): 407–417. https://doi.org/10.1016/j.cmet.2014.02.006.

Li, Y., Saldanha, S.N., and Tollefsbol, T.O. (2014). Impact of epigenetic dietary compounds on transgenerational prevention of human diseases. *The AAPS Journal 16* (1): 27–36. https://doi.org/10.1208/s12248-013-9538-7.

Li, D., Chen, L., Zhao, W. et al. (2016). MicroRNA-let-7f-1 is induced by lycopene and inhibits cell proliferation and triggers apoptosis in prostate cancer. *Molecular Medicine Reports 13* (3): 2708–2714. https://doi.org/10.3892/mmr.2016.4841.

Li, Y., Li, S., Meng, X. et al. (2017). Dietary natural products for prevention and treatment of breast cancer. *Nutrients 9* (7): 1–38. https://doi.org/10.3390/nu9070728.

Li, K., Hong, S., Lin, S., and Chen, K. (2020). Genistein inhibits the proliferation, migration and invasion of the squamous cell carcinoma cells via inhibition of MEK/ERK and JNK signalling pathways. *Journal of BU ON.: Official Journal of the Balkan Union of Oncology 25* (2): 1172–1177.

Liang, G., Tang, A., Lin, X. et al. (2010). Green tea catechins augment the antitumor activity of doxorubicin in an in vivo mouse model for chemoresistant liver cancer. *International Journal of Oncology 37* (1): 111–123.

Liang, D., Qin, Y., Zhao, W. et al. (2011). S-allylmercaptocysteine effectively inhibits the proliferation of colorectal cancer cells under in vitro and in vivo conditions. *Cancer Letters 310* (1): 69–76. https://doi.org/10.1016/j.canlet.2011.06.019.

Liao, H., Wang, Z., Deng, Z. et al. (2015). Curcumin inhibits lung cancer invasion and metastasis by attenuating GLUT1/MT1-MMP/MMP2 pathway. *International Journal of Clinical and Experimental Medicine 8* (6): 8948–8957.

Liguori, I., Russo, G., Curcio, F. et al. (2018). Oxidative stress, aging, and diseases. *Clinical Interventions in Aging 13*: 757.

Lin, J., Cook, N.R., Lee, I.M. et al. (2006). Total magnesium intake and colorectal cancer incidence in women. *Cancer Epidemiology, Biomarkers and Prevention 15* (10): 2006–2009. https://doi.org/10.1158/1055-9965.EPI-06-0454.

Lo, A.H., Liang, Y.C., Lin-Shiau, S.Y. et al. (2002). Carnosol, an antioxidant in rosemary, suppresses inducible nitric oxide synthase through down-regulating nuclear factor-κB in mouse macrophages. *Carcinogenesis 23* (6): 983–991. https://doi.org/10.1093/carcin/23.6.983.

Loh, C.Y., Chai, J.Y., Tang, T.F. et al. (2019). The E-Cadherin and N-Cadherin switch in epithelial-to-mesenchymal transition: signaling, therapeutic implications, and challenges. *Cell* 8 (10): https://doi.org/10.3390/cells8101118.

López-Lázaro, M., Willmore, E., and Austin, C.A. (2007). Cells lacking DNA topoisomerase IIβ are resistant to genistein. *Journal of Natural Products 70* (5): 763–767. https://doi.org/10.1021/np060609z.

López-Lázaro, M., Willmore, E., and Austin, C.A. (2010). The dietary flavonoids myricetin and fisetin act as dual inhibitors of DNA topoisomerases I and II in cells. *Mutation Research, Genetic Toxicology and Environmental Mutagenesis 696* (1): 41–47. https://doi.org/10.1016/j.mrgentox.2009.12.010.

López-Lázaro, M., Calderón-Montaño, J.M., Burgos-Morón, E., and Austin, C.A. (2011). Green tea constituents (-)-epigallocatechin-3-gallate (EGCG) and gallic acid induce topoisomerase I- and topoisomerase II-DNA complexes in cells mediated by pyrogallol-induced hydrogen peroxide. *Mutagenesis 26* (4): 489–498. https://doi.org/10.1093/mutage/ger006.

Łuczak, M. and Jagodziński, P.P. (2006). The role of DNA methylation in cancer development. *Folia Histochemica et Cytobiologica 44* (3): 143–154.

MacLennan, M. and Ma, D.W. (2010). Role of dietary fatty acids in mammary gland development and breast cancer. *Breast Cancer Research 12* (5): 211.

Mag, P., Samarghandian, S., Azimi-nezhad, M. et al. (2016). Inhibitory and cytotoxic activities of chrysin on human breast adenocarcinoma cells by induction of apoptosis. *Pharmacognosy Magazine* 436–440. https://doi.org/10.4103/0973-1296.191453.

Mahady, G.B., Parrot, J., Lee, C. et al. (2003). Botanical dietary supplement use in peri-and postmenopausal women. *Menopause 10* (1): 65–72. https://doi.org/10.1097/01.GME.0000029028.95924.F9.

Martín-Cordero, C., López-Lázaro, M., Gálvez, M., and Ayuso, M.J. (2003). Curcumin as a DNA topoisomerase II poison. *Journal of Enzyme Inhibition and Medicinal Chemistry 18* (6): 505–509. https://doi.org/10.1080/14756360310001613085.

Mateo Anson, N., van den Berg, R., Havenaar, R. et al. (2009). Bioavailability of ferulic acid is determined by its bioaccessibility. *Journal of Cereal Science 49* (2): 296–300. https://doi.org/10.1016/j.jcs.2008.12.001.

Mawson, A., Lai, A., Carroll, J. S., Sergio, C. M., Mitchell, C. J., & Sarcevic, B. (2005). Estrogen and insulin/IGF-1 cooperatively stimulate cell cycle progression in MCF-7 breast cancer cells through differential regulation of c-Myc and cyclin D1. *Molecular and Cellular Endocrinology, 229*(1–2), 161–173. doi:https://doi.org/10.1016/j.mce.2004.08.002

Mazzanti, G., Menniti-Ippolito, F., Moro, P.A. et al. (2009). Hepatotoxicity from green tea: a review of the literature and two unpublished cases. *European Journal of Clinical Pharmacology 65* (4): 331–341. https://doi.org/10.1007/s00228-008-0610-7.

McCubrey, J.A., Lertpiriyapong, K., Steelman, L.S. et al. (2017). Effects of resveratrol, curcumin, berberine and other nutraceuticals on aging, cancer development, cancer stem cells and microRNAs. *Aging 9* (6): 1477–1536. https://doi.org/10.18632/aging.101250.

Mecocci, P., Tinarelli, C., Schulz, R.J., and Polidori, M.C. (2014). Nutraceuticals in cognitive impairment and Alzheimer's disease. *Frontiers in Pharmacology* 5: 1–11. https://doi.org/10.3389/fphar.2014.00147.

Melstrom, L.G., Salabat, M.R., Ding, X.Z. et al. (2008). Apigenin inhibits the GLUT-1 glucose transporter and the phosphoinositide 3-kinase/Akt pathway in human pancreatic cancer cells. *Pancreas 37* (4): 426–431.

Meng, Q., Goldberg, I.D., Rosen, E.M., and Fan, S. (2000). Inhibitory effects of indole-3-carbinol on invasion and migration in human breast cancer cells. *Breast Cancer Research and Treatment 63* (2): 147–152.

Messina, M.J. and Wood, C.E. (2008). Soy isoflavones, estrogen therapy, and breast cancer risk: analysis and commentary. *Nutrition Journal 7* (1): 1–11. https://doi.org/10.1186/1475-2891-7-17.

Metzler, M., Pfeiffer, E., Schulz, S.I., and Dempe, J.S. (2012). Curcumin uptake and metabolism. *BioFactors 39* (1): 14–20. https://doi.org/10.1002/biof.1042.

Middha, P., Weinstein, S. J., Männistö, S., Albanes, D., & Mondul, A. M. (2019). β-Carotene supplementation and lung cancer incidence in the alpha-tocopherol, beta-carotene cancer prevention study: the role of tar and nicotine. *Nicotine & Tobacco Research, 21*(8), 1045–1050. doi:https://doi.org/10.1093/ntr/nty115

Min, Y.D., Choi, C.H., Bark, H. et al. (2007). Quercetin inhibits expression of inflammatory cytokines through attenuation of NF-κB and p38 MAPK in HMC-1 human mast cell line. *Inflammation Research 56* (5): 210–215. https://doi.org/10.1007/s00011-007-6172-9.

Misaka, S., Müller, F., and Fromm, M.F. (2013). Clinical relevance of drug efflux pumps in the gut. *Current Opinion in Pharmacology 13* (6): 847–852. https://doi.org/10.1016/j.coph.2013.08.010.

Mizushina, Y., Shiomi, K., Kuriyama, I. et al. (2013). Inhibitory effects of a major soy isoflavone, genistein, on human DNA topoisomerase II activity and cancer cell proliferation. *International Journal of Oncology 43* (4): 1117–1124. https://doi.org/10.3892/ijo.2013.2032.

Moelants, K.R.N., Lemmens, L., Vandebroeck, M. et al. (2012). Relation between particle size and carotenoid bioaccessibility in carrot- and tomato-derived suspensions. *Journal of Agricultural and Food Chemistry 60* (48): 11995–12003. https://doi.org/10.1021/jf303502h.

Monagas, M., Urpi-Sarda, M., Sánchez-Patán, F. et al. (2010). Insights into the metabolism and microbial biotransformation of dietary flavan-3-ols and the bioactivity of their metabolites. *Food & Function 1* (3): 233–253. https://doi.org/10.1039/c0fo00132e.

Monsuez, J.J., Charniot, J.C., Vignat, N., and Artigou, J.Y. (2010). Cardiac side-effects of cancer chemotherapy. *International Journal of Cardiology 144* (1): 3–15. https://doi.org/10.1016/j.ijcard.2010.03.003.

Na, H.K. and Surh, Y.J. (2008). Modulation of Nrf2-mediated antioxidant and detoxifying enzyme induction by the green tea polyphenol EGCG. *Food and Chemical Toxicology 46* (4): 1271–1278. https://doi.org/10.1016/j.fct.2007.10.006.

Nachshon-Kedmi, M., Yannai, S., and Fares, F.A. (2004). Induction of apoptosis in human prostate cancer cell line, PC3, by 3,3′-diindolylmethane through the mitochondrial pathway. *British Journal of Cancer 91* (7): 1358–1363. https://doi.org/10.1038/sj.bjc.6602145.

Nasri, H., Baradaran, A., Shirzad, H., and Rafieian-Kopaei, M. (2014). New concepts in nutraceuticals as alternative for pharmaceuticals. *International Journal of Preventive Medicine 5* (12): 1487–1499.

Niemeyer, E.D. and Brodbelt, J.S. (2007). Isomeric differentiation of green tea catechins using gas-phase hydrogen/deuterium exchange reactions. *Journal of the American Society for Mass Spectrometry 18* (10): 1749–1759. https://doi.org/10.1016/j.jasms.2007.07.009.

Nikhil, K., Sharan, S., Chakraborty, A., and Roy, P. (2014a). Pterostilbene-isothiocyanate conjugate suppresses growth of prostate cancer cells irrespective of androgen receptor status. *PLoS One 9* (4): https://doi.org/10.1371/journal.pone.0093335.

Nikhil, K., Sharan, S., Singh, A.K. et al. (2014b). Anticancer activities of pterostilbene-isothiocyanate conjugate in breast cancer cells: involvement of PPARγ. *PLoS One 9* (8): 1–17. https://doi.org/10.1371/journal.pone.0104592.

Nosrati, N., Bakovic, M., and Paliyath, G. (2017). Molecular mechanisms and pathways as targets for cancer prevention and progression with dietary compounds. *International Journal of Molecular Sciences 18* (10): 2050. https://doi.org/10.3390/ijms18102050.

Nussbaumer, S., Bonnabry, P., Veuthey, J.L., and Fleury-Souverain, S. (2011). Analysis of anticancer drugs: a review. *Talanta 85* (5): 2265–2289. https://doi.org/10.1016/j.talanta.2011.08.034.

Oda, Y., Hidaka, M., and Suzuki, A. (2017). Caffeine has a synergistic anticancer effect with cisplatin via inhibiting fanconi anemia group D2 protein monoubiquitination in hepatocellular carcinoma cells. *Biological and Pharmaceutical Bulletin 40* (11): 2005–2009. https://doi.org/10.1248/bpb.b17-00457.

Omenn, G.S., Goodman, G.E., Thornquist, M.D. et al. (1996). Effects of a combination of beta carotene and vitamin A on lung cancer and cardiovascular disease. *New England Journal of Medicine 334* (18): 1150–1155. https://doi.org/10.1056/NEJM199605023341802.

Ottaviani, J.I., Momma, T.Y., Heiss, C. et al. (2011). The stereochemical configuration of flavanols influences the level and metabolism of flavanols in humans and their biological activity in vivo. *Free Radical Biology and Medicine 50* (2): 237–244. https://doi.org/10.1016/j.freeradbiomed.2010.11.005.

Panieri, E., & Santoro, M. M. (2016). ROS homeostasis and metabolism: a dangerous liason in cancer cells. *Cell Death and Disease*, 7(6), e2253–e2253. doi:https://doi.org/10.1038/cddis.2016.105.

Parada, J. and Aguilera, J.M. (2007). Food microstructure affects the bioavailability of several nutrients. *Journal of Food Science 72* (2): 21–32. https://doi.org/10.1111/j.1750-3841.2007.00274.x.

Park, K.D., Lee, S.G., Kim, S.U. et al. (2004). Anticancer activity of 3-O-acyl and alkyl-(-)-epicatechin derivatives. *Bioorganic and Medicinal Chemistry Letters 14* (20): 5189–5192. https://doi.org/10.1016/j.bmcl.2004.07.063.

Park, Y., Leitzmann, M.F., Subar, A.F. et al. (2009). Dairy food, calcium, and risk of cancer in the NIH-AARP diet and health study. *Archives of Internal Medicine 169* (4): 391–401. https://doi.org/10.1001/archinternmed.2008.578.

Párrizas, M., Saltiel, A.R., and LeRoith, D. (1997). Insulin-like growth factor 1 inhibits apoptosis using the phosphatidylinositol 3'-kinase and mitogen-activated protein kinase pathways. *Journal of Biological Chemistry 272* (1): 154–161. https://doi.org/10.1074/jbc.272.1.154.

Pereyra-Vergara, F., Olivares-Corichi, I.M., Perez-Ruiz, A.G. et al. (2020). Apoptosis induced by (−)-epicatechin in human breast cancer cells is mediated by reactive oxygen species. *Molecules 25* (5): 1–13. https://doi.org/10.3390/molecules25051020.

Petri, N., Tannergren, C., Holst, B. et al. (2003). Absorption/metabolism of sulforaphane and quercetin, and regulation of phase II enzymes, in human jejunum in vivo. *Drug Metabolism and Disposition 31* (6): 805–813. https://doi.org/10.1124/dmd.31.6.805.

Phuah, N.H. and Nagoor, N.H. (2014). Regulation of microRNAs by natural agents: new strategies in cancer therapies. *BioMed Research International 2014*: 1–17.

Planas, J.M., Alfaras, I., Colom, H., and Juan, M.E. (2012). The bioavailability and distribution of trans-resveratrol are constrained by ABC transporters. *Archives of Biochemistry and Biophysics 527* (2): 67–73. https://doi.org/10.1016/j.abb.2012.06.004.

Pommier, Y. (2006). Topoisomerase I inhibitors: camptothecins and beyond. *Nature Reviews Cancer 6* (10): 789–802. https://doi.org/10.1038/nrc1977.

Porter, C.J.H., Wasan, K.M., and Constantinides, P. (2008). Lipid-based systems for the enhanced delivery of poorly water soluble drugs. *Advanced Drug Delivery Reviews 60* (6): 615–616. https://doi.org/10.1016/j.addr.2007.10.009.

Qin, S. and Hou, D.X. (2016). Multiple regulations of Keap1/Nrf2 system by dietary phytochemicals. *Molecular Nutrition & Food Research 60* (8): 1731–1755. https://doi.org/10.1002/mnfr.201501017.

Rahal, A., Kumar, A., Singh, V. et al. (2014). Oxidative stress, prooxidants, and antioxidants: the interplay. *BioMed Research International 2014*: 1–19.

Raina, K., Rajamanickam, S., Deep, G. et al. (2008). Chemopreventive effects of oral gallic acid feeding on tumor growth and progression in TRAMP mice. *Molecular Cancer Therapeutics 7* (5): 1258–1267. https://doi.org/10.1158/1535-7163.MCT-07-2220.

Rein, M.J., Renouf, M., Cruz-Hernandez, C. et al. (2013). Bioavailability of bioactive food compounds: a challenging journey to bioefficacy. *British Journal of Clinical Pharmacology 75* (3): 588–602. https://doi.org/10.1111/j.1365-2125.2012.04425.x.

Riddle, S.R., Ahmad, A., Ahmad, S. et al. (2000). Hypoxia induces hexokinase II gene expression in human lung cell line A549. *American Journal of Physiology. Lung Cellular and Molecular Physiology 278* (2): L407–L416.

Ronis, M.J., Gomez-acevedo, H., Blackburn, M.L. et al. (2016). Uterine responses to feeding soy protein isolate and treatment with 17 β -estradiol differ in ovariectomized female rats. *Toxicology and Applied Pharmacology 297*: 68–80. https://doi.org/10.1016/j.taap.2016.02.019.

Ronis, M.J.J., Pedersen, K.B., and Watt, J. (2018). Adverse effects of nutraceuticals and dietary supplements. *Annual Review of Pharmacology and Toxicology 58* (1): 583–601. https://doi.org/10.1146/annurev-pharmtox-010617-052844.

Russo, G.L. (2007). Ins and outs of dietary phytochemicals in cancer chemoprevention. *Biochemical Pharmacology 74* (4): 533–544. https://doi.org/10.1016/j.bcp.2007.02.014.

Rysman, E., Brusselmans, K., Scheys, K. et al. (2010). De novo lipogenesis protects cancer cells from free radicals and chemotherapeutics by promoting membrane lipid saturation. *Cancer Research 70* (20): 8117–8126. https://doi.org/10.1158/0008-5472.CAN-09-3871.

Saini, S., Arora, S., Majid, S. et al. (2011). Curcumin modulates microRNA-203-mediated regulation of the Src-Akt axis in bladder cancer. *Cancer Prevention Research 4* (10): 1698–1709. https://doi.org/10.1158/1940-6207.CAPR-11-0267.

Salami, A., Seydi, E., and Pourahmad, J. (2013). Use of nutraceuticals for prevention and treatment of cancer. *Iranian Journal of Pharmaceutical Research 12* (3): 219–220. https://doi.org/10.22037/ijpr.2013.1371.

Saldanha, S.N. and Tollefsbol, T.O. (2012). The role of nutraceuticals in chemoprevention and chemotherapy and their clinical outcomes. *Journal of Oncology 2012*: https://doi.org/10.1155/2012/192464.

Salti, G.I., Grewal, S., Mehta, R.R. et al. (2000). Genistein induces apoptosis and topoisomerase II-mediated DNA breakage in colon cancer cells. *European Journal of Cancer 36* (6): 796–802.

Samanta, S.K., Bhattacharya, K., Mandal, C., and Pal, B.C. (2010). Identification and quantification of the active component quercetin 3-O-rutinoside from Barringtonia racemosa, targets mitochondrial apoptotic pathway in acute lymphoblastic leukemia. *Journal of Asian Natural Products Research 12* (8): 639–648. https://doi.org/10.1080/10286020.2010.489040.

Samarghandian, S., Nezhad, M., and Mohammadi, G. (2014). Role of caspases, bax and Bcl-2 in chrysin-induced apoptosis in the A549 human lung adenocarcinoma epithelial cells. *Anti-Cancer Agents in Medicinal Chemistry 14* (6): 901–909. https://doi.org/10.2174/1871520614666614 0209144042.

Sang, S., Lee, M.J., Hou, Z. et al. (2005). Stability of tea polyphenol (-)-epigallocatechin-3-gallate and formation of dimers and epimers under common experimental conditions. *Journal of Agricultural and Food Chemistry 53* (24): 9478–9484. https://doi.org/10.1021/jf0519055.

Sanjoaquin, M.A., Allen, N., Couto, E. et al. (2005). Folate intake and colorectal cancer risk: a meta-analytical approach. *International Journal of Cancer 113* (5): 825–828. https://doi.org/10.1002/ijc.20648.

Saw, C.L.L., Yang, A.Y., Cheng, D.C. et al. (2012). Pharmacodynamics of ginsenosides: antioxidant activities, activation of Nrf2, and potential synergistic effects of combinations. *Chemical Research in Toxicology* 25 (8): 1574–1580. https://doi.org/10.1021/tx2005025.

Schug, Z.T., Peck, B., Jones, D.T. et al. (2015). Acetyl-CoA synthetase 2 promotes acetate utilization and maintains cancer cell growth under metabolic stress. *Cancer Cell* 27 (1): 57–71. https://doi.org/10.1016/j.ccell.2014.12.002.

Seki, T., Harada, S., Hosoya, O. et al. (2008). Evaluation of the establishment of a tight junction in caco-2 cell monolayers using a pore permeation model involving two different sizes. *Biological and Pharmaceutical Bulletin* 31 (1): 163–166. https://doi.org/10.1248/bpb.31.163.

Selhub, J. and Rosenberg, I.H. (1996). Folic acid. In: *Present Knowledge in Nutrition* (ed. E.E. Ziegler and L.J. Filer), 206–219. Washington, DC: 7th International Life Sciences Institute Press.

Semenza, G.L. (2010). HIF-1: upstream and downstream of cancer metabolism. *Current Opinion in Genetics and Development* 20 (1): 51–56. https://doi.org/10.1016/j.gde.2009.10.009.

Shankar, E., Kanwal, R., Candamo, M., and Gupta, S. (2016). Dietary phytochemicals as epigenetic modifiers in cancer: promise and challenges. *Seminars in Cancer Biology* https://doi.org/10.1016/j.semcancer.2016.04.002.

Shao, Z.M., Shen, Z.Z., Liu, C.H. et al. (2002). Curcumin exerts multiple suppressive effects on human breast carcinoma cells. *International Journal of Cancer* 98 (2): 234–240. https://doi.org/10.1002/ijc.10183.

Sharma, R. (2009). Nutraceuticals and nutraceutical supplementation criteria in cancer: a literature survey. *The Open Nutraceuticals Journal* 2 (1).

Shiomi, K., Kuriyama, I., Yoshida, H., and Mizushina, Y. (2013). Inhibitory effects of myricetin on mammalian DNA polymerase, topoisomerase and human cancer cell proliferation. *Food Chemistry* 139 (1–4): 910–918. https://doi.org/10.1016/j.foodchem.2013.01.009.

Shishodia, S., Majumdar, S., Banerjee, S., and Aggarwal, B.B. (2003). Ursolic acid inhibits nuclear factor-κB activation induced by carcinogenic agents through suppression of IκBα kinase and p65 phosphorylation: correlation with down-regulation of cyclooxygenase 2, matrix metalloproteinase 9, and cyclin D1. *Cancer Research* 63 (15): 4375–4383.

Shishodia, S., Amin, H.M., Lai, R., and Aggarwal, B.B. (2005). Curcumin (diferuloylmethane) inhibits constitutive NF-κB activation, induces G1/S arrest, suppresses proliferation, and induces apoptosis in mantle cell lymphoma. *Biochemical Pharmacology* 70 (5): 700–713. https://doi.org/10.1016/j.bcp.2005.04.043.

Siles, L., Cela, J., and Munné-bosch, S. (2013). Phytochemistry Vitamin E analyses in seeds reveal a dominant presence of tocotrienols over tocopherols in the Arecaceae family. *Phytochemistry* 95: 207–214. https://doi.org/10.1016/j.phytochem.2013.07.008.

Singh, A. and Settleman, J. (2010). EMT, cancer stem cells and drug resistance: an emerging axis of evil in the war on cancer. *Oncogene* 29 (34): 4741–4751. https://doi.org/10.1038/onc.2010.215.

Singh, S.V., Warin, R., Xiao, D. et al. (2009). Sulforaphane inhibits prostate carcinogenesis and pulmonary metastasis in TRAMP mice in association with increased cytotoxicity of natural killer cells. *Cancer Research* 69 (5): 2117–2125. https://doi.org/10.1158/0008-5472.CAN-08-3502.

Sita, G., Hrelia, P., Graziosi, A., and Morroni, F. (2018). Sulforaphane from cruciferous vegetables: recent advances to improve glioblastoma treatment. *Nutrients* 10 (11): 1755. https://doi.org/10.3390/nu10111755.

Slatore, C.G., Littman, A.J., Au, D.H. et al. (2008). Long-term use of supplemental multivitamins, vitamin C, vitamin E, and folate does not reduce the risk of lung cancer. *American Journal of Respiratory and Critical Care Medicine* 177 (5): 524–530. https://doi.org/10.1164/rccm.200709-1398OC.

Snyder, R.D. and Arnone, M.R. (2002). Putative identification of functional interactions between DNA intercalating agents and topoisomerase II using the V79 in vitro micronucleus assay. *Mutation Research, Fundamental and Molecular Mechanisms of Mutagenesis 503* (1-2): 21–35.

Soerjomataram, I., Oomen, D., Lemmens, V. et al. (2010). Increased consumption of fruit and vegetables and future cancer incidence in selected European countries. *European Journal of Cancer 46* (14): 2563–2580. https://doi.org/10.1016/j.ejca.2010.07.026.

Solaini, G., Landi, L., Pasquali, P., and Rossi, C.A. (1987). Protective effect of endogenous coenzyme Q on both lipid peroxidation and respiratory chain inactivation induced by an adriamycin-iron complex. *Biochemical and Biophysical Research Communications 147* (2): 572–580.

Sood, M.M. and Sood, A.R. (2007). Dietary vitamin D and decreases in cancer rates: Canada as the national experiment. *The American Journal of Clinical Nutrition 86* (5): 1549–1549.

Stepien, M., Chajes, V., and Romieu, I. (2016). The role of diet in cancer: the epidemiologic link. *Salud Pública de México 58*: 261–273.

Stevenson, D.E., Scheepens, A., and Hurst, R.D. (2011). Bioavailability and metabolism of dietary flavonoids – much known – much more to discover. *Nutrition and Diet Research: Appetite and Weight Loss 16* (3): 49–100.

Strogantsev, R. and Ferguson-Smith, A.C. (2012). Proteins involved in establishment and maintenance of imprinted methylation marks. *Briefings in Functional Genomics 11* (3): 227–239. https://doi.org/10.1093/bfgp/els018.

Sun, L.P., Chen, A.L., Hung, H.C. et al. (2012). Chrysin: a histone deacetylase 8 inhibitor with anticancer activity and a suitable candidate for the standardization of chinese propolis. *Journal of Agricultural and Food Chemistry 60* (47): 11748–11758. https://doi.org/10.1021/jf303261r.

Sun, H., Zhang, T., Liu, R. et al. (2020). Resveratrol inhibition of renal cancer stem cell characteristics and modulation of the Sonic Hedgehog pathway. *Nutrition and Cancer* 1–11. https://doi.org/10.1080/01635581.2020.1784966.

Surh, Y.J., Chun, K.S., Cha, H.H. et al. (2001). Molecular mechanisms underlying chemopreventive activities of anti-inflammatory phytochemicals: down-regulation of COX-2 and iNOS through suppression of NF-κB activation. *Mutation Research, Fundamental and Molecular Mechanisms of Mutagenesis 480–481*: 243–268. https://doi.org/10.1016/S0027-5107(01)00183-X.

Suzuki, K., Yahara, S., Hashimoto, F., and Uyeda, M. (2001). Inhibitory activities of (-)-epigallocatechin-3-O-gallate against topoisomerases I and II. *Biological and Pharmaceutical Bulletin 24* (9): 1088–1090. https://doi.org/10.1248/bpb.24.1088.

Talalay, P. and Fahey, J.W. (2001). Phytochemicals from cruciferous plants protect against cancer by modulating carcinogen metabolism. *The Journal of Nutrition 131* (11): 3027S–3033S.

Thomasset, S.C., Berry, D.P., Garcea, G. et al. (2007). Dietary polyphenolic phytochemicals – promising cancer chemopreventive agents in humans? A review of their clinical properties. *International Journal of Cancer 120* (3): 451–458. https://doi.org/10.1002/ijc.22419.

Tosetti, F., Ferrari, N., De Flora, S., and Albini, A. (2002). 'Angioprevention': angiogenesis is a common and key target for cancer chemopreventive agents. *The FASEB Journal 16* (1): 2–14. https://doi.org/10.1096/fj.01-0300rev.

Tosetti, F., Noonan, D.M., and Albini, A. (2009). Metabolic regulation and redox activity as mechanisms for angioprevention by dietary phytochemicals. *International Journal of Cancer 125* (9): 1997–2003. https://doi.org/10.1002/ijc.24677.

Tripathi B. Yamini, T. P. and A. H. B. (2005). Nutraceutical and cancer management. *Frontiers in Bioscience, 10*, 1607–1618. doi:https://doi.org/10.1016/s0741-5214(05)00111-4

Tsao, R. (2010). Chemistry and biochemistry of dietary polyphenols. *Nutrients 2* (12): 1231–1246. https://doi.org/10.3390/nu2121231.

Tso, P., Nauli, A., and Lo, C.M. (2004). Enterocyte fatty acid uptake and intestinal fatty acid-binding protein. *Biochemical Society Transactions 32* (1): 75–78. https://doi.org/10.1042/BST0320075.

Tsutsumi, K., Li, S.K., Hymas, R.V. et al. (2008). Systematic studies on the paracellular permeation of model permeants and oligonucleotides in the rat small intestine with chenodeoxycholate as enhancer. *Journal of Pharmaceutical Sciences 97* (1): 350–367. https://doi.org/10.1002/jps.21093.

Turati, F., Rossi, M., Pelucchi, C. et al. (2015). Fruit and vegetables and cancer risk: a review of southern European studies. *British Journal of Nutrition 113* (S2): S102–S110. https://doi.org/10.1017/S0007114515000148.

Vardi, A., Bosviel, R., Rabiau, N. et al. (2010). Soy phytoestrogens modify DNA methylation of GSTP1, RASSF1A, EPH2 and BRCA1 promoter in prostate cancer cells. *Vivo 24* (4): 393–400.

Vasudevan, A., Yu, Y., Banerjee, S. et al. (2014). Omega-3 fatty acid is a potential preventive agent for recurrent colon cancer. *Cancer Prevention Research 7* (11): 1138–1148. https://doi.org/10.1158/1940-6207.CAPR-14-0177.

Vega, F.M. and Ridley, A.J. (2008). Rho GTPases in cancer cell biology. *FEBS Letters 582* (14): 2093–2101. https://doi.org/10.1016/j.febslet.2008.04.039.

Walle, T., Wen, X., and Walle, U.K. (2007). Improving metabolic stability of cancer chemoprotective polyphenols. *Expert Opinion on Drug Metabolism & Toxicology 3* (3): 379–388.

Walsh, K.R., Zhang, Y.C., Vodovotz, Y. et al. (2003). Stability and bioaccessibility of isoflavones from soy bread during in vitro digestion. *Journal of Agricultural and Food Chemistry 51* (16): 4603–4609. https://doi.org/10.1021/jf0342627.

Wang, X.F., Wu, D.M., Li, B.X. et al. (2009). Synergistic inhibitory effect of sulforaphane and 5-fluorouracil in high and low metastasis cell lines of salivary gland adenoid cystic carcinoma. *Phytotherapy Research: An International Journal Devoted to Pharmacological and Toxicological Evaluation of Natural Product Derivatives 23* (3): 303–307. https://doi.org/10.1002/ptr.

Warburg, O. (1925). The metabolism of carcinoma cells 1. *The Journal of Cancer Research 9* (1): 148–163. https://doi.org/10.1158/jcr.1925.148.

WHO health topic for cancer (2020). https://www.who.int/health-topics/cancer#tab=tab_1 (accessed 30 June 2020).

Wiczk, A., Hofman, D., Konopa, G., and Herman-Antosiewicz, A. (2012). Sulforaphane, a cruciferous vegetable-derived isothiocyanate, inhibits protein synthesis in human prostate cancer cells. *Biochimica et Biophysica Acta-Molecular Cell Research 1823* (8): 1295–1305. https://doi.org/10.1016/j.bbamcr.2012.05.020.

Williams, C.D., Satia, J.A., Adair, L.S. et al. (2010). Associations of red meat, fat, and protein intake with distal colorectal cancer risk. *Nutrition and Cancer 62* (6): 701–709. https://doi.org/10.1080/01635581003605938.

Wilson, M.M., Weinberg, R.A., Lees, J.A., and Guen, V.J. (2020). Emerging mechanisms by which EMT programs control stemness. *Trends in Cancer* 1–6. https://doi.org/10.1016/j.trecan.2020.03.011.

Wiseman, M. (2008). The second world cancer research fund/american institute for cancer research expert report. food, nutrition, physical activity, and the prevention of cancer: a global perspective. *Proceedings of the Nutrition Society 67* (3): 253–256. https://doi.org/10.1017/S002966510800712X.

Woo, H.M., Kang, J.H., Kawada, T. et al. (2007). Active spice-derived components can inhibit inflammatory responses of adipose tissue in obesity by suppressing inflammatory actions of macrophages and release of monocyte chemoattractant protein-1 from adipocytes. *Life Sciences 80* (10): 926–931. https://doi.org/10.1016/j.lfs.2006.11.030.

World Cancer Research Fund, & American Institute for Cancer Research (2007). *Food, Nutrition, Physical Activity, and the Prevention of Cancer: A Global Perspective*, vol. 1. American Institute for Cancer Research.

Wu, B., Yao, X., Nie, X., and Xu, R. (2013). Epigenetic reactivation of RANK in glioblastoma cells by curcumin: involvement of STAT3 inhibition. *DNA and Cell Biology 32* (6): 292–297. https://doi.org/10.1089/dna.2013.2042.

Wu, C., Yang, M., and Wang, C. (2019). Quercetin-3-O-glucuronide inhibits doxorubicin resistance by reducing endoplasmic reticulum stress in hepatocellular carcinoma cells. *Journal of Functional Foods 54* (110): 301–309. https://doi.org/10.1016/j.jff.2019.01.015.

Xu, G., Chen, J., Wang, G. et al. (2020). Resveratrol inhibits the tumorigenesis of follicular thyroid cancer via ST6GAL2-regulated activation of the hippo signaling pathway. *Molecular Therapy: Oncolytics 16* (March): 124–133. https://doi.org/10.1016/j.omto.2019.12.010.

Yang, C.S. and Wang, H. (2011). Mechanistic issues concerning cancer prevention by tea catechins. *Molecular Nutrition & Food Research 55* (6): 819–831. https://doi.org/10.1002/mnfr.201100036.

Yang, C.S., Wang, X., Lu, G., and Picinich, S.C. (2009a). Cancer prevention by tea: animal studies, molecular mechanisms and human relevance. *Nature Reviews Cancer 9* (6): 429–439. https://doi.org/10.1038/nrc2641.

Yang, Q., Bostick, R.M., Friedman, J.M., and Flanders, W.D. (2009b). Serum folate and cancer mortality among U.S. adults: findings from the third national health and nutritional examination survey linked mortality file. *Cancer Epidemiology, Biomarkers and Prevention 18* (5): 1439–1447. https://doi.org/10.1158/1055-9965.EPI-08-0908.

Yang, S., Zhang, H., Yang, X. et al. (2015). Evaluation of antioxidative and antitumor activities of extracted flavonoids from Pink Lady apples in human colon and breast cancer cell lines. *Food & Function 6* (12): 3789–3798. https://doi.org/10.1039/c5fo00570a.

Yang, B., Zhang, W., Zhang, M. et al. (2020). KRT6A promotes EMT and cancer stem cell transformation in lung adenocarcinoma. *Technology in Cancer Research & Treatment 19* (Iii): 1–8. https://doi.org/10.1177/1533033820921248.

Yao, M., Xie, C., Constantine, M. et al. (2012). How can food extracts consumed in the Mediterranean and East Asia suppress prostate cancer proliferation? *British Journal of Nutrition 108* (3): 424–430. https://doi.org/10.1017/S0007114511005770.

Yin, L., Zhang, R., Hu, Y. et al. (2020). Gastric-cancer-derived mesenchymal stem cells: a promising target for resveratrol in the suppression of gastric cancer metastasis. *Human Cell 33* (3): 652–662. https://doi.org/10.1007/s13577-020-00339-5.

Yu, W., Simmons-Menchaca, M., Gapor, A. et al. (1999). Induction of apoptosis in human breast cancer cells by tocopherols and tocotrienols. *Nutrition and Cancer 33* (1): 26–32. https://doi.org/10.1080/01635589909514744.

Yu, J., Peng, Y., Wu, L.C. et al. (2013). Curcumin down-regulates DNA methyltransferase 1 and plays an anti-leukemic role in acute myeloid leukemia. *PLoS One 8* (2): e55934. https://doi.org/10.1371/journal.pone.0055934.

Zamani, M., Sadeghizadeh, M., Behmanesh, M., and Najafi, F. (2015). Dendrosomal curcumin increases expression of the long non-coding RNA gene MEG3 via up-regulation of epi-miRs in hepatocellular cancer. *Phytomedicine 22* (10): 961–967. https://doi.org/10.1016/j.phymed.2015.05.071.

Zhai, Y.J., Cheng, F., Wang, T.M. et al. (2011). in vitro anticancer activity of taxifolin on human cervical cancer Hela cells and its mechanism. *Chinese Traditional Patent Medicine 12*.

Zhang, S. M., Cook, N. R., Albert, C. M., Gaziano, J. M., Buring, J. E., & Manson, J. E. (2008). Effect of combined folic acid, vitamin B6, and vitamin B12 on cancer risk in women: a randomized trial. *JAMA*, 300(17), 2012–2021. Doi:https://doi.org/10.1001/jama.2008.555.

Zhang, Z.R., Al Zaharna, M., Wong, M.M. et al. (2013). Taxifolin enhances andrographolide-induced mitotic arrest and apoptosis in human prostate cancer cells via spindle assembly checkpoint activation. *PLoS One 8* (1): https://doi.org/10.1371/journal.pone.0054577.

Zhang, Y.J., Gan, R.Y., Li, S. et al. (2015). Antioxidant phytochemicals for the prevention and treatment of chronic diseases. *Molecules 20* (12): 21138–21156. https://doi.org/10.3390/molecules201219753.

Zhang, W.L., Zhao, Y.N., Shi, Z.Z. et al. (2018). Lutein inhibits cell growth and activates apoptosis via the PI3K/AKT/mTOR signaling pathway in A549 human non-small-cell lung cancer cells. *Journal of Environmental Pathology, Toxicology and Oncology 37* (4): https://10.1615/JEnvironPatholToxicolOncol.2018027418.

Zhang, X., Zhang, C., Ren, Z. et al. (2020). Curcumin affects gastric cancer cell migration, invasion and cytoskeletal remodeling through gli1-β-catenin. *Cancer Management and Research 12*: 3795–3806.

Zhao, W., Zhou, X., Qi, G., and Guo, Y. (2018). Curcumin suppressed the prostate cancer by inhibiting JNK pathways via epigenetic regulation. *Journal of Biochemical and Molecular Toxicology 32* (5): e22049. https://doi.org/10.1002/jbt.22049.

Zheng, J., Zhou, Y., Li, Y. et al. (2016). Spices for prevention and treatment of cancers. *Nutrients 8* (8): https://doi.org/10.3390/nu8080495.

Zhou, H.B., Chen, J.M., Cai, J.T. et al. (2008). Anticancer activity of genistein on implanted tumor of human SG7901 cells in nude mice. *World Journal of Gastroenterology: WJG 14* (4): 627.

Zhuo, H., Tang, J., Lin, Z. et al. (2016). The aberrant expression of MEG3 regulated by UHRF1 predicts the prognosis of hepatocellular carcinoma. *Molecular Carcinogenesis 55* (2): 209–219. https://doi.org/10.1002/mc.22270.

Zu, K. and Ip, C. (2003). Synergy between selenium and vitamin E in apoptosis induction is associated with activation of distinctive initiator caspases in human prostate cancer cells. *Cancer Research 63* (20): 6988–6995.

Zunino, F., Pratesi, G., Micheloni, A. et al. (1989). Protective effect of reduced glutathione against cisplatin-induced renal and systemic toxicity and its influence on the therapeutic activity of the antitumor drug. *Chemico-Biological Interactions 70* (1–2): 89–101. https://doi.org/10.1016/0009-2797(89)90065-3.

3

Pro-Angiogenic and Anti-Angiogenic Effects of Phytochemicals as Nutraceuticals

Viney Kumar[1], Souvik Ghosh[1,2], Saakshi Saini[1], Himanshu Agrawal[1], Deo Paranav Milind[1], Debabrata Sircar[3], and Partha Roy[1]

[1] *Molecular Endocrinology Laboratory, Department of Biotechnology, Indian Institute of Technology Roorkee, Roorkee, Uttarakhand, India*
[2] *Tissue Engineering Laboratory, Centre of Nanotechnology, Indian Institute of Technology Roorkee, Roorkee, Uttarakhand, India*
[3] *Plant Molecular Biology Laboratory, Department of Biotechnology, Indian Institute of Technology Roorkee, Roorkee, Uttarakhand, India*

3.1 Introduction

The circulatory system, also known as cardiovascular system, comprising the blood vessels and the heart is responsible for the transportation of nutrients, oxygen, carbon dioxide, hormones, and blood cells to provide nourishment and help fight diseases. It is also responsible for stabilizing temperature and pH and maintaining homeostasis. The blood vessels form a network within the body. Unless it is a severe damage caused to this network, as it happens in case of third-degree burns, localized damages heal by regeneration of blood vessels from the surrounding cells. This process is called angiogenesis. Although angiogenesis is important to the body, if it gets uncontrolled, it can cause many diseases. Angiogenesis is a highly regulated process, the smooth execution of which is dependent on many factors and signaling pathways. Disturbances in the levels of these factors or the signaling pathways can lead to severe consequences, such as metastatic cancer. The equilibrium between the pro- (when blood vessels are formed) and anti- (when formation of blood vessels is prevented) angiogenic processes is crucial for normal functioning of the body. However, under abnormal conditions, this healthy balance is disturbed, consequently, leading to various disease conditions. Treatments currently used to restore this balance are associated with undesirable side effects. Nutraceuticals, food with medicinal benefits, are being actively explored as an alternative to the existing treatments for restoring the angiogenic homeostasis (Souyoul et al. 2018). The key focus of this chapter will be on these nutraceuticals and the mechanism through which they are capable of maintaining angiogenic homeostasis. But, prior to that, it is pertinent to have a recapitulation of the angiogenic process as a whole and the steps involved in it, which is the topic discussed in the next section.

3.1.1 Origin and Key Steps in the Process of Angiogenesis

Angiogenesis is a multifaceted process of formation of new blood vessels from preexisting ones, thus making it indispensable for wound healing, tissue regeneration and bone growth processes, and tissue engineering (Augustine et al. 2019). First ever insight into angiogenic process was studied by Dr. John Hunter (a Scottish surgeon and anatomist) in 1794 (Folkman 2006).

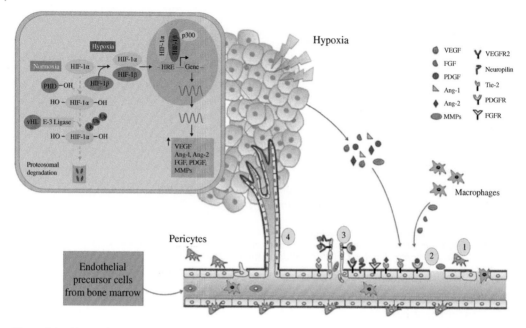

Figure 3.1 Mechanism involved in the progression of angiogenesis. *Source:* Rajasekar et al. (2019). Reproduced with permission of Elsevier.

The steps involved in angiogenesis are mentioned below (see Figure 3.1) (Rajasekar et al. 2019).

1) Pericyte dissociation promoted by vascular endothelial growth factor (VEGF) and angiopoietin-2 (ang-2).
2) Degradation of basement membrane assisted by matrix metalloproteinases (MMPs).
3) Migration of endothelial cells.
4) Blood vessel sprouting mediated by endothelial cell differentiation.

In 1971, Judah Folkman hypothesized the concept of angiogenic switch, which involves ensuing imbalance between anti-angiogenic (inhibitory factors) and pro-angiogenic factors, which in turn

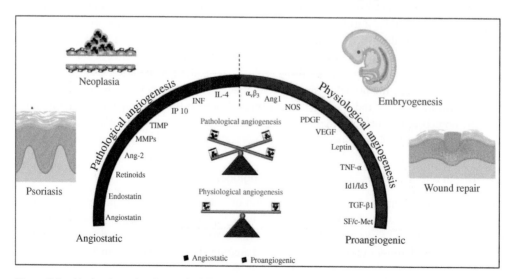

Figure 3.2 Mechanism of action underlying the regulation of pathological and physiological angiogenesis in response to changes in the anti-angiogenic and pro-angiogenic balance of the tissue.

could lead to tumor growth (Folkman 1971). The altered balance between the anti-angiogenic and pro-angiogenic factors during tumor progression is depicted in Figure 3.2.

3.1.2 Types of Angiogenesis

Two types of angiogenesis occur in almost all organs and tissues of both adults and in utero: these are intussusceptive angiogenesis, first described by Burri and Tarek (1990), and sprouting angiogenesis, described nearly 200 years earlier (see Figure 3.3).

Sprouting angiogenesis occurs in the tissues devoid of blood to reestablish the blood supply. New blood vessels originate as sprouts and grow further into mature vessels through stimulation from vascular endothelial growth factor type A (VEGF-A). In intussusceptive angiogenesis, existing blood vessels get interrupted and split apart to form transvascular pillars of tissue (Aldair and Montani 2010). Under normal circumstances, angiogenesis is the outcome of a fine balance between the angiogenic and the inhibitory factors. Dys-homeostasis in this process is responsible for various disease conditions, which are discussed in detail in the following section.

Overall, this chapter will be comprehensively focusing on understanding the angiomodulatory potentials of nutraceuticals, especially phytochemicals and their targeted pathways, through which angiogenic homeostasis is maintained. A separate section on *in vitro* and *in vivo* experimental techniques used to study angiogenesis is also included at the end of this chapter to provide an idea on the methodologies used to generate the current knowledge base on angiogenic process.

3.2 Angiogenesis in Health and Diseases

3.2.1 Angiogenesis in Normal Physiology

Under normal physiological conditions, blood vessel development involves vasculogenesis and angiogenesis. Through vasculogenesis, primary plexus develops during embryonic development by vasculature arising from angioblast, the precursor of endothelial cells. Primary plexus is then remodeled through angiogenesis. The primary difference between vasculogenesis and angiogenesis is that blood vessels arise from existing ones, in case of latter while they develop from angioblast *de novo* in case of former (Papetti and Herman 2002). One of the most crucial role of angiogenesis in normal physiology is the development of cardiovascular system during embryonic development (Carmeliet 2005). In general, formation of new blood vessels stops after birth, except for few established adulthood processes that require regular and controlled involvement of angiogenesis. One

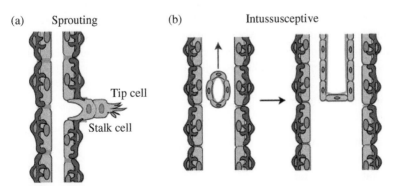

(a) Sprouting   (b) Intussusceptive

Tip cell

Stalk cell

Figure 3.3 Diagrammatic representation of angiogenesis types. *Source:* Lugano et al. (2019). Under Creatives Common (CCBY) License.

such processes is the menstrual cycle during which the highly vascularized endometrial wall sheds at a regular period and gets rebuilt through extensive angiogenesis for the next cycle (Smith 2001; Folkman 2006). Angiogenesis is required for wound healing when it occurs after birth and later in life. Scarring is a regular step in wound healing wherein collagen deposition occurs in the ensuing granulation tissue formation on the wound bed and comes off with the existing intricate network of blood vessels only to be replaced by the fresh ones through controlled angiogenesis (Tonnesen et al. 2000). Another rare type is compensatory angiogenesis observed in diseases that tend to create a heavy functional burden on the vasculature, such as cardiac failure where reperfusion is required to improve the condition (Carmeliet 2003).

Thus, under normal physiological conditions angiogenesis, though indispensable for some biological processes, is tightly regulated. In fact, certain natural inhibitors are involved in preventing neovascularization to ensure surveillance over unwanted sprouting of blood vessels. All these observations suggest the existence of a dynamic equilibrium between inhibitors and stimulators (growth factors) of angiogenesis. This implies the significance of the process and importance of keeping it under control (Folkman and Shing 1992).

3.2.2 Angiogenesis in Diseases

Uncontrolled angiogenesis has been associated with several inflammatory diseases (Carmeliet 2003). The balance between angiogenic stimulators and inhibitors that exist in normal conditions skews toward stimulators during disease pathogenesis in multiple sclerosis, cancer, obesity, warts, vascular malformations, psoriasis, allergic dermatitis, primary pulmonary hypertension (PPH), diabetic retinopathy, Kaposi's sarcoma in AIDS, asthma, inflammatory bowel disease, cystic fibrosis, liver cirrhosis, uterine bleeding, endometriosis, arthritis, ovarian cysts, diabetic nephropathy, osteomyelitis, periodontal disease, etc. (Carmeliet 2005). Among these diseases, this chapter has focused on cancer, arthritis, obesity, PPH, psoriasis, and ocular diseases due to their high occurrence rate in humans. Remarkably, angiogenesis inhibition therapy can be an option to treat these disorders.

3.2.2.1 Angiogenesis in Cancer

Tumor growth and metastasis depend wholly on angiogenesis as well as lymphogenesis. From tumor cells chemical signals are produced in a rapid growth phase to trigger angiogenesis (Folkman 1971). In a preliminary study, behavior of cancer cells with respect to angiogenesis was scrutinized. For this, the cancer cells were injected in two regions: one traversed with blood circulation (toward iris) and another devoid of circulation (toward anterior chamber). The tumor grew $1-2\,mm^3$ in diameter where blood circulation was absent but on the contrary tumor grew beyond $2\,mm^3$ in diameter where blood circulation was present, thus confirming the fact that angiogenesis positively regulates tumor growth (Muthukkaruppan et al. 1982). Without angiogenesis, the tumor became necrotic or apoptotic after certain growth (Holmgren et al. 1995; Parangi et al. 1996), which precisely demonstrated that angiogenesis plays a pivotal role in cancer progression.

The process of angiogenesis is executed by four distinct steps.

The steps are as follows:

1) Local injury of tissue basement membrane and creation of hypoxic condition.
2) Angiogenic factors propagate to activate the endothelial cells.
3) Endothelial cells proliferate and get stabilized.
4) Angiogenic factors influence the process of angiogenesis.

The purpose of angiogenesis is to provide required nutrients and oxygen to the tumor for its survival. Angiogenesis in disease condition depends not only on the over-activation of the activator but also inactivation of their respective inhibitors (Dameron et al. 1994). In angiogenesis, more than 12 activator proteins (APs), i.e. VEGF; angiogenin; tumor necrosis factor-α (TNF-α); basic fibroblast growth factor (bFGF); platelet-derived endothelial growth factor (PDEGF); transforming growth factor (TGF)-α, β; granulocyte colony-stimulating factor (GCSF); hepatocyte growth factor (HGF); placental growth factor (PlGF); epidermal growth factor (EGF); fibroblast growth factor (FGF); and interleukin-8 (IL-8), are involved. Among all these proteins VEGF family and VEGFR acquire maximum attention among researchers working on neoplastic vascularization. A crucial role is played by VEGF in normal and neoplastic tissues as an angiogenesis-promoting protein. In cancerous tissue and the adjacent stroma, neovascularization is mainly regulated by this protein, under the influence of certain growth factors and cytokines (Folkman 1990, 1995a, b). In cancerous tissues, angiogenesis commences when the size of the tumor increases and existing capillaries fail to support the growing tumor. Increasing size of the tumor causes hypoxia, thus inducing the expression of VEGF and its receptor through hypoxia-inducible factor-1α (HIF-1α) (Bottaro and Liotta 2003). By producing VEGF, tumor cells feed on the new blood vessels and subsequently secrete it into the surrounding tissue. The cancer cells, followed by the cross talk with endothelial cells, secrete VEGF which then binds to its receptor present on the membrane of endothelial cells. After the receptor–ligand interaction the relay proteins get activated and that in turn transmits signal to nucleus of endothelial cells. This activates several genes to translate into proteins required for new endothelial cell growth. Following this, endothelial cells secrete MMPs, which snap the extracellular matrix (ECM), allowing endothelial cells to propagate. The endothelial cells start dividing while migrating to surrounding tissues. Soon after, by virtue of adhesion factors, i.e. α/β integrins, they form hollow tubes which eventually grow into an extensive mesh of matured blood vessels (Mizejewski 1999; Nelson et al. 2017). Angiotensin-1,2 and their receptor Tie-2 direct and stabilize the growth of the newly formed vascular tissues (Suri et al. 1996; Maisonpierre et al. 1997; Tournaire et al. 2004), thereby ensuring their maturation.

3.2.2.2 Angiogenesis in Obesity

Almost one billion adults worldwide are overweight and major chronic diseases are associated with obesity. Obesity is mainly caused due to the over-intake of calorie-dense diets and sedentary lifestyle. Implementing behavioral modifications in lifestyle for promoting weight loss, involving a healthy diet and physical activity, is considered to be a paramount clinical challenge that still remains a difficult goal to achieve. Likewise, the safety and potential complexities in long run, concerned with caloric restriction via bariatric surgery, remains a debatable issue. A novel pathway for expansion of adipose tissue during obesity was explained by Cutchins et al. (2012). In their study, inhibitor of differentiation-3 (Id3) was found to be overexpressed in adipose tissue during obesity (Cutchins et al. 2012). The deletion of Id3 was found to prevent the expansion of adipose tissue during obesity in mice. It was thus speculated that Id3 is primarily a rate limiting protein needed for mass accumulation of adipose tissue in obesity that is induced by diet. Increasing adipose tissue also requires angiogenesis like other tissues. For the expansion of the adipose tissue during increased caloric intake, angiogenesis is required. Cutchins et al. established a link between diet-induced adipose tissue and angiogenesis prevention in Id3 gene deleted mice. It was observed that in Id3 deleted mice, microvascular blood volume is decreased. In the study, an explicit mechanism of Id3-directed angiogenesis was established. Obesity-linked expansion of adipose tissue causes tissue hypoxia (Kabon et al. 2004). Hypoxic condition induces the expressions of VEGF in adipocytes (Claffey et al. 1992; Zhang et al. 1997), which in turn induces angiogenesis. Inhibition of VEGF attenuates the expansion of adipose tissue in diet-induced obesity (Tam et al. 2009). Cutchins et al. reported that VEGF secretion was inhibited in diet-induced obesity in Id3-deficient mice. In this context, Id3 is perceived to be repressing transcriptional activity of VEGF by virtue of E-protein-E12 and thereby regulating the expression patterns of VEGF. This is caused by direct protein binding and inhibiting interaction between E-proteins and the target DNA. The extent of Id3-mediated VEGF repression by E-proteins and a cross talk between Id3 expressions in obesity actually provides a basis for establishing a connection between obesity and angiogenesis regulation during adipose tissue expansion.

3.2.2.3 Angiogenesis in Pulmonary Arterial Hypertension

Mean pulmonary artery pressure above 25 mmHg is considered as pulmonary arterial hypertension (PAH) (Voelkel and Tuder 2002). The pressure in pulmonary artery increases due to the pulmonary vascular resistance, which in turn is enhanced due to pulmonary vasoconstriction or lung vessel remodeling, or both (Rabinovitch 2008). Pulmonary vascular remodeling takes place in PAH. To elucidate the drivers of this pulmonary vascular remodeling, mechanical concepts of shear stress, flow, and pressure as well as cell phenotype plasticity, cell growth, and cell death have been implicated (Rabinovitch 2012). In PAH, a substantial number of genes and proteins correspond to its pathobiology. Two particular proteins are found to be crucially involved among the pool of proteins in both human and experimental animal models of PAH. These two proteins are VEGF and the bone morphogenetic protein receptor (BMPR). VEGF is the key protein for angiogenic growth and maintenance in the development of PAH. VEGF is extensively present in lungs, and it has numerous roles and actions in maintaining the lung structure (Voelkel et al. 2006). Patients with severe PAH have elevated plasma level of VEGF (Eddahibi et al. 2000; Papaioannou et al. 2009; Selimovic et al. 2009; Kümpers et al. 2010). Both VEGF and VEGF receptor type 2 (VEGFR2) are highly expressed in the multiplex vascular lesions in lungs of PAH patients (Hirose et al. 2000). An increase in the expression of VEGF, VEGFR1, and VEGFR2 in lungs (Tuder et al. 1995) due to acute and chronic hypoxia sets the pace for studies of experimental pulmonary hypertension (PH) in mice and rats. In all the experimental PAH cases, studies depicted increased expression of VEGF and its receptors were observed within lungs under hypoxic condition. In human form of PAH, the expression of VEGF and its receptors are upregulated conferring to pulmonary arteriolar endothelial cell growth (Tuder et al. 2001). Assessment of lung tissue of infants with PAH associated with congenital diaphragmatic hernia enumerated an elevated VEGF expression in pressure-regulating small pulmonary arteries, thereby appearing to play a part in vascular remodeling process (Shehata et al. 1999). The high expression of VEGF and VEGFR1 was observed in tracheal aspirates of infants having persistent PAH (Lassus et al. 2001), and VEGF-C (isoform of VEGF) and VEGFR3 were significantly upregulated in the lung tissue of fetuses and neonates with bronchopulmonary dysplasia which is associated with PAH.

3.2.2.4 Angiogenesis in Psoriasis

One of the most common inflammatory skin diseases is psoriasis, affecting almost 1–2% of the American population. Multiple other diseases, e.g. type 2 diabetes mellitus, inflammatory bowel disease, obesity, hepatitis C, coronary artery disease, and arthritis, are associated with psoriasis. In a study, T-cell subsets (preliminary TH17 and TH1) were considered as the drivers of chronic inflammatory psoriasis which eventually resulted in classic epidermal manifestations

(Nickoloff et al. 2007; Asarch et al. 2008). Angiogenesis is intricately associated with psoriatic lesions. They show lightly proliferating endothelial cells, dilated capillary bed, augmented blood flow, tortuosity of capillary loops through the skin and increased capillary permeability (Nickoloff 2000). The cytokine milieu of psoriasis is pro-angiogenic (by TNF-α, IL-8, IL-15, IL-17, IL-20, and IL-23); however, IL-12 is also involved in psoriasis despite being an anti-angiogenic cytokine (Nickoloff et al. 1999; Numasaki et al. 2003; Villadsen et al. 2003; Langowski et al. 2006). In psoriasis, increased vascular permeability is detected. Hypoxia-inducible factor 2-alpha (HIF-2α)- ang-2 pathway is responsible for this (Kuroda et al. 2001; Daly et al. 2006; Perry et al. 2006). In psoriasis, non-lesional skin and psoriatic plaque, markers of angiogenesis, are overexpressed. The key component of angiogenesis, i.e. VEGF, is elevated in plasma and tissues in patients suffering from psoriasis. The endothelial cells are induced by VEGF to produce pro-inflammatory cytokines, e.g. IL-6, IL-8, and GRO-alpha (Hao et al. 2009). These cytokines help in the activation and recruitment of neutrophil and lymphocyte from the blood to psoriatic site. Significantly, IL-8 is observed to promote the expression of VEGF in endothelial cells ultimately leading to activation of VEGFR2 in autocrine manner which is HIF-independent. IL-8 independently transactivates VEGFR2, without VEGF by binding to cytokines of CXC chemokine receptors (CXCR1 and CXCR2) (Petreaca et al. 2007). This perhaps establishes a signaling loop, where the VEGF from keratinocytes induces its own receptor expression in endothelial cells via IL-8 causing extensive vascular permeability and inflammation.

Receptors for VEGF, VEGFR1, and VEGFR2 expressions are induced in lesional and non-lesional psoriatic epidermis. In keratinocytes, VEGF itself can induce the autocrine expression of VEGFR (Man et al. 2008; Zhang et al. 2008). In a study with mice, the epidermal barrier of skin was seen to be disrupted, which resulted in increased expression of VEGF in keratinocyte cells. This ultimately led to skin angiogenesis (Elias et al. 2008). However, epidermal barrier disruption of skin does not exactly mimic the psoriasis scenario. Stretch has also been perceived to induce the VEGF expression, which accounts for the common location of psoriasis in body parts such as elbow and knees (Shrader et al. 2008).

3.2.2.5 Angiogenesis in Rheumatoid Arthritis

Rheumatoid arthritis (RA) is a systemic disorder associated with high rate of angiogenesis. In this arthritis, angiogenesis allows the infiltration of inflammatory cells into the joints resulting in synovial hyperplasia and ultimately leading to progressive destruction of bone (Koch 1998; Veale and Fearon 2006; Lainer-Carr and Brahn 2007; Szekanecz and Koch 2008). The process involves a chain of several events in a deregulated manner along with synthesis of new capillary sprouts from preexisting blood vessels. This deregulation occurs due to the dominance of pro-angiogenic factors over anti-angiogenic ones. Several earlier studies documented the factors involved in arthritic angiogenesis. These include growth factors (VEGF, Ang-2, FGF, and platelet-derived growth factor [PDGF]), chemokines and their receptors (chemokine (C-X-C motif) ligand [CXCL] (1, 5, 7, 8, 12, 13, 16), chemokine (C-C motif) ligand [CCL] (2, 3, 5, 20, 21, 23), chemokine (C-X-C motif) receptor [CXCR] (4, 5), and chemokine (C-C motif) receptor [CCR] (10)), ECM components (type I collagen, fibronectin, and vitronectin), cytokines (TNF-α, IL-6, IL-11, and IL-15), and proteases (MMPs and plasminogen activator [PA]). The pivotal factors for inflammatory arthritis-associated angiogenesis are HIF-VEGF-Ang-1-receptor tyrosine kinase (Tie2) system. Angiogenesis in RA starts with hypoxia which occurs in the joint with RA. Hypoxia is a condition of cellular demand for oxygen which exceeds the vascular supply leading to a bioenergetic crisis. Hypoxia creates immature and unstable microvasculature.

In RA also, angiogenic factors such as VEGF and HIF are induced by hypoxia. In this case, HIF plays a preliminary role in initiating the angiogenesis process. During the angiogenesis process, HIF-1α (one of the partners of HIF heterodimer) translocates to the nucleus and dimerizes with HIF-1β (another partner of HIF heterodimer) which then binds to the hypoxic response element (HRE) and thereby activates the transcription of HIF-dependent genes. The most significant HRE-containing gene is VEGF. In normal condition where hypoxia is absent, the HIF-1α undergoes proteasomal degradation after prolyl hydroxylases hydroxylation. But hypoxia inhibits hydroxylation of HIF-1α, and as a consequence, HIFα gets activated and dimerizes with HIF-1β and results in the transcription of HRE-containing gene. HIFα is extensively expressed in RA synovium. However, there are HIF-independent pathways as well which act through peroxisome-proliferator-activated receptor (PPAR), nuclear factor kappa-light-chain-enhancer of activated B-cells (NF-κB), Notch, and Janus kinases/signal transducer and activator of transcription proteins (JAK/STAT) pathways. After the initiation of angiogenesis, vessel stabilization is one of the primary factors. Ang-1–Tie-2 complex interacts with VEGF to stabilize the vessel in neo-angiogenesis. In RA, synovium, both Ang-1 and Tie-2 along with VEGF have been detected even in very early stage of the disease. Chemokines such as CXCL12, which is a major chemokine involved in RA angiogenesis, are produced by RA fibroblasts (Asahara et al. 1998; Taylor and Sivakumar 2005; Szekanecz and Koch 2007; Shibuya 2008; Gao et al. 2015; McGarry et al. 2018).

3.2.2.6 Angiogenesis in Ocular Diseases

Angiogenesis is the process by which new blood vessels are generated from existing capillaries in both normal and pathologic condition. The process of angiogenesis involves a large pool of factors, namely pro- and anti-angiogenic factors. Enhanced vascular permeability, choroidal neovascularization, and VEGF play a significant role in proliferative retinal diseases, such as proliferative diabetic retinopathy and age-related macular degeneration, causing loss of vision. Retinal pigment epithelium cells are the primary source of VEGF in the eye. The expression of VEGF is induced by hypoxia. There are four major isoforms of VEGF present in humans. Among the four isoforms, VEGF165 is predominant in human eye and it is the pivotal factor to be responsible for ocular neovascularization in pathologic condition. VEGF is an extremely specific and potent mitogen for endothelial cells. Besides being a mitogen for endothelial cells, it prevents the endothelial cells from apoptosis. It also functions as a chemoattractant for the precursors of endothelial cells. Along with these, VEGF increases the vascular permeability. Several other factors such as angiopoietins, bFGF, pigment epithelium-derived factor (PEDF), and cell-adhesion molecules are also linked to ocular neovascularization. All these factors together induce the process of neovascularization during ocular diseases (Dreyfuss et al. 2015).

3.3 Existing Anti-Angiogenic Treatments and Their Drawbacks

Preventing tumor angiogenesis is challenging because, unlike the balanced hierarchical network of venules, arterioles and capillaries are maintained by the natural anti-angiogenic factors, such as angiostatin, endostatin, and thrombospondin (TSP), that involve a complex interaction between several pathways and adopt alternative strategies in case of specific target blockades. For example, if VEGF signaling is blocked, bFGF molecule is activated to induce angiogenesis as evidenced by the formation of disorganized blood vessel networks that eventually leads to tumor formation (Huang and Bao 2004).

Avastin[TM] is the synthetically designed VEGF-targeting anti-angiogenic drug approved by Food and Drug Administration (FDA) (Neufeld and Kessler 2006). Many anti-angiogenic drugs such as endostar, bevacizumab, axitinib, aflibercept, ranibizumab, regorafenib, pazopanib, and sorafenib are now commercially available. However, despite being effective as anti-angiogenic agents during early phases of treatment, over time the patients stop responding, which in fact, often, leads to revascularization. Most likely, this is due to adjustment in favor of expression of pro-angiogenic genes, a response mounted by cancer pathogenesis against the treatment (Augustine et al. 2019). Moreover, only a few types of tumors such as hepatocellular, renal cell (advanced stage), and colorectal carcinomas are targeted by these agents and remain ineffective toward pancreatic adenocarcinoma, breast cancer, prostate cancer, and melanoma (Vasudev and Reynolds 2014). There is an additional issue of vascular mimicry observed in gliomas in which the tumors develop new vessels to adapt to the hypoxic conditions created by anti-angiogenic treatments (Lugano et al. 2019). There are reports of increase in death and relapse rates post bevacizumab treatment in colorectal cancer cases (de Gramont et al. 2012). Anti-angiogenic resistance can be innate or acquired, depending on the operative right at the beginning of the treatment or after an initial positive response (Bergers and Hanahan 2008).

3.4 Factors Involved in Pro-Angiogenesis

The bFGF, isolated from a chondrosarcoma, is the first pro-angiogenic factor to be identified (Huang and Bao 2004). Out of several such pro-angiogenic factors, VEGF has been thoroughly studied with respect to tumor angiogenesis (Neufeld and Kessler 2006). Other pro-angiogenic genes such as endothelial nitric oxide synthase (eNOS) (Park et al. 2015), vascular endothelial cadherin (VE-cadherin), cadherin 5 (CDH5) (Du et al. 2016), and forkhead box M1 (FOXM1) (Gartel 2010) are also known to play important role in angiogenesis.

During cancer pathogenesis, several angiogenic factors are released by the cancer cells that eventually trigger the release of MMPs by binding to their respective receptors. Being proteolytic in nature, MMPs degrade ECM of the existing blood vessels surrounding the tumor to facilitate intravasation and migration of metastatic cells from primary site. Likewise, MMPs also facilitate extravasation of the circulating cancer cells from blood vessels at the secondary site. Besides, through ECM degradation, MMPs allow adherence of endothelial cells to the surrounding matrix, proliferation, lumen formation, and sprouting, which ultimately results in the formation of well-organized 3D structure of blood vessel (Folkman 2006; Chung and Ferrara 2011). Being the source of energy for developing blood vessels, the role of lipoproteins is implicated in impaired angiogenesis (Kalaivani and Jaleel 2020). Angiogenesis begins with the primary capillary plexuses expanding into vascular tree that matures through astrogenesis (Teleanu et al. 2019). Pro-angiogenic factors released by tumorigenic tissues communicate with their receptors present on the endothelial cells and activate several receptor molecules, consequently, triggering extracellular signal-regulated kinase (ERK)/mitogen-activated protein kinases (MAPK) and phosphatidylinositol 3'-kinase-protein kinase B (PI3K-Akt) signaling pathways that in turn activate the intracellular proteins involved in endothelial cell proliferation, sprouting, and migration. Figure 3.4 represents the mechanism of action of some of the major pro-angiogenic factors.

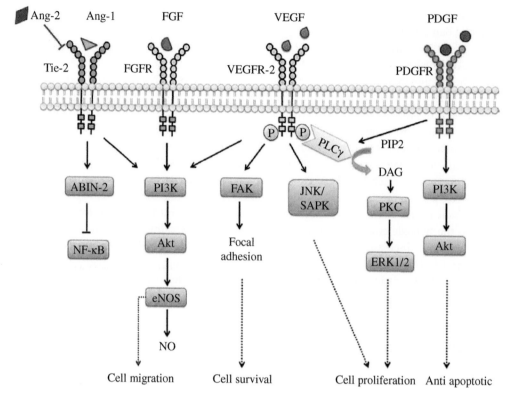

Figure 3.4 Mechanism of action of pro-angiogenic factors in endothelial cells. ABIN, A20 binding inhibitor of NF-κB; Ang-2, angiopoietin-2; Ang 1, angiopoietin 1; eNOS, endothelial nitric oxide synthase; DAG, diacylglycerol; ERK, extracellular signal-regulated kinases; JNK/SAPK, c-Jun N-terminal protein kinase/stress-activated protein kinase; FGF, fibroblast growth factor; FGFR, fibroblast growth factor receptor; NF-κB, nuclear factor kappa-light-chain-enhancer of activated B-cells; FAK, focal adhesion kinase; NO, nitric oxide; PIP2, phosphatidylinositol 4,5-bisphosphate; PI3K, phosphatidylinositol 3′-kinase; PKC, protein kinase C; PDGFR, platelet-derived growth factor receptor; PDGF, platelet-derived growth factor; PLC-γ, phospholipase C gamma; VEGFR-2, vascular endothelial growth factor receptor-2; VEGF, vascular endothelial growth factor. *Source:* Rajasekar et al. (2019). Reproduced with permission of Elsevier.

3.5 Factors Involved in Anti-Angiogenesis

Anti-angiogenic therapy is based on the principle of disrupting blood vessels that supply nutrition to the tumor, thus inhibiting proliferation and subsequent metastasis. Naturally, drugs with ability to inhibit neovascularization are focused on as a promising option for treating cancer. Angiostatin, endostatin, and TSPs – TSP-1, TSP-2, TSP-3, TSP-4, and TSP-5 – are among the main anti-angiogenic factors that balance out with the pro-angiogenic ones under normal conditions (see Table 3.1) (Park et al. 2015). Tumor progression is characterized by the overexpression of VEGF-A (isoform of VEGF) and consequential facilitation of invasion and metastasis. Hence, most common anti-angiogenic drugs are either VEGF-A or VEGFR2 inhibitors and act by inhibiting tyrosine kinases, known to promote the expressions of the former. Antibodies against VEGF-A and VEGFR2 are also

Table 3.1 List of pro- and anti-angiogenic factors.

Types	Pro-angiogenic factors	Anti-angiogenic factors
Growth factors	PLGF-152/131, VEGF, FGF 1-9, Ang-1, EGF, PDGF, HGF, insulin-like growth factor (IGF)-1,2, GCSF, platelet-derived endothelial cell growth factor (PD-ECGF)	Natural splice variant of hepatocyte growth factor (NK) 1,2,4 Transforming growth factor-β (TGF-β)
Hormones	Tissue factor, androgen, leptin estrogen, kallikrein, angiogenin factor XIII, integrins	NA
Cytokines	Tumor necrosis factor-α (TNF-α) Interleukin (IL)-1β, IL-6, IL-8 Stromal cell-derived factor 1 (SDF-1)	PR-39 Interferon (IFN)-α, β, γ Platelet factor (PF)-4
Proteases/ protease inhibitors	NA	Pigment epithelium-derived factor (PEDF), prothrombin, tissue inhibitor of metalloproteinase (TIMP)-1,2,3, maspin Endostatin, plasminogen activator inhibitor (PAI)-1, cleaved AT-III, Angiostatin
Matrix proteins	Cysteine-rich angiogenic inducer (CYR61), fibrin, connective tissue growth factor (CTGF), thrombin, MMP-2, MMP-9, urokinase plasminogen activators (uPA), aminopeptidase (APN)	NA
miRNAs	miR-130a, miR-210, Let-7f, miR-17-92 cluster, miR-378, miR-27b	miR-15, miR-16, miR20a, miR-20b, miR-221, miR-222

Source: Urbich et al. (2008) and Rajasekar et al. (2019). Reproduced with permission from Elsevier.

used for this purpose. The strategy used for designing anti-angiogenesis drugs depends on the factors listed below (Teleanu et al. 2019).

1) Targeting the endogenous factors that help in blood vessel formation.
2) Based on wound healing properties, using natural anti-angiogenic compounds.
3) Targeting molecules facilitating metastases of the surrounding tissues.
4) Factors inhibiting active proliferation of endothelial cells.

3.6 Nutraceuticals

The term *nutraceutical* is an amalgamation of the two words, *nutrition* and *pharmaceuticals*. The term was first coined by Dr. Stephen Defelice in the year 1989. Nutraceuticals may be obtained from plants, microbes, or animals and consist all those food products which have medicinal applications in maintaining and improving human health, in addition to providing nutrition. Nutraceuticals are also called as functional foods and besides serving as the basic food source, they also provide protective effects against a wide range of disorders. Being a broad category, nutraceutical comprises of phytochemicals such as alkaloids, polyphenols, flavonoids, non-flavonoids, diterpenes, phenolic acids, and so on.

In pharmacology and molecular biology, organic compounds weighing <900 Daltons are considered as small molecules (Thangarasu et al. 2019). They can be artificial or natural. According to metabolomics, acceptable mass range of small molecules is 50–1500 Daltons. Weights of some nutraceuticals fall within the range that defines small molecules. These are called small natural molecules. They are organic compounds of low molecular weight from natural sources that possess an array of biological activities with potential application as medicinal drug or cell signaling molecule. They are produced by a variety of plants, bacteria, and fungi. Some examples of small natural molecules are glycosides, lipids, alkaloids, flavonoids, phenazines, polyketide, triterpenoids, terpenes, tetrapyrroles, and saponins (Atta-ur-Rahman 2018).

3.6.1 Nutraceuticals and Their Role in Angiogenesis

A food item with medicinal values is considered to be nutraceutical and is the amalgamation of "nutrition" and "pharmaceutical." Nutraceuticals are a group of substances which are more than food but less than pharmaceuticals. Unfortunately, there is still no internationally accepted definition of these products, therefore their judgment varies from country to country. But in general terms, it could be considered as food or part of food that imparts beneficial health effects. Global nutraceutical market has experienced a boost due to changes in the trend and outlook toward health management. Nutraceuticals include dietary fiber, prebiotics, probiotics, polyunsaturated fatty acids, antioxidants, and other different types of herbal/natural foods. Nutraceuticals have been found to be very effective against managing serious health issues of the century, such as obesity, cardiovascular diseases, cancer, osteoporosis, arthritis, and diabetes. Growing demands for nutraceuticals has turned food industry into a research-oriented sector (Das et al. 2012). Food components in general are known to affect angiogenic pathways and thus impart beneficial health effects. This makes screening and identification of angiogenic agents from natural resources possible. List of different bioactive compounds with their bioavailability and concentrations used *in vitro* and *in vivo* to analyze their angiogenic potential in some experimental models are depicted in Table 3.2.

3.6.2 Importance of Nutraceuticals as Angiogenic Inhibitors

As discussed earlier, similar to that of angiogenic agents that induce angiogenesis, there are also a class of both synthetic and natural compounds which act like anti-angiogenic agents. They function opposite to that of angiogenic agents. They also have potential role in prevention of various diseases including cancer. Available synthetic anti-angiogenic agents either target VEGF, the most dominant pro-angiogenic factor and its receptors, VEGFR, or the tyrosine kinases involved in angiogenic pathways. Some of the FDA-approved anti-angiogenic agents are VEGF aptamer, pegaptanib, VEGF neutralizing antibody, bevacizumab, and anti-VEGF Fab antibody, ranibizumab (see Table 3.3). However, such drugs have been reported to induce acquired tumor resistance due to the use of alternative pro-angiogenic factors or the vascularization mechanism of specific tumor cells (Bergers and Hanahan 2008; Azam et al. 2010). There are also clinical evidences of adverse effects associated with these drugs, such as hypertension, cardiac toxicity, hemorrhage, clots in the arteries, endocrine dysfunction, and thrombosis in cancer patients (Hutson et al. 2008; Chen and Cleck 2009). These drugs are risky to be administered intravitreally as there are reports of increased bleeding and cardiovascular toxicity in age-related macular degeneration (AMD) patients (Thulliez et al. 2014). Therefore, safer alternatives for anti-angiogenic agents with least side effects are the real need of the hour.

Table 3.2 Experimental doses and bioavailability of angiogenesis modulating phytochemicals.

Active compounds		Plant species	In vivo dose and models used	In vitro concentration and cell lines used	Bioavailability	References
Polyphenols	Resveratrol	Grapes and all berry family	5.7 µg/ml on T241 fibrosarcoma xenografts	50 µM on A2780/CP70 and OVCAR-3 cells	<1%	Bråkenhielm et al. (2001), Cao et al. 2004 and Walle (2011)
	Catechin derivatives	Tea	1.5 mg of epigallocatechin gallate (EGCG) on HT29 xenografts, 10 mg/kg of EGCG on 4T1 breast cancer xenografts	40 mg/l EGCG on MDA-MB231 cells, 30 µM EGCG on HT29 cells 0.75~25 µM EGCG on neutrophils	<1%	Jung and Ellis (2001), Sartippour et al. (2002), Donà et al. (2003), Jang et al. (2013) and Cai et al. (2018)
	Curcumin	Curcumin longa	10 mg of curcumin in HACAT-derived mouse corneal model	0.5~10 µM on human intestinal microvascular endothelial cells (HIMEC)	1%	Arbiser et al. (1998), Binion et al. (2008) and Prasad et al. (2014)
	Quercetin	Fruits, vegetables, onion, red wine, apples	75 mg/kg of quercetin on human prostate cancer PC3 cell xenograft	100 µM on human umbilical vein endothelial cells (HUVEC) and prostate cancer cells (PC3) cells	Poor	Kasikci and Bagdatlioglu (2016) and Yang et al. (2016b)
Alkaloids	Sanguinarine	Sanguinaria canadensis	100 ng on CAM assay	10~300 nM on HUVECs	Poor	Eun and Koh (2004) and Hu et al. (2019)
	Piperine	Black pepper	50 µM on MDA-MB-231-induced angiogenesis in the CAM assay	100 µM on HUVECs	24%	Doucette et al. (2013) and Sahu et al. (2014)
	Caffeine	Coffee	1 mM on CAM assay	500 µM on HUVECs	99–100%	Li et al. (2013) and Teekachunhatean et al. (2013)
Carotenoid	Lycopene	Tomato	5 mg/kg body weight in BALB/c mice	10 µM HUVEC	2%	Azam et al. (2010) and Chen et al. (2012)
	β-Carotene	Vegetables	60 mg/kg C57BL/6 mice	10 µg/ml HUVEC	14%	van het Hof et al. (2000) and Guruvayoorappan and Kuttan (2007)

(Continued)

Table 3.2 (Continued)

Active compounds		Plant species	In vivo dose and models used	In vitro concentration and cell lines used	Bioavailability	References
Terpenoids and tannins	Ginsenosides	*Panax ginseng*	10 μg/mouse i.v. or 100~1000 μg/mouse p.o. on lung metastasis model	Unknown	<10%	Katsuaki et al. (1994), Mochizuki et al. (1995) and Won et al. (2019)
	Taxol	*Taxus brevifolia*	Unknown	25~100 nM on 1A9 and MDA-MB-231 cells	30%	Foa et al. (1994), Escuin et al. (2005) and Zyting Zyting Chu et al. (2008)
	Zerumbone	Ginger	200 μM on mouse matrigel plug assay in C57BL/6 mice	500 nM or 1 μM on HUVECs	68–93%	Tsuboi et al. (2014) and Kalantari et al. (2017)
	Thymoquinone	Black cumin seed oil	10 μM in matrigel plug assays *in vivo*	80–100 nM on HUVECs	58%	Yi et al. (2009) and Alkharfy et al. (2014)
	Ursolic acid	Apple, berry, guava, basil, rosemary	12.5 mg/kg on HT29-induced colorectal cancer (CRC) xenograft mice	40 μM on HUVECs	Poor	Lin et al. (2013) and Mlala et al. (2019)

Table 3.3   FDA-approved angiogenesis inhibitors.

Scientific name	Trade name
Axitinib	Inlyta
Ziv-aflibercept	Zaltrap
Cabozantinib	Cometriq
Everolimus	Afinitor
Regorafenib	Stivarga
Lenvatinib mesylate	Lenvima
Ramucirumab	Cyramza
Bevacizumab	Avastin
Vandetanib	Caprelsa
Thalidomide	Synovir, Thalomid
Lenalidomide	Revlimid
Sunitinib	Sutent
Pazopanib	Votrient

Source: Rajasekar et al. (2019). Reproduced with permission from Elsevier.

3.7   Angiogenic Modulation Through Nutraceuticals

Epidemiological studies have shown that prolonged consumption of fruit- and vegetable-rich diets reduces the incidences of cancer, cardiovascular diseases, and type 2 diabetes (Wang et al. 2014, 2016). These observed health benefits are scientifically attributed to the phytochemicals such as carotenoids, phenols, alkaloids, and terpenoids present in these foods (Liu et al. 2012; Weng and Yen 2012; Van Dam et al. 2013; Kaulmann and Bohn 2014; Ng et al. 2015). Since unregulated angiogenesis is associated with many diseases and the currently used anti-angiogenic agents have severe side effects, food-based anti-angiogenic approach is being explored worldwide (Albini et al. 2007). Following section of this chapter will review these bioactive small molecules which have the potential to manage several diseases through modulation of angiogenesis. Since these phytochemicals are available through food, they are also called nutraceuticals. However, some of these phytochemicals acting as nutraceuticals are <900 Daltons and therefore, by definitions are included under the group of small molecules. Interestingly, while the phytochemicals weighing >900 Daltons are reported to be anti-angiogenic, these small molecules can be both pro- and anti-angiogenic in function. The molecules that will be discussed in the subsequent sections of this chapter for their angiogenic modulatory properties are classified in Figure 3.5 and their chemical structures provided in Figure 3.6.

3.7.1   Nutraceuticals/Natural Products as Anti-Angiogenic Agent

Several bioactive compounds present in plants are found to possess anti-angiogenic activity. Therefore, insight into the molecular mechanisms responsible for this activity is required for deciding the necessary course of action to harvest their anti-angiogenic potentials in the form of therapeutics.

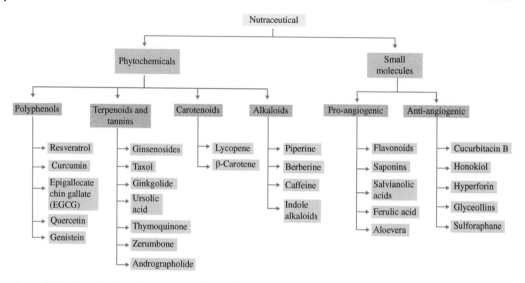

Figure 3.5 Classification of nutraceuticals involved in angiogenesis.

3.7.1.1 Polyphenols

3.7.1.1.1 Resveratrol

Resveratrol, a polyphenolic stilbene, is known to inhibit HIF-1α accumulation and downregulate VEGF to exert its anti-angiogenic effect (Cao et al. 2004; Chen et al. 2006; Garvin et al. 2006; Park et al. 2007; Wu et al. 2008). Actually, resveratrol-mediated VEGF inhibition has been found to be operational at an upstream stage, such as JAK-STAT and MAP-kinase and NF-κB pathways in human retinal pigment epithelial cells (HRPE cells) (Nagineni et al. 2012, 2014). VEGFR-2 is also reported to be suppressed by resveratrol (Alex et al. 2010). Through the downregulation of VEGF and VEGFR-2, resveratrol has been reported to be effective against diabetic neuropathy as evident from inhibition of HIF-1α/VEGF/VEGFR-2 signaling axis in HRPE cells (Wen et al. 2013; Zhang et al. 2015). Resveratrol showed anti-angiogenic potency at 1–2.5 μmol/l in HUVEC as manifested by significantly reduced VEGF-mediated migration and tube formation but not cell proliferation (Lin et al. 2003). At the same concentration, resveratrol prevented VEGF-mediated tyrosine phosphorylation of VE-cadherin and its complex partner, β-catenin. VEGF-induced endogenous Src-kinase activation is also prevented by resveratrol (Lin et al. 2003).

3.7.1.1.2 Curcumin

Curcumin is a low-molecular weight polyphenolic compound isolated from a commonly used Indian spice, *Curcuma longa* (turmeric). It has potent anti-cancer and anti-inflammatory activities (Aggarwal et al. 2013; Naksuriya et al. 2014). Curcumin is known to inhibit bFGF-induced endothelial cell proliferation in a dose-dependent manner (Arbiser et al. 1998). However, anti-angiogenic effect of curcumin was not always experimentally evident. It has been shown that 10 mg curcumin inhibited 80 ng bFGF-mediated corneal vascularization in mice but failed to prevent phorbol ester-stimulated VEGF mRNA production (Arbiser et al. 1998). However, the reports showed that inhibitory effects of curcumin on VEGFR, EGFR, and amino peptidase eventually prevented angiogenesis process (Furness et al. 2005; Yance and Sagar 2006). Curcumin can negatively target MMP-2 and MMP-6 to exert its anti-angiogenic effect while upregulating tissue inhibitor of MMP-1 (TIMP-1). Through reduced inducible nitric oxide synthase (iNOS) expression in endothelial cells,

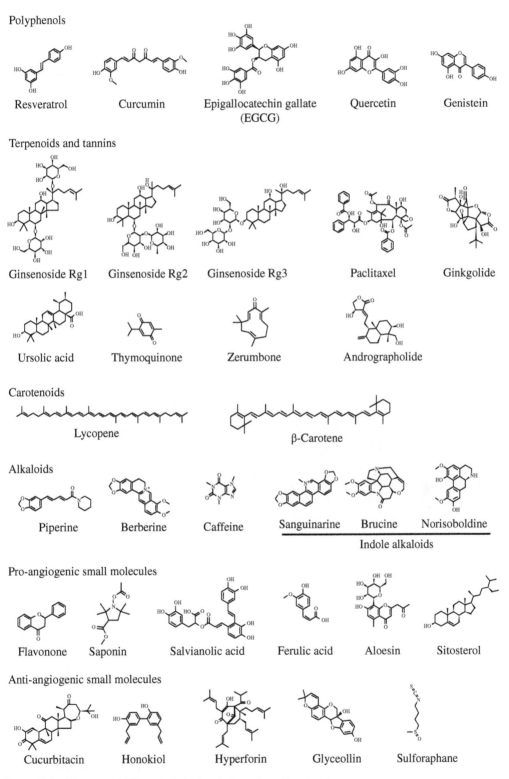

Figure 3.6 Structure of different phytochemicals and small molecules.

curcumin ensures less NO production and consequent angiogenesis (Yance and Sagar 2006; Singh and Agarwal 2007). Curcumin has also been reported to target cyclooxygenase (COX-1 and COX-2) that results in the inhibition of TNF-α-induced NF-κB activation (Anand et al. 2008). Tumor neo-capillary density in nude mice xenografted with hepatocarcinoma was significantly reduced on oral treatment with curcumin (Granci et al. 2010). Curcumin also targets HIF-1 in mice bearing Hep3B hepatoma (Choi et al. 2006). Suppression of NF-κB and mechanistic target of rapamycin (mTOR) pathways and VEGF-A and MMP-9 expressions are also regulated by curcumin (Bimonte et al. 2013; Kalinski et al. 2014; Yoysungnoen-chintana et al. 2014; Zhang et al. 2014). So, curcumin prevents angiogenesis by inhibiting VEGF secretion, VEGFR2 activation, and its downstream signaling pathways (Fu et al. 2015).

3.7.1.1.3 Epigallocatechin Gallate

In vivo, in vitro, and chemical assays have shown that epigallocatechin gallate (EGCG) has potent anti-cancer activity due to its antioxidant, anti-inflammatory, photoprotective, and anti-photocarcinogenic effects. EGCG is the most common phytochemical belonging to the catechin group present in green tea. Catechins in one way were found to be effective in downregulating the expressions of MMPs (zinc-dependent proteinases, type IV collagenases involved in matrix turnover) and VEGF, while at the same time promoted the expression of TIMP1 (Demeule et al. 2002; Katiyar et al. 2007). EGCG inhibits MMP expression to prevent degradation of basement membrane and consequential cell invasion in tumor cells. Mechanistically, EGCG suppresses the expression of membrane type 1 MMP (MT1-MMP) to downregulate MMP-2. MT1-MMP generates the active form of MMP-2 from proMMP-2 (El Sayed 2005). The MAP-kinase family members, Erk-1 and Erk-2, facilitate VEGF expression. EGCG is thought to chelate divalent cations essential for the facilitative activities of certain receptor kinases upstream of Erk-1 and 2. Consequently, Erk 1 and 2 expressions are reduced. Besides, EGCG can also downregulate VEGF expression by interfering with the VEGF promoter binding activity of AP-1. In addition, EGCG is also reported to be inhibitory toward VEGFR-1 and VEGFR-2 tyrosine phosphorylation (Ann Beltz et al. 2006). COX-2, whose own expression is under the influence of NF-κB and AP-1, in turn activates the expressions of MMP and angiogenic PGE2. It has been reported that EGCG interferes with NF-κB and AP-1 binding to COX-2 promoter in order to reduce the expression of the latter to prevent angiogenesis (Ann Beltz et al. 2006). In addition, there are also other pathways that EGCG targets as an anti-angiogenic agent which includes the levels of iNOS by increasing IκB kinase activity (Ann Beltz et al. 2006; Singh and Agarwal 2007), downregulating the vascular endothelial cell antigens, such as CD31, and suppressing protein kinase C (PKC) activity and EGFR signaling (Jung and Ellis 2001; Yance and Sagar 2006; Yang et al. 2009).

3.7.1.1.4 Quercetin

Quercetin is a flavone found in citrus fruits, red grapes, apples, raspberries, onions, cherries, leafy greens, and broccoli. Quercetin multi-targets lipoxygenase (LOX)-5 and COX-2 interaction, EGF receptor, and HER-2-mediated NF-κB signaling pathway to inhibit angiogenesis (Igura et al. 2001; Banerjee et al. 2002). Experimentally, quercetin was shown to completely inhibit hypoxia-induced VEGF expression and STAT-3 tyrosine phosphorylation in NCI-H157 cells. STAT-3 signaling is involved in VEGF expression and therefore, its targeting by quercetin is implicated in anti-angiogenic activities (Yance and Sagar 2006; Ansó et al. 2010; Noori-Daloii et al. 2011). In breast cancer, quercetin modulates VEGFR-2-regulated signaling pathways by targeting COX-2 expression in choroid-retinal endothelial cells (Xiao et al. 2011; Li et al. 2015a). In human prostate cancer, quercetin downregulated VEGFR-2-mediated Akt/mTOR/P70S6K pathway activation while enhancing the level of anti-angiogenic factor, TSP-1 (Pratheeshkumar et al. 2012; Yang et al. 2016b). Studies have also reported the anti-invasive activity of quercetin by reducing the levels of VEGF, MMP-2, and MMP-9 proteins in human glioblastoma cells. Further, quercetin was also reported to inhibit Akt signaling and thus prevent cell survival and angiogenesis in murine T-cell lymphoma (Maurya and Vinayak 2017).

3.7.1.1.5 Genistein

Genistein is an isoflavonic phytoestrogen mainly available in soybeans. It can downregulate VEGF expression and inhibit bFGF-induced neovascularization, migration, and proliferation of endothelial cells (Paper 1998; Singh and Agarwal 2007). In fact, under *in vitro* experimental set up, quercetin, at as low as 30 μM concentration, prevented endothelial cell tube formation by suppressing plasminogen activator inhibitor-1 (PAI-1) and PA and prevented angiogenesis in renal cell carcinoma (Fotsis et al. 1993; Koroma and de Juan 1994). In a recent report, quercetin was also shown to upregulate the expression of TIMP-1 and TIMP-2, thus inhibiting cell migration and angiogenesis (El Sayed 2005).

3.7.1.2 Terpenoids and Tannins
3.7.1.2.1 Ginsenosides

Ginsenosides are triterpene saponins and a class of natural product steroid glycosides found in *Panax* (ginseng) plant. It is used as the most popular herbal supplement and its major bioactive component is ginseng. Ginsenosides, such as ginsenoside-Rg3 and ginsenoside-Rb2 from the roots of red ginseng, can significantly decrease the number of neovessels in murine B16 melanomas (Katsuaki et al. 1994; Mochizuki et al. 1995). Rb1 suppressed the formation of endothelial tube-like structures through modulation of PEDF via ER-β in HUVECs (Lu et al. 2017). Inhibitory effect of ginsenoside-Rg3 on the growth of the ectopic endometrium in rats might occur through the blocking of the VEGFR-2-mediated PI3K/Akt/mTOR signaling pathway, thus halting angiogenesis and promoting the apoptosis of ectopic endometrial cells (Cao et al. 2017).

3.7.1.2.2 Taxol

Taxol, the complex polyoxygenated diterpene, obtained from the bark of *Taxus brevifolia*, is anti-angiogenic and has been reported to act by inhibiting HIF-1α expression and VEGF production as evident in human leukemia cell lines (Kadioglu 2013). Taxol-induced cytotoxic effects are mediated by microtubule network disturbance, G2-M arrest, increase in Bax/Bcl-2 ratio, and mitochondria permeabilization in HUVECs. This leads to a decrease in angiogenic survival factors such as Ang-1 and VEGF in human ovarian cancer cell lines (Bocci et al. 2013).

3.7.1.2.3 Ginkgolide

Yet another diterpene, Ginkgolide B present in *Ginkgo biloba* is known to downregulate VEGF expressions (Yance and Sagar 2006). The diterpene, *G. biloba* extract (EGb 761) isolated from Ginkgo leaf, suppresses angiogenesis by targeting VEGF, T-lymphocytes, PDGF, iNOS, and TGF-β2 (without influencing iNOS-mediated NO production) (DeFeudis et al. 2003). Ginkgolide B has been reported to significantly inhibit the level of pro-angiogenic cytokines IL-1β and TNF-α which may contribute to angiogenesis in murine chronic granulomatous air pouch model (Ou-Yang et al. 2005). In another study, the Ginkgo extract EGb 761 was found to inhibit a major population of splenic T-lymphocyte which is involved in inducing angiogenesis (DeFeudis et al. 2003).

3.7.1.2.4 Ursolic Acid

Ursolic acid is a triterpene isolated from rosemary (*Rosmarinus officinalis*). The levels of VEGF, NO, and pro-inflammatory cytokine were found to be reduced in response to ursolic acid treatment (Kanjoormana and Kuttan 2010). It has been reported that B16-F10 melanoma cells bearing C57BL/6 mice showed reduced capillary formation when treated with ursolic acid (Kanjoormana and Kuttan 2010). In addition, ursolic acid prevented proliferation of bovine aortic endothelial cells (BAEC) and induction of COX-2 and iNOS (El Sayed 2005; Shanmugam et al. 2011a). Anti-angiogenic activity of ursolic acid is attributed to its ability to inhibit canonical NF-κB signaling and STAT3 phosphorylation pathways by impeding JAK2 and Src activation upstream (Shanmugam et al. 2011b). Likewise, ursolic acid has also been reported to target VEGF-A and FGF-2 as anti-angiogenic agent in colorectal cancer. VEGF-A along with HIF-1α inhibition by ursolic acid in these cells prevented tumor growth and metastasis (Lin et al. 2013; Gao et al. 2016).

3.7.1.2.5 Thymoquinone

Thymoquinone is a monoterpene molecule and is found in the seed of *Nigella sativa* also known as black cumin or black seed. It can suppress NF-κB signaling and VEGF expression which concomitantly interferes with tube formation and angiogenesis of endothelial cells (Peng et al. 2013). Besides NF-κB, PI3K/Akt pathway is also targeted by thymoquinone in cholangiocarcinoma cells in order to downregulate VEGF and COX-2 expressions to exert anti-angiogeneic activity (Xu et al. 2014).

3.7.1.2.6 Zerumbone

Zerumbone is a sesquiterpenoid and cyclic ketone obtained by steam distillation from a type of edible ginger. Recently, it has gained interest as a potent anti-angiogenic agent and has been found to act by targeting NF-κB pathway in gastric and pancreatic cancers and retina of diabetic rats (Shamoto et al. 2014; Tsuboi et al. 2014; Tzeng et al. 2016). It also prevented phosphorylation-mediated activation of VEGF/VEGFR-2 and FGF/FGFR1 signaling pathways which are the crucial proteins involved in angiogenesis (Park et al. 2015). In hepatocellular carcinoma, zerumbone prevented migration of cancer cells through downregulation of MMP-9, VEGF, and VEGFR-2 and concomitantly raising the levels of anti-angiogenic endostatin and TSP (Samad et al. 2018).

3.7.1.2.7 Andrographolide

Andrographolide is a diterpenoid isolated from a medicinal plant called *Andrographis paniculata* (Burm. f.) Nees. Its anti-angiogenic abilities have been recently established through blood vessel formation in chick chorioallantoic membrane (CAM) model and inhibition of endothelial tube formation in HUVEC model. Effects of andrographolides have been found to be mechanistically multifaceted. It was shown to suppress MMP-8 by targeting TIMP3 through decreasing miR-21 (a short noncoding RNA) levels (Dai et al. 2017). It also inhibited other MMPs, such as MMP2 and MMP-9, and consequently prevented the MMP-mediated metastasis *in vitro*. Besides, andrographolide is likely to modulate angiogenesis by targeting the nuclear translocation of various transcription factors such as NF-κB, p65, p50, activated transcription factor-2 (ATF-2), c-fos, and cyclic adenosine monophosphate (cAMP) response element-binding (CREB) protein (Pratheeshkumar et al. 2012). Andrographolide-mediated anti-angiogenic effects were also evident in nude mice xenografted with Hep3B cancer cells. This effect is mediated through inhibition of VEGF-A/VEGFR2 and subsequent MAPK signaling (Shen et al. 2014).

3.7.1.3 Carotenoids

3.7.1.3.1 Lycopene

Lycopene is a naturally occurring red carotenoid pigment found in tomatoes, pink grape fruit, watermelon, papaya, guava, and also in other fruits. Lycopene was found to reduce the risk of prostate cancer by preventing angiogenesis (Zu et al. 2014). Anti-angiogenic activity of lycopene is attributed to its ability to target multiple pathways involved in angiogenesis. It modulates VEGFR-2-mediated PI3K-Akt and ERK-1/2-p38 axes and inhibits expressions of MMP-9, MMP-2, and HIF-1α (Chen et al. 2012; Bhatia et al. 2015; Treggiari et al. 2018). Lycopene is also capable of immunomodulation through IL-12 and interferon (IFN)-γ to promote pro-angiogenic cytokine secretion (Huang et al. 2013).

3.7.1.3.2 β-Carotene

β-*Carotene* is a yellow/orange pigment that gives their color to vegetables and fruits and is a powerful antioxidant. β-carotene is a fat-soluble vitamin and is found in sweet potatoes, carrots, dark leafy greens, butternut squash, cantaloupe, lettuce, red bell peppers, apricots, broccoli, and peas. β-carotene acts as an anti-angiogenic agent by blocking cellular migration, proliferation, and tube formation of endothelial cells. It facilitates all these by downregulating MMPs (MMP-2 and MMP-9), lysyl oxidase, and prolyl hydroxylase and upregulating TIMP1 and TIMP2. After treatment with β-carotene, B16F-10 tumor-bearing mice showed significantly reduced capillaries supplying the tumors. Not only that, serum cytokine levels were altered in favor of anti-angiogenic activity in addition to a distinct decrease in nuclear translocation of pro-angiogenic transcription factors such as NF-κB, p65, p50, ATF-2, c-fos, and CREB protein (Guruvayoorappan and Kuttan 2007).

3.7.1.4 Alkaloids

3.7.1.4.1 Piperine

Black pepper is rich in the dietary alkaloid piperine which has been associated with anti-angiogenesis and its mode of actions has been worked out in recent years. Through its anti-angiogenic activity, piperine prevents invasiveness of the tumors. Piperine targets PI3K/Akt pathway by impeding the Akt phosphorylation (Doucette et al. 2013). In addition to the PI3K/Akt pathway, it also suppresses the ERK-1/2 signaling pathway to inhibit proliferation and migration of HER+ breast cancer cells. Downregulation of PI3K/Akt and ERK-1/2 pathways by piperine leads to a decrease in NF-κB-induced MMP-9 expression (Do et al. 2013).

3.7.1.4.2 Berberine

Berberine, a quaternary ammonium salt belonging to the protoberberine class, is present in many occidental and oriental medicinal plants such as *Hydrastis canadensis* L.(Ranunculaceae) and *Coptis chinensis franch* var. chinensis (Ranunculaceae), commonly known as Goldenseal and Huanglian, respectively (Grycová et al. 2007). Berberine was shown to disrupt the cross talk between HUVEC and cells of hepatocarcinogenic (HCC) and gastric adenocarcinogenic (SC-M1) origins, which are necessary for triggering the former to differentiate into endothelial tube. At the cellular level, these outcomes are attributed to its ability to decrease HIF-1α-mediated transcription of VEGF in these cancer cell lines with a significant resultant decrease in its extracellular secretion to cue the HUVECs for angiogenesis (Jie et al. 2011; Lopes et al. 2013).

3.7.1.4.3 Caffeine

Caffeine is a bitter, white crystalline purine, a methylxanthine alkaloid, and is chemically related to the adenine and guanine bases of deoxyribonucleic acid (DNA) and ribonucleic acid (RNA). It is found in the seeds, nuts, or leaves of a number of plants native to Africa, East Asia, and South America and helps to protect them against predator insects and to prevent germination of nearby seeds. The most well-known source of caffeine is the coffee bean, seed of the plant belonging to the genus *Coffea*. Caffeine and its derivative cafestol are potent anti-angiogenic agents. Caffeine reduced STAT3-mediated HIF-1α-induced VEGF expression in a Caki-I renal carcinoma murine model and also affected the levels of MMPs. Cafestol, a bioactive compound present in unfiltered coffee, suppresses VEGF signaling in order to inhibit endothelial cell proliferation, migration, and capillary tube formation (Jung et al. 2007; Wang et al. 2012; Abduljawad et al., 2013). Thus, caffeine seems to have a potential role in inhibiting angiogenesis.

3.7.1.4.4 Indole Alkaloids

Different indole alkaloids, such as sanguinarine, brucine, tylophorine, norisoboldine, and 6′-debromohamacanthin A, derivable from different natural sources, namely, medicinal plants, such as *Sanguinaria canadensis*, *Strychnos nux-vomica*, *Tylophora indica*, *Radix linderae*, and marine sponges, respectively, have been associated with anti-angiogenic activities. All these alkaloids target VEGF through Src, FAK, Erk, Akt, and mTOR signaling pathways. Brucine, in addition to all these, showed inhibitory effects on IL-6, IL-8, NO, TNF-α, and IFN-γ in human umbilical vein cells. Norisoboldine can also target Notch-1 signaling to downregulate angiogenesis (Eun and Koh 2004; Lu et al. 2012; Saraswati and Agrawal 2013; Saraswati et al. 2013).

3.7.2 Natural Small Molecules as Anti-Angiogenic Agents

3.7.2.1 Cucurbitacin B

The triterpenoid cucurbitacin B, available in plants of the Cucurbitaceae family, such as pumpkins and gourds, have been reported to downregulate VEGF/FAK/MMP-9 signaling pathways as evident from decrease in the neovasculature marker, i.e. CD31 in 4T1-syngeneic mouse mammary cancer (Sinha et al. 2016). HUVECs treated with cucurbitacin B showed reduced cell migration, invasion, and tube formation. This phytochemical also reduced preexisting vasculature in a CAM and matrigel plug mice model (Shukla et al. 2016; Sinha et al. 2016).

3.7.2.2 Honokiol

Magnolia officinalis, a popular Chinese medicinal plant, is the richest source of honokiol. Honokiol has been shown to suppress JAK2/STAT3, Akt, and Erk pathways in human oral squamous cells and inhibited IL-6-mediated endothelial cell migration in mice xenograft model. The levels of pro-angiogenic markers such as proliferative cell nuclear antigen (PCNA) and CD31 were reduced upon honokiol treatment (Huang et al. 2016). A derivative of honokiol, 5-formylhonokiol, is also a potent inhibitor of cell migration, invasion, and tube formation in HUVECs *in vitro* and *in vivo* in zebra fish model. It has been reported that 5-formylhonokiol targets ERK signaling pathway to abolish the process of angiogenesis (Zhu et al. 2011).

3.7.2.3 Hyperforin

Hyperforin is a phloroglucinol derivative of St. John's wort. It was shown to completely abrogate cell growth, invasion, and tube formation in endothelial cells. This anti-angiogenic activity of hyperforin has been reported to be associated with its efficient inhibition of urokinase and MMP-2 suppression. Its anti-angiogenic activity was also reflected in the reduced level of CD31-positive microvessels in tumor stroma (Martínez-Poveda et al. 2005; Schempp et al. 2005).

3.7.2.4 Glyceollins

Glyceollins belong to the family of prenylated pterocarpan and are found in ineffective types of nodule in soybean in response to symbiotic infection and hence are called soy phytoalexins. Glyceollins are found to reduce microvessel densities in mice xenografted with Lewis lung carcinoma. *In vitro*, glyceollins, like other natural anti-angiogenic agents, were found to down-regulate bFGF/FGFR-1 and VEGF/VEGFR2, ERK-1/2, JNK, p38 MAPK, and FAK signaling pathways (Lee et al. 2013).

3.7.2.5 Sulforaphane

Cruciferous vegetables such as broccoli and cabbages contain a bioactive small molecule called sulforaphane. It is found to be a highly efficient anti-angiogenic agent. Sulforaphane attenuated proliferation, migration, adhesion, and tube formation in HepG2-induced HUVECs. The pathway analysis showed that this phytochemical inhibited STAT3/HIF-1α/VEGF signaling in these cells (Liu et al. 2017).

Some of the major bioactive natural compounds of plant origin that possess anti-angiogenic activity are listed below along with their respective mechanisms of actions (see Table 3.4).

3.7.3 Natural Small Molecules as Pro-Angiogenic Agents

Like the wide variety of small molecules acting as anti-angiogenic agents, there are equally numerous natural molecules that are known to be pro-angiogenic or simply angiogenic and are facilitative for processes such as wound healing. Nut oil from *Pouteria lucuma* that contains oleic acid, linoleic acid, palmitic acid, γ-linolenic acid, and stearic acid is a potent wound healing agent owing to its angiogenic property (Rojo et al. 2010). Nutraceuticals facilitate vascular development through improved capillary structure formation as evident from *in vivo* pharmacological studies involving ginseng (Fan et al. 2006; Diniz et al. 2017), pseudo-ginseng (Yang et al. 2016a), *Carthamiflos* (Zhou et al. 2014), *Radix achyranthis bidentatae* (Zhou et al. 2017), *Radix cyathulae* (Zhou et al. 2017), *Radix salviae miltiorrhizae* (Li et al. 2010), *Angelica sinensis* (Lam et al. 2008), *Astragalus membranaceus bunge* (Lai et al. 2014), *Radix rehmannia glutinosa* (Liu et al. 2011), *Panax notoginseng* (Hong et al. 2009), and *Radix angelicae sinensis* (Tereza et al. 2011). The following section discusses the role of certain plant-based small molecules for their role in angiogenesis process.

3.7.3.1 Flavonoids

Flavonoids such as calycosin, formononetin, and puerarin are potent angiogenic stimulators. Mechanistically, they vary from each other although having a common generic source from *Radix* species: calycosin and formononetin obtained from *Radix astragali* and puerarin from *Radix puerariae*. Studies using zebrafish model revealed that calycosin promotes VEGF, FGF, and Erb signaling pathways (Li et al. 2011). Phosphorylations of PI3K and basal Flt1 tyrosine kinase were also involved in calycosin-induced angiogenesis process (Tang et al. 2010). Estrogen receptor (ER) modulation through VEGF/VEGFR2, ER, and MAPK signaling pathways are also found to be associated with calycosin-mediated angiogenesis. In case of formononetin-mediated angiogenesis, ERα-modulated ROCK-II–MMP-2/-9 signaling pathway was found to be involved (Li et al. 2015c). Puerarin could induce angiogenesis in the ischemic and non-ischemic myocardium and efficiently prevent myocardial infarction. In this process, VEGF, HIF-1α, Ang-1, Ang-2, and eNOS were found to be upregulated (Zhang et al. 2006; Ai et al. 2015).

Table 3.4 Anti-angiogenic natural compounds and their biological mechanisms of actions.

Compound	Biological mechanisms of actions	References
Genistein	Suppressed HGF/SF-activated ERK-1/2, Akt, VEGF, CD31, and HIF-1α	Guo et al. (1995), Myoung et al. (2003), Sengupta et al. (2003) and Wang et al. (2005)
Quercetin	Suppressed ribosomal protein S6 kinase, VEGF/VEGFR2, AKT/mTOR/P70S6K, ERK, and calcineurin/NFATc3	Pratheeshkumar et al. (2012), Zhao et al. (2014, 2016) and Maurya and Vinayak (2017)
Kahweol	Inhibited uPA and extracellular matrix molecules MMP-2	Cárdenas et al. (2011)
Andrographolide	Downregulated miR21 expression, targets TIMP3 and suppresses MMP-9 expression	Dai et al. (2017)
EGCG	Activated FOXO transcription factors and TRPV1-Ca^{2+} signaling pathway; inhibits MEK/ERK, AMPK, HIF-1α, PCNA, NF-κB, VEGF, Akt, Ki67, MMP-2, -7 and -9, CD31, neutrophil, IL-6 and 8, N-cadherin, Zeb1, and PI3K/AKT and eNOS activation and NO production	Shankar et al. (2008), Gu et al. (2013), Shankar et al. (2013) and Guo et al. (2015)
Curcumin	Blocked c-Met/Akt/mTOR, VEGF/Ang-2/TSP1, and PI3K/Akt/mTOR signaling pathways; reduces vimentin, CD34, and VEGF expression and induces E-cadherin expression	Jiao et al. (2016) and Zhang et al. (2017)
Ginsenosides Rb1	Inhibited ERβ-mediated PEDF; PEDF/PPARγ and miR33a pathway	Leung et al. (2007) and Lu et al. (2017)
Ginsenoside Rg3	Decreased the expression of MMP-2 and -9, EPHB-2 and 4; mTOR/AKT/PI3K/VEGF/VEGFR2 signaling pathway	Kim et al. (2012), Keung et al. (2016) and Cao et al. (2017)
Caffeine	Downregulated expression of VE-cadherin(+), IGF-2, PlGF, VEGF, VEGFR2, NRP1, and upregulated Ang-1 and -2 expression	Ma et al. (2016)
Lycopene	Downregulate the expression of MMP-2, Rac1, VEGF, and uPA and MMP-2; increased protein expression of TIMP2 and plasminogen activator inhibitor-1; attenuated AKT/PI3K/VEGFR2 and MAPK (ERK and p38 MAPK) signaling pathways	Yang et al. (2011) and Chen et al. (2012)
β-Carotene	Downregulated expression of MMP-2 and -9, lysyl oxidase and prolyl hydroxylase, and upregulated TIMP1 and TIMP2 expressions	Guruvayoorappan and Kuttan (2007)
Cucurbitacin B	Downregulated CD31, FAK/VEGF/MMP-9, and Wnt/β-catenin signaling pathway	Shukla et al. (2016) and Sinha et al. (2016)
Honokiol	Reduced JAK2/STAT3/AKT/Erk pathways and CD31, proliferative cell nuclear antigen (PCNA) expression	Huang et al. (2016)
Shikonin	Decreased HIF-1α, integrin subunit alpha-V β3 (ITGAV-β3) expression, and its downstream eIF4E/mTOR/p70S6K/4EBP1 signaling pathway	Li et al. (2017)
Hyperforin	Suppressed MMP-2 and CD31 and inhibited urokinase activity	Martínez-Poveda et al. 2005 and Schempp et al. (2005)
Glyceollins	Downregulated bFGF/FGFR1 and VEGF/VEGFR2 and their corresponding signaling pathways such as ERK-1/2, MAPK, JNK and FAK, p38	Lee et al. (2013)
Sulforaphane	Inhibited VEGF/STAT3/HIF-1α signaling	Liu et al. (2017)

3.7.3.2 Saponins

Saponins from *Panax ginseng* and *P. notoginseng* are noted to have pro-angiogenic activities. Saponins isolated from *P. ginseng*, ginsenosides Rg1, and Re have been evaluated for their pro-angiogenic activity *in vitro* and *in vivo* (Sengupta et al. 2004; Yu et al. 2007). In an *in vivo* matrigel plug assay, a seven-day implantation showed that Rg1 and Re significantly increased the density of neovessels compared to the blank control (matrigel alone). Activated PI3K-Akt signaling pathways and enhanced expression of NOS are inferred to be involved in improved neovasculization due to Rg1 and Re. Pro-angiogenic saponin fractions from *P. notoginseng* were functionally tested in zebra fish model and were found to exert their angiogenic activity through activation of PI3K-Akt-eNOS and vascular endothelial growth factor-kinase insert domain receptor (VEGF-KDR) signaling pathways (Hong et al. 2009). One of the notoginsenosides, R1, was found to promote angiogenesis is a way similar to its structural alikes, Rg1 and Re ginsenosides, in a chemical-induced blood vessel loss model of zebrafish (Yang et al. 2016a). Astragaloside IV, yet another saponin from *R. astragali*, facilitated cell proliferation, migration, and tube formation in HUVECs. Activation of KDR/Akt/Flk1/VEGF/VEGFR2/JAK2/STAT3 and ERK-1/2 signaling pathways was found to be involved in the process in addition to upregulation of eNOS expression and NO productions (Zhang et al. 2011). Angiogenic property of astragaloside IV was confirmed in a transgenic zebrafish model *in vivo* (Zhang et al. 2012).

3.7.3.3 Salvianolic Acids

The popular traditional Chinese medicinal herb *Radix Salviae miltiorrhizae* (*danshen* in Chinese) is a rich source of salvianolic acids A and B. The angiogenic activity of water-soluble fraction of salvianolic acid A was found to be due to stimulated VEGF, VEGFR2, and MMP-9 activations. This helped it to induce neovascularization in the ischemic rat myocardium *in vivo*. *In vitro*, it could stimulate angiogenesis in endothelial progenitor cells (EPCs) and the CAM model (Li et al. 2010; Li et al. 2014). Likewise, salvianolic acid B promoted angiogenesis through VEGF and VEGFR2, but instead of MMP-9, as in salvianolic acid A, MMP-2 was involved in this case (Lay et al. 2003).

3.7.3.4 Ferulic Acid

Ferulic acid is a hydroxycinnamic acid, an abundant phenolic phytochemical found in plant cell walls, covalently bonded as side chains to molecules such as arabinoxylans. Medicinal herbs such as *A. sinensis*, *Cimicifuga heracleifolia*, and *Ligusticum chuang xiong*, vegetables such as spinach and parsley, and processed foods such as rice bran oil and cooked sweet corn contain ferulic acid. The observed ferulic acid-induced angiogenesis in CAM and HUVEC models was due to enhanced HIF-1α expression and its target molecules, VEGF and PDGF. Interestingly, ERK-1/2, PI3K, and MAPK signaling pathways are also implicated in this process (Lin et al. 2010).

3.7.3.5 *Aloe vera*

β-Sitosterol and aloesin are the two potent angiogenic small natural molecules isolated from *Aloe vera* gel. Angiogenic potential and vascularization efficiency of β-sitosterol were established through skin wound, CAM, and matrigel plug assay in mice in the presence of heparin (Moon et al. 1999; Choi et al. 2002). The β-sitosterol-mediated vascularization in the ischemia/reperfusion-damaged brain of Mongolian gerbil was through VEGF, VEGF receptor Flk1, von Wille brand factors, and blood vessel matrix laminin (Choi et al. 2002). Aloesin modulated MAPK/Rho and Smad (Smad2 and Smad3) signaling pathways and migration-related proteins such as Rac1, Cdc42, and α-Pak to heal skin wounds as well (Wahedi et al. 2017).

Some of the well-known small natural compounds with pro-angiogenic activities are listed along with their experimentally determined mechanisms of action in Table 3.5.

Thus, angiogenic modulation through phytochemicals is a complex process that targets multiple signaling pathways (see Figure 3.7).

Table 3.5 Pro-angiogenic small natural compounds and their biological mechanisms.

Compound	Biological mechanisms	References
Calycosin	Regulated VEGF-VEGFR2, FGF, basal Flt1 tyrosine kinase, ErbB, PI3K, MAPK, and ER	Tang et al. (2010), Li et al. (2011) and Li et al. (2015b)
Puerarin	Improved VEGF, VEGF-A, HIF-1α, Ang-1and -2, and eNOS	Zhang et al. (2006) and Ai et al. (2015)
Ginsenoside Rg1	Increases NOS expression and activates Akt-PI3K signaling pathway	Sengupta et al. (2004) and Yu et al. (2007)
Ginsenoside Re	Increases NOS expression and activates Akt-PI3K signaling pathway	Sengupta et al. (2004) and Yu et al. (2007)
Notoginsenoside R1	Activated PI3K-Akt-eNOS and KDR-VEGF pathways	Yang et al. (2016a)
Salvianolic acid A	Increased formation of MMP-9, VEGF, and VEGFR2	Li et al. (2014)
Salvianolic acid B	Upregulated MMP-2, VEGFR, and VEGF	Lay et al. (2003)
Ferulic acid	Activated VEGF, HIF-1α, PDGF, PI3K, and Erk-1/2	Lin et al. (2010)
β-Sitosterol	Regulated VEGF, VEGF receptor Flk1, von Willebrand factors, and blood vessel matrix laminin	Moon et al. (1999)
Aloesin	Modulated migration-related proteins (Cdc42, Rac1, and α-Pak), MAPK/Rho, and Smad (Smad2 and Smad3)	Wahedi et al. (2017)

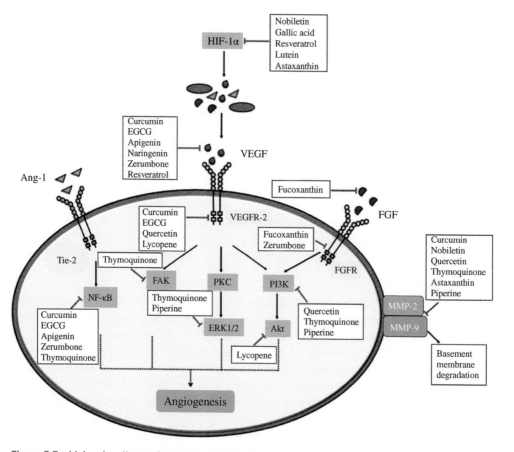

Figure 3.7 Major signaling pathways targeted by dietary phytochemicals in angiogenesis. *Source:* Rajasekar et al. (2019). Under CCBY license.

3.8 Nutraceutical Targeting MicroRNAs

MicroRNAs (miRNAs) play an important role in regulating gene expression. This class of noncoding single-stranded RNA molecules (22 nucleotides) regulate gene expression posttranscriptionally by either degrading or silencing the target mRNA, and thus coordinate cell physiology such as proliferation and apoptosis (Bushati and Cohen 2007). Their dysregulation in human pathologies, including cancer, heart disease, and neuropathy, is known and is likely to cause them (Esquela-Kerscher and Slack 2006; Chang and Mendell 2007; Van Rooij and Olson 2007; Bushati and Cohen 2008). These new molecular regulators, collectively termed as Angio-miRs, have been identified in endothelial cells, and their role has recently been examined in several laboratories in regulating various aspects of the angiogenic process (Poliseno et al. 2006; Kuehbacher et al. 2007; Fish et al. 2008; Wang et al. 2008; Tiwari et al. 2017). There are many pathways regulating angiogenesis, but the main trigger is hypoxia-induced activation of HIF-1α resulting in upregulation of VEGF expression. miRNA can have dual (pro- or anti-angiogenic) effects during angiogenic modulation (Tiwari et al. 2017).

Since its first report in 2006 by Poliseno, there have been several evidences on the angiogenic regulatory role of miRNA (Poliseno et al. 2006). miRNA-21, which plays an important role in tumor angiogenesis and is associated with poor prognosis in triple negative breast cancer (TNBC), has been found to be frequently upregulated in some cancers (Dong et al. 2014). Cardamonin, a chalconoid present in many *Alpinia* spp. from *Zingiberaceae* family, was found to be effectively suppressing VEGF-induced angiogenesis in a dose-dependent manner. It could decrease the phosphorylation of ERK and AKT (Jiang et al. 2015). Resveratrol can downregulate oncogenic miRNA-155 that acts as a pro-angiogeneic miRNA in HUVECs (Tili et al. 2010). Silibinin, a flavonoid isolated from milk thistle (*Silybum marianum*), in combination with EGCG has been shown to downregulate miR-17-92 cluster, thereby decreasing VEGF-VEGFR2 expression in HUVECs (Zadeh et al. 2015). miRNA-21 and miRNA-27 that regulate glycolytic pathways are targeted by EGCG. miR-221/222 promotes angiogenesis by targeting c-KIT and eNOS. Genestein efficiently inhibits miR-221/222 in MDA-MB 435 cells thereby decreasing metastasis and improving focal adhesion connections (De La Parra et al. 2016). Betulinic acid (BA), a pentacyclic triterpene, suppresses oncogenic miR-27a. This, consequently, inhibits breast cancer metastasis through β-catenin-mediated glycolysis. Besides, cell proliferation is also affected while apoptosis is induced (Talcott et al. 2020).

3.9 *In vivo* Assays for Angiogenesis

All the data as presented above involved a set of experimental parameters tested in response to various nutraceuticals/phytochemicals. These experimental parameters are an array of test models involving both *in vitro* and *in vivo* systems that mimic the (anti)angiogenic system that is observed in *in vivo* physiological system. In general, *in vitro* assays are performed to examine the behavior of the endothelial cells in a regulated manner but cannot imitate the actual steps of blood vessel formation. Conversely, *in vivo* assay represents a complete depiction of the angiogenesis process by involving all the steps of angiogenesis and vessel maturation. *In vivo* assays are also supportive in the validation of the proposed molecular mechanism of test substances (Irvin et al. 2014). In the following section, some commonly used *in vivo* angiogenesis assays are described.

3.9.1 Chick Chorioallantoic Membrane (CAM) Assay

The CAM assay uses a complete biological living system and closer to a physiological system as compared to *in vitro* system. This assay involves epithelial surface enclosing a stromal compartment that contains a complete vascular system and various cell types such as inflammatory and fibroblast cells. CAM system is quite simple in nature and a widely used model for angiogenesis study. Similar to immune-deficient mice, chick embryo has deficient immune response toward the exogenous materials such as cancer cells and tumors that allow easier xenografting (Staton et al. 2009; Irvin et al. 2014). The CAM assay can be performed in two different ways (Figure 3.8). The first one is *in ovo*, where test substances may be positioned to the CAM by making a minor cut in eggshell and allows the development of the embryo in the eggshell. Another method is *ex ovo*, where embryos along with CAM are cultured in a petri dish. *In ovo* method needs less maintenance and angiogenesis may be analyzed until the advanced embryonic development. Second method (*ex ovo*) on the other hand is advantageous over *in ovo*, as it allows easier access to test sites and test molecules can be added frequently. Additionally, several test sites per embryo are also available. A test substance can be pro- and anti-angiogenesis molecules, tissue samples, or cancerous cell lines. Test substance can be encapsulated or immobilized using an air-dried filter, polymer pellet, and gelatin sponges. These processes mediate the sustained release of test substances. For angiogenesis analysis, CAM is removed from the area surrounding the filter disc or xenograft. Vascular density can be scored semi-quantitatively by giving a score (0–4) or alternately determine

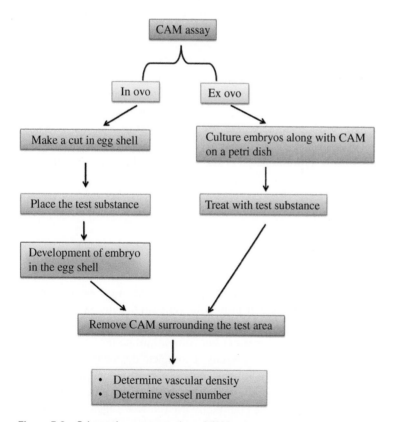

Figure 3.8 Schematic representation of CAM assay.

the vessel number using the microscope (Auerbach et al. 2003; Staton et al. 2004; Irvin et al. 2014). Recently, florescent-labeled dyes and nanoparticle are also injected in the vasculature for the identification of parent vessels and enhanced resolving of sprouts (Zijlstra et al. 2006; Palmer et al. 2011).

3.9.2   *In vivo* Matrix Invasion Assay

This assay analyzes the capabilities of a test substance to enhance/inhibit the host-mediated angiogenic responses. In this assay, synthetic scaffold or ECM component (matrigel) are used for the delivery of test substances. Synthetic scaffolds are generally made up of polyvinyl acid, polyethylene, or polyurethane. Test substances are enclosed into these scaffolds or matrigel and delivered subcutaneously into the animal model, i.e. mice, rats, and rabbits (Akhtar et al. 2002). The test substances could be a growth factor, a new drug, cancerous cells, or tumor. These substances are examined for their impact on the recruitment of host endothelial cells. After 7–10 days post-delivery, matrigel plug or synthetic scaffold is removed and sectioned. Immunostaining is performed for different markers specific for the endothelial cell types. Apart from this, amount of hemoglobin is also measured, which provides an indirect clue about the angiogenesis (Figure 3.9) (Staton et al. 2009; Irvin et al. 2014).

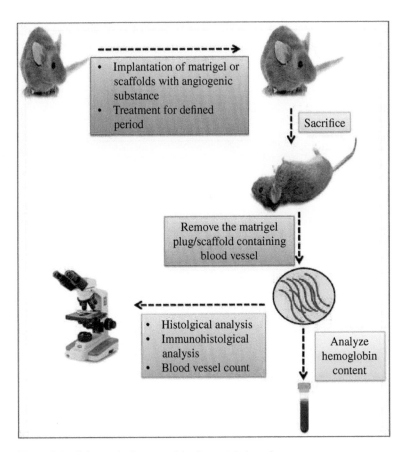

Figure 3.9   Schematic diagram of *in vivo* matrix invasion assay.

3.9.3 Tumor-Associated Angiogenesis

Tumor-associated angiogenesis is another *in vivo* method for analyzing pathological changes associated with angiogenesis. After a certain limit, tumor growth needs initiation of angiogenesis that support the tumor growth by providing nutrient and oxygen and eliminating the waste products. Therefore, anti-angiogenic potential of a novel drug can be examined using the tumor model system. In this method, tumor cells are injected into mice by several means such as subcutaneous, intra-bone, intra-spleen, and orthotopic. After that the mice are treated with test substances or left untreated. These mice are sacrificed after a defined time period that is based on the type of tumor and injection site (Amano et al. 2003). After tumor retrieval, histological and immunohistological assays are performed to examine the impact of test substance on tumor allied angiogenesis. In the case of subcutaneous injection of tumor cells, anesthetized mice can be examined to determine the impact of test substance on the quantity of blood flow and capillary network (Figure 3.10) (Staton et al. 2009; Irvin et al. 2014). The use of green fluorescent protein (GFP)-tagged tumor cells also permits continuous monitoring of tumor growth and metastasis (Cross et al. 2008). Nowadays transgenic mice are used, where targeted oncogenes are expressed under a regulatory system to form tumor in a defined time period (Staton et al. 2009; Irvin et al. 2014).

3.9.4 Zebrafish Angiogenesis Assay

Zebrafish is also utilized to study the function of test substances during angiogenesis *in vivo*. Molecular mechanism of angiogenesis in zebrafish is quite similar to mammals. This model provides the opportunity of large-scale screening of test substances, as a huge number of transparent embryos are

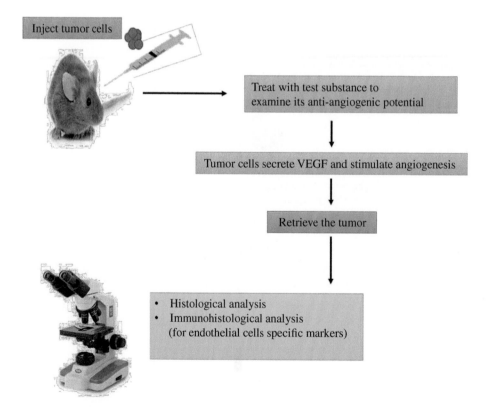

Figure 3.10 Diagrammatic representation of tumor-associated angiogenesis assay.

generated in single mating and can be maintained inexpensively. This characteristic makes this method attractive for the study of vasculature and angiogenesis development (Staton et al. 2004; Staton et al. 2009). The chemical nature of the test substance determines the mode of insertion. Small lipophilic substances are easily taken up by the fish embryo after the addition into the water, whereas protein/peptide needs direct injection into the fish embryo (Irvin et al. 2014). Antisense morpholinos nucleotide and mutagenic compounds could be used for genetic modifications and to analyze their impact on specific gene functions related to angiogenesis (Schütte et al. 2010). Zebrafish embryo develops externally and their transparent nature permits a visual monitoring of progressing angiogenesis. Vasculature development can be examined either through alkaline phosphatase staining or through fluorescent dye/beads followed by microscopic examination (Figure 3.11). Recently, different transgenic zebrafish models have been engineered for easier visualization of vasculature and used extensively in angiogenesis studies. These fish express GFP from native promoters of endothelial genes (Fli-GFP, mTie2-GFP, and Flk-GFP). The transgenic fish model offers a better visualization of vasculature in developing embryos and can also be analyzed over a period of time (Young and Weinstein 2007). However, there are concerns regarding the suitability of embryonic zebrafish as a model for studying and understanding the process of angiogenesis in adult humans. In zebrafish

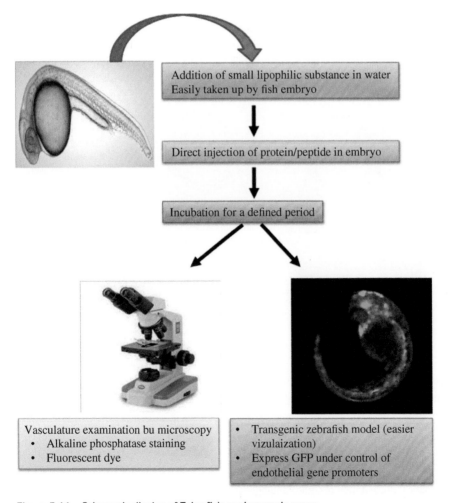

Figure 3.11   Schematic display of Zebrafish angiogenesis assay.

embryo, neovascularization involves both vasculogenesis and angiogenesis. Distinguishing these two processes at the embryonic stage is difficult. Furthermore, the exact region that participates in angiogenesis is ill identified. However, subintestinal veins are recognized to be formed through angiogenesis and hence, preferred while using embryonic zebrafish model while studying angiogenesis (Zheng et al. 2007; Staton et al. 2009; Irvin et al. 2014).

3.9.5 Cornea Angiogenesis Assay

The cornea is considered as an appropriate model for the *in vivo* angiogenesis because of its avascular nature and therefore, any vascular development occurs due to test substance under examination. This model was first developed for the rabbit, now it is widely used in mice and rats. In this assay, a pocket is created in the corneal stroma of an experimental animal, followed by the insertion of the test substance into it (Auerbach et al. 2003). The test substance could be tumor tissue or cells, drugs, growth factors, cytokines, conditioned media, etc. Various types of slow-release polymer pellets are also used for the controlled delivery of test substances. To test the anti-angiogenic potential of the compound, experimental animals can be treated either through systematic administration or through an eye drop applied directly. Angiogenic response and neovascularization are analyzed visually; the cornea is perfused with either florescent dye or India ink that helps in the visualization of the blood vessel. Then, corneas are extracted and certain parameters are used for the determination of neovascularization that includes counting of vessel number and determining the length and density of new vessels (Sarayba et al. 2005; Staton et al. 2009). This assay offers reliable and measurable readouts. Use of transgenic mice also allows the study of molecular mechanisms (Figure 3.12).

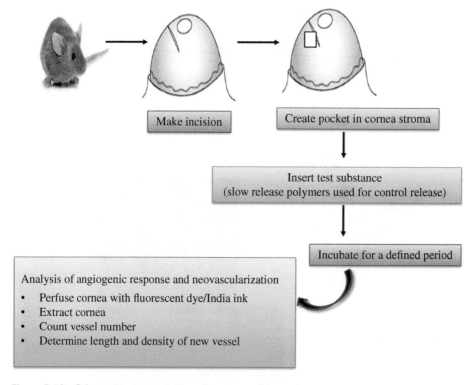

Figure 3.12 Schematic representation of cornea angiogenesis assay.

However, ease of use of this assay is limited by its specific requirement for technical perfection in surgery. Besides, corneal angiogenesis provides two-dimensional environments, whereas human angiogenesis naturally occurs in three dimensions. Thus, certain level of uncertainty exists as to how closely this angiogenic model can represent overall process. Ethical concerns are also raised against the invasive usage of a main sensory organ (Irvin et al. 2014).

3.10 Conclusion

The aberrations in the equilibrium between pro- and anti-angiogenic molecules play a significant role in various pathological complications. A number of drugs are available to treat angiogenesis, but because of their adverse side effects alternative approach must be looked for which there will be lesser or no side effects. Many phytochemicals have been reported to have potentials to treat angiogenesis. In this chapter, we mainly emphasized such angiogenic potentials of phytochemical, dietary bioactive compounds, nutraceuticals, and their mechanism of actions as potent anti/pro-angiogenic agents. Generally, most of them seems to target and subsequently downregulate the angiogenic factors (FGF, Ang, VEGF, and MMPs), block phosphorylation of the receptors, or inhibit receptor-mediated signaling pathways (PI3K/Akt and ERK pathways). In addition, these phytochemicals also target oncogenic miRNAs, involved in cancer-related angiogenesis. Such multi-targeting by phytochemicals during angiogenic modulation can be a plausible reason behind their cyto-safety. Just like a coin has two sides, a minor drawback with these phytochemicals is their low bioavailability. However, this flaw can be resolved with the help of biodegradable nano-carriers. Extensive preclinical researches have paved the way for clinical trials on these phyto-chemicals. In the context of cancer treatment (if not angiogenesis in particular), many such phytochemicals have entered into prospective clinical trials with even some being already in clinical use. Thus, angiogenesis-specific clinical trials of phytochemicals/nutraceuticals are possible and they might be in the pipeline and soon be reported.

References

Abduljawad, S. H., El-Refaei, M. F. and El-Nashar, N. N. (2013) Protective and anti-angiopathy effects of caffeic acid phenethyl ester against induced type 1 diabetes in vivo, *International Immunopharmacology*. 17(2), pp. 408–414. doi:https://doi.org/10.1016/j.intimp.2013.06.019.

Aggarwal, B. B., Gupta, S. C. and Sung, B. (2013) 'Curcumin: an orally bioavailable blocker of TNF and other pro-inflammatory biomarkers', *British Journal of Pharmacology*, 169(8), pp. 1672–1692. doi:https://doi.org/10.1111/bph.12131.

Ai, F., Chen, M., Yu, B. et al. (2015). Puerarin accelerate scardiac angiogenesis and improves cardiac function of myocardial infarction by upregulating VEGFA, Ang-1 and Ang-2 in rats. *International Journal of Clinical and Experimental Medicine* 8 (11): 20821–20828.

Akhtar, N., Dickerson, E. B. and Auerbach, R. (2002) 'The sponge/Matrigel angiogenesis assay', *Angiogenesis*, 5(1–2), pp. 75–80. doi:https://doi.org/10.1023/A:1021507031486.

Albini, A., Noonan, D. M. and Ferrari, N. (2007) 'Molecular pathways for cancer angioprevention', *Clinical Cancer Research*, 13(15), pp. 4320–4325. doi: https://doi.org/10.1158/1078-0432. CCR-07-0069.

Aldair, T. and Montani, J. (2010). Chapter 1. Overview of angiogenesis. *Angiogenesis* 2: 1–10.

Alex, D., Leong, E. C., Zhang, Z. J. et al. (2010) 'Resveratrol derivative, trans-3,5,4′-trimethoxystilbene, exerts antiangiogenic and vascular-disrupting effects in zebrafish through the downregulation of VEGFR2 and cell-cycle modulation', *Journal of Cellular Biochemistry*, 109(2), pp. 339–346. doi: https://doi.org/10.1002/jcb.22405.

Alkharfy, K. M., Ahmad, A., Khan, R. M., and Al-Shagha, W. M. (2014) 'Pharmacokinetic plasma behaviors of intravenous and oral bioavailability of thymoquinone in a rabbit model', *European Journal of Drug Metabolism and Pharmacokinetics*, 40(3), pp. 319–323. doi: https://doi.org/10.1007/s13318-014-0207-8.

Amano, H., Hayashi I., Endo H. et al. (2003) 'Host prostaglandin E2-EP3 signaling regulates tumor-associated angiogenesis and tumor growth', *Journal of Experimental Medicine*, 197(2), pp. 221–232. doi: https://doi.org/10.1084/jem.20021408.

Anand, P., Thomas, S. G., Kunnumakkara, A. B. et al. (2008) 'Biological activities of curcumin and its analogues (Congeners) made by man and mother nature', *Biochemical Pharmacology*, 76(11), pp. 1590–1611. doi: https://doi.org/10.1016/j.bcp.2008.08.008.

Ann Beltz, L., Kay Bayer, D., Lynn Moss, A., and Mitchell Simet, I. (2006) 'Mechanisms of cancer prevention by green and black tea polyphenols', *Anti-Cancer Agents in Medicinal Chemistry*, 6(5), pp. 389–406. doi: https://doi.org/10.2174/187152006778226468.

Ansó, E., Zuazo, A., Irigoyen, M. et al. (2010) 'Flavonoids inhibit hypoxia-induced vascular endothelial growth factor expression by a HIF-1 independent mechanism', *Biochemical Pharmacology*, 79(11), pp. 1600–1609. doi: https://doi.org/10.1016/j.bcp.2010.02.004.

Arbiser, J. L., Klauber, N., Rohan, R. et al. (1998) 'Curcumin is an in vivo inhibitor of angiogenesis', *Molecular Medicine*, 4(6), pp. 376–383. doi: https://doi.org/10.1007/BF03401744.

Asahara, T., Chen, D., Takahashi, T. et al. (1998) Tie2 receptor ligands, angiopoietin-1 and angiopoietin-2, modulate VEGF-induced postnatal neovascularization. *Circulation Research*, 83(3), pp. 233–240. doi: https://doi.org/10.1093/oxfordjournals.aje.a116359.

Asarch, A., Barak, O., Loo, D. S., and Gottlieb, A. B. (2008) 'Th17 cells: a new paradigm for cutaneous inflammation', *Journal of Dermatological Treatment*, 19(5), pp. 259–266. doi: https://doi.org/10.1080/09546630802206686.

Atta-ur-Rahman (2018) Studies in Natural Products Chemistry. Vol. 56, pp. 1–478. San Diego: Elsevier Science. doi: https://doi.org/10.1016/B978-0-444-64058-1.00006-6.

Auerbach, R., Lewis, R., Shinners, B. et al. (2003) 'Angiogenesis assays: a critical overview', *Clinical Chemistry*, 49(1), pp. 32–40. doi: https://doi.org/10.1373/49.1.32.

Augustine, R., Prasad, P. and Khalaf, I. M. N. (2019) Therapeutic angiogenesis: from conventional approaches to recent nanotechnology-based interventions, *Materials Science and Engineering C*. 97, pp. 994–1008. doi: https://doi.org/10.1016/j.msec.2019.01.006.

Azam, F., Mehta, S. and Harris, A. L. (2010) Mechanisms of resistance to antiangiogenesis therapy *European Journal of Cancer*. 46(8), pp. 1323–1332. doi: https://doi.org/10.1016/j.ejca.2010.02.020.

Banerjee, T., Van der Vliet, A. and Ziboh, V. A. (2002) 'Downregulation of COX-2 and iNOS by amentoflavone and quercetin in A549 human lung adenocarcinoma cell line', *Prostaglandins Leukotrienes and Essential Fatty Acids*, 66(5–6), pp. 485–492. doi: https://doi.org/10.1054/plef.2002.0387.

Bergers, G. and Hanahan, D. (2008) 'Modes of resistance to anti-angiogenic therapy', *Nature Reviews Cancer*, 8(8), pp. 592–603. doi: https://doi.org/10.1038/nrc2442.

Bhatia, N., Gupta, P., Singh, B., and Koul, A. (2015) 'Lycopene enriched tomato extract inhibits hypoxia, angiogenesis, and metastatic markers in early stage *N*-nitrosodiethylamine induced hepatocellular carcinoma', *Nutrition and Cancer*, 67(8), pp. 1270–1277. doi: https://doi.org/10.1080/01635581.2015.1087040.

Bimonte, S., Barbieri, A., Palma, G. et al. (2013) 'Curcumin inhibits tumor growth and angiogenesis in an orthotopic mouse model of human pancreatic cancer', *BioMed Research International*, 2013:810423. doi: https://doi.org/10.1155/2013/810423.

Binion, D. G., Otterson, M. F. and Rafiee, P. (2008) 'Curcumin inhibits VEGF-mediated angiogenesis in human intestinal microvascular endothelial cells through COX-2 and MAPK inhibition', *Gut*, 57(11), pp. 1509–1517. doi: https://doi.org/10.1136/gut.2008.152496.

Bocci, G., Di Paolo, A. and Danesi, R. (2013) 'The pharmacological bases of the antiangiogenic activity of paclitaxel', *Angiogenesis*, 16(3), pp. 481–492. doi: https://doi.org/10.1007/s10456-013-9334-0.

Bottaro, D. P. and Liotta, L. A. (2003) 'Out of air is not out of action', *Nature*, 423(6940), pp. 593–595. doi: https://doi.org/10.1038/423593a.

Bråkenhielm, E., Cao, R. and Cao, Y. (2001) 'Suppression of angiogenesis, tumor growth, and wound healing by resveratrol, a natural compound in red wine and grapes', *The FASEB Journal*, 15(10), pp. 1798–1800. doi: https://doi.org/10.1096/fj.01-0028fje.

Burri, P. H. and Tarek, M. R. (1990) 'A novel mechanism of capillary growth in the rat pulmonary microcirculation', *The Anatomical Record*, 228(1), pp. 35–45. doi: https://doi.org/10.1002/ar.1092280107.

Bushati, N. and Cohen, S. M. (2007) 'microRNA functions', *Annual Review of Cell and Developmental Biology*, 23(1), pp. 175–205. doi: https://doi.org/10.1146/annurev.cellbio.23.090506.123406.

Bushati, N. and Cohen, S. M. (2008) 'microRNAs in neurodegeneration', *Current Opinion in Neurobiology*, 18(3), pp. 292–296. doi: https://doi.org/10.1016/j.conb.2008.07.001.

Cai, Z. Y., Li, X. M., Liang, J. P. et al. (2018) 'Bioavailability of tea catechins and its improvement', *Molecules*, 23(9), pp. 2346. doi: https://doi.org/10.3390/molecules23092346.

Cao, Z., Fang, J., Xia, C. et al. (2004) 'Trans-3,4,5′-Trihydroxystibene inhibits hypoxia-inducible factor 1α and vascular endothelial growth factor expression in human ovarian cancer cells', *Clinical Cancer Research*, 10(15), pp. 5253–5263. doi: https://doi.org/10.1158/1078-0432.CCR-03-0588.

Cao, Y., Ye, Q., Zhuang, M. et al. (2017) 'Ginsenoside Rg3 inhibits angiogenesis in a rat model of endometriosis through the VEGFR-2-mediated PI3K/Akt/mTOR signaling pathway', *PLoS ONE*, 12(11), pp. e0186520. doi: https://doi.org/10.1371/journal.pone.0186520.

Cárdenas, C., Quesada, A. R. and Medina, M. A. (2011) 'Anti-angiogenic and anti-inflammatory properties of kahweol, a coffee diterpene', *PLoS ONE*, 6(8). e23407 doi: https://doi.org/10.1371/journal.pone.0023407.

Carmeliet, P. (2003) 'Angiogenesis in health and disease', *Nature Medicine*, 9(6), pp. 653–660. doi: https://doi.org/10.1016/S0306-3623(01)00111-2.

Carmeliet, P. (2005) 'Angiogenesis in life, disease and medicine', *Nature*, 438(7070), pp. 932–936. doi: https://doi.org/10.1038/nature04478.

Chang, T.-C. and Mendell, J. T. (2007) 'microRNAs in vertebrate physiology and human disease', *Annual Review of Genomics and Human Genetics*, 8(1), pp. 215–239. doi: https://doi.org/10.1146/annurev.genom.8.080706.092351.

Chen, H. X. and Cleck, J. N. (2009) Adverse effects of anticancer agents that target the VEGF pathway, *Nature Reviews Clinical Oncology*, 6(8), pp. 465–477. doi: https://doi.org/10.1038/nrclinonc.2009.94.

Chen, J.C., Chen, Y., Lin, J.H. et al. (2006). Resveratrol suppresses angiogenesis in gliomas: evaluation by color Doppler ultrasound. *Anticancer Research* 26 (2A): 1237–1245.

Chen, M. L., Lin, Y. H., Yang, C. M., and Hu, M. L. (2012) 'Lycopene inhibits angiogenesis both in vitro and in vivo by inhibiting MMP-2/uPA system through VEGFR2-mediated PI3K-Akt and ERK/p38 signaling pathways', *Molecular Nutrition and Food Research*, 56(6), pp. 889–899. doi: https://doi.org/10.1002/mnfr.201100683.

Choi, S., Kim, K. W., Choi, J. S. et al. (2002) 'Angiogenic activity of β-sitosterol in the ischaemia/reperfusion-damaged brain of Mongolian gerbil', *Planta Medica*, 68(4), pp. 330–335. doi: https://doi.org/10.1055/s-2002-26750.

Choi, H., Chun, Y. S., Kim, S. W. *et al.* (2006) 'Curcumin inhibits hypoxia-inducible factor-1 by degrading aryl hydrocarbon receptor nuclear translocator: a mechanism of tumor growth inhibition', *Molecular Pharmacology*, 70(5), pp. 1664–1671. doi: https://doi.org/10.1124/mol.106.025817.

Zyting Chu, Jen-Shi Chen, Chi-Ting Liau, Hung-Ming Wang, Yung-Chang Lin, Muh-Hwa Yang, Po-Min Chen, Erin R. Gardner, William D. Figg, A. S. (2008) 'Oral bioavailability of a novel paclitaxel formulation (Genetaxyl) administered with cyclosporin A in cancer patients', *Anticancer Drugs*, 19(3), pp. 275. doi: https://doi.org/10.1038/jid.2014.371.

Chung, A. S. and Ferrara, N. (2011) 'Developmental and pathological angiogenesis', *Annual Review of Cell and Developmental Biology*, 27(1), pp. 563–584. doi: https://doi.org/10.1146/annurev-cellbio-092910-154002.

Claffey, K.P., Wilkison, W.O., and Spiegelman, B.M. (1992). Vascular endothelial growth factor. Regulation by cell differentiation and activated second messenger pathways. *Journal of Biological Chemistry* 267 (23): 16317–16322.

Cross, N. A., Fowles, A., Reeves, K. et al. (2008) 'Imaging the effects of castration on bone turnover and hormone-independent prostate cancer colonization of bone', *The Prostate*, 68(15), pp. 1707–1714. doi: https://doi.org/10.1002/pros.20833.

Cutchins, A., Harmon, D. B., Kirby, J. et al. (2012) 'Inhibitor of differentiation-3 mediates high fat diet-induced visceral fat expansion', *Arteriosclerosis, Thrombosis, and Vascular Biology*, 32(2), pp. 317–324. doi: https://doi.org/10.1161/ATVBAHA.111.234856.

Dai, J., Lin, Y., Duan, Y. et al. (2017) 'Andrographolide inhibits angiogenesis by inhibiting the Mir-21-5p/TIMP3 signaling pathway', *International Journal of Biological Sciences*, 13(5), pp. 660–668. doi: https://doi.org/10.7150/ijbs.19194.

Daly, C., Pasnikowski, E., Burova, E. *et al.* (2006) 'Angiopoietin-2 functions as an autocrine protective factor in stressed endothelial cells', *Proceedings of the National Academy of Sciences of the United States of America*, 103(42), pp. 15491–15496. doi: https://doi.org/10.1073/pnas.0607538103.

Dameron, K. M., Volpert, O. V., Tainsky, M. A., & Bouck, N. (1994) 'Control of angiogenesis in fibroblasts by p53 regulation of thrombospondin-1', *Science*, 265(5178), pp. 1582–1584. doi: https://doi.org/10.1126/science.7521539.

Das, S., Dey, K. K., Dey, G. et al. (2012) 'Antineoplastic and apoptotic potential of traditional medicines thymoquinone and diosgenin in squamous cell carcinoma', *PLoS ONE*, 7(10), pp. e46641. doi: https://doi.org/10.1371/journal.pone.0046641.

De La Parra, C., Castillo-Pichardo, L., Cruz-Collazo, A. et al. (2016) 'Soy isoflavone genistein-mediated downregulation of miR-155 contributes to the anticancer effects of genistein', *Nutrition and Cancer*, 68(1), pp. 154–164. doi: https://doi.org/10.1080/01635581.2016.1115104.

DeFeudis, F. V., Papadopoulos, V. and Drieu, K. (2003) 'Ginkgo biloba extracts and cancer: a research area in its infancy', *Fundamental and Clinical Pharmacology*, 17(4), pp. 405–417. doi: https://doi.org/10.1046/j.1472-8206.2003.00156.x.

Demeule, M., Michaud-Levesque, J., Annabi, B. et al. (2002) 'Green tea catechins as novel antitumor and antiangiogenic compounds', *Current Medicinal Chemistry – Anti-Cancer Agents*, 2(4), pp. 441–463. doi: https://doi.org/10.2174/1568011023353930.

Diniz, C., Suliburska, J. and Ferreira, I. M. P. L. V. O. (2017) 'New insights into the antiangiogenic and proangiogenic properties of dietary polyphenols', *Molecular Nutrition and Food Research*, 61(6), pp. 1–38. doi: https://doi.org/10.1002/mnfr.201600912.

Do, M. T., Kim, H. G., Choi, J. H. et al. (2013) Antitumor efficacy of piperine in the treatment of human HER2-overexpressing breast cancer cells. *Food Chemistry*. 141(3), pp. 2591–2599. doi: https://doi.org/10.1016/j.foodchem.2013.04.125.

Donà, M., Dell'Aica, I., Calabrese, F. et al. (2003) 'Neutrophil restraint by green tea: inhibition of inflammation, associated angiogenesis, and pulmonary fibrosis', *The Journal of Immunology*, 170(8), pp. 4335–4341. doi: https://doi.org/10.4049/jimmunol.170.8.4335.

Dong, G., Liang, X., Wang, D. et al. (2014) 'High expression of miR-21 in triple-negative breast cancers was correlated with a poor prognosis and promoted tumor cell in vitro proliferation', *Medical Oncology*, 31(7).57 doi: https://doi.org/10.1007/s12032-014-0057-x.

Doucette, C. D., Hilchie, A. L., Liwski, R., and Hoskin, D. W. (2013) 'Piperine, a dietary phytochemical, inhibits angiogenesis', *Journal of Nutritional Biochemistry*, 24(1), pp. 231–239. doi: https://doi.org/10.1016/j.jnutbio.2012.05.009.

Dreyfuss, J. L., Giordano, R. J. and Regatieri, C. V. (2015) 'Ocular angiogenesis', *Journal of Ophthalmology*, 2015, pp. 2–4. doi: https://doi.org/10.1155/2015/892043.

Du, J., Yang, Q., Luo, L., & Yang, D. (2016) C1qr and C1qrl redundantly regulate angiogenesis in zebrafish through controlling endothelial Cdh5. *Biochemical and Biophysical Research Communications*. 483(1), pp. 482–487. doi: https://doi.org/10.1016/j.bbrc.2016.12.118.

Eddahibi, S., Humbert, M., Sediame, S. et al. (2000) Imbalance between platelet vascular endothelial growth factor and platelet-derived growth factor in pulmonary hypertension: effect of prostacyclin therapy. *American Journal of Respiratory and Critical Care Medicine*, 162(4), pp. 1493–1499. doi: https://doi.org/10.1164/ajrccm.162.4.2003124.

El Sayed, K. A. (2005) 'Natural products as angiogenesis modulators', *Mini-Reviews in Medicinal Chemistry*, 5, pp. 971–993. doi: https://doi.org/10.1055/s-2006-957559.

Elias, P. M., Arbiser, J., Brown, B. et al. (2008) 'Epidermal vascular endothelial growth factor production is required for permeability barrier homeostasis, dermal angiogenesis, and the development of epidermal hyperplasia: implications for the pathogenesis of psoriasis: *American Journal of Pathology*, 173(3), pp. 689–699. doi: https://doi.org/10.2353/ajpath.2008.080088.

Escuin, D., Kline, E. R. and Giannakakou, P. (2005) 'Both microtubule-stabilizing and microtubule-destabilizing drugs inhibit hypoxia-inducible factor-1α accumulation and activity by disrupting microtubule function', *Cancer Research*, 65(19), pp. 9021–9028. doi: https://doi.org/10.1158/0008-5472.CAN-04-4095.

Esquela-Kerscher, A. and Slack, F. J. (2006) 'Oncomirs – microRNAs with a role in cancer', *Nature Reviews Cancer*, 6(4), pp. 259–269. doi: https://doi.org/10.1038/nrc1840.

Eun, J. P. and Koh, G. Y. (2004) 'Suppression of angiogenesis by the plant alkaloid, sanguinarine', *Biochemical and Biophysical Research Communications*, 317(2), pp. 618–624. doi: https://doi.org/10.1016/j.bbrc.2004.03.077.

Fan, T. P., Yeh, J. C., Leung, K. et al. (2006) 'Angiogenesis: from plants to blood vessels', *Trends in Pharmacological Sciences*, 27(6), pp. 297–309. doi: https://doi.org/10.1016/j.tips.2006.04.006.

Fish, J. E., Santoro, M. M., Morton, S. U. et al. (2008) 'miR-126 regulates angiogenic signaling and vascular integrity', *Developmental Cell*, 15(2), pp. 272–284. doi: https://doi.org/10.1016/j.devcel.2008.07.008.

Foa, R., Norton, L. and Seidman, A. D. (1994) 'Taxol (paclitaxel): a novel anti-microtubule agent with remarkable anti-neoplastic activity', *International Journal of Clinical and Laboratory Research*, 24(1), pp. 6–14. doi: https://doi.org/10.1007/BF02592403.

Folkman, J. (1971) 'Tumor angiogenesis:therapeutic implications', *The New England Journal of Medicine*, 285(21), pp. 1182–1186. doi: https://doi.org/10.1056/NEJM196006162622401.

Folkman, J. (1990) 'What is the evidence that tumors are angiogenesis dependent?', *Journal of the National Cancer Institute*, 82(1), pp. 4–7. doi: https://doi.org/10.1093/jnci/82.1.4.

Folkman, J. (1995a) 'Angiogenesis in cancer, vascular, rheumatoid and other disease', *Nature Medicine*, 1(1), pp. 27–30. doi: https://doi.org/10.1038/nm0195-27.

Folkman, J. (1995b). Clinical Applications of Research on Angiogenesis. *The New England Journal of Medicine* 333 (26): 1757–1763.

Folkman, J. (2006) 'Ngiogenesis Judah Folkman', *Vascular*, 57, pp. 1–18. doi: https://doi.org/10.1146/annurev.med.57.121304.131306.

Folkman, J. and Shing, Y. (1992). Angiogenesis. *Journal of Biological Chemistry* 267 (16): 10931–10934.

Fotsis, T., Pepper, M., Adlercreutz, H. et al. (1993) 'Genistein, a dietary-derived inhibitor of in vitro angiogenesis', *Proceedings of the National Academy of Sciences of the United States of America*, 90(7), pp. 2690–2694. doi: https://doi.org/10.1073/pnas.90.7.2690.

Fu, Z., Chen, X., Guan, S. et al. (2015) 'Curcumin inhibits angiogenesis and improves defective hematopoiesis induced by tumor-derived VEGF in tumor model through modulating VEGF-VEGFR2 signaling pathway', *Oncotarget*, 6(23), pp. 19469–19482. doi: https://doi.org/10.18632/oncotarget.3625.

Furness, M., Robinson, T., Ehlers, T. et al. (2005) 'Antiangiogenic agents: studies on fumagillin and curcumin analogs', *Current Pharmaceutical Design*, 11(3), pp. 357–373. doi: https://doi.org/10.2174/1381612053382142.

Gao, W., McCormick, J., Connolly, M. et al. (2015) 'Hypoxia and STAT3 signalling interactions regulate pro-inflammatory pathways in rheumatoid arthritis', *Annals of the Rheumatic Diseases*, 74(6), pp. 1275–1283. doi: https://doi.org/10.1136/annrheumdis-2013-204105.

Gao, J. L., Shui, Y. M., Jiang, W. et al. (2016) 'Hypoxia pathway and hypoxia-mediated extensive extramedullary hematopoiesis are involved in ursolic acid's anti-metastatic effect in 4T1 tumor bearing mice', *Oncotarget*, 7(44), pp. 71802–71816. doi: https://doi.org/10.18632/oncotarget.12375.

Gartel, A. L. (2010) 'A new target for proteasome inhibitors: FoxM1', *Expert Opinion on Investigational Drugs*, 19(2), pp. 235–242. doi: https://doi.org/10.1517/13543780903563364.

Garvin, S., Öllinger, K. and Dabrosin, C. (2006) 'Resveratrol induces apoptosis and inhibits angiogenesis in human breast cancer xenografts in vivo', *Cancer Letters*, 231(1), pp. 113–122. doi: https://doi.org/10.1016/j.canlet.2005.01.031.

de Gramont, A., Van Cutsem, E., Schmoll, H. J. et al. (2012) Bevacizumab plus oxaliplatin-based chemotherapy as adjuvant treatment for colon cancer (AVANT): a phase 3 randomised controlled trial. *The Lancet Oncology*, 13(12), pp. 1225–1233. doi: https://doi.org/10.1016/S1470-2045(12)70509-0.

Granci, V., Dupertuis, Y. M. and Pichard, C. (2010) 'Angiogenesis as a potential target of pharmaconutrients in cancer therapy', *Current Opinion in Clinical Nutrition and Metabolic Care*, 13(4), pp. 417–422. doi: https://doi.org/10.1097/MCO.0b013e3283392656.

Grycová, L., Dostál, J. and Marek, R. (2007) 'Quaternary protoberberine alkaloids', *Phytochemistry*, 68(2), pp. 150–175. doi: https://doi.org/10.1016/j.phytochem.2006.10.004.

Gu, J. W., Makey, K. L., Tucker, K. B. et al. (2013) 'EGCG, a major green tea catechin suppresses breast tumor angiogenesis and growth via inhibiting the activation of HIF-1α and NFκB, and VEGF expression', *Vascular Cell*, 5(1), pp. 1–10. doi: https://doi.org/10.1186/2045-824X-5-9.

Guo, D., Jia, Q., Song, H. Y. et al. (1995) 'Vascular endothelial cell growth factor promotes tyrosine phosphorylation of mediators of signal transduction that contain SH2 domains. Association with endothelial cell proliferation. *Journal of Biological Chemistry*, 270(12): pp. 6729–6733. doi: https://doi.org/10.1074/jbc.270.12.6729.

Guo Bei-chia, Wei, J., Su, K. H. et al. (2015) Transient receptor potential vanilloid type 1 is vital for (−)-epigallocatechin-3-gallate-mediated activation of endothelial nitric oxide synthase. *Molecular Nutrition & Food Research*, 59(4): pp. 646–657. doi: https://doi.org/10.1002/mnfr.201400013.

Guruvayoorappan, C. and Kuttan, G. (2007) 'β-Carotene inhibits tumor-specific angiogenesis by altering the cytokine profile and inhibits the nuclear translocation of transcription factors in B16F-10 melanoma cells', *Integrative Cancer Therapies*, 6(3), pp. 258–270. doi: https://doi.org/10.1177/1534735407305978.

Hao, Q., Wang, L. and Tang, H. (2009) 'Vascular endothelial growth factor induces protein kinase D-dependent production of proinflammatory cytokines in endothelial cells', *American Journal of Physiology – Cell Physiology*, 296(4). C821–C827 doi: https://doi.org/10.1152/ajpcell.00504.2008.

Hirose, S., Hosoda, Y., Furuya, S. et al. (2000) 'Expression of vascular endothelial growth factor and its receptors correlates closely with formation of the plexiform lesion in human pulmonary hypertension', *Pathology International*, 50(6), pp. 472–479. doi: https://doi.org/10.1046/j.1440-1827.2000.01068.x.

Holmgren, L., O'reilly, M. S. and Folkman, J. (1995) 'Dormancy of micrometastases: balanced proliferation and apoptosis in the presence of angiogenesis suppression', *Nature Medicine*, 1(2), pp. 149–153. doi: https://doi.org/10.1038/nm0295-149.

Hong, S.-J., Wan, J.-B., Zhang, Y. et al. (2009) 'Angiogenic effect of saponin extract from *Panax notoginseng* on HUVECs in vitro and zebrafish in vivo', *Phytotherapy Research*, 23, pp. 677–686. doi: https://doi.org/10.1002/ptr.

Hu, N. X., Chen, M., Liu, Y. S. et al. (2019) 'Pharmacokinetics of sanguinarine, chelerythrine, and their metabolites in broiler chickens following oral and intravenous administration', *Journal of Veterinary Pharmacology and Therapeutics*, 42(2), pp. 197–206. doi: https://doi.org/10.1111/jvp.12729.

Huang, Z. and Bao, S. D. (2004) 'Roles of main pro- and anti-angiogenic factors in tumor angiogenesis', *World Journal of Gastroenterology*, 10(4), pp. 463–470. doi: https://doi.org/10.3748/wjg.v10.i4.463.

Huang, C. S., Chuang, C. H., Lo, T. F., and Hu, M. L. (2013) 'Anti-angiogenic effects of lycopene through immunomodualtion of cytokine secretion in human peripheral blood mononuclear cells', *Journal of Nutritional Biochemistry*, 24(2), pp. 428–434. doi: https://doi.org/10.1016/j.jnutbio.2012.01.003.

Huang, J. S., Yao, C. J., Chuang, S. E. et al. (2016) 'Honokiol inhibits sphere formation and xenograft growth of oral cancer side population cells accompanied with JAK/STAT signaling pathway suppression and apoptosis induction. *BMC Cancer*, 16(1), pp. 1–13. doi: https://doi.org/10.1186/s12885-016-2265-6.

Hutson, T. E., Figlin, R. A., Kuhn, J. G., and Motzer, R. J. (2008) 'Targeted therapies for metastatic renal cell carcinoma: an overview of toxicity and dosing strategies', *The Oncologist*, 13(10), pp. 1084–1096. doi: https://doi.org/10.1634/theoncologist.2008-0120.

Igura, K., Ohta, T., Kuroda, Y., and Kaji, K. (2001) 'Resveratrol and quercetin inhibit angiogenesis in vitro', *Cancer Letters*, 171(1), pp. 11–16. doi: https://doi.org/10.1016/S0304-3835(01)00443-8.

Irvin, M. W., Zijlstra, A., Wikswo, J. P., and Pozzi, A. (2014) 'Techniques and assays for the study of angiogenesisa', *Experimental Biology and Medicine*, 239(11), pp. 1–7. doi: https://doi.org/10.1038/jid.2014.371.

Jang, J. Y., Lee, J. K., Jeon, Y. K., and Kim, C. W. (2013) 'Exosome derived from epigallocatechin gallate treated breast cancer cells suppresses tumor growth by inhibiting tumor-associated macrophage infiltration and M2 polarization', *BMC Cancer*, 13:421. doi: https://doi.org/10.1186/1471-2407-13-421.

Jiang, F. S., Tian, S. S., Lu, J. J. et al. (2015) 'Cardamonin regulates miR-21 expression and suppresses angiogenesis induced by vascular endothelial growth factor', *BioMed Research International*, 2015:501581. doi: https://doi.org/10.1155/2015/501581.

Jiao, D., Wang, J., Lu, W. et al. (2016) Curcumin inhibited HGF-induced EMT and angiogenesis through regulating c-Met dependent PI3K/Akt/mTOR signaling pathways in lung cancer', *Molecular Therapy – Oncolytics*, 3, p. 16018. doi: https://doi.org/10.1038/mto.2016.18.

Jie, S., Li, H., Tian, Y. et al. (2011) 'Berberine inhibits angiogenic potential of Hep G2 cell line through VEGF down-regulation in vitro', *Journal of Gastroenterology and Hepatology (Australia)*, 26(1), pp. 179–185. doi: https://doi.org/10.1111/j.1440-1746.2010.06389.x.

Jung, Y. D. and Ellis, L. M. (2001) 'Inhibition of tumour invasion and angiogenesis by epigallocatechin gallate (EGCG), a major component of green tea', *International Journal of Experimental Pathology*, 82(6), pp. 309–316. doi: https://doi.org/10.1046/j.1365-2613.2001.00205.x.

Jung, J. E., Kim, H. S., Lee, C. S. et al. (2007) 'Caffeic acid and its synthetic derivative CADPE suppress tumor angiogenesis by blocking STAT3-mediated VEGF expression in human renal carcinoma cells', *Carcinogenesis*, 28(8), pp. 1780–1787. doi: https://doi.org/10.1093/carcin/bgm130.

Kadioglu, O., Seo, E. J., and Efferth, T. (2013) 'Targeting angiogenesis by phytochemicals', *Medicinal and Aromatic Plants*, 02(05). doi: https://doi.org/10.4172/2167-0412.1000134.

Kabon, B., Nagele, A., Reddy, D. et al. (2004) 'Obesity decreases perioperative tissue oxygenation', *Anesthesiology*, 100(2), pp. 274–280. doi: https://doi.org/10.1097/00000542-200402000-00015.

Kalaivani, V. and Jaleel, A. (2020) Apolipoprotein(a), an enigmatic anti-angiogenic glycoprotein in human plasma: a curse or cure?, *Pharmacological Research*. 158, p. 104858. doi: https://doi.org/10.1016/j.phrs.2020.104858.

Kalantari, K., Moniri, M., Moghaddam, A. B. et al. (2017) 'A review of the biomedical applications of zerumbone and the techniques for its extraction from ginger rhizomes', *Molecules*, 22(10). doi: https://doi.org/10.3390/molecules22101645.

Kalinski, T., Sel, S., Hütten, H. et al. (2014) 'Curcumin blocks interleukin-1 signaling in chondrosarcoma cells', *PLoS ONE*, 9(6) e99296. doi: https://doi.org/10.1371/journal.pone.0099296.

Kanjoormana, M. and Kuttan, G. (2010) 'Antiangiogenic activity of ursolic acid', *Integrative Cancer Therapies*, 9(2), pp. 224–235. doi: https://doi.org/10.1177/1534735410367647.

Kasikci, M.B. and Bagdatlioglu, N. (2016). Bioavailability of quercetin. *Current Research in Nutrition and Food Science* 4 (Special Issue 2): 146–151. https://doi.org/10.12944/CRNFSJ.4. Special-Issue-October.20.

Katiyar, S., Elmets, C. A. and Katiyar, S. K. (2007) 'Green tea and skin cancer: photoimmunology, angiogenesis and DNA repair', *Journal of Nutritional Biochemistry*, 18(5), pp. 287–296. doi: https://doi.org/10.1016/j.jnutbio.2006.08.004.

Katsuaki, S., Mochizuki, M., Ikuo, S. et al. (1994). Inhibition of tumor angiogenesis and metastasis by a saponin of *Panax ginseng*, ginsenoside-Rb2. *Biological and Pharmaceutical Bulletin* 17 (5): 635–639. http://www.mendeley.com/research/geology-volcanic-history-eruptive-style-yakedake-volcano-group-central-japan/.

Kaulmann, A. and Bohn, T. (2014) 'Carotenoids, inflammation, and oxidative stress-implications of cellular signaling pathways and relation to chronic disease prevention. *Nutrition Research*, 34(11), pp. 907–929. doi: https://doi.org/10.1016/j.nutres.2014.07.010.

Keung, M. H., Chan, L. S., Kwok, H. H. et al. (2016) Role of microRNA-520h in 20(R)-ginsenoside-Rg3-mediated angiosuppression. *Journal of Ginseng Research*, 40(2), pp. 151–159. doi: https://doi.org/10.1016/j.jgr.2015.07.002.

Kim, J. W., Jung, S. Y., Kwon, Y. H. et al. (2012) 'Ginsenoside Rg3 attenuates tumor angiogenesis via inhibiting bioactivities of endothelial progenitor cells', *Cancer Biology and Therapy*, 13(7), pp. 504–515. doi: https://doi.org/10.4161/cbt.19599.

Koch, A. E. (1998) 'Angiogenesis: Implications for rheumatoid arthritis', *Arthritis and Rheumatism*, 41(6), pp. 951–962. doi: https://doi.org/10.1002/1529-0131(199806)41:6<951::AID-ART2>3.0.CO;2-D.

Koroma, B. M. and de Juan, E. (1994) 'Phosphotyrosine inhibition and control of vascular endothelial cell proliferation by genistein', *Biochemical Pharmacology*, 48(4), pp. 809–818. doi: https://doi.org/10.1016/0006-2952(94)90060-4.

Kuehbacher, A., Urbich, C., Zeiher, A. M., and Dimmeler, S. (2007) 'Role of dicer and drosha for endothelial microRNA expression and angiogenesis', *Circulation Research*, 101(1), pp. 59–68. doi: https://doi.org/10.1161/CIRCRESAHA.107.153916.

Kümpers, P., Nickel, N., Lukasz, A. et al. (2010) 'Circulating angiopoietins in idiopathic pulmonary arterial hypertension', *European Heart Journal*, 31(18), pp. 2291–2300. doi: https://doi.org/10.1093/eurheartj/ehq226.

Kuroda, K., Sapadin, A., Shoji, T. et al. (2001) 'Altered expression of angiopoietins and Tie2 endothelium receptor in psoriasis', *Journal of Investigative Dermatology*, 116(5), pp. 713–720. doi: https://doi.org/10.1046/j.1523-1747.2001.01316.x.

Lai, P., Chan, J., Kwok, H. F. et al. (2014) Induction of angiogenesis in zebrafish embryos and proliferation of endothelial cells by an active fraction isolated from the root of astragalus membranaceus using bioassay-guided fractionation. *Journal of Traditional and Complementary Medicine*, 4(4), pp. 239–245. doi: https://doi.org/10.4103/2225-4110.139109.

Lainer-Carr, D. and Brahn, E. (2007) 'Angiogenesis inhibition as a therapeutic approach for inflammatory synovitis', *Nature Clinical Practice Rheumatology*, 3(8), pp. 434–442. doi: https://doi.org/10.1038/ncprheum0559.

Lam, H. W., Lin, H. C., Lao, S. C. et al. (2008) 'The angiogenic effects of *Angelica sinensis* extract on HUVEC in vitro and zebrafish in vivo', *Journal of Cellular Biochemistry*, 103(1), pp. 195–211. doi: https://doi.org/10.1002/jcb.21403.

Langowski, J. L., Zhang, X., Wu, L. et al. (2006) 'IL-23 promotes tumour incidence and growth', *Nature*, 442(7101), pp. 461–465. doi: https://doi.org/10.1038/nature04808.

Lassus, P., Turanlahti, M., Heikkilä, P. et al. (2001) Pulmonary vascular endothelial growth factor and Flt-1 in fetuses, in acute and chronic lung disease, and in persistent pulmonary hypertension of the newborn *American Journal of Respiratory and Critical Care Medicine*, 164, pp. 1981–1987. doi: https://doi.org/10.1164/rccm2012036.

Lay, I. S., Chiu, J. H., Shiao, M. S. et al. (2003) 'Crude extract of *Salvia miltiorrhiza* and salvianolic acid B enhance in vitro angiogenesis in murine SVR endothelial cell line', *Planta Medica*, 69(1), pp. 26–32. doi: https://doi.org/10.1055/s-2003-37034.

Lee, S. H., Lee, J., Jung, M. H., and Lee, Y. M. (2013) 'Glyceollins, a novel class of soy phytoalexins, inhibit angiogenesis by blocking the VEGF and bFGF signaling pathways', *Molecular Nutrition and Food Research*, 57(2), pp. 225–234. doi: https://doi.org/10.1002/mnfr.201200489.

Leung, K. W., Cheung, L. W. T., Pon, Y. L. et al. (2007) 'Ginsenoside Rb1 inhibits tube-like structure formation of endothelial cells by regulating pigment epithelium-derived factor through the oestrogen β receptor', *British Journal of Pharmacology*, 152(2), pp. 207–215. doi: https://doi.org/10.1038/sj.bjp.0707359.

Li, Y. J., Duan, C. L., Liu, J. X., and Xu, Y. G. (2010) Pro-angiogenic actions of Salvianolic acids on in vitro cultured endothelial progenitor cells and chick embryo chorioallantoic membrane model *Journal of Ethnopharmacology*. 131(3), pp. 562–566. doi: https://doi.org/10.1016/j.jep.2010.07.040.

Li, S., Lou, S., Lei, B. U. W. et al. (2011) 'Transcriptional profiling of angiogenesis activities of calycosin in zebrafish', *Molecular BioSystems*, 7(11), pp. 3112–3121. doi: https://doi.org/10.1039/c1mb05206c.

Li, H., Jin, S.-Y., Son, H.-J. et al. (2013) 'Caffeine-induced endothelial cell death and the inhibition of angiogenesis', *Anatomy & Cell Biology*, 46(1), p. 57. doi: https://doi.org/10.5115/acb.2013.46.1.57.

Li, Y. J., Duan, C. L. and Liu, J. X. (2014) Salvianolic acid A promotes the acceleration of neovascularization in the ischemic rat myocardium and the functions of endothelial progenitor cells. *Journal of Ethnopharmacology*. 151(1), pp. 218–227. doi: https://doi.org/10.1016/j.jep.2013.10.019.

Li, F., Bai, Y., Zhao, M. et al. (2015a) 'Quercetin inhibits vascular endothelial growth factor-induced choroidal and retinal angiogenesis in vitro', *Ophthalmic Research*, 53(3), pp. 109–116. doi: https://doi.org/10.1159/000369824.

Li, S., Zhou, X. L., Dang, Y. Y. et al. (2015b) Basal Flt1 tyrosine kinase activity is a positive regulator of endothelial survival and vascularization during zebrafish embryogenesis *Biochimica et Biophysica Acta – General Subjects*. 1850(2), pp. 373–384. doi: https://doi.org/10.1016/j.bbagen.2014.10.023.

Li, S., Dang, Y., Zhou, X. et al. (2015c) Formononetin promotes angiogenesis through the estrogen receptor alpha-enhanced ROCK pathway, *Scientific Reports*, 5, pp. 1–17. doi: https://doi.org/10.1038/srep16815.

Li, M. Y., Mi, C., Wang, K. S. et al. (2017) Shikonin suppresses proliferation and induces cell cycle arrest through the inhibition of hypoxia-inducible factor-1α signaling *Chemico-Biological Interactions*. 274, pp. 58–67. doi: https://doi.org/10.1016/j.cbi.2017.06.029.

Lin, M. T., Yen, M. I., Lin, C. Y., and Kuo, M. L. (2003) 'Inhibition of vascular endothelial growth factor-induced angiogenesis by resveratrol through interruption of src-dependent vascular endothelial cadherin tyrosine phosphorylation', *Molecular Pharmacology*, 64(5), pp. 1029–1036. doi: https://doi.org/10.1124/mol.64.5.1029.

Lin, C. M., Chiu, J. H., Wu, I. H. et al. (2010) 'Ferulic acid augments angiogenesis via VEGF, PDGF and HIF-1α', *Journal of Nutritional Biochemistry*, 21(7), pp. 627–633. doi: https://doi.org/10.1016/j.jnutbio.2009.04.001.

Lin, J., Chen, Y., Wei, L. et al. (2013) 'Ursolic acid inhibits colorectal cancer angiogenesis through suppression of multiple signaling pathways', *International Journal of Oncology*, 43(5), pp. 1666–1674. doi: https://doi.org/10.3892/ijo.2013.2101.

Liu, C. L., Cheng, L., Kwok, H. F. et al. (2011) Bioassay-guided isolation of norviburtinal from the root of Rehmannia glutinosa, exhibited angiogenesis effect in zebrafish embryo model *Journal of Ethnopharmacology*. 137(3), pp. 1323–1327. doi: https://doi.org/10.1016/j.jep.2011.07.060.

Liu, Y., Whelan, R. J., Pattnaik, B. R. et al. (2012) 'Terpenoids from *Zingiber officinale* (Ginger) induce apoptosis in endometrial cancer cells through the activation of p53', *PLoS ONE*, 7(12). e53178 doi: https://doi.org/10.1371/journal.pone.0053178.

Liu, P., Atkinson, S. J., Akbareian, S. E. et al. (2017) Sulforaphane exerts anti-angiogenesis effects against hepatocellular carcinoma through inhibition of STAT3/HIF-1α/VEGF signalling. *Scientific Reports* 7(1), pp. 1–11. doi: https://doi.org/10.1038/s41598-017-12855-w.

Lopes, F. C. M., Regasini L.O., de Magalhães Pinheiro Alçada M.N., and Soares R. (2013) Antiangiogenic alkaloids from plants. Ramawat, K. G. and Merillon, J. M. (eds) *Natural Products: Phytochemistry, Botany and Metabolism of Alkaloids, Phenolics and Terpenes*. Berlin, Heidelberg: Springer. doi: https://doi.org/10.1007/978-3-642-22144-6_48.

Lu, Q., Lu, S., Gao, X. et al. (2012) 'Norisoboldine, an alkaloid compound isolated from *Radix linderae*, inhibits synovial angiogenesis in adjuvant-induced arthritis rats by moderating Notch1 pathway-related endothelial tip cell phenotype', *Experimental Biology and Medicine*, 237(8), pp. 919–932. doi: https://doi.org/10.1258/ebm.2012.011416.

Lu, H., Zhou, X., Kwok, H. H. et al. (2017) Ginsenoside-Rb1-mediated anti-angiogenesis via regulating PEDF and miR-33a through the activation of PPAR-γ pathway. *Frontiers in Pharmacology*, 8(NOV), pp. 1–9. doi: https://doi.org/10.3389/fphar.2017.00783.

Lugano, R., Ramachandran, M. and Dimberg, A. (2019) Tumor angiogenesis: causes, consequences, challenges and opportunities. *Cellular and Molecular Life Sciences*. 77(9), pp. 1745–1770. doi:https://doi.org/10.1007/s00018-019-03351-7.

Ma, Z. L., Wang, G., Lu, W. H. et al. (2016) Investigating the effect of excess caffeine exposure on placental angiogenesis using chicken "functional" placental blood vessel network', *Journal of Applied Toxicology*, 36(2), pp. 285–295. doi: https://doi.org/10.1002/jat.3181.

Maisonpierre, P. C., Suri, C., Jones, P.F. et al. (1997) 'Angiopoietin-2, a natural antagonist for Tie2 that disrupts in vivo angiogenesis', *Science*, 277(5322), pp. 55–60. doi: https://doi.org/10.1126/science.277.5322.55.

Man, X. Y., Yang, X. H., Cai, S. Q. et al. (2008) Overexpression of vascular endothelial growth factor (VEGF) receptors on keratinocytes in psoriasis: regulated by calcium independent of VEGF. *Journal of Cellular and Molecular Medicine*, 12(2), pp. 649–660. doi: https://doi.org/10.1111/j.1582-4934.2007.00112.x.

Martínez-Poveda, B., Quesada, A. R. and Medina, M. Á. (2005) Hyperforin, a bio-active compound of St. John's Wort, is a new inhibitor of angiogenesis targeting several key steps of the process *International Journal of Cancer*, 117(5), pp. 775–780. doi: https://doi.org/10.1002/ijc.21246.

Maurya, A. K. and Vinayak, M. (2017) Quercetin attenuates cell survival, inflammation, and angiogenesis via modulation of AKT signaling in murine T-cell lymphoma. *Nutrition and Cancer*. 69(3), pp. 470–480. doi: https://doi.org/10.1080/01635581.2017.1267775.

McGarry, T., Biniecka, M., Veale, D. J., and Fearon, U. (2018) Hypoxia, oxidative stress and inflammation. *Free Radical Biology and Medicine*. 125, pp. 15–24. doi: https://doi.org/10.1016/j.freeradbiomed.2018.03.042.

Mizejewski, G. J. (1999) 'Role of integrins in cancer: survey of expression patterns', *Proceedings of the Society for Experimental Biology and Medicine*, 222(2), pp. 124–138. doi: https://doi.org/10.1046/j.1525-1373.1999.d01-122.x.

Mlala, S., Oyedeji, A. O., Gondwe, M., and Oyedeji, O. O. (2019) 'Ursolic acid and its derivatives as bioactive agents', *Molecules (Basel, Switzerland)*, 24(15), pp. 1–25. doi: https://doi.org/10.3390/molecules24152751.

Mochizuki, M., Yoo, Y.C., Matsuzawa, K. et al. (1995). Inhibitory effect of tumor metastasis in mice by saponins,ginsenoside-Rb2,20(*R*)- and 20(*S*)-ginsenoside-Rg3, of red ginseng. *Biological and Pharmaceutical Bulletin* 18 (9): 1197–1202. http://www.mendeley.com/research/geology-volcanic-history-eruptive-style-yakedake-volcano-group-central-japan/.

Moon, E., Lee, Y. M., Lee, O. et al. (1999) A novel angiogenic factor derived from Aloe vera gel: β-sitosterol, a plant sterol. *Angiogenesis* 3, pp. 117–123. doi:https://doi.org/10.1023/A:1009058232389.

Muthukkaruppan, V. R., Kubai, L. and Auerbach, R. (1982) 'Tumor-induced neovascularization in the mouse eye.', *Journal of the National Cancer Institute*, 69(3), pp. 699–708. doi: https://doi.org/10.1093/jnci/69.3.699.

Myoung, H., Hong, S. P., Yun, P. Y. et al. (2003) 'Anti-cancer effect of genistein in oral squamous cell carcinoma with respect to angiogenesis and in vitro invasion', *Cancer Science*, 94(2), pp. 215–220. doi: https://doi.org/10.1111/j.1349-7006.2003.tb01422.x.

Nagineni, C. N., Kommineni, V. K., William, A. et al. (2012) 'Regulation of VEGF expression in human retinal cells by cytokines: implications for the role of inflammation in age-related macular degeneration', *Journal of Cellular Physiology*, 227(1), pp. 116–126. doi: https://doi.org/10.1002/jcp.22708.

Nagineni, C. N., Raju, R., Nagineni, K. K. et al. (2014) 'Resveratrol suppresses expression of VEGF by human retinal pigment epithelial cells: potential nutraceutical for age-related macular degeneration', *Aging and Disease*, 5(2), pp. 88–100. doi: https://doi.org/10.14366/AD.2014.050088.

Naksuriya, O., Okonogi, S., Schiffelers, R. M., and Hennink, W. E. (2014) Curcumin nanoformulations: a review of pharmaceutical properties and preclinical studies and clinical data related to cancer treatment. *Biomaterials*, 35(10), pp. 3365–3383. doi: https://doi.org/10.1016/j.biomaterials.2013.12.090.

Nelson, A. R., Fingleton, B., Rothenberg, M. L., and Matrisian, L. M. (2017) Biology of neoplasia matrix metallo proteinases: biologic activity and clinical implications', *Journal of Clinical Oncology*, 18(5), pp. 1135–1149. doi: https://doi.org/10.1200/JCO.2000.18.5.1135.

Neufeld, G. and Kessler, O. (2006) Pro-angiogenic cytokines and their role in tumor angiogenesis. *Cancer and Metastasis Reviews*, 25(3), pp. 373–385. doi: https://doi.org/10.1007/s10555-006-9011-5.

Ng, Y. P., Or, T. C. T. and Ip, N. Y. (2015) Plant alkaloids as drug leads for Alzheimer's disease. *Neurochemistry International*, 89, pp. 260–270. doi: https://doi.org/10.1016/j.neuint.2015.07.018.

Nickoloff, B. J. (2000) 'Characterization of lymphocyte-dependent angiogenesis using a SCID mouse: human skin model of psoriasis', *Journal of Investigative Dermatology Symposium Proceedings*, 5(1), pp. 67–73. doi: https://doi.org/10.1046/j.1087-0024.2000.00006.x.

Nickoloff, B. J., Wrone-Smith, T., Bonish, B., and Porcelli, S. A. (1999) Response of murine and normal human skin to injection of allogeneic blood-derived psoriatic immunocytes *Archives of Dermatology*, 135(5), pp. 546–552. doi: https://doi.org/10.1001/archderm.135.5.546.

Nickoloff, B. J., Qin, J. Z. and Nestle, F. O. (2007) 'Immunopathogenesis of psoriasis', *Clinical Reviews in Allergy and Immunology*, 33(1–2), pp. 45–56. doi: https://doi.org/10.1007/s12016-007-0039-2.

Noori-Daloii, M. R., Momeny, M., Yousefi, M. et al. (2011) Multifaceted preventive effects of single agent quercetin on a human prostate adenocarcinoma cell line (PC-3): implications for nutritional transcriptomics and multi-target therapy. *Medical Oncology*, 28(4), pp. 1395–1404. doi: https://doi.org/10.1007/s12032-010-9603-3.

Numasaki, M., Fukushi, J. I., Ono, M. et al. (2003) 'Interleukin-17 promotes angiogenesis and tumor growth', *Blood*, 101(7), pp. 2620–2627. doi: https://doi.org/10.1182/blood-2002-05-1461.

Ou-Yang, X.Y., Wang, W.J., Liao, W.H., and Chen, X.H. (2005). Inhibitory effect of ginkgolide B on angiogenesis in chronic inflammation. *Acta Pharmaceutica Sinica* 40 (4): 311–315.

Palmer, T. D., Lewis, J. and Zijlstra, A. (2011) 'Quantitative analysis of cancer metastasis using an avian embryo model.', *Journal of Visualized Experiments: JoVE*, (51), pp. 3–8. doi: https://doi.org/10.3791/2815.

Papaioannou, A. I., Zakynthinos, E., Kostikas, K. et al. (2009) 'Serum VEGF levels are related to the presence of pulmonary arterial hypertension in systemic sclerosis', *BMC Pulmonary Medicine*, 9, pp. 1–8. doi: https://doi.org/10.1186/1471-2466-9-18.

Paper, D. H. (1998) 'Natural products as angiogenesis inhibitors', *Planta Medica*, 64(8), pp. 686–695. doi: https://doi.org/10.1055/s-2006-957559.

Papetti, M. and Herman, I. M. (2002) Mechanisms of normal and tumor-derived angiogenesis. *American Journal of Physiology – Cell Physiology*, 282(5): 51–55. doi: https://doi.org/10.1152/ajpcell.00389.2001.

Parangi, S., O'Reilly, M., Christofori, G. et al. (1996) 'Antiangiogenic therapy of transgenic mice impairs de novo tumor growth', *Proceedings of the National Academy of Sciences of the United States of America*, 93(5), pp. 2002–2007. doi: https://doi.org/10.1073/pnas.93.5.2002.

Park, S. Y., Jeong, K. J., Lee, J. et al. (2007) 'Hypoxia enhances LPA-induced HIF-1α and VEGF expression: their inhibition by resveratrol', *Cancer Letters*, 258(1), pp. 63–69. doi: https://doi.org/10.1016/j.canlet.2007.08.011.

Park, S., Sorenson, C. M. and Sheibani, N. (2015) 'PECAM-1 isoforms, eNOS and endoglin axis in regulation of angiogenesis', *Clinical Science*, 129(3), pp. 217–234. doi: https://doi.org/10.1042/CS20140714.

Peng, L., Liu, A., Shen, Y. et al. (2013) 'Antitumor and anti-angiogenesis effects of thymoquinone on osteosarcoma through the NF-κB pathway', *Oncology Reports*, 29(2), pp. 571–578. doi: https://doi.org/10.3892/or.2012.2165.

Perry, B. N., Govindarajan, B., Bhandarkar, S. S. et al. (2006) 'Pharmacologic blockade of angiopoietin-2 is efficacious against model hemangiomas in mice', *Journal of Investigative Dermatology*, 126(10), pp. 2316–2322. doi: https://doi.org/10.1038/sj.jid.5700413.

Petreaca, M. L., Yao, M., Liu, Y. et al. (2007) 'Transactivation of vascular endothelial growth factor receptor-2 by interleukin-8 (IL-8/CXCL8) is required for IL-8/CXCL8-induced endothelial permeability', *Molecular Biology of the Cell*, 18, pp. 5014–5023. doi: https://doi.org/10.1091/mbc.E07.

Poliseno, L., Tuccoli, A., Mariani, L. et al. (2006) MicroRNAs modulate the angiogenic properties of HUVECs. *Blood*, 108(9), pp. 3068–3071. doi: https://doi.org/10.1182/blood-2006-01-012369.

Prasad, S., Tyagi, A. K. and Aggarwal, B. B. (2014) 'Recent developments in delivery, bioavailability, absorption and metabolism of curcumin: the golden pigment from golden spice', *Cancer Research and Treatment*, 46(1), pp. 2–18. doi: https://doi.org/10.4143/crt.2014.46.1.2.

Pratheeshkumar, P., Budhraja, A., Son, Y. et al. (2012) 'Quercetin inhibits angiogenesis mediated human prostate tumor growth by targeting VEGFR-2 regulated AKT/mTOR/P70S6K signaling pathways', *PLoS ONE*, 7(10), pp. 1–10. doi: https://doi.org/10.1371/journal.pone.0047516.

Rabinovitch, M. (2008) 'Molecular pathogenesis of pulmonary arterial hypertension', *The Journal of Clinical Investigation*, 118(7), pp. 2372–2379. doi: https://doi.org/10.1007/978-3-319-31407-5_26.

Rabinovitch, M. (2012) 'Molecular pathogenesis of pulmonary arterial hypertension find the latest version: science in medicine molecular pathogenesis of pulmonary arterial hypertension', *Journal of Clinical Investigation*, 122(12), pp. 4306–4313. doi: https://doi.org/10.1172/JCI60658DS1.

Rajasekar, J., Perumal, M. K. and Vallikannan, B. (2019) 'A critical review on anti-angiogenic property of phytochemicals', *Journal of Nutritional Biochemistry*, 71, pp. 1–15. doi: https://doi.org/10.1016/j.jnutbio.2019.04.006.

Rojo, L. E., Villano, C. M., Joseph, G. et al. (2010) 'Wound-healing properties of nut oil from *Pouteria lucuma*', *Journal of Cosmetic Dermatology*, 9(3), pp. 185–195. doi: https://doi.org/10.1111/j.1473-2165.2010.00509.x.

Sahu, P. K., Sharma, A., Rayees, S. et al. (2014) Pharmacokinetic study of piperine in wistar rats after oral and intravenous administration, *International Journal of Drug Delivery*, 6(1), pp. 82–87. doi: https://doi.org/10.5138/ijdd.v6i1.1353.

Samad, N. A., Abdul, A. B., Rahman, H. S. et al. (2018) Zerumbone suppresses angiogenesis in HepG2 cells through inhibition of matrix metalloproteinase-9, vascular endothelial growth factor, and vascular endothelial growth factor receptor expressions. *Pharmacognosy Magazine*, 13 (Suppl 62), pp. 179–188. doi: https://doi.org/10.4103/pm.pm.

Saraswati, S. and Agrawal, S. S. (2013) 'Brucine, an indole alkaloid from *Strychnos nux-vomica* attenuates VEGF-induced angiogenesis via inhibiting VEGFR2 signaling pathway in vitro and in vivo', *Cancer Letters*, 332(1), pp. 83–93. doi: https://doi.org/10.1016/j.canlet.2013.01.012.

Saraswati, S., Kanaujia, P. K., Kumar, S. et al. (2013) Tylophorine, a phenanthraindolizidine alkaloid isolated from *Tylophora indica* exerts antiangiogenic and antitumor activity by targeting vascular endothelial growth factor receptor 2-mediated angiogenesis. *Molecular Cancer* 12(1), p. 1. doi: https://doi.org/10.1186/1476-4598-12-82.

Sarayba, M. A., Li, L., Tungsiripat, T. et al. (2005) 'Inhibition of corneal neovascularization by a peroxisome proliferator-activated receptor-γ ligand', *Experimental Eye Research*, 80(3), pp. 435–442. doi: https://doi.org/10.1016/j.exer.2004.10.009.

Sartippour, M. R., Shao, Z.-M., Heber, D. et al. (2002) 'Green tea inhibits vascular endothelial growth factor (VEGF) induction in human breast cancer cells', *The Journal of Nutrition*, 132(8), pp. 2307–2311. doi: https://doi.org/10.1093/jn/132.8.2307.

Schempp, C. M., Kiss, J., Kirkin, V. et al. (2005) 'Hyperforin acts as an angiogenesis inhibitor in vitro and in vivo', *Planta Medica*, 71(11), pp. 999–1004. doi: https://doi.org/10.1055/s-2005-871303.

Schütte, A., Hedrich, J., Stöcker, W., and Becker-Pauly, C. (2010) 'Let it flow: morpholino knockdown in zebrafish embryos reveals a pro-angiogenic effect of the metalloprotease meprin α2', *PLoS ONE*, 5(1), pp. 1–6. doi: https://doi.org/10.1371/journal.pone.0008835.

Selimovic, N., Bergh, C. H., Andersson, B. et al. (2009) 'Growth factors and interleukin-6 across the lung circulation in pulmonary hypertension', *European Respiratory Journal*, 34(3), pp. 662–668. doi: https://doi.org/10.1183/09031936.00174908.

Sengupta, S., Gherardi, E., Sellers, L. A. et al. (2003) 'Hepatocyte growth factor/scatter factor can induce angiogenesis independently of vascular endothelial growth factor', *Arteriosclerosis, Thrombosis, and Vascular Biology*, 23(1), pp. 69–75. doi: https://doi.org/10.1161/01. ATV.0000048701.86621.D0.

Sengupta, S., Toh, S. A., Sellers, L. A. et al. (2004) 'Modulating angiogenesis: the yin and the yang in ginseng', *Circulation*, 110(10), pp. 1219–1225. doi: https://doi.org/10.1161/01. CIR.0000140676.88412.CF.

Shamoto, T., Matsuo, Y., Shibata, T. et al. (2014) 'Zerumbone inhibits angiogenesis by blocking NF-κB activity in pancreatic cancer', *Pancreas*, 43(3), pp. 396–404. doi: https://doi.org/10.1097/ MPA.0000000000000039.

Shankar, S., Chen, Q. and Srivastava, R. K. (2008) 'Inhibition of PI3K/AKT and MEK/ERK pathways act synergistically to enhance antiangiogenic effects of EGCG through activation of FOXO transcription factor', *Journal of Molecular Signaling*, 3, pp. 1–11. doi: https://doi. org/10.1186/1750-2187-3-7.

Shankar, S., Marsh, L. and Srivastava, R. K. (2013) 'EGCG inhibits growth of human pancreatic tumors orthotopically implanted in Balb C nude mice through modulation of FKHRL1/FOXO3a and neuropilin', *Molecular and Cellular Biochemistry*, 372(1–2), pp. 83–94. doi: https://doi.org/10.1007/ s11010-012-1448-y.

Shanmugam, M. K., Manu, K. A., Ong, T. H. *et al.* (2011a) 'Inhibition of CXCR4/CXCL12 signaling axis by ursolic acid leads to suppression of metastasis in transgenic adenocarcinoma of mouse prostate model', *International Journal of Cancer*, 129(7), pp. 1552–1563. doi: https://doi.org/10.1002/ijc.26120.

Shanmugam, M. K., Rajendran, P., Li, F. *et al.* (2011b) 'Ursolic acid inhibits multiple cell survival pathways leading to suppression of growth of prostate cancer xenograft in nude mice', *Journal of Molecular Medicine*, 89(7), pp. 713–727. doi: https://doi.org/10.1007/s00109-011-0746-2.

Shehata, S. M. K., Mooi, W. J., Okazaki, T. et al. (1999) 'Enhanced expression of vascular endothelial growth factor in lungs of newborn infants with congenital diaphragmatic hernia and pulmonary hypertension', *Thorax*, 54(5), pp. 427–431. doi: https://doi.org/10.1136/thx.54.5.427.

Shen, K., Ji, L., Lu, B. et al. (2014) Andrographolide inhibits tumor angiogenesis via blocking VEGFA/ VEGFR2-MAPKs signaling cascade. *Chemico-Biological Interactions*. 218, pp. 99–106. doi: https:// doi.org/10.1016/j.cbi.2014.04.020.

Shibuya, M. (2008) 'Vascular endothelial growth factor-dependent and-independent regulation of angiogenesis', *BMB Reports*, 41(4), pp. 278–286. doi: https://doi.org/10.5483/BMBRep.2008.41.4.278.

Shrader, C. D., Ressetar, H. G., Luo, J. et al. (2008) 'Acute stretch promotes endothelial cell proliferation in wounded healing mouse skin', *Archives of Dermatological Research*, 300(9), pp. 495–504. doi: https://doi.org/10.1007/s00403-008-0836-3.

Shukla, S., Sinha, S., Khan, S. et al. (2016) Cucurbitacin B inhibits the stemness and metastatic abilities of NSCLC via downregulation of canonical Wnt/β-catenin signaling axis. *Scientific Reports*, 6, pp. 1–17. doi: https://doi.org/10.1038/srep21860.

Singh, R. P. and Agarwal, R. (2007) Inducible nitric oxide synthase-vascular endothelial growth factor axis: a potential target to inhibit tumor angiogenesis by dietary agents', *Current Cancer Drug Targets*, 7(5), pp. 475–483. doi: https://doi.org/10.2174/156800907781386632.

Sinha, S., Khan, S., Shukla, S. et al. (2016) Cucurbitacin B inhibits breast cancer metastasis and angiogenesis through VEGF-mediated suppression of FAK/MMP-9 signaling axis. *International Journal of Biochemistry and Cell Biology*. 77, pp. 41–56. doi: https://doi.org/10.1016/j.biocel.2016.05.014.

Smith, S. K. (2001) 'Angiogenesis and reproduction', *British Journal of Obstetrics and Gynaecology*, 108(8), pp. 777–783. doi: https://doi.org/10.1016/S0306-5456(00)00211-4.

Souyoul, S. A., Saussy, K. P. and Lupo, M. P. (2018) Nutraceuticals: a review. *Dermatology and Therapy*, 8(1), pp. 5–16. doi: https://doi.org/10.1007/s13555-018-0221-x.

Staton, C. A., Stribbling, S. M., Tazzyman, S. et al. (2004) 'Current methods for assaying angiogenesis in vitro and in vivo', *International Journal of Experimental Pathology*, 85(5), pp. 233–248. doi: https://doi.org/10.1111/j.0959-9673.2004.00396.x.

Staton, C. A., Reed, M. W. R. and Brown, N. J. (2009) 'A critical analysis of current in vitro and in vivo angiogenesis assays', *International Journal of Experimental Pathology*, 90(3), pp. 195–221. doi: https://doi.org/10.1111/j.1365-2613.2008.00633.x.

Suri, C., Jones, P. F., Patan, S. et al. (1996) 'Requisite role of angiopoietin-1, a ligand for the TIE2 receptor, during embryonic angiogenesis', *Cell*, 87(7), pp. 1171–1180. doi: https://doi.org/10.1016/S0092-8674(00)81813-9.

Szekanecz, Z. and Koch, A. E. (2007) 'Mechanisms of disease: angiogenesis in inflammatory diseases', *Nature Clinical Practice Rheumatology*, 3(11), pp. 635–643. doi: https://doi.org/10.1038/ncprheum0647.

Szekanecz, Z. and Koch, A. E. (2008) Vascular involvement in rheumatic diseases: cascular rheumatology, *Arthritis Research and Therapy*, 10(5). 224 doi: https://doi.org/10.1186/ar2515.

Talcott, S.U., Li, X., Chintharlapalli, S., and Safe, S. (2020). The effects of betulinic acid on microRNA – 27a regulated target genes in MDA – MB – 231 breast cancer cells. *Experimental Biology* 22: 26–28.

Tam, J., Duda, D. G., Perentes, J. Y. et al. (2009) 'Blockade of VEGFR2 and not VEGFR1 can limit diet-induced fat tissue expansion: role of local versus bone marrow-derived endothelial cells', *PLoS ONE*, 4(3), pp. 1–6. doi: https://doi.org/10.1371/journal.pone.0004974.

Tang, J. Y., Li, S., Li, Z. H. *et al.* (2010) 'Calycosin promotes angiogenesis involving estrogen receptor and mitogen-activated protein kinase (MAPK) signaling pathway in zebrafish and HUVEC', *PLoS ONE*, 5(7), pp. 1–14. doi: https://doi.org/10.1371/journal.pone.0011822.

Taylor, P. C. and Sivakumar, B. (2005) 'Hypoxia and angiogenesis in rheumatoid arthritis', *Current Opinion in Rheumatology*, 17(3), pp. 293–298. doi: https://doi.org/10.1097/01.bor.0000155361.83990.5b.

Teekachunhatean, S., Tosri, N., Rojanasthien, N. et al. (2013) Pharmacokinetics of caffeine following a single administration of coffee enema versus oral coffee consumption in healthy male subjects. *ISRN Pharmacology*, 2013, pp. 1–7. doi: https://doi.org/10.1155/2013/147238.

Teleanu, R. I., Chircov, C., Grumezescu, A. M., and Teleanu, D. M. (2019) 'Tumor angiogenesis and anti-angiogenic strategies for cancer treatment', *Journal of Clinical Medicine*, 9(1), p. 84. doi: https://doi.org/10.3390/jcm9010084.

Tereza, J. Y., Belleri, C. M., Morbidelli, L. et al. (2011) The natural compound *n*-butylidenephthalide derived from the volatile oil of *Radix angelica* sinensis inhibits angiogenesis in vitro and in vivo. *Angiogenesis* 14 pp. 187–197. doi: https://doi.org/10.1007/s10456-011-9202-8.

Thangarasu, P., Manikandan, A. and Thamaraiselvi, S. (2019) Discovery, synthesis and molecular corroborations of medicinally important novel pyrazoles; drug efficacy determinations through in silico, in vitro and cytotoxicity validations. *Bioorganic Chemistry*. 86, pp. 410–419. doi: https://doi.org/10.1016/j.bioorg.2019.02.003.

Thulliez, M., Angoulvant, D., Le Lez, M. L. et al. (2014) 'Cardiovascular events and bleeding risk associated with intravitreal antivascular endothelial growth factor monoclonal antibodies: systematic review and meta-analysis', *JAMA Ophthalmology*, 132(11), pp. 1317–1326. doi: https://doi.org/10.1001/jamaophthalmol.2014.2333.

Tili, E., Michaille, J. J., Adair, B. et al. (2010) 'Resveratrol decreases the levels of miR-155 by upregulating miR-663, a microRNA targeting JunB and JunD', *Carcinogenesis*, 31(9), pp. 1561–1566. doi: https://doi.org/10.1093/carcin/bgq143.

Tiwari, A., Mukherjee, B. and Dixit, M. (2017) 'MicroRNA key to angiogenesis regulation: MiRNA biology and therapy', *Current Cancer Drug Targets*, 18(3), pp. 266–277. doi: https://doi.org/10.2174/1568009617666170630142725.

Tonnesen, M.G., Feng, X., and Clark, R.A. (2000). Angiogenesis in wound healing (supplement). *The Society for Investigative Dermatology, Inc.* 5: 40–46.

Tournaire, R., Simon, M. P., le Noble, F. et al. (2004) 'A short synthetic peptide inhibits signal transduction, migration and angiogenesis mediated by Tie2 receptor', *EMBO Reports*, 5(3), pp. 262–267. doi: https://doi.org/10.1038/sj.embor.7400100.

Treggiari, D., Dalbeni, A., Meneguzzi, A. et al. (2018) Lycopene inhibits endothelial cells migration induced by vascular endothelial growth factor A increasing nitric oxide bioavailability, *Journal of Functional Foods*, 42, pp. 312–318. doi: https://doi.org/10.1016/j.jff.2018.01.020.

Tsuboi, K., Matsuo, Y., Shamoto, T. et al. (2014) 'Zerumbone inhibits tumor angiogenesis via NF-κB in gastric cancer', *Oncology Reports*, 31(1), pp. 57–64. doi: https://doi.org/10.3892/or.2013.2842.

Tuder, R. M., Flook, B. E. and Voelkel, N. F. (1995) 'Increased gene expression for VEGF and the VEGF receptors KDR/Flk and Flt in lungs exposed to acute or to chronic hypoxia: modulation of gene expression by nitric oxide', *Journal of Clinical Investigation*, 95(4), pp. 1798–1807. doi: https://doi.org/10.1172/JCI117858.

Tuder, R. M., Chacon, M., Alger, L. et al. (2001) 'Expression of angiogenesis-related molecules in plexiform lesions in severe pulmonary hypertension: evidence for a process of disordered angiogenesis', *Journal of Pathology*, 195(3), pp. 367–374. doi: https://doi.org/10.1002/path.953.

Tzeng, T. F., Liou, S. S., Tzeng, Y. C., and Liu, I. M. (2016) 'Zerumbone, a phytochemical of subtropical ginger, protects against hyperglycemia-induced retinal damage in experimental diabetic rats', *Nutrients*, 8(8):449. doi: https://doi.org/10.3390/nu8080449.

Urbich, C., Kuehbacher, A. and Dimmeler, S. (2008) 'Role of microRNAs in vascular diseases, inflammation, and angiogenesis', *Cardiovascular Research*, 79(4), pp. 581–588. doi: https://doi.org/10.1093/cvr/cvn156.

Van Dam, R. M., Naidoo, N. and Landberg, R. (2013) 'Dietary flavonoids and the development of type 2 diabetes and cardiovascular diseases: review of recent findings', *Current Opinion in Lipidology*, 24(1), pp. 25–33. doi: https://doi.org/10.1097/MOL.0b013e32835bcdff.

Van Hof, K.H., West, C.E., Weststrate, J.A., and Hautvast, J.G. (2000). Recent advances in nutritional sciences dietary factors that affect the bioavailability of carotenoids. *The Journal of Nutrition* 14: 503–506.

Van Rooij, E. and Olson, E. N. (2007) 'MicroRNAs: powerful new regulators of heart disease and provocative therapeutic targets', *Journal of Clinical Investigation*, 117(9), pp. 2369–2376. doi: https://doi.org/10.1172/JCI33099.

Vasudev, N. S. and Reynolds, A. R. (2014) 'Anti-angiogenic therapy for cancer: current progress, unresolved questions and future directions', *Angiogenesis*, 17(3), pp. 471–494. doi: https://doi.org/10.1007/s10456-014-9420-y.

Veale, D. J. and Fearon, U. (2006) 'Inhibition of angiogenic pathways in rheumatoid arthritis: potential for therapeutic targeting', *Best Practice and Research: Clinical Rheumatology*, 20(5), pp. 941–947. doi: https://doi.org/10.1016/j.berh.2006.05.004.

Villadsen, L. S., Schuurman, J., Beurskens, F. et al. (2003) Resolution of psoriasis upon blockade of IL-15 biological activity in a xenograft mouse model. *Journal of Clinical Investigation*, 112(10), pp. 1571–1580. doi: https://doi.org/10.1172/JCI200318986.

Voelkel, N.F. and R.M. Tuder. (2002) Angiogenesis and pulmonary hypertension: a unique process in a unique disease. *Antioxidants & Redox Signaling*, 4, pp. 883–843. doi: https://doi.org/10.1111/j.1475-4959.2010.00371.x.

Voelkel, N. F., Vandivier, R. W. and Tuder, R. M. (2006) 'Vascular endothelial growth factor in the lung', *American Journal of Physiology – Lung Cellular and Molecular Physiology*, 290(2):L209–L221. doi: https://doi.org/10.1152/ajplung.00185.2005.

Wahedi, H. M., Jeong, M., Chae, J. K. et al. (2017) Aloesin from *Aloe vera* accelerates skin wound healing by modulating MAPK/Rho and Smad signaling pathways in vitro and in vivo. *Phytomedicine*. 28, pp. 19–26. doi: https://doi.org/10.1016/j.phymed.2017.02.005.

Walle, T. (2011) 'Bioavailability of resveratrol', *Annals of the New York Academy of Sciences*, 1215(1), pp. 9–15. doi: https://doi.org/10.1111/j.1749-6632.2010.05842.x.

Wang, B., Zou, Y., Li, H. et al. (2005) 'Genistein inhibited retinal neovascularization and expression of vascular endothelial growth factor and hypoxia inducible factor 1α in a mouse model of oxygen-induced retinopathy', *Journal of Ocular Pharmacology and Therapeutics*, 21(2), pp. 107–113. doi: https://doi.org/10.1089/jop.2005.21.107.

Wang, S., Aurora, A. B., Johnson, B. A. et al. (2008) The endothelial-specific microRNA miR-126 governs vascular integrity and angiogenesis. *Developmental Cell* 15(2), pp. 261–271. doi: https://doi.org/10.1016/j.devcel.2008.07.002.

Wang, S., Yoon, Y. C., Sung, M. J. et al. (2012) Antiangiogenic properties of cafestol, a coffee diterpene, in human umbilical vein endothelial cells. *Biochemical and Biophysical Research Communications*. 421(3), pp. 567–571. doi:https://doi.org/10.1016/j.bbrc.2012.04.046.

Wang, Q., Chen, Y., Wang, X. et al. (2014) Consumption of fruit, but not vegetables, may reduce risk of gastric cancer: results from a meta-analysis of cohort studies. *European Journal of Cancer*. 50(8), pp. 1498–1509. doi:https://doi.org/10.1016/j.ejca.2014.02.009.

Wang, P. Y., Fang, J. C., Gao, Z. H. et al. (2016) 'Higher intake of fruits, vegetables or their fiber reduces the risk of type 2 diabetes: a meta-analysis', *Journal of Diabetes Investigation*, 7(1), pp. 56–69. doi:https://doi.org/10.1111/jdi.12376.

Wen, D., Huang, X., Zhang, M. et al. (2013) 'Resveratrol attenuates diabetic nephropathy via modulating angiogenesis', *PLoS ONE*, 8(12), pp. 1–12. doi:https://doi.org/10.1371/journal.pone.0082336.

Weng, C. J. and Yen, G. C. (2012) 'Flavonoids, a ubiquitous dietary phenolic subclass, exert extensive in vitro anti-invasive and in vivo anti-metastatic activities', *Cancer and Metastasis Reviews*, 31(1–2), pp. 323–351. doi:https://doi.org/10.1007/s10555-012-9347-y.

Won, H. J., Kim, H. II, Park, T. et al. (2019) Non-clinical pharmacokinetic behavior of ginsenosides. *Journal of Ginseng Research*, 43(3), pp. 354–360. doi:https://doi.org/10.1016/j.jgr.2018.06.001.

Wu, H., Liang, X., Fang, Y. *et al.* (2008) Resveratrol inhibits hypoxia-induced metastasis potential enhancement by restricting hypoxia-induced factor-1α expression in colon carcinoma cells. *Biomedicine and Pharmacotherapy*. 62(9), pp. 613–621. doi:https://doi.org/10.1016/j.biopha.2008.06.036.

Xiao, X., Shi, D., Liu, L. et al. (2011) 'Quercetin suppresses cyclooxygenase-2 expression and angiogenesis through inactivation of P300 signaling', *PLoS ONE*, 6(8). e22934 doi:https://doi.org/10.1371/journal.pone.0022934.

Xu, D., Ma, Y., Zhao, B. et al. (2014) 'Thymoquinone induces G2/M arrest, inactivates PI3K/Akt and nuclear factor-κB pathways in human cholangiocarcinomas both in vitro and in vivo', *Oncology Reports*, 31(5), pp. 2063–2070. doi:https://doi.org/10.3892/or.2014.3059.

Yance, D. R. and Sagar, S. M. (2006) 'Targeting angiogenesis with integrative cancer therapies', *Integrative Cancer Therapies*, 5(1), pp. 9–29. doi:https://doi.org/10.1177/1534735405285562.

Yang, C. S., Wang, X., Lu, G., and Picinich, S. C. (2009) Cancer prevention by tea: animal studies, molecular mechanisms and human relevance. *Nature Reviews Cancer* 9(6), pp. 429–439. doi:https://doi.org/10.1038/nrc2641.Cancer.

Yang, C., Yen, Y., Huang, C., and Hu, M. (2011) Growth inhibitory efficacy of lycopene and β-carotene against androgen-independent prostate tumor cells xenografted in nude mice. *Molecular Nutrition and Food Research* 55:pp. 606–612. doi:https://doi.org/10.1002/mnfr.201000308.

Yang, B. R., Hong, S. J., Lee, S. M. et al. (2016a) 'Pro-angiogenic activity of notoginsenoside R1 in human umbilical vein endothelial cells in vitro and in a chemical-induced blood vessel loss model of zebra fish in vivo', *Chinese Journal of Integrative Medicine*, 22(6), pp. 420–429. doi: https://doi.org/10.1007/s11655-014-1954-8.

Yang, F., Jiang, X., Song, L. et al. (2016b) Quercetin inhibits angiogenesis through thrombospondin-1 upregulation to antagonize human prostate cancer PC-3 cell growth in vitro and in vivo. *Oncology Reports*. 35 pp. 1602–1610. doi:https://doi.org/10.3892/or.2015.4481.

Yi, T., Cho, S., Yi, Z. *et al.* (2009) 'Thymoquinone inhibits tumor angiogenesis and tumor growth through suppressing AKT and ERK signaling pathways', *Molecular Cancer Therapeutics*, 7(7), pp. 1789–1796. doi:https://doi.org/10.1158/1535-7163.MCT-08-0124.Thymoquinone.

Young, R. C. and Weinstein, B. M. (2007) 'Visualization and experimental analysis of blood vessel formation using transgenic zebrafish', *Birth Defects Research Part C – Embryo Today: Reviews*, 81(4), pp. 286–296. doi:https://doi.org/10.1002/bdrc.20103.

Yoysungnoen-chintana, P., Bhattarakosol, P., and Patumraj, S. (2014). Antitumor and antiangiogenic activities of curcumin in cervical cancer xenografts in nude mice. *Biomed Research International* 2014: 817972.

Yu, L., Chen, S., Chang, W. et al. (2007) 'Stability of angiogenic agents, ginsenoside Rg 1 and Re, isolated from *Panax ginseng*: in vitro and in vivo studies', *International Journal of Pharmaceutics*, 328, pp. 168–176. doi:https://doi.org/10.1016/j.ijpharm.2006.08.009.

Zadeh, M. M., Ranji, N. and Motamed, N. (2015) 'Deregulation of miR-21 and miR-155 and their putative targets after silibinin treatment in T47D breast cancer cells', *Iranian Journal of Basic Medical Sciences*, 18(12), pp. 1209–1214. doi:https://doi.org/10.22038/ijbms.2015.6273.

Zhang, Q.-X., Mangovern, C.J., Mack, C.A. et al. (1997). Vascular endothelial growth factor is the major angiogenic factor in omentum: mechanism of the omentum-mediated angiogenesis. *Journal of Surgical Research* 154 (67): 147–154.

Zhang, S., Chen, S., Shen, Y. et al. (2006). Puerarin induces angiogenesis in myocardium of rat with myocardial. *Biological and Pharmaceutical Bulletin* 29: 945–950.

Zhang, Y., Zhang, Y., Furumura, M. et al. (2008) 'Distinct signaling pathways confer different vascular responses to VEGF 121 and VEGF 165', *Growth Factors*, 26, pp. 125–131. doi:https://doi.org/10.1080/08977190802105909.

Zhang, L., Liu, Q., Lu, L. et al. (2011) Astragaloside IV stimulates angiogenesis and increases hypoxia-inducible factor-1α accumulation via phosphatidylinositol 3-kinase/Akt pathway. *Journal of Pharmacology and Experimental Therapeutics* 338(2), pp. 485–491. doi:https://doi.org/10.1124/jpet.111.180992.ever.

Zhang, Y. I., Hu, G., Li, S. et al. (2012) Pro-angiogenic activity of astragaloside IV in HUVECs in vitro and zebrafish in vivo. *Medicine Reports* 5: pp. 805–811. doi:https://doi.org/10.3892/mmr.2011.716.

Zhang, F., Zhang, Z., Chen, L. et al. (2014) Curcumin attenuates angiogenesis in liver fibrosis and inhibits angiogenic properties of hepatic stellate cells. *Journal of Cellular and Molecular Medicine* 18(7), pp. 1392–1406. doi:https://doi.org/10.1111/jcmm.12286.

Zhang, H., He, S., Spee, C. et al. (2015) SIRT1 mediated inhibition of VEGF/VEGFR2 signaling by resveratrol and its relevance to choroidal neovascularization. *Cytokine*. 76: pp. 6–9. doi:https://doi.org/10.1016/j.cyto.2015.06.019.

Zhang, J., Feng, Z., Wang, C. et al. (2017). Curcumin derivative WZ35 efficiently suppresses colon cancer progression through inducing ROS production and ER stress-dependent apoptosis. *American Journal of Cancer Research* 7 (2): 275–288.

Zhao, D., Qin, C., Fan, X. et al. (2014) Inhibitory effects of quercetin on angiogenesis in larval zebra fish and human umbilical vein endothelial cells. *European Journal of Pharmacology*, 723, pp. 360–367. doi:https://doi.org/10.1016/j.ejphar.2013.10.069.

Zhao, X., Wang, Q., Yang, S. et al. (2016) Quercetin inhibits angiogenesis by targeting calcineurin in the xenograft model of human breast cancer, *European Journal of Pharmacology*. 781:60–68 doi:https://doi.org/10.1016/j.ejphar.2016.03.063.

Zheng, L., Ling, P., Wang, Z. et al. (2007) 'A novel polypeptide from shark cartilage with potent anti-angiogenic activity', *Cancer Biology and Therapy*, 6(5), pp. 775–780. doi:https://doi.org/10.4161/cbt.6.5.4002.

Zhou, X., Siu, W., Fung, C., and Cheng, L. (2014) Phytomedicine pro-angiogenic effects of carthami flos whole extract in human microvascular endothelial cells in vitro and in zebrafish in vivo. *European Journal of Integrative Medicine*. 21(11), pp. 1256–1263. doi:https://doi.org/10.1016/j.phymed.2014.06.010.

Zhou, X., Siu, W. S. U. M., Zhang, C. et al. (2017) Whole extracts of *Radix achyranthis bidentatae* and *Radix cyathulae* promote angiogenesis in human umbilical vein endothelial cells in vitro and in zebrafish in vivo. *Experimental and Therapeutic Medicine* 13: pp. 1032–1038. doi:https://doi.org/10.3892/etm.2017.4053.

Zhu, W., Fu, A., Hu, J. et al. (2011) 5-Formylhonokiol exerts anti-angiogenesis activity via inactivating the ERK signaling pathway. *Experimental and Molecular Medicine* 43(3), pp. 146–152. doi:https://doi.org/10.3858/emm.2011.43.3.017.

Zijlstra, A., Seandel, M., Kupriyanova, T. A. et al. (2006) 'Proangiogenic role of neutrophil-like inflammatory heterophils during neovascularization induced by growth factors and human tumor cells', *Blood*, 107(1), pp. 317–327. doi:https://doi.org/10.1182/blood-2005-04-1458.

Zu, K., Mucci, L., Rosner, B. A. et al. (2014) Dietary lycopene, angiogenesis, and prostate cancer: a prospective study in the prostate-specific antigen era, *JNCI: Journal of the National Cancer Institute*, 106(2):djt430. doi:https://doi.org/10.1093/jnci/djt430.

4

Nutraceuticals and Natural-Product Derivatives for Disease Prevention

Neetu Kumra Taneja[1], Amritpal Singh[1], D.P. Shivaprasad[1,3], Pankaj Taneja[2], and Divya Sachdev[1]

[1] *Department of Basic and Applied Sciences, National Institute of Food Technology, Entrepreneurship and Management, Sonipat, Haryana, India*
[2] *Department of Biotechnology, Sharda University, Greater Noida, Uttar Pradesh, India*
[3] *Department of Grain Science & Industry, Kansas State University, Manhattan, KS, USA*

4.1 Introduction

The term *nutraceutical* is a combination of words *nutrition* and *pharmaceutical* and was coined by Dr. Stephen L. DeFelice (MD, founder and chairman of the Foundation for Innovation in Medicine) in 1989. Nutraceuticals can be defined as food or part of food that provides medical and health benefits such as prevention and treatment of disease (Andlauer and Fürst 2002; Chauhan et al. 2013; Ghaffari and Roshanravan 2020; Kalra 2003). Nutraceuticals upgrade the well-being status of individuals by regulating the body functions. It is due to the nutritional, safety, and therapeutic effect that nutraceuticals have attracted significant interest (Swaroopa and Srinath 2017). Nutraceuticals can assist in preventing certain disorders such as allergies, Alzheimer's disease, cardiovascular diseases, cancer, diabetes, eye disorders, inflammation, obesity, and Parkinson's disease (Nasri et al. 2014). Nutraceuticals possess several advantages over prophylactic conventional medicines/pharmaceuticals, such as negligible or no adverse health effects, economically affordable, and easily available and reliable (Golla 2018). The nutraceutical industry consists of three parts: herbal or natural products, dietary supplements, and functional parts (Das et al. 2012). Out of these three segments, herbal or natural products (11.6% per year) and dietary supplements (19.5% per year) are the most quickly growing areas (Chauhan et al. 2013; Das et al. 2012). According to a report by Global Research Future, the nutraceutical market will reach USD 407650 million globally with an expected compound annual growth rate (CAGR) of 7.37%. Primary players in nutraceutical market include Perrigo Company Plc (Ireland), Glanbia Plc (Ireland), Danone SA (US), GlaxoSmithKline Plc (UK), Abbott Laboratories (US), Daflorn Ltd (Bulgaria), Bactolac Pharmaceutical Inc (US), Yakult Honsha Co., Ltd (Japan), Meiji Holdings Co., Ltd (Japan), and E.I.D. – Parry (India) Limited (India) (global nutraceuticals market: information by type (vitamins and minerals; probiotics, proteins, and peptides; omega fatty acids, and so on), source (plant, animal, and microbial), form (capsules, tablets, and softgels, powder, and liquid and gummies), distribution channel (store-based [supermarkets and hypermarkets, specialty stores, and so on], and non-store based), and region (North America, Europe, Asia-Pacific, and rest of the world) – forecast till 2025, 2020).

The food sources utilized as nutraceuticals are all natural and are classified as products procured from plants, animals, minerals, or microbial sources (Figure 4.1) (Chauhan et al. 2013). Plant

Handbook of Nutraceuticals and Natural Products: Biological, Medicinal, and Nutritional Properties and Applications,
Volume 2, First Edition. Edited by Preetha Balakrishnan and Sreerag Gopi.
© 2022 John Wiley & Sons, Inc. Published 2022 by John Wiley & Sons, Inc.

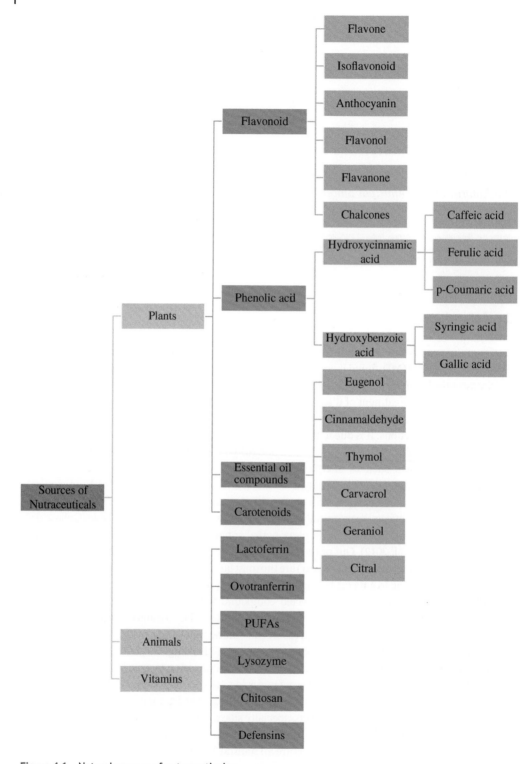

Figure 4.1 Natural sources of nutraceuticals

chemicals or phytochemicals are nonessential and nonnutritive chemicals synthesized by plants to provide them protection and are known to possess disease-protective properties. Various foods such as whole grains, beans, fruits, vegetables, and herbs contain phytonutrients or phytochemicals that either alone or in combination have the potential to cure various diseases. Phytochemicals with nutraceutical properties offer protection against diseases such as cancers, heart diseases, diabetes, high blood pressure, inflammation, osteoporosis, and microbial infections (Table 4.1). Polyphenols, flavonoids, isoflavonoids, anthocyanidins, terpenoids, and carotenoids are some of the phytochemicals/phytonutrients that are antimicrobials and are known to provide health benefits (Prakash et al. 2012). Significant attention has been received by the plant-based nutraceuticals owing to their safety and potential nutritional and therapeutic impact (Pandey et al. 2011).

There has been extensive research with respect to intake of polyphenols and human health in terms of incidence of chronic diseases such as cardiovascular diseases (CVDs), hypertension, diabetes, cancer, and obesity. Polyphenols are categorized into two main groups: flavonoid polyphenols such as flavones, flavonones, and anthocyanins; and non-flavonoid polyphenols such as phenolic acids, xanthones, lignans, and tannins (Durazzo et al. 2019).

Flavonoids (Figure 4.2), a significant group of naturally occurring phytochemicals belonging to secondary metabolites having phenolic structure (Hayat et al. 2017; Panche et al. 2016), are primarily found in fruits, vegetables, tea, and cocoa (Egert and Rimbach 2011). Though all the flavonoids have the same C_6-C_3-C_6 carbon skeleton, there is a variation in the structure surrounding the heterocyclic oxygen ring. All the flavonoids are derived from the 2-phenylchromone parent compound consisting of three phenolic rings that are both hydroxylated and methoxylated in varying degrees (Yao et al. 2004). They are produced by the plant in order to protect itself from microbial infection and the plant tissues in abiotic and biotic stress by acting as secondary antioxidant defense system (Kumar and Pandey 2013; Panche et al. 2016). With respect to human health, a broad variety of pharmacological properties such as anti-allergenic, anti-inflammatory, antiviral, prevention of CVDs, anticarcinogenic, antidiabetic, and antiproliferative have been demonstrated by flavonoids. Flavonoids are classified into different groups which include flavanones (citrus fruits, cumin, oranges, and grapefruits), flavones (herbs, fruits, parsley, and thyme), isoflavones (soyabean), flavonols (apples, tea, beer, and black tea), anthocyanin (fruits and vegetables), and flavonols (onions, cherries, apples, broccoli, tea, and red wine), which are the most commonly found flavonoids in the diet (Yao et al. 2004).

Phenolic acids (Figure 4.3), non-flavonoid polyphenolic compounds that contain carboxyl group attached to benzene rings, are derived from benzoic and cinnamic acids. They are further classified as gallic, vanillic, syringic, caffeic, ferulic, and p-coumaric acids. They are present in red fruits, vegetables, coffee, tea, cocoa, and whole grains (Durazzo et al. 2019).

Essential oils (EOs) also known as "volatile oils" are secondary metabolites produced by aromatic and medicinal plants and consists of terpenic hydrocarbons such as monoterpenes and sesquiterpenes, alcoholic compounds such as menthol and linalool, acidic compounds such as cinnamic and benzoic, aldehydes such as cinnamaldehyde, and ketones such as eugenol and phenols (Figure 4.4) (Dagli et al. 2015; Pandey et al. 2017). They can be found in buds, flowers, leaves, seeds, stems, roots, wood, or bark of a plant. EOs are known to possess antimicrobial, antioxidant, and immunomodulatory properties (Table 4.2) make them suitable in food preservation and ingredients in functional foods (Valdivieso-Ugarte et al. 2019).

Table 4.1 Natural compounds, their sources, and therapeutic benefits.

No.	Category	Molecule	Sources	Therapeutic benefits	References
1	Flavone	Luteolin	Celery, parsley, broccoli, onion leaves, apple skins, cabbages, carrots, and peppers (Lin et al. 2008)	Immune system stimulator, antioxidant, anti-inflammatory, anticancer, and cardiovascular protection (Sun et al. 2015a)	Lin et al. (2008), Sun et al. (2015a)
		Apigenin	Grapes, apples, chamomile teas, and red wine	Antioxidant, anticancer, anti-inflammatory, antibacterial, and antiviral	Ai et al. (2017), Shukla et al. (2015), Yan et al. (2017)
		Tangeretin	Peel of sweet and mandarin oranges	Anti-inflammation, anticancer, and antiadipogenesis	Funaro et al. (2016)
		Chrysin	Plants, honey, and bee propolis	Antioxidant, anti-inflammatory, antiapoptotic, neuroprotective, antidepressant, and antianxiety	Rashno et al. (2020)
		Baicalein	*Scutellaria baicalensis*	Anti-inflammation, antihypertension, cardioprotective, antibacterial, and anticancer	Zhang et al. (2017b)
2	Flavanones	Hesperetin	Citrus peel (oranges, lemons, and grapes)	Anti-inflammatory, antioxidant, antiapoptotic, and antitumor	Chen et al. (2019b)
		Naringenin	Citrus fruits, tomatoes, and grapes	Antidepressant (Wu et al. 2016a), antidiabetic, anti-inflammatory, antioxidative (Nguyen-Ngo et al. 2019), and antitumor	Wu et al. (2016a)
		Eriodictyol	Citrus fruits	Antioxidant, anti-inflammatory, and antiosteoclastogenic	Wang et al. (2018c)
3	Flavonols	Quercetin	Apples, berries, onions, and tea	Antioxidant, antiviral, anti-inflammatory, neuroprotective, cardioprotective, anticancer, and antiaging	Wei et al. (2018)
		Kaempferol	Onion, tea, grapes, strawberry, lettuce, and medicinal plants such as *Cerbera manghas*	Antioxidative, anticancer, antiaging, and anti-inflammatory	Kim et al. (2015)
		Myricetin	Teas, wines, berries, fruits, and medicinal plants	Anti-inflammatory, antioxidant, antiviral, antimicrobial, cytoprotective, and anticancer	Ci et al. (2018)

#	Class	Compound	Source	Activities	Reference
4	Isoflavonoids	Biochanin A	*Trifolium pratense L., Cicer arietinum L., and Lupinus termis L*	Anti-inflammatory, lipid lowering, anticancer, and antidiabetic	Oza and Kulkarni (2018a)
		Formononetin	Green peas, red clover, soybeans, astragalus roots, and liquorice roots	Anti-inflammatory, antidiabetic, and cardioprotective	Oza and Kulkarni (2018b)
		Genistein	Soybean	Anti-inflammatory, antioxidant, anticancer, and bone-protective	Du et al. (2018)
		Daidzein	Soybean	Anti-inflammatory, anticancer, and antioxidant	Peng et al. (2017)
5	Anthocyanins	Pelargonidin and malvidin	Berries, currants, grapes, red- to purplish-blue-colored leafy vegetables, grains roots, and tubers	Antidiabetic, anticancer, antimicrobial, anti-inflammatory, anti-CVDs, and anti-obesity	Khoo et al. (2017)
6	Chalcones	Butein	*Toxicodendron vernicifluum* or *Rhus verniciflua*	Antidiabetic, antioxidant, and anti-inflammatory	Lee and Jeong (2016)
		Flavokavain A	Kava	Anticancer	Wang et al. (2020)
7	Hydroxycinnamic acid	Caffeic acid	Propolis (Dai et al. 2020)	Antibacterial, antioxidant, antidiabetic, anticancer, and anti-inflammatory	Salem et al. (2019)
		p-Coumaric acid	Apples, pears, and grapes; vegetables such as carrots, onions, tomatoes, potatoes, and beans; cereals such as corn, rice, oats, and wheats; and mushrooms	Antioxidant, antimicrobial, antiviral, anti-inflammatory, anticancer, antidiabetic, and antihyperlipidemic	Shen et al. (2019)
		FA	Grapes, bananas, and oranges; vegetables such as bamboo shoots, tomatoes, and peanuts; whole grains; and coffee (Qi et al. 2020)	Antioxidant, antihyperlipidemic, antidiabetic, antimicrobial, anticancer, neuroprotective, and antiatherogenic (Mir et al. 2018)	Mir et al. (2018), Qi et al. (2020)
		Sinapic acid	Citrus fruits, strawberries, broccoli, turnip, kale, or tronchuda cabbage	Antioxidant and anticancer	Eroğlu et al. (2018)

(Continued)

Table 4.1 (Continued)

No.	Category	Molecule	Sources	Therapeutic benefits	References
8	Hydroxybenzoic acid	Syringic acid	Grapes, acai palm, honey, red wine, dates, pumpkin, olives, and spices	Antioxidant, anti-inflammatory, antimicrobial, antiadipogenic, antidiabetic, hepatoprotective, neuroprotective, cardioprotective, and anticancer	Ren et al. (2019)
		Gallic acid	Gallnut, pineapple, grapes, green tea, oak's bark, lemon, banana, pine apple, and apple's peel	Cardioprotective, hepatoprotective, neuroprotective, antioxidant, and anticancer	Liao et al. (2018)
9	Stilbene	Resveratrol	Grapes, blueberries, plums, peanuts, and apples	Diabetes mellitus, CVDs, obesity, inflammatory, neurogenerative, and age-related disorders	Koushki et al. (2018)
10	Carotenoids	Lycopene	Tomatoes and red fruits such as watermelons, pink grapefruits, guava, red peppers, and papayas	Anti-inflammatory, anticancer, cardioprotective, and detoxification	Xu et al. (2017)
		Fucoxanthin	Brown alga (Phaeophyceae) and diatoms (Bacillariophyta)	Antioxidant, anti-obesity, antidiabetic, anticancer, and antimicrobial	Karpiński and Adamczak (2019)

(a) (b) (c)

(d) (e) (f)

(g) (h) (i)

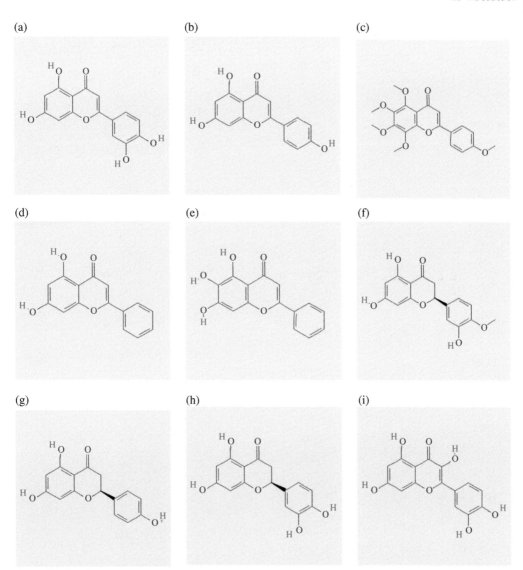

Figure 4.2 Structure of flavonoids: (a) structure of luteolin, (b) structure of apigenin, (c) structure of tangeretin, (d) structure of chrysin, (e) structure of baicalein, (f) structure of hesperetin, (g) structure of naringenin, (h) structure of eriodictyol, (i) structure of quercetin, (j) structure of kaempferol, (k) structure of myricetin, (l) structure of biochanin A, (m) structure of formononetin, (n) structure of genistein, (o) structure of daidzein, (p) structure of butein, (q) structure of cyanidin, (r) structure of pelargonidin, and (s) structure of malvidin. *Source:* PubChem.

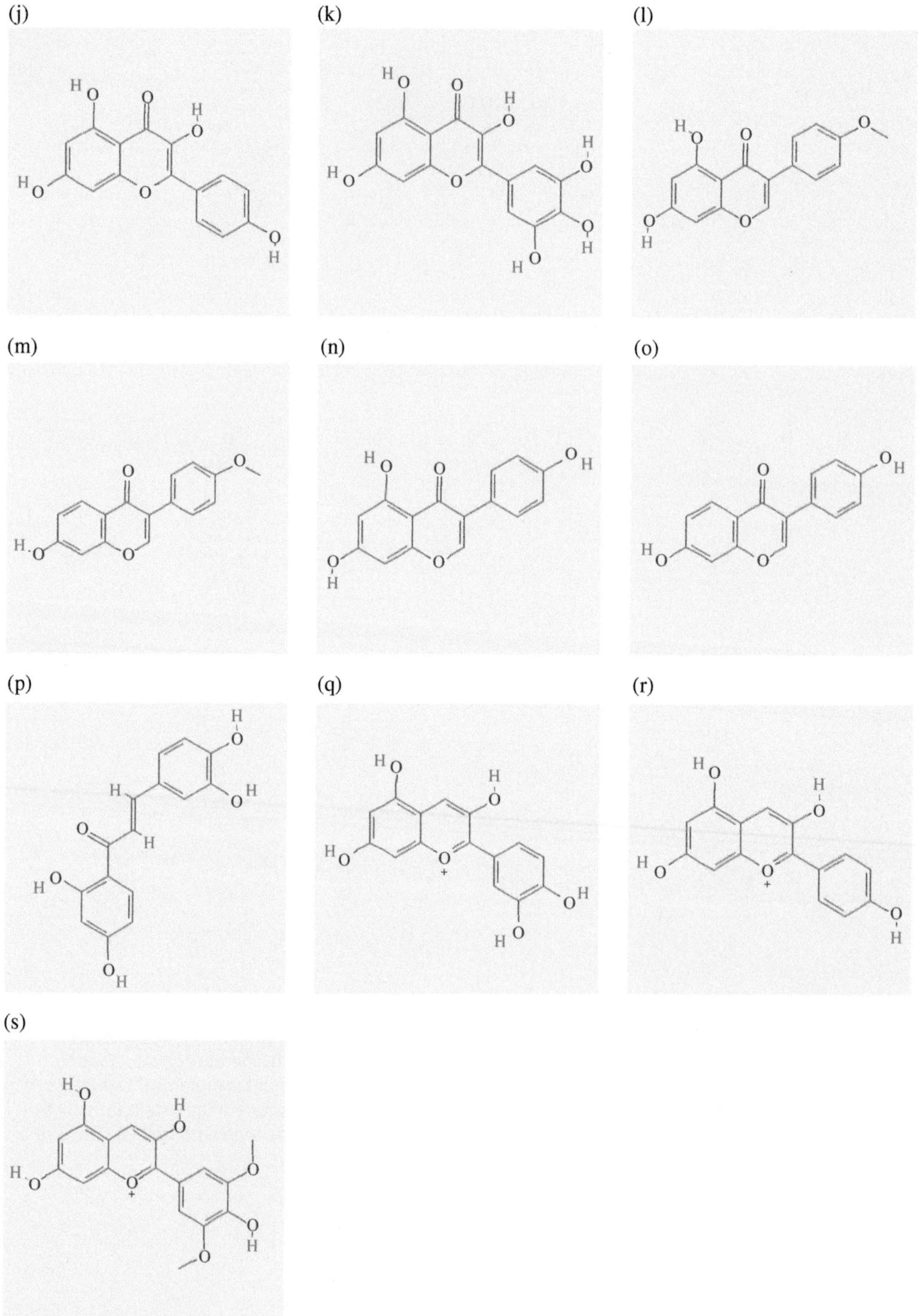

(j)

(k)

(l)

(m)

(n)

(o)

(p)

(q)

(r)

(s)

Figure 4.2 (Continued)

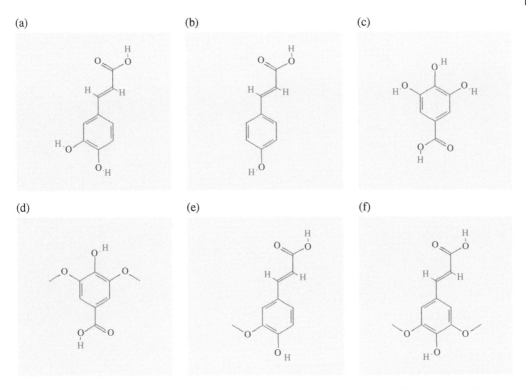

Figure 4.3 Structure of phenolic acids: (a) structure of Caffeic acid, (b) structure of p-coumaric acid, (c) structure of gallic acid, (d) structure of syringic acid, (e) structure of ferulic acid (FA), and (f) structure of sinapic acid. *Source:* PubChem.

Other natural sources of nutraceuticals used for the prevention of diseases include animals (lactoferrin, ovotransferrin, lysozyme, polyunsaturated fatty acids (PUFAs), chitosan, and defensins) and vitamins (Table 4.3).

4.2 Natural-Product Derivatives and Cancer Prevention

Cancer, the primary cause of mortality and morbidity in the past few decades, is characterized by uncontrolled growth and spread of transformed cells. Each year, about 3.5 million deaths associated with cancer are recorded globally (Hashemzaei et al. 2017). The global figures are expected to rise to 17.5 million per year by 2050 (Prakash et al. 2020). Natural products such as plant extracts and its active components are the foundation of cancer chemotherapeutics and contribute about 70% to the formation of anticancer compounds (Hashemzaei et al. 2017). Some of the natural anticancer compounds, their dose and mode of action are listed in Table 4.4 and discussed below:

Flavonoids: Anticancer efficacy of apigenin was demonstrated as it binds with IKKα (inhibitory-kB kinase), a primary regulator of oncogenesis, resulting in the weakening of IKKα kinase activity and therefore suppressing nuclear factor-κB (NF-κB) activation in human prostate cancer PC-3 and 22Rv1 cells (Shukla et al. 2015). Expression and translation of one of the major components in Notch signaling, *Notch-1*, and other genes in the pathway such as *Hes-1, Hey-1, Hey-2,* and

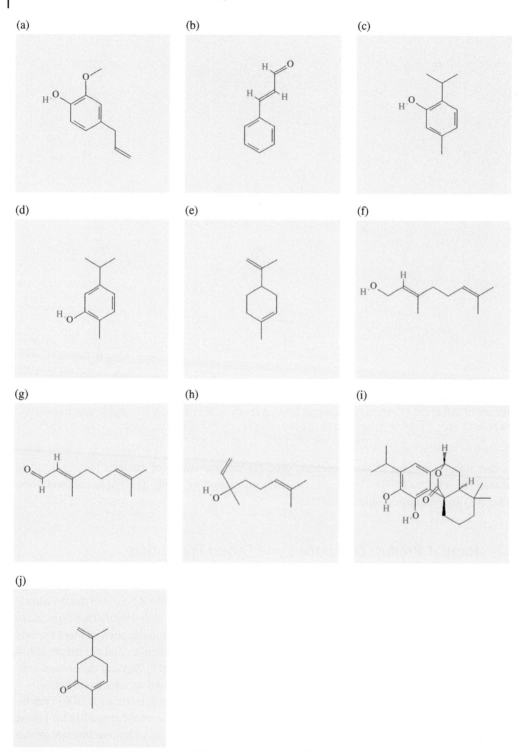

Figure 4.4 Structure of essential oil compounds: (a) structure of eugenol, (b) structure of cinnamaldehyde, (c) structure of thymol, (d) structure of carvacrol, (e) structure of limonene, (f) structure of geraniol, (g) structure of citral, (h) structure of linalool, (i) structure of carnosol, (j) and structure of carvone. *Source:* PubChem.

Table 4.2 Essential oil compounds, their sources, and therapeutic benefits.

No.	Compound	Sources	Therapeutic benefits	References
1	Eugenol	Clove and cinnamon	Pain reliver, antioxidant, anti-inflammatory, and anticancer	Islam et al. (2018)
2	Cinnamaldehyde	Bark of *Cinnamomum cassia*	Antibacterial, immunomodulatory, and antitumor	Li et al. (2016b)
3	Thymol	*Thymus, Ocimum, Origanum, Satureja, Thymra,* and *Monarda* (Marchese et al. 2016)	Anti-inflammatory, anticancer, antioxidant, antibacterial, and antimicrobial (Kang et al. 2016)	Kang et al. (2016), Marchese et al. (2016)
4	Carvacrol	*Origanum vulgare, Thymus vulgaris, Lepidium flavum,* and *Citrus aurantium bergamia*	Antimicrobial, antioxidant, and anticancer	Sharifi-Rad et al. (2018)
5	Limonene	Lemon tree, orange, neroli, bergamot, and tangerine	Anti-inflammatory, antioxidant, anticancer, and antidiabetic	Soulimani et al. (2019)
6	Geraniol	Geranium, lemon, and medicinal plants	Antioxidative, antimicrobial, antitumor, and anti-inflammatory	Xue et al. (2016)
7	Citral	*Cymbopogon citratus*	Antioxidants, antifungal, antiviral, and anti-inflammation	Devi and Ashokkumar (2018)
8	Linalool	Coriander, basil, oregano, and grapevine	Anti-inflammatory, antioxidant, antimicrobial, and antitumor	Rodenak-Kladniew et al. (2018)
9	Carnosol	Rosemary, sage, and oregano	Antioxidant, anti-inflammatory, antidiabetic, and anticancer	Wang et al. (2018b)
10	Carvone	Caraway seed, spearmint, and dill	Antihyperlipidemic, antimicrobial, anticancer, and antihypertensive	Zhao and Du (2019)

Table 4.3 Animal- and vitamin-based nutraceuticals, their sources, and therapeutic benefits.

No.	Category	Molecule	Sources	Therapeutic benefits	References
1	Animal	Lactoferrin	Colostrum, breast milk, and mucosal (saliva and tears), nasal, and bronchial secretions (bile and gastrointestinal fluids)	Antimicrobial, antioxidant, anti-inflammatory, and anticancer	Giansanti et al. (2016)
		Ovotransferrin	Avian plasma and egg whites	Antibacterial, antiviral, anti-inflammatory, and anticancer	Giansanti et al. (2015)
		Polyunsaturated fatty acids	ω-3 PUFAs: cod-liver oil, oily fish, and algal oils. ω-6 PUFAs: meat, egg yolk, and dairy products	Anti-inflammatory properties, reduce atherosclerosis, and CVDs	Simonetto et al. (2019)
		Chitosan	Shellfish and crustaceans (contain about 15–40% chitin) such as crabs, lobster, shrimp, oysters, and squid	Antioxidant, antibacterial, hypocholesterolemia, anti-inflammatory, and immune stimulating	Je and Kim (2012)
2	Vitamins	Ascorbic acid	Citrus fruits, green and red peppers, Indian gooseberry, tomatoes, turnip, broccoli, and leafy vegetables	Antioxidant, antimicrobial anticancer, antiatherosclerosis, antidiabetic, neuroprotective, and cardioprotective agent	Chambial et al. (2013)
		Tocopherol	Coconut, maize, palm, olives, peanuts, and sunflower	Antioxidant, cardioprotective, anticancer, cataract preventive, and Alzheimer's disease preventive and immunity improving agent	Rizvi et al. (2014)
		Cholecalciferol	Fish such as salmon, mackerel, and tune; cod-liver oil; beef; egg yolk; and milk and milk products	Anti-inflammatory, antiapoptotic, antifibrotic, and immunomodulatory effects	Anandabaskar et al. (2018)

Table 4.4 Natural anticancer compounds, their dose, and mode of action.

No.	Natural compounds	Dose	Mode of action	Studied on	References
1	Genistein	IC$_{50}$: 50 μm	Activation of capase-3 and reduction of p38 *MAPK* gene expression	HT29 colon cancer cell	Shafiee et al. (2016)
2	Daidzein	IC$_{50}$: 20 μm	Inducing mitochondrial apoptosis and cell arrest at G2/M and inhibition of Raf/MEK (mitogen-activated protein kinase)/ERK cascade	SKOV3 cells and mouse	Hua et al. (2018)
3	Butein	IC$_{50}$: 185 ± 23.48 μm (SiHa) IC$_{50}$: 79.88 ± 7.45 μm (C-33A)	Suppression of antiapoptotic Bcl-xL and inhibitor of apoptosis (IOP) protein, increased cytochrome c levels, and caspase activities	C-33A and SiHa cell lines	Yang et al. (2018)
4	Flavokavain A	IC$_{50}$: 198.80 μm for 24 hours	Cell apoptosis, cell arrest at G2/M phase, interference with tubulin polymerization, and inhiation of survinin expression	PC3 cell line	Wang et al. (2020)
5	Epicatechin	IC$_{50}$: 350 μm	Increase in ROS production and upregulation of proapoptotic protein	MDA-MB-231 and MCF-7 cells	Pereyra-vergara et al. (2020)
6	Sinapic acid	IC$_{50}$: 1000 μm	For PC-3 cells: upregulation of *BAX, caspase-3, caspase-8, CYCS, FAS, TIMP-1*, and *CDH1* and downregulation of *MMP-9* For LNCaP cells: upregulated *Bax, caspase-3, caspase-7,* and *CYCS* and downregulation of *CDH2, MMP-2,* and *MMP-9*	PC-3 and LNCaP cancer cells	Eroğlu et al. (2018)
7	Gingerol	Dose dependent	Blocking cyclins, cell arrest at G1 phase, inhibiting AKT and p38^{MAPK} activity, and blocking epidermal growth factor receptor (EGFR)	MDA-MB-231 breast cancer cells	Joo et al. (2016)
8	Ellagic acid	5, 10, and 20 μm	Inhibition of PI3k and AKT phosphorylation, suppression of cell proliferation, cell cycle arrest at G1 phase, upregulation of p21 and Bax, and suppression of Bcl-2 and cyclin D1	A549 cells	Liu et al. (2018)

(Continued)

Table 4.4 (Continued)

No.	Natural compounds	Dose	Mode of action	Studied on	References
9	Gallic acid (GA) and curcumin (curc)	IC_{50} (GA): 150 μm IC_{50} (curc.): 80 μm for 24 hours	Decreased cell growth, suppressed GSH, increased ROS, decreased Bcl-2 level and promoted Bax, caspase-3, and PARP levels	MDA-MB-231 cells	Moghtaderi et al. (2018)
10	Citral	IC_{50}: 145.32 μm (HCT116) IC_{50}: 181.21 μm (HT29) for 24 hours	Apoptosis via p53 Activation, upregulation of ROS level and Bax, and downregulation of Bcl-2 and Bcl-xL	HCT116 and HT29 cells	Sheikha et al. (2017)
11	Zingiberene	IC_{50}: 20 μm	Inhibition of mTOR/PI3K/AKT signaling pathway and deactivation of capsase-2	HT-29 colon cancer cells	Chen et al. (2019a)
12	Linalool	Dose dependent	Induction of G0/G1 arrest and apoptosis involving pathways of Ras, MAPKs, and AKT/mTOR	Hepatocellular carcinoma HepG2 cells	Rodenak-Kladniew et al. (2018)
		IC_{50}: 10 μm	Loss of mitochondrial membrane potential and inhibition of PI3K/AKT signaling pathway	Oral cancer cell line OECM-1	Pan and Zhang (2019)
13	Carvone	IC_{50}: 20 μm	Induction of apoptosis, cell cycle arrest at G2/M phase, and suppression of p38MAPK signaling pathway	Myeloma KMS-5 cells	Ding and Chen (2018)
14	Thymoquinone	IC_{50}: 55 μmol/l	Antimetastatic via activation of AMPK/mTOR pathway	Renal cancer cell lines, 786-O and ACHN	Zhang et al. (2018d)

Cyclin D1 mRNAs in breast cancer cell was reduced using luteolin. Introduction of Notch-1 siRNA and mRNA mimics MDA-MB-231 cells, which exhibited changes in miRNA levels which led to a decrease in Notch signaling proteins and reduced tumor survival (Sun et al. 2015a).

Tangeretin also exhibited anticancer effect against the drug-resistant MDA-MB-231 breast cancer cell line with IC_{50} as 9 µm by increasing and decreasing the BCL2-associated X (Bax) and B-cell lymphoma 2 (Bcl-2) expression, respectively. It caused induction of arrest at G2/M phase of colorectal cancer cells through upregulation of p21 and p27 and also arrested MDA-MB-231 cells at G2/M checkpoint along with a decrease in cycline B1 and D expression (Fan et al. 2019). Anticancer effects in ovarian cancer cell lines ES2 and OV90 were demonstrated by the inhibition of cell proliferation, induction of cell death by promoting reactive oxygen species (ROS) production, suppression of matrix metalloproteinase (MMP), and activation of mitogen-activated protein kinases (MAPK) and phosphoionositide 3-kinase (PI3/AKT) pathways (Lim et al. 2018). Baicalein also demonstrated anticancer effect in MCF-7 and MDA-MB-231 breast cancer cells by inducing apoptosis and autophagy in vitro and in vivo. It also suppressed the expressions of p-AKT, p-mTOR, NFκB), and p-IκB; suppressed the ratio of p-AKT/AKT and p-mTOR/mTOR; and upregulated the expression of IκB (Yan et al. 2018).

The anticancer effect of hesperetin extracted from *Cordia sebestena* was found out using in silico molecular docking study which has shown interactions with E6 protein of human papillomavirus (HPV16) cervical carcinoma with substantial binding energy (Prakash et al. 2020). SGC7901 gastric cancer cell line was used to investigate the combined and individual anticancer effects of naringenin and Bcl-2 inhibitor, ABT-737. It was found that the cell growth and colony growth was inhibited by both, individually as well as in combination with increase in cleavage of caspase-3, ADP ribose polymerase, and p53 expression and decrease in AKT activation (Zhang et al. 2016a). The anticancer activity of quercetin in vitro and in vivo was depicted by inducing apoptosis and phenomenally reducing the volume of tumor in estrogen receptor-positive breast cancer cells (MCF-7) and colon cancer cells (CT-26) in mice, respectively (Hashemzaei et al. 2017). Kaempferol exhibited its potential in treating cervical cancer by causing cell apoptosis in HeLa cancer cells and upregulating genes such as *p53, p21, caspase 3, caspase 9, Bax*, and *PTEN* and aging by suppressing the PI3K/AKT and hTERT (telomerase) pathways (Kashafi et al. 2017).

Myricetin demonstrated its anticancer therapeutic property by decreasing the cell viability and inducing apoptosis by activating caspases 3, 8, and 9 and thereby inducing the release of apoptosis-inducing factor from mitochondria to cytosol, which further alters the mitochondrial membrane potential and Bax expression in SNU-790 HPTC cell lines (Ha et al. 2017). Biochanin A also demonstrated its anticancer effects in A549 and 95D cells by inhibiting cell proliferation and inducing S-phase cell arrest and apoptosis owing to the activation of P21, caspase-3, and Bcl-2 pathways (Li et al. 2018b). Formononetin also demonstrated its anticancer potential by decreasing cell proliferation via cell arrest at G0/G1 phase, enhancing apoptosis, causing loss of MMP, producing ROS, downregulating extracellular signal regulated kinase (ERK1/2), P90RSK, AKT, P70S6K, and S6 proteins, and enhancing the phosphorylation of P38 proteins in ES2 and OV90 ovarian cancer cells (Park et al. 2018). Purple sweet potato anthocyanin demonstrated its antitumor capacity by decreasing the viability of bladder cancer by inducing the expression of proapoptotic genes such as *caspase-3, Fas, Fasl, Bax*, suppressing the expression of anti-apoptotic *Bcl-2* gene and suppressing the activation of the phosphatidylinositol 4,5-bisphosphate 3-kinase/AKT (PI3K/AKT) signaling pathway (Li et al. 2018a).

Non-Flavonoids: Caffeic acid phenethyl ester (CAPE) showed its therapeutic potential to combat against colitis-associated cancer by reducing activation of NLRP3 inflammasome by suppressing ROS production in mouse having azoxymethane and dextran sulfate sodium-induced colon cancer (Dai et al. 2020). Recent evidences also demonstrated the potential effect of p-CA as an anticancer agent by suppressing the expression of glucose-regulated protein (GRP 78), involved in oncogenic progression and deactivating the unfolded protein response and downregulating the expression of cyclooxygenase (COX)-2, interleukin (IL)-6, tumor necrosis factor (TNF)-α, prostaglandin E2 (PGE2), p-p65, and p-IκBα in Ht-29 and SW-480 cancer cell lines (Sharma et al. 2018). Gallic acid demonstrated its anticancer property in human urinary bladder cancer cell (TSGH-8301) by suppressing the expression of Skp2 protein and weakening the Skp2-p27 association, blocking transition at G2/M phase and by further inhibiting the FAS-(fatty acid synthase) supported ER alpha pathway, ERK and AKT phosphorylation (Liao et al. 2018). Recent evidences suggest the potential of this FA as an anticancer agent at 40.54 μm IC$_{50}$ as it provides cytotoxic effect by increasing the expression of apoptotic markers such as casepase-3 and caspase-9, cytochrome c, Apaf-1, Bax, and p53 and by suppressing the Bcl-2 expression (which further declines MMP) and cell growth in HepG2 cell line (Gheena and Ezhilarasan 2019).

Curcumin, a yellow-colored nontoxic phenolic pigment, also demonstrated its potential as an anticancer agent in human cervical cancer cell line Hella by inhibiting the proliferative and invasive activities, suppressing Wnt/β-catenin and NF-κB pathways, and arresting the cell at G2/M followed by sub-G1 apoptosis (Ghasemi et al. 2019). Resveratrol demonstrated its anticancer cancer effect by binding (as suggested by in silico screening) to AKT serine/threonine kinase 1 (AKT1) and AKT2 (which assists in the inhibition of cell proliferation), suppressing the expression of cyclin D1, cyclin E2, and BCL2, upregulating Bax and p53, and inducing apoptosis with cell cycle arrest at phase G1 in DLD1 and HCT15 colon cancer cells (Li et al. 2019a).

Essential Oil Compounds: Eugenol displayed anticancer effects when combined with cisplatin (a metal-based anticancer drug) and demonstrated cytotoxic and proapoptotic effects by blocking aldehyde dehydrogenase (ALDH) enzyme activity, ALDH-positive cells, and NF-κB pathway in breast cancer stem cells (Islam et al. 2018). Similar combination consisting of eugenol and cisplatin demonstrated anticancer activity by blocking the growth and survival by inducing apoptosis, inhibiting the Notch-Hes1 pathway, and downregulating the drug-resistant *ABC* transporter genes on ovarian cancer cell line SKOV3 and OV2774 (Islam and Aboussekhra 2019). Cinnamaldehyde exhibited its anticancer property to combat colon cancer by upregulating the E-cadherin expression and suppressing the MMP-2 and MMP-9, inducing apoptosis and inhibiting the PI3K/AKT signaling pathway (Li et al. 2016b). Thymol exhibits anticancer effects by inhibiting cell growth, inducing apoptosis, generating ROS, and depolarizing mitochondrial membrane potential (activating caspases, Bax expression, and poly-ADP ribose polymer (PARP)) (Kang et al. 2016). Thymol also demonstrates its anticancer effects in oral cancer cells (Cal27 and HeLa) by establishing a direct and inverse relation with apoptosis and mitochondrial membrane potential, respectively (De La Chapa et al. 2018).

Carvacrol combated cancer by downregulating the expression of Bcl-2 and Cox2 and upregulating the level of Bax, suppressing the phosphorylation of focal adhesion kinase (FAK), plummeting the levels of MMP-9 and MMP-2, reducing the transcription factors such as ZEB1, and blocking the expression of β-catenin proteins caused by the inhibitive response in migration and invasion in Tca-8113 cell lines (Dai et al. 2016). The anticancer activity of limonene was demonstrated by promoting apoptosis (caused by substantial nuclear fragmentation, chromatic condensation, and break the apoptotic cascade), increasing the level of Bax and upregulating the caspase-3 expression, decreasing the Bcl-2 expression, arresting the cell at G2/M phase and inhibiting the cell migration, and providing cytotoxic effects and reduction in cell viability in human bladder cancer cells T24 (Ye et al. 2020). Geraniol also exhibited its anticancer property by downregulating the expression of E2F8 (a primary governor of prostate cancer) and suppressing the growth of cells by inducing G2/M cell arrest (Lee et al. 2016) and by inducing apoptosis which is governed by upregulation of expression of Bax and downregulation of Bcl-2 expression in Colo-205 cancer cells (Qi et al. 2018).

Carotenoids: Lycopene exhibited anticancer effect in PANC-1 cells by suppressing the levels of intracellular and mitochondrial ROS, mitochondrial functions, and NK-κB and upregulating the level of caspase-3 and ratio of Bax to Bcl-2 (Jeong et al. 2019). A study by Yu et al. Liu et al. (2018) demonstrated the anticancer effect of fucoxanthin when administered at a certain dose (50 or 75 μm) by arresting the cell cycle at S and G2/M phase and suppressing the Mcl-1, signal transducer and activator of transcription 3 (STAT3), and p-STAT3 in SGC-7901 or BGC-823 cells (Yu et al. 2018).

Animals: Various studies have been conducted demonstrating the role of lactoferrin in fighting cancer by inhibiting proliferation; inducing apoptosis, intracellular acidification, and disturbing the lysosomal acidification in PC-3 and MG-63 cell lines (Guedes et al. 2018); and inducing apoptosis and reducing the cell viability by 53 and 80% after 20 and 62 hours, respectively, when administered at a concentration of 500 μg/ml in esophageal cancer cell line KYSE-30 (Farziyan et al. 2016). Alpha linolenic acid (ALA), an ω-3 PUFA, also demonstrated its anticancer effect by reducing the cell migration, expression of VEGF (vascular endothelial growth factor), MMP-2, and MMP-9 protein; decreasing phosphorylated p38, pERK1/2, c-JUN, NF-κB, and COX2; proteins expression; and reducing the HPV oncoprotein E6 and E7 expression which induces the restoration of tumor-inhibiting proteins such as p53 and Rb in cancer cell lines, SiHa and HeLa (Deshpande et al. 2016). Another ω-3 PUFA, docosahexaenoic acid (DHA), also exerted its anticancer activity in HT-29 cell lines by inhibiting its cell proliferation activity and by downregulating proteasome particles (Ortea et al. 2018).

Vitamins: Vitamin C demonstrated its anticancer effect when administered at a defined dose (2 μm for 2 hours) in thyroid cancer therapy by suppressing the activity of ATP-dependent MARPK/ERK signaling and by inducing degradation of AKT through ROS-governed pathways and inhibition of PI3/AKT pathway both in vivo and in vitro (Su et al. 2019). A study conducted by Bazzaz in 2019 demonstrated the anticancer activity of γ-tocopherol (IC$_{50}$- 14.4 ± 2.6 μm) by increasing the expression or level of Bax, downregulating the expression of Bcl-2 and cyclin levels (cyclin D1 and cycline E), and accumulating cell population in phase sub-G1 (apoptotic cells) in HT-29 colon cancer cells.

4.3 Natural-Product Derivatives and CVDs Prevention

CVD is responsible for about 17.3 million deaths per year globally and its one form or the other can be seen in majority of people aged above 60 years. The factors responsible for the development of CVD include unhealthy diet, obesity, hypertension, hyperlipidemia, and diabetes mellitus. Various foods and dietary supplements have been shown to plummet the risk of CVDs. CVDs can be treated or prevented by using various classes of nutraceuticals such as plant sterol/stanols (by lowering low-density lipoprotein-cholesterol (LDL-C) or treating dyslipidemia with negligible effect on high-density lipoprotein-cholesterol (HDL-C), thus preventing the risk of CVD), polyphenols (intake of cocoa flavonols assists in reduction in LDL-C and total cholesterol (TC) with increase in HDL-C, tea polyphenols also assists in lowering TC and LDL-C with no effect on HDL-C, and olive oil polyphenols 30 mg/day for 2 months helps in decreasing blood pressure (Moreno-luna et al. 2012)), and spirulina (1 g spirulina taken for 3 months helps in reducing TC, LDL-C, and triglyceride levels (Mazokopakis et al. 2014)) (Sosnowska et al. 2017).

Flavonoids: Hesperetin demonstrated its effect against cardiac inflammation when administered at a certain dose (30 mg/kg/day for 8 weeks) by decreasing the expression of TNF-α, IL-1β and IL-6 (inflammatory markers), and collagen I and III (cardiac fibrosis markers) and by suppressing the NF-κB signaling pathway (Wang et al. 2017a). Quercetin exerted its cardioprotective effects in mice suffering from lipopolysaccharide (LPS)-induced cardiac abnormalities by suppressing TNF-α and IL-1β and by inhibiting the I-κB phosphorylation (Wei et al. 2018). Kaempferol reduced the inflammation by inhibiting the release of TNF-α, IL-1β, IL-6, and IL-18 and by suppressing the activation of NF-κB and AKT pathways in LPS-ATP-induced cardiac fibroblasts at the concentrations of 12.5 and 25 μg/ml (Tang et al. 2014). Fisetin treatment has also demonstrated therapeutic effect in treating hypertension and cardiac deterioration by inhibiting cardiac hypertrophy which was further demonstrated by the activation of p-P38 and the upregulation of ANP (atrial natriuretic peptide), BNP (B-type natriuretic peptide), NFATC3 (nuclear factor of activated T cells 3), and GATA-4 both in vivo and in vitro (Lin et al. 2019). Biochanin A induces cardioprotective effects by decreasing the serum glutamic oxaloacetic transaminase, lactate dehydrogenase (LDH), serum glutamic pyruvic transaminase, creatine kinase-MB (CK-MB), and cardiac troponin and by enhancing the antioxidant enzymes such as superoxide dismutase (SOD), catalase, glutathione peroxidase, glutathione-S-transferase, and glutathione reductase (Govindasami et al. 2020).

Non-flavonoids: Syringic acid exhibited its cardioprotective effect in rats having myocardial infection owing to downregulation of CK-MB, LDH, aspartate transaminase (AST), ALT, lipid peroxidation, protein carbonyl TNF-α, and IL-6 and upregulation of GSH and antioxidant enzymes(Shahzad et al. 2019). A study by Manjunatha et al. (2020) revealed that resveratrol along with syringic acid could be used to provide cardioprotective effect by decreasing serum CK-MB, LDH, alkaline phosphatase (AKP), TC, triglycerides, LDL-C, very LDL-C, thiobarbutyric acids, NF-kB, and TNF-α and by upregulating the cardiac tissue CK-MB, SOD, and catalase. A study by Aswar et al. (2019) demonstrated that FA provides cardioprotective effect in rats suffering from myocardial toxicity by reducing IL-1β, IL-6, calcium, normalizing heart rate, Ca^{2+}, Mg^{2+}, Na^+, and K^+ adenosine triphosphatase (ATPase) and by elevating GSH level.

Essential Oil: A study by El-Bassossy et al. (2017) revealed the potential of geraniol to combat diabetes-induced cardiac dysfunction when administered at a certain dose (150 mg/kg for 7 weeks) by suppressing the oxidative stress by inhibiting the increase in 8-isoprotane, arresting the inhibiting in catalase activity, and reducing the hyperglycemia and hypercholesterolemia. Another research demonstrated the cardioprotective effect of carvacrol by increasing the levels of SOD, decreasing the levels of MDA, upregulating the p-ERK (phosphorylated-ERK), and activating the signaling pathways such as MAPK/ERK and AKT/endothelial nitric oxide synthase (eNOS) (Chen et al. 2017)

Carotenoids: Lycopene has the potential to combat diclofenac sodium- and tulathromycin-induced cardiotoxicity in mice by upregulating antioxidant enzymes, scavenging free radicals of oxygen, and suppressing nitric oxide (NO) production, caspase-3, and Bax expression (Abdel-Daim et al. 2018).

Vitamin: Vitamin C, when administered at 50 mg/kg in rats suffering from doxorubicin-induced cardiomyopathy, provided cardioprotective effect by improving the systolic and diastolic function; restoring the structural damage; decreasing ROS, apoptotic protein expression, inflammation, superoxide, protein carbonyl formation, lipid peroxidation, NO and its synthase activity, inducible NO synthase (iNOS), IL-1β, TNF-α, and IL-6; and upregulation of antioxidant enzyme activities and vitamin C-transported proteins such as sodium ascorbate cotransporter 2 and glucose transporter 4 (Akolkar et al. 2017).

Some of the natural cardioprotective compounds, their dose and mode of action are discussed in Table 4.5.

Table 4.5 Natural cardioprotective compounds, their dose, and mode of action.

No.	Natural compounds	Dose	Mode of action	Studied on	References
1	Epicatechin	1 mg/kg body weight/day	Activation of SP1/SIRT1 signaling pathway	Mouse ventricular myocytes	Dong et al. (2017)
2	Sinapic acid	20mg/kg	Reduction of LDH, CK -MB, NF-κB p65, TNF-α, and IL-1β, endothelin (ET)-1 levels, Bax, and caspase-3; and upregulation of Bcl-2	Rats having cardiotoxicity induced by doxorubicin	Bin Jardan et al. (2020)
3	Ellagic acid	30 mg/kg for 14 days	Decrease in MDA and NO; and upregulation of catalase, SOD, and glutathione peroxidase	Rats having cardio- and hematotoxicity	Goudarzi et al. (2018)
4	Gingerol	10–40 μm	Suppression of expression of HMGB2 and JNK pathway and inhibited NF-κB nuclear translocation	AC16 cardiomyocytes	Zhang et al. (2019)
5	Vitamin C and vitamin E	1.7 mg vitamin C/50/ml water and chow diet with 2000 IU vitamin E/kg	Improvement in HDL antioxidant function and suppressed TNF-α, reduced serum cholesterol by suppressing apolipoprotein B (apoB)-48-containing lipoproteins	Atherogenic diet-fed mice	Contreras-Duarte et al. (2018)

4.4 Natural-Product Derivatives and Diabetes Prevention

Globally, around 300 million people are affected by type 2 diabetes which is characterized by insulin resistance in liver and muscles and lack of insulin secretion (Ramírez-Espinosa et al. 2018). Because of the development of vascular complications, the life expectancy of a person suffering from this disorder falls by 15 years (Oza and Kulkarni 2018a). Natural products may play a pivotal role in developing the required drugs for preventing diabetic disorders (Ramírez-Espinosa et al. 2018).

Polyphenols: Biochanin A is effective in decreasing type 2 diabetes mellitus when administered at 10, 20, and 40 mg/kg for 28 days to diabetic animals. It demonstrated a reduction in blood glucose (10, 20, and 40 mg/kg), reduction in glucose tolerance (40 mg/kg), reduction in insulin resistance (all doses), improvement in lipid profile (all doses), reduced formation of glycohemoglobin (all doses), and improvement in glycogen level of liver and increase in SIRT1 expression (40 mg/kg) (Oza and Kulkarni 2018a). Formononetin also exhibited its antidiabetic properties by reducing the levels of glucose in blood and glycohemoglobin content and enhancing the glucose tolerance, insulin sensitivity, lipid profile, and hepatic glycogen level along with a rise in SIRT1 expression when administered at 10, 20, and 40 mg/kg body weight to diabetic rats (Oza and Kulkarni 2018b). Syringic acid demonstrated its therapeutic role in closing the wounds fastly in diabetic rats by inhibiting NF-κB, p65, TNF-α, IL-1β, IL-8, IL-2, protein expression of CD 31 and 68, oxidative stress, MMP-2, MMP-8, and MMP-9 while upregulating SOD, CAT, GPx, GST, GR, IL-10, tissue inhibitors of metalloproteinases (TIMP)-1, and TIMP-2 (Ren et al. 2019). FA, 100 mg/kg once a day for 8 weeks, suppressed the oxidative stress, inflammation, and fibrosis in diabetic rats by increasing the kidney organ coefficient, SOD, CAT, GPx, and proteins such as nephrin and podocin and downregulating urinary protein, BUN, creatinine, fast blood glucose, TC, triglycerides, p-NF-κB p65, TNF-α, transforming growth factor (TGF)-β1, and collagen IV proteins (Qi et al. 2020). Curcumin exhibited its potential as an antidiabetic agent when administered at 100 mg/kg body weight for 8 weeks by increasing the expression of proliferating cell nuclear antigen (PCNA), SOD, and Bcl-2 and by downregulating the expressions of Bax and MDA in diabetic rats (Zhao et al. 2017).

Essential Oil Compounds: Eugenol is known to exert antihyperglycemic potential by dropping the blood glucose, glycosylated hemoglobin; increasing the level of plasma insulin; and restoring the activity of principle enzymes involved in carbohydrate metabolism (hexokinase, pyruvate kinase), liver marker enzymes, CK, and blood urea nitrogen present in serum and blood of rats when a dose of 10 mg/kg body weight was administered to streptozotocin-induced diabetic rats (Srinivasan and Sathish 2014). A recent evidence by Oskouei et al. (2019) suggests that thymol can also display antihypoglycemic and antihypolipidemic effect when administered at a certain dose (20 and 40 mg/kg) by decreasing the creatinine levels, reducing the cholesterols levels (LDL-C), and suppressing the enzymes related to the functioning of liver, such as aspartate aminotransferase and alanine aminotransferase in diabetic rats. Bacanli et al. (2017) proposed the antidiabetic effect of limonene by reducing the DNA damage, glutathione reductase, and MDA levels and increasing total glutathione, catalase activities, SOD, and glutathione peroxidase in diabetic rats. Another study by El-Bassossy et al. (2017) revealed the potential of geraniol to combat diabetes-induced cardiac dysfunction when administered at a certain dose (150 mg/kg for 7 weeks) by suppressing the oxidative stress by inhibiting the increase in 8-isoprotane, arresting the inhibition in catalase activity and reducing hyperglycemia and hypercholesterolemia.

Carotenoid: Lycopene showed its antidiabetic effects when administered at 4 mg/kg for 3 months by reducing MDA, total oxidative status, oxidative stress index, NK-κB, and TNF-α and by increasing total glutathione and total antioxidative status in alloxan-administered rats (Icel et al. 2019). Fucoxanthin demonstrated its potential as an antidiabetic agent to counter type 2 diabetes mellitus when administered at 0.2 and 0.4% for 6 weeks by suppressing the blood glucose (by increasing glucokinase (GK) and decreasing phosphoenolpyruvate carboxy kinase (PEPCK) mRNA expression); decreasing the lipid levels (by regulating PPAR α [peroxisome proliferator activated receptor alpha], p-ACC [p-acetyl CoA carboxylase], CPT [carnitine palmitoyl transferase]-1 and FAS), insulin resistance, reducing body weight and epididymal fat weight; and regulating the expression of signaling proteins such as IRS-1/PI3K/AKT and activated AMPK (Zhang et al. 2018b).

Animals: Chitosan oligosaccharides exhibited their role as antidiabetic agent when administered at a certain dose (200mg/kg/day for 3 months) for the treatment of type 2 diabetes by decreasing the blood glucose, reversing the resistance of insulin, suppressing the inflammation mediators, downregulating the lipogenesis, inhibiting the adipocyte differentiation, and restoring the damaged metabolic pathways which helped in reshaping the destructed gut microbiota by promoting *Akkermansia* and suppressing *Helicobacter* in mice (Zheng et al. 2018). Low-molecular weight chitosan, less than 1000 kDa, also demonstrated antidiabetic effects by inhibiting the suppression of intestinal α-glucosidase enzyme and glucose transporters such as SGLT1 and GLUT2 and by increasing the glucose uptake and the adipocyte differentiation via activation of PPARγ expression (Yu et al. 2017c).

Some of the naturally occurring anti-diabetic compounds, their dose and mode of action are discussed in Table 4.6.

Table 4.6 Natural antidiabetic compounds, their dose, and mode of action.

No.	Natural compounds	Dose	Mode of action	Studied on	References
1	Gallic acid (GA)	20mg/kg body weight for 6 weeks	Suppressed expression of TNF-α and upregulation of expression of PPARγ, mRNA, and adiponectin	Type 2 diabetic rat	Abdel-moneim et al. (2018)
	p-Coumaric acid (p-CA)	40 mg/kg body weight for 6 weeks			
2	Ellagic acid	15 and 30 μm	Upregulation of glucose consumption, IRS1, SOD, Nrf2, Heme oxygenase-1 (HO-1), miR-223, and phosphorylation of AKT and ERK expression; downregulation of ROS and keap1 protein level	HepG2 cell	Ding et al. (2019)
3	Carnasol	1, 5, and 10 mg/kg/day for 4 weeks	Decrease in IL-6, TNF-α, MDA, triglycerides, total cholesterol, LDL-C, serum glucose, and elevation in glutathione-s-transferase, SOD, catalase activity, and HDL-C	Streptozotocin-induced diabetic Rats	Samarghandian et al. (2017)
4	Vitamin C	100 μm	Reduction of NOS protein, inhibition of eNOS and iNOS mRNA expression	Human umbilical vein endothelial cells (HUVECs)s	Ghaffari et al. (2016)
	Vitamin E	200 μm			

4.5 Natural-Product Derivatives and Inflammation Prevention

Inflammation is the immune response or defense of the body against injury, infection, and irritation to remove the causative agents and promote healing (Barboza et al. 2018). Such a response comprises pain, heat, swelling, and redness. At a molecular level, the release of TNF-α, toxic molecules (NO and ROS), activation of NF-κB, and increased expression of certain inflammatory encoding genes such as COX-2 and iNOS have been observed. The increased level of inflammation can ultimately lead to organ failure, cancer, diabetes, and atherosclerosis (Kim et al. 2015). Immunosuppressive drugs such as anti-TNF-α antibodies and 5-aminosalicylates exert limited efficacy and side effects while curing the inflammation. Therefore, an increased interest is seen in curing or alleviating inflammation by natural products or bioactive compounds (Wang et al. 2017d).

Flavonoids: Luteolin exerted anti-inflammatory and antioxidant effect by introducing Heme oxygenase-1 (HO-1) expression along with reduction of NF-κB pathway activation that protected mice with severe acute pancreatitis (SAP) (Xiong et al. 2017). Apigenin effectively inhibited ulcerative colitis, a type of inflammatory bowel disease and colitis-associated cancer by suppressing NF-κB and STAT3 activity (Ai et al. 2017). Study demonstrated that luteolin and tangeretin together worked in synergy to show anti-inflammatory effects by inducing a great suppression of pro-inflammatory mediators such as PGE2, IL-1β, and IL-6 induced by LPSs. Decrease in LPS-induced protein and mRNA expression of iNOS and COX-2 using the combination was shown by real-time

PCR analysis (Funaro et al. 2016). Naringenin also demonstrated anti-inflammatory activity by inhibiting the NO release and expression of iNOS and COX-2, which was mediated via suppressors of cytokine signaling-3 which was further regulated by adenosine monophosphate-activate protein kinase α and protein kinase C δ (Wu et al. 2016a).

Quercetin also exerted its anti-inflammatory effect in microglial cells by suppressing LPS-induced NO production and enhancing the Nrf2/HO-1 protein expression (Sun et al. 2015b). Kaempferol demonstrated its anti-inflammatory capabilities by inhibiting the kinase activities of Src, Syk (spleen tyrosine kinase), IRAK (interleukin-1 receptor-associated kinase 1) 1, and IRAK4 which were involved in the activation of NF-κB and AP-1 both in vivo and in vitro. The flavonoid also inhibited the downstream pathways of NF-κB and AP-1 comprising IκBα or MKK3/4, JNK, and p38 (Kim et al. 2015). Myricetin also demonstrated its potential to combat against inflammation and inflammation-induced tumorigenesis by plummeting the levels of inflammatory factors such as TNF-α, IL-1β, IL-6, NF-κB, p-NF-κB, COX-2, PCNA, and Cyclin D1 (Zhang et al. 2018a). Pelargonidin-3-O-glucoside, an anthocyanin extracted from strawberry, exhibited its anti-inflammatory properties by suppressing IkB-α activation and reduction in JNK^{MAPK} phosphorylation (Jeremias et al. 2017).

Non-flavonoids: The hydroxycinnamic acid, p-coumaric acid, when administered at 100 mg/kg also displayed anti-inflammatory effects in acute liver injury by suppressing TNF-α and IL-6 (Kheiry et al. 2019). Gallic acid also showed its potential to combat inflammation in ulcerative colitis and by upregulating the expressions of IL-4 and IL-10 and suppressing the level of apoptosis, IL-1, IL-6, IL-12, IL-17, IL-23, TGF-β and TNF-α, and NF signaling pathway (Zhu et al. 2019). Curcumin is also effective in combating LPS-induced inflammation by suppressing the expression of inflammatory cytokine and microRNA-155 (due to suppression of PI3K/AKT signaling pathway) and decreasing the levels of AST, blood urea nitrogen, histological damage, and macrophages in spleen in Raw264.7 (IC50: 21.8 µm) and THP-1 (IC50: 22.3 µm) cells (Maa et al. 2017). Recent evidences prove that RA has the potential to fight inflammation by increasing the expression of Nrf2 and HO-1 and by suppressing the ASC (inflammasome adaptor protein), caspase-1, IL-1β, and NLRP3-inflammasome in UVB-exposed HaCat keratinocytes (Rodríguez-Luna et al. 2019).

Essential Oil Compounds: Recent studies suggest that eugenol (at a concentration of 150 mg/kg) can prevent lung damage by providing anti-inflammatory and antioxidant effects by blocking the release of inflammatory cytokines such as TNF-α, IL-1β, and IL-6; inhibiting the activity of NADPH oxidase; suppressing the activity of antioxidant enzymes such as catalase, glutathione peroxidase, and SOD; and reducing LPS-induced protein oxidation (Magalhães et al. 2019). Thymol also demonstrated its capacity to lower acetic acid-induced inflammation in rat colon tissue by blocking the production of myeloperoxidase (MPO) and TNF-α and by inhibiting the NF-κB signaling pathway (Chamanara et al. 2019). Recent evidences also demonstrate the potential of carvacrol to act as anti-inflammatory agent by suppressing activity of muscle MPO and edema, and inhibiting the activity of IL-1β, IL-6, MIP-2 (macrophage inflammatory protein), and TNF-α (Souza et al. 2018). Limonene also proved its potential as an anti-inflammatory agent by suppressing the MMP-2 and MMP-9 expression, increasing antioxidant expression levels of iNOS and COX-2 protein, decreasing the production of prostaglandin E2, and suppressing the expression of TGF-β and ERK½ in ulcerative colitis rat model (Yu et al. 2017b).

Animals: Lactoferrin exhibited its anti-inflammatory, antioxidant, and hepatoprotective property by decreasing the expression of IL-1β and by upregulating the expression of both IL-10 and hepatic paraoxonase-1 (PON1) (Farid et al. 2019). The dipeptides ((Cys-Arg), (Phe-Leu), (His-Cys), (Leu-Leu), and (Met-Lys)) derived from ovotransferrin demonstrated their anti-inflammatory effects by inhibiting the expression of genes in cytokines such as TNF-α, IL-8, IL-6, IL-1β, and

IL-12 and by upregulating the expression of anti-inflammatory cytokines (IL-10) in Caco-2 cells (Wang et al. 2017d). Trans-11, cis-12 conjugated linoleic acid (t10,c12 CLA), α-linolenic acid, and linoleic acids demonstrated their anti-inflammatory activity by upregulating the expression of PPARγ which helped in inhibiting the transcription of pro-inflammatory cytokines (Dipasquale et al. 2018). Eicosapentaenoic acid (EPA) and DHA also demonstrated their potential as an anti-neuroinflammatory agent by suppressing the expression or level of TNF, MPO activity, ATF-3 (Activation transcription factor) and by improving the SFI (Sciatic Functional Index) which further promoted the increase in expression of GAP-45 and myelinated fibers in sciatic nerve in mice having peripheral nerve injury (Silva et al. 2017). Vitamin D demonstrated antioxidative and anti-inflammatory effects by suppressing the level of MDA and by inhibiting the expression of all the pro-inflammatory cytokines, promoting the antioxidant activity and expression of anti-inflammatory markers in rats suffering from hepatorenal injuries induced by paracetamol (El-boshy et al. 2019).

Some of the natural anti-inflammatory compounds, their dose, and mode of action are discussed in Table 4.7.

Table 4.7 Natural anti-inflammatory compounds, their dose, and mode of action.

No.	Natural compounds	Dose	Mode of action	Studied on	References
1	Genistein	—	G protein-coupled estrogen activation, inhibition of inflammatory mediators, and activation of MAPKs and NF-κB	BV2 microglial cell line	Du et al. (2018)
2	Daidzein derivatives	0.01, 1, and 100 μm	Inhibition of TNF-α-induced phosphorylation of JNK	Caco-2 cells	Peng et al. (2017)
3	Epicatechin	—	Inhibition of TNF-α, IL-6, IL-1β, Bax, and caspase-3 Downregulation of mitochondrial apoptotic pathway and increased Bcl-2	Liver injured mice	Wu et al. (2020)
4	Caffeic acid and FA	—	Suppressing iNOS, COX-2, IL-6, IL-1β, phosphorylation of STAT3, AKT, and IκB and NF-κB expression	BV2 and RAW264.7 cells	Kwon et al. (2019)
5	Gingerol	200,150, 100, 50, and 25 μg/ml	Suppression of IL-1β, TNF-α, iNOS, COX-2, IL-6, p-p65, and p-IκB expression	RAW 264.7 cells	Liang et al. (2018)
6	Citral	3, 6, and 12 μm	Activation of PPAR-γ and suppressing NF-κB activation	Human umbilical vein endothelial cells (HUVECs)	Song et al. (2016)
7	Linalool	15 or 30 mg/kg	Activation of AKT, suppression of iNOS expression, MAPKs, and NK-κB pathways	Mice with allergic asthma	Kim et al. (2019)
8	Carnosol	100 μl of 10 μm of carnosol in 0.05% DMSO	Activation of STAT3 (regulates inflammatory genes) and inhibition of iNOS and COX-2	Mice	Yeo et al. (2019)
9	Carvone	25 and 50 mg/kg	Reduction of TNF-α, IL-1β, and IL-6	LPS-induced lung injury in Mice	Zhao and Du (2019)

4.6 Natural-Product Derivatives and Neurogenerative Diseases Prevention

One of the factors promoting the neurogenerative disease is oxidative stress (caused by neuroinflammation (Lee and Jeong 2016)) or lipid peroxidization which can be prevented using the enzymatic antioxidant defense system of the body. This mechanism contains antioxidants such as SOD and glutathione peroxidase (Haq et al. 2018). Recently, natural and herbal products such as flavonoids and their derivatives and other herbal products having medicinal values are getting significant attention as therapeutic agents against neurogenerative diseases such as Alzheimer's and Parkinson's diseases (Motaghinejad et al. 2017).

Flavonoids: Baicalein induces a neuroprotective effect against rotenone-induced Parkinson's disease model by attenuating depletion of dopaminergic neurons thereby restoring mitochondrial function and improving mitobiogenesis. Improvement in mitobiogenesis was facilitated by CREB (cAMP-responsive element-binding protein) and glycogen synthase kinase-3β (GSK-3β) pathways in SH-SY5Y cells (Zhang et al. 2017b). Fisetin induces a neuroprotective effect against lead (Pb)-induced neuroinflammation and neurodegeneration by reducing the levels of Bax, toll-like receptor (TLR) 4, myeloid differentiation factor 88 (MyD88), NF-κB, and cleaved caspase-3 and by inactivating the inflammatory factors such as IL-6 and TNF-α. It also restores the lead-induced synaptic dysfunction by promoting the levels of SNAP (synaptosomal-associated protein)-25, postsynaptic density (PSD)-95, CREB phosphorylation, and CaMKII (calcium or calmodulin kinase II) phosphorylation (Yang et al. 2019). Butein, a chalcone, demonstrated its neuroprotective effect in HT-22 cell lines by the inhibition of IL-6, IL-1β and TNF-α and the upregulation of Nrf2/ARE-promoted HO1 via PI3K/AKT pathways (Lee and Jeong 2016).

Non-flavonoids: CAPE exhibited neuroprotective effect against memory disorder (Alzheimer's disease) by reducing oxidative stress via upregulation of Nrf2 and HO-1 fueled by modulating GSK-3β and downregulating neural apoptosis and suppressing neuroinflammation along with improvement in learning, when administered at a dose of 10mg/kg (Morroni et al. 2018). p-Coumaric acid also worked as an antidepressant by reducing inflammatory cytokines, increasing BDNF (brain-derived neurotrophic factor) and playing a role in improving despair-related behavior in forced swim test, tail suspension test and sucrose splash test (Lee et al. 2018b). Gallic acid exhibited neuroprotective effect in 6-OHDA-induced neurotoxic SH-SY5Y cell line by preventing the depolarization of MMP, decreasing cell death, suppressing the ROS, caspase-3 and keap-1, decreasing the ratio of Bax to Bcl-2 and upregulating the Nrf2, BDNF, and p-CREB (Chandrasekhar et al. 2018). FA also exhibited neuroprotective role by blocking the glial cell activation, phosphor-C-jun N-terminal kinase (p-JNK), NFκB, iNOS, COX-2, TNF-α, IL-1β, Bax, cytochrome C, caspase-3 and PARP-1 and upregulating the proteins such as PSD-95, synaptophysin, SNAP-25 and SNAP-23 (Rehman et al. 2019).

Recent studies demonstrated that curcumin at a defined concentration (10, 20, 40, and 60 mg/kg for 21 days) can act as a promising agent for neuroprotection against nicotine-induced inflammation, apoptosis, and oxidative stress by suppressing LPO, GSH, IL-1β, TNF-α, and Bax levels and by upregulating the levels of Bcl-2, SOD, P-CREB, and BDNF (Motaghinejad et al. 2017). Resveratrol exhibited neuroprotective effect by upregulating the expression of choline acetyltransferase, SOD, glutathione, and Sirt1 and by downregulating the acetylcholinesterase, MDA, IL-1β, IL-6 levels, thereby preventing the memory impairment in rat suffering from diabetes and Alzheimer's disease (Ma et al. 2020). Rosmarinic acid is also known to combat memory disorder (Alzheimer's disease) by decreasing aggregation of amyloid β (Aβ) in mice, upregulating monoamines (norepinephrine, 3,4-dihydoxypehnnylacetic acid, levodopa, and dopamine), and downregulating monoamine oxidase B (a dopamine degrading enzyme) (Hase et al. 2019).

Essential Oil Compounds: Cinnamaldehyde demonstrated its capacity to counter neuroinflammation-induced memory impairment in mice by decreasing the production of NO which was fueled by the degradation of iNOS mRNA which was further caused by the suppression of MEK1/2-ERK1/2 signaling pathway (Zhang et al. 2016b). Limonene also exhibited its neuroprotective and antidepressant effect by suppressing the level or production of MDA, NO, activities involving NADPH, pro-inflammatory markers' expression (iNOS, COX-2, IL-6 and IL-1β), TNF-α, and proapoptotic protein expression and by cleaving the caspase-3, activating the AMPKα signaling pathways and suppressing NK-κB in PC12 cell lines (Tang et al. 2019b).

Carotenoids: Fucoxanthin showed its neuroprotective effect when administered at a defined dose (0.3 to 3 µM for 2 hours) against H_2O_2-induced neurotoxicity by decreasing the activity of ERK pathway and by upregulating the P13-K/AKT pathways in SH-SY5Y cells (Yu et al. 2017a).

Vitamins: α-tocopherol also displayed a potential to counter cognitive impairment and oxidative stress when used at a concentration of 100 mg/kg for 2 weeks as indicated by improvement in behavior tests, decrease in mRNA level of VEGF, and upregulation in mRNA expression levels of BDNF, TrkB (tyrosine receptor kinase B), and CREB (Nagib et al. 2019). The molecule exhibited similar effect when administered at a certain dose (10 µm for 1 hour) along with an increase in reduced glutathione and decreased lipid peroxidation level in brain tissue of sheep having H_2O_2-induced oxidative stress (Haq et al. 2018). α-tocopherol demonstrated neuroprotective effect when administered at a defined dose (100–300 mg/kg) in rats suffering from epilepsy induced by pentylenetetrazole by inducing improvement in cognitive performance and reducing the oxidative stress (Patil et al. 2017).

Some of the naturally occurring neuroprotectice compounds, their dose and mode of action are discussed in Table 4.8.

4.7 Natural-Product Derivatives and Obesity Prevention

Obesity is recognized as one of the most prevalent chronic diseases in the world and promotor of certain chronic and fatal diseases such as diabetes mellitus, dyslipidemia, coronary heart disease, hypertension, and cancer. The primary reason for the onset of obesity includes high-fat and high-energy diet which causes abnormal body fat accumulation causing the lipid levels of the body to rise (Si et al. 2017). Many anti-obesity drugs are available in the market, but they are associated with side effects such as liver damage, abdominal pain, and bloating (Wu et al. 2016b).

Flavonoids: Quercetin demonstrated its potential to be used as an anti-obesity agent by inhibiting MAPK signaling factors such as ERK1/2, JNK, and p38MAPK; suppressing the inflammatory cytokines such as IL-1β and IL-6; promoting the anti-inflammatory cytokine IL-10; and ultimately reducing the body weight by almost 40% (Seo et al. 2015). Cherry and mulberry anthocyanins demonstrated their potential as an anti-inflammatory and anti-obesity agent by improving the lipid profile and by decreasing the oxidative stress and inflammation in diet-induced obesity by reducing the glucose and leptin levels in serum; decreasing the MDA (malondialdehyde) production and expression of TNFα, IL-6, iNOS, and NF-κB genes; and promoting activities of SOD and GP_x (glutathione peroxidase activity) (Wu et al. 2016c). A study conducted by Wu et al. (2016b) demonstrated that administration of blueberry anthocyanin at doses of 200 mg/kg for 8 weeks in the daily food of obese mice decreased their weight by 19.4% due to the reduction of glucose in serum and fall in epididymal adipocytes, downregulation of TNFα, IL-6, PPARγ, and FAS genes expression, and improvement in lipid profile.

Table 4.8 Natural neuroprotective compounds, their dose, and mode of action.

No.	Natural compounds	Dose	Neurogenerative disease	Mode of action	Studied on	References
1	Quercetin	30 mg per kg per day for 14 days	Alzheimer's disease	Inhibition of lipid peroxidation and formation of NO, and improvement in memory and cognitive abilities	$A\beta_{25-35}$-injected Alzheimer's disease mice model	Hyun et al. (2016)
2	Chrysin	200 mg/kg	Parkinson's disease	Upregulated hepatic glutathione (GSH), SOD, suppressed lipid peroxidase (LPO) levels, improved muscular activity, and locomotion	Parkinson's disease mouse model	Krishnamoorthy et al. (2019)
3	Linalool	25 mg/kg/2days for 3 months	Alzheimer's disease	Suppression in pro-inflammatory p38 MAPK, NOS2, COX2, and IL-1β	Mice	Sabogal-Guáqueta et al. (2016)
4	FA (-)-Epigallocatechin-3-gallate	30 mg/kg each, once a day for 3 months	Alzheimer's disease	Upregulation of APP-α and α-secretase and downregulation of expression of APP-β, β-carboxyl-terminal APP fragment, and β-secretase	Mice	Mori et al. (2019)

Non-Flavonoids: A study conducted by Ding et al. (2016) proved the role of curcumin in preventing obesity and insulin resistance by suppressing the expression of SREBP (sterol regulatory element-binding protein) in vitro in Huh-7/SRE-Luc cells and ameliorating the level of serum lipids and insulin sensitivity in high fat diet (HFD)-induced mice. Lycopene demonstrated antiobesity effect when administered at 0.03% w/w for 10 weeks by inhibiting lipid accumulation and lipogenesis of genes' expression (via increased thermogenic and mitochondrial genes' mRNA expression), improving insulin resistance, downregulating circulating insulin and leptin, and inflammation expression in obese mice with high fructose and fat diet (Wang et al. 2019a). Clove extract containing 42.27% eugenol exhibited anti-obesity property by inhibiting FAS (a potential target in cancer and obesity), arresting S-phase DNA replication of HepG2 cells, inhibiting OP9 cell differentiation, and suppressing the high-fat diet-induced obesity (Ding et al. 2017)

Animal: Chitosan oligosaccharide capsules were administered for eight weeks on high-fat diet rats which caused inhibition of synthesis of hepatic lipid by increasing SREBP-1c, FAS, ACC, 3-hydroxy-3-methylglutaryl-CoA reductase (HMGCR), adiponectin, PPARγ, CCAAT-enhancer binding protein α (C/EBPα), and adipose differentiation-related protein (ADRP) expression and by reducing leptin resistance and lipid accumulation via activation of Jak2 and STAT3 signaling pathways (Pan et al. 2018). The combination of chitosan-starch complex was more successful than individual components in controlling the body weight, proving its hypolipidemic effect, along with enhancement in concentration of HDL-C and suppression of oxidative stress owing to the antioxidant capacity. The complex led to downregulation of genes such as *SREBP-1* (metabolism gene), *PPARγ*, *HMGCR* (cholesterol synthesis gene), and *GAPDH* (gluconeogenesis gene) and upregulation of genes such as *Acox1* (lipid oxidation gene)and liver functional genes such as *Gstm2* and *Gclc* (Si et al. 2017).

Vitamins: Ascorbic acid also demonstrated suppression in visceral obesity induced by high-fat diet when administered at a dose (1% w/w for 15 weeks) by decreasing gain in body weight, mass of adipose tissues, and size of visceral adipocyte; upregulating the concentration of mRNAs of PPARα; and increasing its target enzymes which involved oxidation of fatty acids in visceral tissues, decreasing hepatic inflammation, fibrosis, and apoptosis (Lee et al. 2019).

Some of the natural anti-obesity compounds, their dose and mode of action are discussed in Table 4.9.

Table 4.9 Natural anti-obesity compounds, their dose, and mode of action.

No.	Natural compounds	Dose	Mode of action	Studied on	References
1	Secoisolariciresinol	100 μm	Inhibition of PPARγ and C/EBPα, decreased lipid accumulation, adipocyte fatty acid binding protein, adiponectin and resistin, and upregulation of AMPK α	3T3-L1 cell line	Kang et al. (2018)
2	Citral	30, 40, and 50 μm	Suppression of PI3K/AKT, transcription factors (PPARγ, Sterol regulatory element-binding proteins (SREBP)-1c, FAS, CPD), inflammatory genes (*TNF-α, IL-6,* and *MCP-1*)	Mouse fibroblast 3T3-L1 cells	Devi and Ashokkumar (2018)
3	Cinnamaldehyde	40 mg/kg body weight for 8 weeks	Increasing insulin sensitivity and increasing the peroxisome proliferator-activated receptor (PPAR) γ, PR domain-containing 16, and PPARγ coactivator 1α proteins	Mice	Zuo et al. (2017)

4.8 Natural-Product Derivatives and Microbial Disease Prevention

Natural products derived from plants and animals are known to act against various microbial diseases and infections (Table 4.10) caused by various pathogenic microbes (bacteria, fungi, and viruses). Various foodborne pathogens such as *Listeria monocytogenes* are known to threaten people's health by causing meningitis, sepsis, and premature birth (Han et al. 2020). Another foodborne pathogen *Staphylococcus aureus* is known to be one of the primary cause of gastroenteritis globally (Rúa et al. 2019). *Salmonella typhimurium*, a gram-negative foodborne pathogen, is also associated with gastrointestinal infections in humans (Giovagnoni et al. 2020). Different bacterial strains such as *Pseudomonas aeruginosa, Streptococcus pneumoniae, S. aureus, Acinetobacter baumannii,* and *Mycobacterium tuberculosis,* having the potential to cause infections in human, are reported to be multidrug resistant. One such case is the death of a person infected by *Klebsiella pneumoniae,* which was resistant against all the permitted antibiotics in the United States (Reiter et al. 2017). Moreover, the drugs which are utilized in the treatment of diseases are not only expensive but also possess toxicity as well as side effects. There are several studies indicating the use of natural products (which are nontoxic or less toxic and do not cause adverse effects) in developing a novel drug for the treatment of arboviral infections such as chikungunya (Murali et al. 2015).

4.8.1 Quercetin

Quercetin 3-glucoside also known as isoquercetrin or Q3G, a derivative of quercetin isolated from *Dianthus superbus* var. longicalysinus, demonstrated its potent antiviral activity against influenza A and B virus by suppressing the cellular effects such as ROS production and acidic vesicular organelles (AVO) formation and exhibiting more binding affinity, as compared to 7-methylated GTP, by binding to the polymerase basic protein-2 subunit of the virus and ultimately blocking the virus replication (Nile et al. 2020). The flavonoids, consisting of rutin, hyperin, isoquercetrin, and quercetin, extracted from *Houttuynia cordata* Thunb. alleviate influenza-induced acute lung injury by suppressing the levels of TNF-α, IL-8, MDA, monocyte chemotactic protein 1 (MCP-1), TLR, and nuclear transcription factor-κB p65 phosphorylation (NF-κB p65(p)) in the lung tissues. In addition to the study, out of the four flavonoids, two flavonoids (hyperin and quercetin) inhibited the virus replication (Ling et al. 2020). A study conducted by Gaudry et al. (2018) also demonstrated antiviral effect of Q3G against epidemic strains (African and Asian) of Zika virus in different human hepatoma (huh-7), epithelial (A549), and neuroblastoma (SH-SY5Y) cell lines with IC_{90} concentration as 50, 32, and 15 µM, respectively, by preventing the entry of the virus into the host cell.

The flavonoids such as morin, quercitrin, catechin, and quercetin exhibited promising results as antimicrobial compounds by favoring the formation of a more stable compound (which is toxic to the plasmodium) between free and flavonoid (with morin being effective even at a concentration as low as 0.04 mg/ml) and by suppressing the formation of β-hematin (Abu-Lafi et al. 2020). Quercetin also demonstrated its potential to combat pneumococcal infections caused by *S. pneumoniae* by weakening the bacterial ability to form biofilm by suppressing neuraminidase A (NanA) and sortase A (srtA) activity (which plays a crucial role for bacterial colonization) and by acting as a competitive substrate resulting in the loss of srtA transpeptidase activity (Wang et al. 2018a). Recent evidences suggest that the flavonoid can be used to mitigate intestinal infection caused by *Escherichia coli* O157:H7 by suppressing the interaction between the bacteria and the integrin β1

Table 4.10 Natural-product, their category, their dose, their antimicrobial activity, and the disease caused by the pathogen and mechanism.

No.	Compound	Category	Dose	Disease	Pathogen	Mechanism	References
1	Quercetin Kaempferol	Flavonol	MIC: 16 mg/ml MIC: 8 mg/ml	Dental caries	*Streptococcus mutans*	Inhibition of bacterial growth and metabolic activities, suppression of acid production, and inhibition of glucan synthesis	Zeng et al. (2019)
2	Galangin		MIC: 32 µg/ml	Pneumonia, sepsis, and endocarditis	Vancomycin-intermediate *Staphylococcus aureus* (VISA)	Suppression of division of Mu50 cells of VISA, inhibition of murein hydrolase genes such as *atl*, *lytM, and lytN* and regulatory genes such as *cidR, cidA, and cidB*	Ouyang et al. (2018)
3	Isorhamnetin		MIC >1024 µg/ml		*Staphylococcus aureus*	Suppression of *RNAIII* expression and blocking *hla* (gene responsible for making alpha-hemolysin) transcription	Jiang et al. (2016)
4	Hesperetin Naringenin	Flavanone	IC$_{50}$: 8.50 µm IC$_{50}$: 6.818 µm	Chikungunya fever, and lymphadenitis	Chikungunya virus	Inhibiting the RNA replication of the virus (by inhibiting the *Rluc* marker) and reducing the expression of E2 protein	Ahmadi et al. (2016)
5	Hesperetin Ellagic acid	Flavanone Tannin	MIC: 3125 µg/ml MIC: 31.7 µg/ml	Intestinal infections, diarrhea, septicemia, wound infections, and cellulitis	*Aeromonas hydrophila*	Increase in anti-liposaccharide (LPS) IgM expression, suppression in anti-LPS and anti-extracellular protein (ECP) IgA expression	Abuelsaad et al. (2013)

(Continued)

Table 4.10 (Continued)

No.	Compound	Category	Dose	Disease	Pathogen	Mechanism	References
6	Resveratrol	Stilbene	MIC: 70–75 μg/ml	Acne	*Propionibacterium acnes*	Disrupting the cell membrane and cell death	Taylor et al. (2014)
			MIC: 256 μg/ml	Pneumonia, endocarditis, keratitis, and sepsis	*Staphylococcus aureus*	Inhibiting the alpha-hemolysin expression by suppressing *hla* and suppression of transcription of RNA III	Tang *et al.* (2019a)
			MIC: 512 μg/ml			Inhibition of alpha-hemolysin by reducing *hla* and *saeRS*	Duan et al. (2018)
7	Syringic acid	Hydroxybenzoic acid	MIC: 5 mg/ml	Bacteremia, necrotizing enterocolitis, and neonatal meningitis	*Cronobacter sakazakki*	Inhibition of bacterial growth, membrane dysfunction (depolarization of membrane), and changes in cellular morphology	Shi et al. (2016)
8	Benzyl isothiocyanate	Organosulfur compounds	MIC: 200 μg/ml	Gastrointestinal diseases, bloody diarrhea	*E. coli* O157:H7	Disruption of cellular member and release of intracellular content and cell death	Patel et al. (2020)
				Vomiting, gastroenteritis, and salmonellosis	*Salmonella enterica*		
			MIC: 0.5 mmol/l	Pneumonia, sepsis and endocarditis	*S. aureus*	Downregulation of expression of capsular polysaccharide encoding genes (*cp5D* and *cp8F*), thermonuclease (*nuc*), clumping factor (*clf*), and protein A (*spa*)	Wang et al. (2019b)

#	Compound	Class	MIC/value	Disease	Organism	Mechanism	Reference
9	Allicin		MIC_{90}: 128 µg/ml	Urinary tract infections	*Proteus mirabilis*	Diffusion of compound in cytoplasm and inhibition of urease	Ranjbar-Omid et al. (2015)
			250 µm	Bacteremia, UTI, and respiratory infections	*Pseudomonas aeruginosa*	Suppression of quorum-sensing genes (*rhl* and *pqs*), inhibiting factors responsible for pathogenesis such as elastase, pyocyanin, pyoverdine, and rhamnolipids	Xu et al. (2019)
			MIC: 64 µg/ml	Meningitis and bacteremia	*S. pneumoniae*	Passage of allicin via cell membrane	Reiter et al. (2017)
			MIC: 32 µg/ml	Scarlet fever, cellulitis, and pharyngitis	*S. pyogenes*		
10	Berberine	Alkaloid	MIC: 128 µg/ml	Pneumonia, sepsis, and endocarditis	Methicillin-resistant *Staphylococcus aureus* (MRSA)	Inhibition of formation of MRSA amyloid fibrils (as berberine binds with phenol ring (Phe19) of phenol-soluble modulin (PSMα2))	Chu et al. (2016)
			IC_{50}: 16.01±5.0 µm	Diarrhea, UTI, pneumonia, meningitis, bacteremia, and cholecystitis	*Escherichia coli*	Disturbing the FtsZ protofilaments and suppressing its GTPase activity	Domadia et al. (2008)
11	Sanguinarine		MIC: 4 µg/ml	Candidiasis and candidemia	*Candida albicans*	Inhibiting biofilm formation by decreasing protein and polysaccharide	Qian et al. (2020c)
			MIC: 4 µg/ml	Pneumonia, sepsis, and endocarditis	*S. aureus*	Inhibiting biofilm formation by mediating polysaccharides and eDNA level	

(Continued)

Table 4.10 (Continued)

No.	Compound	Category	Dose	Disease	Pathogen	Mechanism	References
12	Piperine and mupirocin (antibiotic)		MIC (piperine alone): >100 µg/ml	Pneumonia, sepsis, and endocarditis	*S. aureus*	Suppression of MdeA efflux pump	Mirza et al. (2011)
13	Caffeic acid	Hydroxycinnamic acid	MIC: 256 to 1024 µg/ml			Increase in cell membrane permeability or membrane impairment/cell damage/ inhibition of α-hemolysin toxic of *S. aureus*	Kępa et al. (2018)
14	Chalcone	Flavonoid	IC_{50}: 28.41±5.34 µm	Listeriosis	*Listeria monocytogenes*	Suppression of sortase A (SrtA) enzyme by binding to an active side of the enzyme	Li et al. (2016a)
15	Eugenol nano emulsion	Phenol	Sub-MIC: 0.2 mg/ml	Bacteremia, UTI, and respiratory infections	*Pseudomonas aeruginosa*	Suppression of *LasI*, *rhlA*, and *rhlI*	Lou et al. (2019)
16	Thymol and carvacrol	Monoterpenoid phenol	MIC: 1.87 µm (both)	Typhoid fever and diarrhea	*Salmonella typhimurium*	Inhibition of virulent genes *hilA*, *prgH*, *invA*, *sipA*, *sipC*, *sipD*, *sopB*, and *sopE2*	Giovagnoni et al. (2020)
			Thymol: 0.005–0.008 mg/ml Carvacrol: 0.007–0.008 mg/ml	Bacteremia, UTI, and respiratory infections	*Pseudomonas aeruginosa*	Disrupting the cell membrane and leakage of intracellular components and cell death	Althunibat et al. (2016)

#	Compound	Class	Concentration	Disease/Symptoms	Organism	Mechanism	Reference
17	Trans-cinnamaldehyde	Aldehyde	Subinhibitory concentration (SIC): 0.005%	Fever, abdominal pain, diarrhea, and Guillain-Barre syndrome	*Campylobacter jejuni*	Downregulation of genes for motility (*fliA*), adhesion (*cadF*) and cytolethal distending toxin (*CDT*) genes (*cdtA*, *cdtB*, and *cdtC*)	Upadhyay et al. (2017)
18	Carvacrol	Monoterpenoid phenol	SIC: 0.001%			Suppressing genes for motility (*motA*), fibronectin adhesion (*cadF*), and *cdtB*	
19	Eugenol	Phenol	SIC: 0.005%			Downregulating *motA*, racR, and *cdtA*	
20	Geraniol	Monoterpene	MIC: 0.25 mg/ml	Pneumonia, sepsis, and endocarditis	*S. aureus*	Cellular death by plasmolysis due to changes in permeability of cell membrane	Pontes et al. (2019)
21	Rosemary extract (carnosol)	Diterpene	5 µm			Suppression of *agr* quorum-sensing expression	Nakagawa et al. (2020)

(a transmembrane glycoprotein receptor) and by interfering with the FAK association resulting in the decrease of focal adhesion proteins (which play a pivotal role in cell adhesion and migration) such as talin, vinculin, and α-actinin (Xue et al. 2019). Quercetin and luteolin along with ceftazidime synergistically demonstrated their antibacterial activity against infections or diseases such as scarlet fever, childbed fever, puerperal sepsis, and pharyngitis causing gram-negative, β-lactamase-producing *Streptococcus pyogenes* by suppressing the production of peptidoglycan, promoting the permeability of cell membranes, and enhancing the amide I protein contents of bacterial cells (Siriwong et al. 2015). Quercetin showed its potential to combat methicillin-resistant *S. aureus* by suppressing the secretion of alpha toxin, a cytotoxic protein which is responsible for the pathogenesis of pneumonia caused by Methicillin-resistant *Staphylococcus aureus* (MRSA) (López and Sánchez 2017).

4.8.2 Kaempferol

Kaempferol demonstrated its ability to combat infections resulting from biofilms of *S. aureus* as it successfully inhibited the *S. aureus* SrtA and suppressed the crucial attachment phase, which is required for the formation of biofilms. From the same study, it was found that the flavonoid at 64 μg/ml reduced the srtA activity and biofilm by 47 and 80%, respectively (Ming et al. 2017). A recent study conducted by Escandón et al. (Escandón et al. 2016) exhibited the antibacterial activity of kaempferol and (−)-epicatechin, both individually and combined, in AGS gastric cancer cells against infections such as gastric ulcers or cancer caused by the gram-negative *Helicobacter pylori*. The flavonoid also displayed anti-inflammatory effect in response to inflammation induced by *H. pylori* by suppressing the level of inflammatory mediators such as TNF-α, IL-8, and IL-1β in AGS cells and reducing the transcription of type IV secretion system (which further reduced the translocation of cytotoxin-associated gene A) and secretion system subunit protein A belonging to type V secretion system (which decreased the vacuolating cytotoxin A) in *H. pylori*.(Yeon et al. 2019). Kaempferol displayed its potential for treating acute liver injury caused by H9N2 influenza virus by reducing the levels of ROS, MDA, TNF-α, IL-6, and IL-1β; inhibiting the TLR4, phosphorylated IκBα, NF-κB, and MAPKs signaling pathways; and upregulating the expression of SOD (Zhang et al. 2017a).

4.8.3 Myricetin

Myricetin (>256 μg/ml) demonstrated its antibacterial and anti-inflammatory property by acting against *Streptococcus suis*, a gram-positive bacterium responsible for a variety of diseases such as arthritis, meningitis, and endocarditis, by inhibiting suilysin (an *S. suis* cytotoxin generated by the bacteria responsible for its virulence) and by suppressing the inflammation caused by infection by reducing the production of pro-inflammatory cytokines such as TNF-α and IL-1β and suppressing the p38 pathway (Li et al. 2019b). The flavonoid also exhibits its potential to combat dental caries which are caused by the biofilms formed by *Streptococcus mutans* and *Candida albicans* as indicated by the reduction in the number of water-soluble exopolysaccharides in the extracellular matrix (Rocha et al. 2018). The flavonoid also demonstrated its antiviral property against herpes simplex virus (HSV) type 1 and type 2 by directly targeting the gD protein (which is required by HSV to enter), resulting in the formation of a more stable myricetin–gd complex and interfering with the adsorption and membrane fusion process and blocking the replication by suppressing the epidermal growth factor receptor (EGFR)/phosphoinositide 3-kinase (PI3k)/protein kinase B (AKT) pathway (Li et al. 2020). A recent study conducted by Daino et al. (2018) revealed that myricetin, with an IC_{50} value of 2.7 μm, can inhibit the recombinant viral protein VP35 in Ebola virus which plays a pivotal role in the lethality of the virus as it blocks the production of interferon type 1, cloaking the dsRNA and preventing its identification by the recognition receptor retinoic acid-inducible gene I (*RIG-I*).

4.8.4 Luteolin

Luteolin exhibits its antibacterial and antibiofilm effect against *S. aureus* and *L. monocytogenes* by partial or entire destruction of the cell membrane and leakage of the intracellular contents (Qian et al. 2020a). Another study by Guo et al. (2017) demonstrated that the flavonoid also reduced the inflammation caused by *S. aureus* by suppressing the expressions of cytokines such as TNF-α, IL-1β, and IL-6; reducing TLR2 and TLR4; decreasing the amount of MMP-2 and MMP-9 and inhibiting NF--κB p65 phosphorylation; and upregulating the expressions of tissue inhibitor of metalloproteinases (TIMP)-1 and TIMP-2. The molecule also alleviates the urinary tract infections caused by uropathogenic *E. coli* by reducing the invasive bacteria which was linked to increased intracellular cAMP levels due to suppressed cAMP-phosphodiesterase activity, thereby activating the protein kinase A and suppressing the activity of Rac1-GTPase-mediated polymerization (Shen et al. 2016). Luteolin also demonstrated its antiviral effect by inhibiting the replication of influenza A virus by interfering with its replication at the initial stage of infection by reducing the expression of β-COP (a component of coat protein I) protein (which prevented or blocked the adsorption of virus) (Yan et al. 2019).

4.8.5 Apigenin

Apigenin extracted from *Aster yomena* (herb for treating inflammation, cold, and asthma) exhibited promising effects as a therapeutic antifungal agent against *C. albicans* by inhibiting its growth mediated by causing stress in cell membrane which leads to the shrinkage of cell and makes the membrane incapable to maintain the osmotic balance (Lee et al. 2018a). Apigenin demonstrated its antiviral activity against hepatitis C virus by inhibiting the expression levels of microRNA122 (miR122), which are responsible for the replication of virus by suppression of TRBP phosphorylation (Shibata et al. 2014). The flavonoid also demonstrated its potential to combat gastric epithelial inflammation induced by *H. pylori* by suppressing the expression or level of NF-κB and inflammatory mediators such as COX-2, intercellular adhesion molecule (ICAM)-1, ROS, IL-6, and IL-8 and by upregulating the expressions of IκBα and mucin (MUC)-2 (suppress the inflammation and prevents development of intestinal tumor) (Wang and Huang 2013).

4.8.6 Chrysin

Chrysin-loaded chitosan nanoparticles exhibited antibiofilm property and a potential to be used as therapeutic drug to combat *S. aureus,* at an MIC and sub-MIC of 1024 μg/ml and 768 μg/ml, respectively, by suppressing the cell hydrophobicity and decreasing the production of exopolysaccharides, which prevents the cell attachment to the substratum (Siddhardha et al. 2020) and prevents pneumonia caused by the *S. aureus* by inhibiting alpha-hemolysin (Wang et al. 2011).

4.8.7 Eriodictyol

Eriodictyol demonstrated its potential to combat *S. aureus* infections or injury with a MIC of 512 μg/ml by targeting or inhibiting alpha-hemolysin (Hla), a critical exotoxin responsible for the pathogenicity of the bacteria (Xuewen et al. 2018).

4.8.8 Naringenin

The flavonoid demonstrated its antimicrobial activity against *S. aureus* (MIC: 1.84 μm or 0.50 g/l), *E. coli, Bacillus cereus, L. monocytogenes*, and *Salmonella enteritidis* (Wang et al. 2017c). The molecule (100 and 200 μg/ml) exhibited its therapeutic potential as an anticaries agent to prevent the dental caries caused by the biofilms of *S. mutans* by suppressing the formation of biofilms by increasing the hydrophobicity of the bacteria, suppressing its aggregation, and decreasing the expression such as gtfB, gtfC, comD, comE, and luxS (Jiaxi Yue et al. 2018). The citrus flavonoid, naringenin, also demonstrated its antibacterial effect against *Salmonella enterica* serovar typhimurium by suppressing genes in *Salmonella* pathogenicity island 1 (SPI-1), which is required for attachment and entry in a pstS/hilD-dependent manner and decreasing class 1 and 2 genes of flagellar operon which reduces the motility of *Salmonella* (Vikram et al. 2011). A study conducted by Cataneo et al. (2019) demonstrated the potential of naringenin for treating Zika virus infections as it acted on the replication of viral particles and interacted, as a noncompetitive inhibitor, with the NS2B-NS3 protease of the virus, as suggested by a molecular docking analysis.

4.8.9   Anthocyanin

Proanthocyanidins excreted from American cranberry demonstrated its antimicrobial effect and potential to combat infections caused by *P. aeruginosa* by inhibiting the N-acyl homoserine lactone (AHL)-mediated quorum sensing by antagonizing its regulators such as *LasR* and *RhlR* and by suppressing its autoinducer synthases *LasI* and *RhlI* (Maisuria et al. 2016). Recent evidences also indicate the effectiveness of wild blueberry anthocyanins against *L. monocytogenes* (MIC: 0.53 mg/ml), *S. aureus* (MIC: 0.27 mg/ml), *Salmonella* enteritidis (MIC: 0.53 mg/ml), and *Vibrio parahaemolyticus* (MIC: 0.13 mg/ml) by disrupting and destroying the membrane integrity (as demonstrated by leakage of nucleic acid and intracellular proteins) and by suppressing the enzyme activity (AKP, ATPase, and SOD) (Sun et al. 2018).

4.8.10   Resveratrol

Resveratrol, with an MIC ranging from 78.12 µg/ml to 156.25 µg/ml (depending on the strain), demonstrated antimicrobial effect to combat biofilms of periodontal disease-causing *Porphyromonas gingivalis* by inhibiting the expressions of genes responsible for its pathogenesis such as fimbriae-encoding genes *fimA* (type II and type IV) and proteinases such as Arg-specific cysteine proteinase (*rgpA*) genes and Lys-specific cysteine proteinase (kgp) genes (Kugaji et al. 2019). Another study conducted by Augustine et al. (2014) also confirmed the antibiofilm activity of resveratrol (in a concentration-dependent manner) at an MIC of 60 µg/ml against cholera-causing *Vibrio cholerae* by targeting the AphB protein. The phytochemical (MIC: 5 µg/ml) can also exhibit antimicrobial activity against typhoid-causing *S. typhimurium* by increasing the cell membrane permeability, DNA damage, and cell death; upregulating the expressions of ROS and MDA; and reducing the levels of reduced form of antioxidant glutathione (GSH) (Lee and Lee 2017).

4.8.11   Gallic Acid

Gallic acid demonstrated its antibiofilm property and therapeutic potential to cure infections caused by *S. aureus,* with an MIC 2 mg/ml for suspension and 4 mg/ml for biofilms, by interfering or changing the expression of *ica* operon (which is responsible for encoding polysaccharide intercellular adhesion) by upregulating the *icaR*, downregulating the expression of *icaA* and *icaD*, and suppressing the formation of slime (Liu et al. 2017). The molecule also exhibited antibiofilm property against the biofilms of *E. coli* and *S. mutans* with an MIC of 8 mg/ml against bacteria (Shao et al. 2015).

4.8.12   Curcumin

Mun et al. (2013) demonstrated the potential of curcumin as an effective natural antibiotic against MRSA with an MIC ranging from 125 to 250 µg/ml. The polyphenolic compound also exhibited antibacterial property against *E. coli,* at a concentration of 24 and 48 µg/ml, by inducing apoptosis as demonstrated by increase in ROS, depolarization of membrane, increase in Ca^{+2}, and increase in *RecA* (a caspase-like protein) (Yun and Lee 2016). Another study by Sethupathy et al. (2016) also demonstrated the antibacterial activity and the potential of curcumin to be used as therapeutic natural drug to treat infections caused by *P. aeruginosa* by inhibiting its quorum-sensing (at a concentration of 5 μg/ml) mediated virulence factors and biofilm formation.

4.8.13 Eugenol

The compound (MIC: 0.2 mg/l) demonstrated its potential to combat carbapenem-resistant *Klebsiella pneumoniae* (CRKP) and a possibility to tackle CRKP-related infections by damaging the cell membrane (which was demonstrated by the suppression of amount of intracellular ATP, decreased pH, and hyperpolarized cell membrane) and by inhibiting the biofilm formation by inhibiting biofilm-associated genes such as *pgA*, *luxS*, *wbbM*, and *wzm* (Qian et al. 2020b). Eugenol also exhibited its antimicrobial property against vancomycin-resistant *S. aureus* by ROS generation and damaging the membrane (Das et al. 2016). Devi et al. (2010) demonstrated the potential antibacterial activity of phenol (MIC: 0.0125% and MBC: 0.025%) against *Salmonella typhi* by promoting membrane permeability, causing the ions and other cellular components such as proteins to leak out and ultimately lead to the disruption of the membrane resulting in cell death. Eugenol also demonstrated its anticaries effect against the biofilms of *S. mutans* by reducing the expression of AgI/II (a protein used by the bacteria to attach to a tooth surface) and downregulating the genes which are related to quorum sensing (*gtfB*, *gtfC*, *comDE*, *smu630*, *vicR*, *brpA*, *ftf*, *relA*, *gbpB*, and *spaP*) (Adil et al. 2014). It also exhibited antibiofilm effect on biofilms formed by enterohemorrhagic *E. coli* O157:H7 by suppressing genes which are crucial for biofilm formation and attachment such as curli genes (*csgA*, *csgB*, *csgD*, *csgF*, and *csgG*), type 1 fimbriae genes (*fimC*, *fimD*, and *fimH*), and ler-controlled toxin genes (*espD*, *escJ*, *escR*, and *tir*) (Kim et al. 2016b). The phenol is also known to act against the infections caused by *L. monocytogenes* in human intestinal cells (Caco-2) by reducing the attachment capability of the pathogen to E-cathedrin, by suppressing the genes responsible for its pathogenesis, and by reducing the pathogenic factors such as motility, cell invasion, and production of listeriolysin (Upadhyay et al. 2016).

4.8.14 Thymol

Thymol demonstrated its potential to combat infections caused by *Salmonella typhimurim* by effectively inhibiting the activity of type III secretion system-1 (T3SS-1), a crucial protein which is responsible for pathogenesis of the bacteria (Zhang et al. 2018c). A study by Wang et al. (2017b) also explained the antibacterial property of the monoterpene phenol against *Actinobacillus pleuropneumoniae* by destroying the integrity of bacterial cell membrane; reducing its biofilm formation; upregulating the expression of *purC*, *tbpB1*, and *clpP*; and downregulating the levels of *ApxI*, *ApxII*, and *Apa1*. Thymol demonstrated its potential for treating infections caused by methicillin-resistance *S. aureus* by inhibiting both biofilm formation and mature biofilms by suppressing the polysaccharide intracellular adhesin (PIA) production (which plays pivotal role in adhesion and assembly), inhibiting the releasing the extracellular DNA (which plays a role in adhesion, assembly, formation of microcolonies and biofilm formation), and reducing the levels of genes responsible for formation of PIA (*icaA*, *sarA*, and *cidA*) (Yuan et al. 2020). Thymol can also protect against female urogenital infections caused by *E. coli* and *S. aureus* by inhibiting the adhesion of bacteria to human vaginal cells (Sasso et al. 2006).

4.8.15 Cinnamaldehyde

Ferro et al. (2016) demonstrated the potential of cinnamaldehyde to be used as antibacterial nutraceutical against the infections caused by *S. aureus* as it successfully suppressed the hemolytic activity of the bacteria, decreased its adhesion to latex (by downregulating the *S. aureus* protein A (spA)), and promoted the lysis in a (freshly isolated human serum) serum-dependent manner. The molecule also demonstrated its capacity to act against infections caused by *M. tuberculosis* by inhibiting its growth and providing bactericidal effects possibly by penetrating the cell wall of mycobacterium and stressing its integrity, as indicated by the overexpression of *clgR* genes (which gets activated or expressed whenever it senses stress on the membrane) (Sawicki et al. 2018). Cinnamaldehyde also provided promising effects against *E. coli* and *S. aureus* at a minimum inhibitory concentration of 0.31 mg/ml by disturbing the cell integrity causing separation of membrane from cell wall, destruction of cell membrane, leakage of cytoplasmic content, cell distortion, and condensation of cytoplasmic components (Shen et al. 2015). Recent evidence has also shown the antibacterial activity of cinnamaldehyde against *Salmonella enterica* serovar *Typhimurium* by inhibiting the SPI-1, which prevents invasion of HeLa cells due to SPI-1 and further suppressing the genes (*sipA* and *sipB*) encoded by SPI-1 (Liu et al. 2019).

Other Essential Oil Compounds: Carvacrol demonstrated its antimicrobial effect at a minimum inhibitory concentration of 450 µg/ml against uropathogenic *E. coli* by upregulating the expression of ROS and by disrupting the membrane, causing the cellular matter to release and ultimately causing cell death (Khan et al. 2017). Limonene inhibited the activity of *L. monocytogenes* at an MIC of 20 ml/l by destructing the membrane integrity and structure of the bacteria, resulting in the leakage of nucleic acid and proteins (Han et al. 2020).

4.8.16 Carotenoids

Fucoxanthin: A study conducted by Karpiński and Adamczak (2019) described the antimicrobial effect of fucoxanthin against *Streptococcus agalactiae* (MIC; ZOI:62.5 µg/ml; 12.2±0.75 mm), *Staphylococcus epidermidis* (MIC; ZOI:125 µg/ml; 11.2±0.75 mm), and *S. aureus* (MIC; ZOI:125 µg/ml; 11.0±0.75 mm).

Lycopene: Lycopene exhibited its antifungal activity against *C. albicans* at a minimum inhibitory concentration of 5 µg/ml by introducing apoptosis by upregulating the production of ROS (promoting DNA damage), increasing Ca^{+2} and mitochondrial dysfunction, and releasing cytochrome c from mitochondria to cytoplasm which leads to caspase activation (Choi and Lee 2015). The carotenoid also demonstrated its potential to combat gastric infections, involving DNA damage, caused by *H. pylori* at a concentration of 2 and 5 µm by suppressing the ROS production, apoptosis by suppressing the ataxia-telangiectasia-mutated (ATM)/checkpoint kinase 2 (Chk2)/p53 and ataxia telangiectasia, and Rad3-related (ATR)/Chk1 activation (Jang et al. 2012). The carotenoid also demonstrated antichlamydial effect against chlamydia infection caused by *Chlamydophila pneumoniae* in volunteers as the level of IgG antibodies against the bacteria dropped significantly, when orally administered with a dose of 7 mg lycopene for 28 days (Zigangirova et al. 2017).

4.8.17 Vitamins

4.8.17.1 Vitamin C

A study by Ran et al. (2018) revealed (using meta-analysis of randomized controlled trials) that extra doses of vitamin C, apart from routine supplementation, can help in reducing the duration of common cold by half a day and decrease the symptoms (sore throat, fever, aching, chest pain, chills, and runny nose) associated with it. Another meta-analysis by Vorilhon et al. (2019) also confirmed that vitamin C can reduce the duration of upper respiratory tract infection in children. Vitamin C, along with red ginseng, demonstrated its therapeutic potential in reducing the lung inflammation caused by influenza A/H1N1 virus by activation of T and natural killer cells' natural cytotoxic receptor NKp46, enhancing the production of interferon (IFN)-γ, suppressing the inflammation, and decreasing the virus replication (Kim et al. 2016a).

A study by Vilchèze et al. (2018) demonstrated that vitamin C (1 µm) has the potential to enhance the efficacy of isoniazid and rifampicin against infections caused by *M. tuberculosis* and reduce the bacterial burden in a more effective way (reduction by seven days) than using the drugs alone (within three to four weeks). The vitamin also demonstrated its potential to dampen acute enterocolitis induced by *Campylobacter jejuni* (MIC: 352-2818 mg/l depending on the strain) by reducing the apoptotic and pro-inflammatory cytokines and upregulating the anti-inflammatory effects in intestine, liver, kidney, and lungs (Mousavi et al. 2020). The molecule also delivered promising results at 5, 10, and 20 mg/ml concentrations against *E. coli* and *K. pneumoniae* which may be due to anti-quorum-sensing activity or structural change (Verghese et al. 2017).

4.8.17.2 Vitamin D
Vitamin D (200 IU/day) and curcumin (200 mg/BB/day) (when administered for five days and maintained for three weeks) demonstrated antimicrobial effect as shown by reduced colonies of *Salmonella typhi* in the intraperitoneal fluid of mice (Febriza et al. 2019). A recent study conducted by Grant et al. (2020) suggests intake of 10000 IU/day of vitamin D3 for a few weeks followed by intake of 5000 IU/day, so as to raise the concentration of 25-hydroxyvitamin D above 46–60 ng/ml, can reduce the risk of influenza/COVID-19. Another study demonstrated the possible role of vitamin D (4000 IU/day for 10 days) in developing innate immunity against dengue virus as the monocyte-derived dendritic cells showed suppressed mRNA expression of TLRs (TLR3, TLR7 and TLR9), decreased level of IL-12/IL-8 generation, and enhanced IL-10 production in response to the virus (Martínez-Moreno et al. 2020).

4.8.17.3 Vitamin E
Both lipophilic and hydrophilic forms of vitamin E demonstrated their potential to be used as a therapeutic drug, along with norfloxacin and ceftazidime, in treating the respiratory infections caused by *Burkholderia cenocepacia* by preventing the binding of BcnA, an extracellular lipocalin protein produced by *B. cenocepacia,* to antibiotics (Naguib and Valvano 2018). Vitamin E and D3 also inhibited the growth of *S. aureus* by inhibiting the efflux pump (Tintino et al. 2016).

4.9 Conclusion

Nutraceuticals are derived from various natural sources such as plants, animals, and microbes and are effective against various diseases, disorders, and infections. Plant-based natural products or phytochemicals include flavonoids such as flavones, flavonols, and anthocyanins; non-flavonoids such as phenolics acids, lignans, and tannins; EOs such as eugenol, thymol, citral, and cinnamaldehyde; and carotenoids such as lycopene. Animal-based natural products include lactoferrin, ovotransferrin, PUFAs, and chitosan. Nutraceuticals derived from the mentioned natural sources have shown their potential to combat various diseases or disorders such as CVDs, inflammation, cancer, obesity, diabetes, and neurogenerative diseases. The natural products also showed their potential to fight against diseases such as dental caries, typhoid, diarrhea, UTI, listeriosis, respiratory infections, pneumonia, and bacteremia caused by different bacteria, fungi, and viruses. Since the already existing synthetic drugs and antibiotics are either quite expensive or cause side effects, the derivatives of natural products can be used to develop drugs which can prevent diseases.

References

Abdel-Daim, M.M., Eltaysh, R., Hassan, A. et al. (2018). Lycopene attenuates tulathromycin and diclofenac sodium-induced cardiotoxicity in mice. *International Journal of Molecular Sciences* 19 (2): 344. doi: 10.3390/ijms19020344.

Abdel-moneim, A., El-twab, S.M.A., Yousef, A.I. et al. (2018). Modulation of hyperglycemia and dyslipidemia in experimental type 2 diabetes by gallic acid and p-coumaric acid: The role of adipocytokines and PPARγ. *Biomedicine & Pharmacotherapy* 105: 1091–1097. doi:10.1016/j.biopha.2018.06.096.

Abuelsaad, A.S.A., Mohamed, I., Allam, G. et al. (2013). Antimicrobial and immunomodulating activities of hesperidin and ellagic acid against diarrheic Aeromonas hydrophila in a murine model. *Life Sciences* 93 (20): 714–722. doi: 10.1016/j.lfs.2013.09.019.

Abu-Lafi, S., Akkawi, M., Al-Rimawi, F. et al. (2020). Morin, quercetin, catechin and quercitrin as novel natural antimalarial candidates. *Pharmacy & Pharmacology International Journal* 8 (3): 184–190. doi: 10.15406/ppij.2020.08.00295.

Adil, M., Singh, K., Verma, P.K. et al. (2014). Eugenol-induced suppression of biofilm-forming genes in Streptococcus mutans: an approach to inhibit biofilms. *Journal of Global Antimicrobial Resistance* 2 (4): 286–292. doi: 10.1016/j.jgar.2014.05.006.

Ahmadi, A., Hassandarvish, P., Lani, R. et al. (2016). Inhibition of chikungunya virus replication by hesperetin and naringenin. *RSC Advances* 6 (73): 69421–69430. doi: 10.1039/C6RA16640G.

Ai, X., Qin, Y., Liu, H. et al. (2017). Apigenin inhibits colonic inflammation and tumorigenesis by suppressing STAT3-NF-κB signaling. *Oncotarget* 8 (59): 100216–100226.

Akolkar, G., Da Silva Dias, D., Ayyappan, P. et al. (2017). Vitamin C mitigates oxidative/nitrosative stress and inflammation in doxorubicin-induced cardiomyopathy. *American Journal of Physiology – Heart and Circulatory Physiology* 313 (4): H795–H809. doi: 10.1152/ajpheart.00253.2017.

Althunibat, O.Y., Qaralleh, H., Al-Dalin, S.Y.A. et al. (2016). Effect of thymol and carvacrol, the major components of Thymus capitatus on the growth of Pseudomonas aeruginosa. *Journal of Pure and Applied Microbiology* 10 (1): 367–374.

Anandabaskar, N., Selvarajan, S., and Kamalanathan, S. (2018). Vitamin D in health and disease – an update. *Journal of Young Pharmacists* 10 (4): 381–387. doi: 10.5530/jyp.2018.10.85.

Andlauer, W. and Fürst, P. (2002). Nutraceuticals: a piece of history, present status and outlook. *Food Research International* 35 (2–3): 171–176. doi: 10.1016/S0963-9969(01)00179-X.

Aswar, U., Mahajan, U., Kandhare, A. et al. (2019). Ferulic acid ameliorates doxorubicin-induced cardiac toxicity in rats. *Naunyn-Schmiedeberg's Archives of Pharmacology* 392 (6): 659–668. doi: 10.1007/s00210-019-01623-4.

Augustine, N., Goel, A.K., Sivakumar, K.C. et al. (2014). Resveratrol – a potential inhibitor of biofilm formation in Vibrio cholerae. *Phytomedicine* 21 (3): 286–289. doi: 10.1016/j.phymed.2013.09.010.

Bacanli, M., Anlar, H.G., Aydın, S. et al. (2017). D-limonene ameliorates diabetes and its complications in streptozotocin-induced diabetic rats. *Food and Chemical Toxicology* 110: 432–442. doi: 10.1016/j.fct.2017.09.020.

Barboza, J.N., Maia, S., Filho, B. et al. (2018). Review article an overview on the anti-inflammatory potential and antioxidant profile of Eugenol. *Oxidative Medicine and Cellular Longevity* 2018: 3957262.

Bazzaz, R. (2019). Adjuvant therapy with γ-tocopherol-induce apoptosis in HT-29 colon cancer via cyclin-dependent cell cycle arrest mechanism. *Journal of Biochemical and Molecular Toxicology* 33 (11): e22399. doi: 10.1002/jbt.22399.

Bin Jardan, Y.A., Ansari, M.A., Raish, M. et al. (2020). Sinapic acid ameliorates oxidative stress, inflammation, and apoptosis in acute doxorubicin-induced cardiotoxicity via the NF-κB-mediated pathway. *BioMed Research International* 2020: doi: 10.1155/2020/3921796.

Cataneo, A.H.D., Kuczera, D., Koishi, A.C. et al. (2019). The citrus flavonoid naringenin impairs the in vitro infection of human cells by Zika virus. *Scientific Reports* 9: 16348. doi: 10.1038/s41598-019-52626-3.

Chamanara, M., Abdollahi, A., Rezayat, S.M. et al. (2019). Thymol reduces acetic acid-induced inflammatory response through inhibition of NF-kB signaling pathway in rat colon tissue. *Inflammopharmacology* 27 (6): 1275–1283. doi: 10.1007/s10787-019-00583-8.

Chambial, S., Dwivedi, S., Shukla, K.K. et al. (2013). Vitamin C in disease prevention and cure: an overview. *Indian Journal of Clinical Biochemistry* 28 (4): 314–328. doi: 10.1007/s12291-013-0375-3.

Chandrasekhar, Y., Kumar, G.P., Ramya, E.M. et al. (2018). Gallic acid protects 6-OHDA induced neurotoxicity by attenuating oxidative stress in human dopaminergic cell line. *Neurochemical Research* 43 (6): 1150–1160. doi: 10.1007/s11064-018-2530-y.

Chauhan, B., Kumar, G., Kalam, N. et al. (2013). Current concepts and prospects of herbal nutraceutical: a review. *Journal of Advanced Pharmaceutical Technology & Research* 4 (1): 4–8. 10.4103/2231-4040.107494.

Chen, Y., Ba, L., Huang, W. et al. (2017). Role of carvacrol in cardioprotection against myocardial ischemia/reperfusion injury in rats through activation of MAPK/ERK and Akt/eNOS signaling pathways. *European Journal of Pharmacology* 796: 90–100. doi: 10.1016/j.ejphar.2016.11.053.

Chen, H., Tang, X., Liu, T. et al. (2019a). Zingiberene inhibits in vitro and in vivo human colon cancer cell growth via autophagy induction, suppression of PI3K/AKT/mTOR Pathway and caspase 2 deactivation. *Journal of BUON* 24 (4): 1470–1475.

Chen, X., Li, X.F., Chen, Y. et al. (2019b). Hesperetin derivative attenuates CCl4-induced hepatic fibrosis and inflammation by Gli-1-dependent mechanisms. *International Immunopharmacology* 76: 105838. doi: 10.1016/j.intimp.2019.105838.

Choi, H. and Lee, D.G. (2015). Lycopene induces apoptosis in Candida albicans through reactive oxygen species production and mitochondrial dysfunction. *Biochimie* 115: 108–115. doi: 10.1016/j.biochi.2015.05.009.

Chu, M., Zhang, M.B., Liu, Y.C. et al. (2016). Role of berberine in the treatment of methicillin-resistant staphylococcus aureus infections. *Scientific Reports* 6: 24747. doi: 10.1038/srep24748.

Ci, Y., Zhang, Y., Liu, Y. et al. (2018). Myricetin suppresses breast cancer metastasis through down-regulating the activity of matrix metalloproteinase (MMP)-2/9. *Phytotherapy Research* 32 (7): 1373–1381. doi: 10.1002/ptr.6071.

Contreras-Duarte, S., Chen, P., Andía, M. et al. (2018). Attenuation of atherogenic apo B-48-dependent hyperlipidemia and high density lipoprotein remodeling induced by vitamin C and E combination and their beneficial effect on lethal ischemic heart disease in mice. *Biological Research* 51 (1): 34. doi: 10.1186/s40659-018-0183-6.

Dagli, N., Dagli, R., Mahmoud, R. et al. (2015). Essential oils, their therapeutic properties, and implication in dentistry: a review. *Journal of International Society of Preventive and Community Dentistry* 5 (5): 335. doi: 10.4103/2231-0762.165933.

Dai, W., Sun, C., Huang, S. et al. (2016). Carvacrol suppresses proliferation and invasion in human oral squamous cell carcinoma. *Oncotargets and Therapy* 9: 2297–2304. doi: 10.2147/OTT.S98875.

Dai, G., Jiang, Z., Sun, B. et al. (2020). Caffeic acid phenethyl ester prevents colitis-associated cancer by inhibiting NLRP3 inflammasome. *Frontiers in Oncology* 10: doi: 10.3389/fonc.2020.00721.

Daino, G.L., Frau, A., Sanna, C. et al. (2018). Identification of myricetin as an Ebola Virus VP35–double-stranded RNA interaction inhibitor through a novel fluorescence-based assay. *Biochemistry* 57 (44): 6367–6378. doi: 10.1021/acs.biochem.8b00892.

Das, L., Bhaumik, E., Raychaudhuri, U. et al. (2012). Role of nutraceuticals in human health. *Journal of Food Science and Technology* 49 (2): 173–183. doi: 10.1007/s13197-011-0269-4.

Das, B., Mandal, D., Dash, S.K. et al. (2016). Eugenol provokes ROS-mediated membrane damage-associated antibacterial activity against clinically isolated multidrug-resistant staphylococcus aureus strains. *Infectious Diseases* 9: 11–19. doi: 10.4137/idrt.s31741.

De La Chapa, J.J., Singha, P.K., Lee, D.R. et al. (2018). Thymol inhibits oral squamous cell carcinoma growth via mitochondria-mediated apoptosis. *Journal of Oral Pathology and Medicine* 47 (7): 674–682. doi: 10.1111/jop.12735.

Deshpande, R., Mansara, P., and Kaul-ghanekar, R. (2016). Alpha-linolenic acid regulates Cox2/VEGF/MAP kinase pathway and decreases the expression of HPV oncoproteins E6/E7 through restoration of p53 and Rb expression in human cervical cancer cell lines. *Tumor Biology* 37 (3): 3295–3305. doi: 10.1007/s13277-015-4170-z.

Devi, S.S. and Ashokkumar, N. (2018). Citral, a monoterpene inhibits adipogenesis through modulation of adipogenic transcription factors in 3T3-L1 cells. *Indian Journal of Clinical Biochemistry* 33 (4): 414–421. doi: 10.1007/s12291-017-0692-z.

Devi, K.P., Nisha, S.A., Sakthivel, R. et al. (2010). Eugenol (an essential oil of clove) acts as an antibacterial agent against Salmonella typhi by disrupting the cellular membrane. *Journal of Ethnopharmacology* 130 (1): 107–115. doi: 10.1016/j.jep.2010.04.025.

Ding, X. and Chen, H. (2018). Anticancer effects of Carvone in myeloma cells is mediated through the inhibition of p38 MAPK signalling pathway, apoptosis induction and inhibition of cell invasion. *Journal of BUON* 23 (3): 747–751.

Ding, L., Li, J., Song, B. et al. (2016). Curcumin rescues high fat diet-induced obesity and insulin sensitivity in mice through regulating SREBP pathway. *Toxicology and Applied Pharmacology* 304: 99–109. doi: 10.1016/j.taap.2016.05.011.

Ding, Y., Gu, Z., Wang, Y. et al. (2017). Clove extract functions as a natural fatty acid synthesis inhibitor and prevents obesity in a mouse model. *Food & Function* 8 (8): 2847–2856. doi: 10.1039/C7FO00096K.

Ding, X., Jian, T., Wu, Y. et al. (2019). Ellagic acid ameliorates oxidative stress and insulin resistance in high glucose-treated HepG2 cells via miR-223/keap1-Nrf2 pathway. *Biomedicine and Pharmacotherapy* 110: 85–94. doi: 10.1016/j.biopha.2018.11.018.

Dipasquale, D., Basiricò, L., Morera, P. et al. (2018). Anti-inflammatory effects of conjugated linoleic acid isomers and essential fatty acids in bovine mammary epithelial cells. *Animal* 12 (10): 2108–2114. doi: 10.1017/S1751731117003676.

Domadia, P.N., Bhunia, A., Sivaraman, J. et al. (2008). Berberine targets assembly of Escherichia coli cell division protein FtsZ. *Biochemistry* 47 (10): 3225–3234. doi: 10.1021/bi7018546.

Dong, Z., Wan, L., Wang, R. et al. (2017). (−)-Epicatechin suppresses Angiotensin II-induced cardiac hypertrophy via the activation of the SP1/SIRT1 signaling pathway. *Cellular Physiology and Biochemistry* 41 (5): 2004–2015. doi: 10.1159/000475396.

Du, Z., Feng, X., Li, N. et al. (2018). G protein-coupled estrogen receptor is involved in the anti-inflammatory effects of genistein in microglia. *Phytomedicine* 43: 11–20. doi: 10.1016/j.phymed.2018.03.039.

Duan, J., Li, M., Hao, Z. et al. (2018). Subinhibitory concentrations of resveratrol reduce alpha-hemolysin production in Staphylococcus aureus isolates by downregulating saeRS. *Emerging Microbes and Infections* 7 (1): 136. doi: 10.1038/s41426-018-0142-x.

Durazzo, A., Lucarini, M., Souto, E.B. et al. (2019). Polyphenols: a concise overview on the chemistry, occurrence, and human health. *Phytotherapy Research* 33 (9): 2221–2243. doi: 10.1002/ptr.6419.

Egert, S. and Rimbach, G. (2011). Which sources of flavonoids: complex diets or dietary supplements? *Advances in Nutrition* 2 (1): 8–14. doi: 10.3945/an.110.000026.

El-Bassossy, H.M., Ghaleb, H., Elberry, A.A. et al. (2017). Geraniol alleviates diabetic cardiac complications: effect on cardiac ischemia and oxidative stress. *Biomedicine and Pharmacotherapy* 88: 1025–1030. doi: 10.1016/j.biopha.2017.01.131.

El-boshy, M., Basalamah, M.A., Ahmad, J. et al. (2019). Vitamin D protects against oxidative stress, inflammation and hepatorenal damage induced by acute paracetamol toxicity in rat. *Free Radical Biology and Medicine* 141: 310–321. doi: 10.1016/j.freeradbiomed.2019.06.030.

Eroğlu, C., Avcı, E., Vural, H. et al. (2018). Anticancer mechanism of Sinapic acid in PC-3 and LNCaP human prostate cancer cell lines. *Gene* 671: 127–134. doi: 10.1016/j.gene.2018.05.049.

Escandón, R.A., del Campo, M., López-Solis, R. et al. (2016). Antibacterial effect of kaempferol and (−)-epicatechin on Helicobacter pylori. *European Food Research and Technology* 242 (9): 1495–1502. doi: 10.1007/s00217-016-2650-z.

Fan, S., Xu, H., Liu, H. et al. (2019). Inhibition of cancer cell growth by Tangeretin flavone in drug-resistant MDA-MB-231 human breast carcinoma cells is facilitated via targeting cell apoptosis, cell cycle phase distribution, cell invasion and activation of numerous Caspases. *Journal of BUON* 24 (4): 1532–1537.

Farid, A.S., El Shemy, M. A., Nafie, E. et al. (2019). Anti-inflammatory, anti-oxidant and hepatoprotective effects of lactoferrin in rats. *Drug and Chemical Toxicology*. Taylor & Francis 1–8. doi: 10.1080/01480545.2019.1585868.

Farziyan, M.A., Moradian, F., and Rafiei, A. (2016). Research in molecular medicine anticancer effect of bovine lactoferrin on human esophagus cancer cell. *Research in Molecular Medicine* 4 (1): 18–23. doi: 10.7508/rmm.2016.01.003.

Febriza, A.M.I., Kasim, V.N.A., Idrus, H.H. et al. (2019). The effects of curcumin and vitamin D combination as inhibitor toward salmonella typhi bacteria growth in vivo. *International Journal of Applied Pharmaceutics* 11 (5): 116–120. doi: https://doi.org/10.22159/ijap.2019.v11s5.T0093.

Ferro, T.A.F., Araújo, J.M.M., do Pinto, B.L.S. et al. (2016). Cinnamaldehyde inhibits staphylococcus aureus virulence factors and protects against infection in a galleria mellonella model. *Frontiers in Microbiology* 7: 2052. doi: 10.3389/fmicb.2016.02052.

Funaro, A., Wu, X., Song, M. et al. (2016). Enhanced anti-inflammatory activities by the combination of luteolin and tangeretin. *Journal of Food Science* 81 (5): H1320–H1327. doi: 10.1111/1750-3841.13300.

Gaudry, A., Bos, S., Viranaicken, W. et al. (2018). The flavonoid isoquercitrin precludes initiation of Zika virus infection in human cells. *International Journal of Molecular Sciences* 19 (4): 1093. doi: 10.3390/ijms19041093.

Ghaffari, S. and Roshanravan, N. (2020). The role of nutraceuticals in prevention and treatment of hypertension: an updated review of the literature. *Food Research International* 128: 108749. doi: 10.1016/j.foodres.2019.108749.

Ghaffari, M.A., Aberumand, M., Roshanmehr, H. et al. (2016). Reduction of high glucose-induced nitric oxide synthase expression in human vascular endothelial cells by ascorbic acid and α-tocopherol. *International Journal Of Pharmaceutical Research And Allied Sciences* 5 (2): 135–143.

Ghasemi, F., Shafiee, M., Banikazemi, Z. et al. (2019). Curcumin inhibits NF-kB and Wnt/β-catenin pathways in cervical cancer cells. *Pathology Research and Practice* 215 (10): 152556. doi: 10.1016/j.prp.2019.152556.

Gheena, S. and Ezhilarasan, D. (2019). Syringic acid triggers reactive oxygen species-mediated cytotoxicity in HepG2 cells. *Human and Experimental Toxicology* 38 (6): 694–702. doi: 10.1177/0960327119839173.

Giansanti, F., Leboffe, L., Angelucci, F., et al. (2015). The nutraceutical properties of ovotransferrin and its potential utilization as a functional food. *Nutrients* 7 (11): 9105–9115. doi: 10.3390/nu7115453.

Giansanti, F., Panella, G., Leboffe, L. et al. (2016). Lactoferrin from Milk: nutraceutical and pharmacological properties. *Pharmaceuticals* 9 (4): 61. doi: 10.3390/ph9040061.

Giovagnoni, G., Rossi, B., Tugnoli, B. et al. (2020). Thymol and carvacrol downregulate the expression of salmonella typhimurium Virulence Genes during an in vitro infection on Caco-2 cells. *Microorganisms* 8 (6): 862. doi: 10.3390/microorganisms8060862.

Global Nutraceuticals Market: Information by Type (2020). *(Vitamins & Minerals, Probiotics, Proteins & Peptides, Omega Fatty Acids, and Others), Source (Plant, Animal, and Microbial), Form (Capsules, Tablets, & Softgels, Powder and Liquid & Gummies), Distribution Channel (Store-Based [Supermarkets & Hypermarkets, Specialty Stores and others] and Non-Store-Based) and Region (North America, Europe, Asia-Pacific and Rest of the World) – Forecast till 2025.* https://www.marketresearchfuture.com/reports/nutraceuticals-market-2181.

Golla, U. (2018). Emergence of nutraceuticals as the alternative medications for pharmaceuticals. *International Journal of Complementary & Alternative Medicine* 11 (3): 155–158. doi: 10.15406/ijcam.2018.11.00388.

Goudarzi, M., Fatemi, I., Siahpoosh, A. et al. (2018). Protective effect of ellagic acid against sodium arsenite-induced cardio- and hematotoxicity in rats. *Cardiovascular Toxicology* 18 (4): 337–345. doi: 10.1007/s12012-018-9446-2.

Govindasami, S., Uddandrao, V.V.S., Raveendran, N. et al. (2020). Therapeutic potential of biochanin-a against isoproterenol-induced myocardial infarction in rats. *Cardiovascular & Hematological Agents in Medicinal Chemistry* 18 (1): 31–36. doi: 10.2174/1871525718666200206114304.

Grant, W.B., Lahore, H., McDonnell, S.L. et al. (2020). Evidence that Vitamin D supplementation could reduce risk of influenza and COVID-19 infections and deaths. *Nutrients* 12 (4): 988. doi: 10.3390/nu12040988.

Guedes, J.P., Pereira, C.S., Rodrigues, L.R. et al. (2018). Bovine milk lactoferrin selectively kills highly metastatic prostate cancer PC-3 and osteosarcoma MG-63 cells in vitro. *Frontiers in Oncology* 8: 200. doi: 10.3389/fonc.2018.00200.

Guo, Y.F., Xu, N.N., Sun, W. et al. (2017). Luteolin reduces inflammation in Staphylococcus aureus-induced mastitis by inhibiting NF-κB activation and MMPs expression. *Oncotarget* 8 (17): 28481–28493. doi: 10.18632/oncotarget.16092.

Ha, T.K., Jung, I., Kim, M.E. et al. (2017). Anti-cancer activity of myricetin against human papillary thyroid cancer cells involves mitochondrial dysfunction–mediated apoptosis. *Biomedicine and Pharmacotherapy* 91: 378–384. doi: 10.1016/j.biopha.2017.04.100.

Han, Y., Sun, Z., and Chen, W. (2020). Antimicrobial susceptibility and antibacterial mechanism of limonene against listeria monocytogenes. *Molecules* 25 (1): 33. doi: 10.3390/molecules25010033.

Haq, S.H., Nounou, H., and Alamro, A.A. (2018). Neuroprotective role of alpha-tocopherol in H2O2 induced oxidative stress in neonatal sheep's brain tissue culture. *Journal of Neurology and Neurobiology* 4 (1).

Hase, T., Shishido, S., Yamamoto, S. et al. (2019). Rosmarinic acid suppresses Alzheimer's disease development by reducing amyloid β aggregation by increasing monoamine secretion. *Scientific Reports* 9 (1): 8711. doi: 10.1038/s41598-019-45168-1.

Hashemzaei, M., Far, A.D., Yari, A. et al. (2017). Anticancer and apoptosis-inducing effects of quercetin in vitro and in vivo. *Oncology Reports* 38 (2): 819–828. doi: 10.3892/or.2017.5766.

Hayat, M., Abbas, M., Munir, F. et al. (2017). Potential of plant flavonoids in pharmaceutics and nutraceutics. *Journal of Biomolecules and Biochemistry* 1 (1): 12–17. https://www.pulsus.com/scholarly-articles/potential-of-plant-flavonoids-in-pharmaceutics-and-nutraceutics-4029.html#17%0Ahttps://www.pulsus.com/scholarly-articles/potential-of-plant-flavonoids-in-pharmaceutics-and-nutraceutics-4029.html.

Hua, F., Li, C.H., Chen, X.G. et al. (2018). Daidzein exerts anticancer activity towards SKOV3 human ovarian cancer cells by inducing apoptosis and cell cycle arrest, and inhibiting the Raf/MEK/ERK cascade. *International Journal of Molecular Medicine* 41 (6): 3485–3492. doi: 10.3892/ijmm.2018.3531.

Hyun, J., Jaemin, K., Sanghyun, L. et al. (2016). Quercetin and quercetin-3-β-D-glucoside improve cognitive and memory function in Alzheimer's disease mouse. *Applied Biological Chemistry* 59 (5): 721–728. doi: 10.1007/s13765-016-0217-0.

Icel, E., Icel, A., Uçak, T. et al. (2019). The effects of lycopene on alloxan induced diabetic optic neuropathy. *Cutaneous and Ocular Toxicology* 38 (1): 88–92. doi: 10.1080/15569527.2018.1530258.

Islam, S.S. and Aboussekhra, A. (2019). Sequential combination of cisplatin with eugenol targets ovarian cancer stem cells through the Notch-Hes1 signalling pathway. *Journal of Experimental & Clinical Cancer Research* 38: 382. doi: 10.1186/s13046-019-1360-3.

Islam, S.S., Al-Sharif, I., Sultan, A. et al. (2018). Eugenol potentiates cisplatin anti-cancer activity through inhibition of ALDH-positive breast cancer stem cells and the NF-κB signaling pathway. *Molecular Carcinogenesis* 57 (3): 333–346. doi: 10.1002/mc.22758.

Jang, S.H., Lim, J.W., Morio, T. et al. (2012). Lycopene inhibits Helicobacter pylori-induced ATM/ATR-dependent DNA damage response in gastric epithelial AGS cells. *Free Radical Biology and Medicine* 52 (3): 607–615. doi: 10.1016/j.freeradbiomed.2011.11.010.

Je, J.Y. and Kim, S.K. (2012). Chitosan as potential marine nutraceutical. *Marine Medicinal Foods: Implications and Applications – Animals and Microbes* 65: 121–135. 1 Elsevier Inc. doi: 10.1016/B978-0-12-416003-3.00007-X.

Jeong, Y., Lim, J.W., and Kim, H. (2019). Lycopene inhibits reactive oxygen species-mediated NF-κB signaling and induces apoptosis in pancreatic cancer cells. *Nutrients* 11 (4): 762. doi: 10.3390/nu11040762.

Jeremias, L., Clasen, V., Vinicius, M. et al. (2017). Molecular mechanism of action of pelargonidin-3-O-glucoside, the main anthocyanin responsible for the anti-inflammatory effect of strawberry fruits. *Food Chemistry* 247: 56–65. doi: 10.1016/j.foodchem.2017.12.015.

Jiang, L., Li, H., Wang, L. et al. (2016). Isorhamnetin attenuates staphylococcus aureus-induced lung cell injury by inhibiting alpha-hemolysin expression. *Journal of Microbiology and Biotechnology* 26 (3): 596–602. doi: http://dx.doi.org/10.4014/jmb.1507.07091.

Joo, J., Hong, S., Cho, Y. et al. (2016). 10-gingerol inhibits proliferation and invasion of MDA-MB-231 breast cancer cells through suppression of Akt and p38MAPK activity. *Oncology Reports* 35 (2): 779–784. doi: 10.3892/or.2015.4405.

Kalra, E.K. (2003). Nutraceutical – definition and introduction. *The AAPS Journal* 5 (3): 1–2. doi: 10.1208/ps050325.

Kang, S., Kim, Y., Kim, E. et al. (2016). Anticancer effect of thymol on AGS human gastric carcinoma cells. *Journal of Microbiology and Biotechnology* 26 (1): 28–37.

Kang, J.W., Park, J., Kim, H.L. et al. (2018). Secoisolariciresinol diglucoside inhibits adipogenesis through the AMPK pathway. *European Journal of Pharmacology* 820: 235–244. doi: 10.1016/j.ejphar.2017.12.038.

Karpiński, T.M. and Adamczak, A. (2019). Fucoxanthin – an antibacterial carotenoid. *Antioxidants* 8 (8): 239.

Kashafi, E., Moradzadeh, M., Mohamadkhani, A. et al. (2017). Kaempferol increases apoptosis in human cervical cancer HeLa cells via PI3K/AKT and telomerase pathways. *Biomedicine and Pharmacotherapy* 89: 573–577. doi: 10.1016/j.biopha.2017.02.061.

Kępa, M., Miklasińska-Majdanik, M., Wojtyczka, R.D. et al. (2018). Antimicrobial potential of caffeic acid against staphylococcus aureus clinical strains. *BioMed Research International* 2018: doi: 10.1155/2018/7413504.

Khan, I., Bahuguna, A., Kumar, P. et al. (2017). Antimicrobial potential of carvacrol against uropathogenic Escherichia coli via membrane disruption, depolarization, and reactive oxygen species generation. *Frontiers in Microbiology* 8: 2421. doi: 10.3389/fmicb.2017.02421.

Kheiry, M., Dianat, M., Badavi, M. et al. (2019). p-Coumaric acid protects cardiac function against lipopolysaccharide-induced acute lung injury by attenuation of oxidative stress. *Iranian Journal of Basic Medical Sciences* 22 (8): 949–955. doi: 10.22038/ijbms.2019.36316.8650.

Khoo, H.E., Azlan, A., Tang, S.T. et al. (2017). Anthocyanidins and anthocyanins: colored pigments as food, pharmaceutical ingredients, and the potential health benefits. *Food & Nutrition Research* 61 (1): 1361779. doi: 10.1080/16546628.2017.1361779.

Kim, S.H., Park, J. G., Lee, J. et al. (2015). The dietary flavonoid kaempferol mediates anti-inflammatory responses via the Src, Syk, IRAK1, and IRAK4 molecular targets. *Mediators of Inflammation* 2015: doi: 10.1155/2015/904142.

Kim, H., Jang, M., Kim, Y. et al. (2016a). Red ginseng and vitamin C increase immune cell activity and decrease lung inflammation induced by influenza A virus/H1N1 infection. *Journal of Pharmacy and Pharmacology* 68 (3): 406–420. doi: 10.1111/jphp.12529.

Kim, Y., Lee, J., Gwon, G. et al. (2016b). Essential Oils and eugenols inhibit biofilm formation and the virulence of Escherichia coli O157:H7. *Scientific Reports* 6: 36377. doi: 10.1038/srep36377.

Kim, M.-G., Kim, S.-M., Min, J.-H. et al. (2019). Anti-inflammatory effects of linalool on ovalbumin-induced pulmonary inflammation. *International Immunopharmacology* 74: 105706. doi: 10.1016/j.intimp.2019.105706.

Koushki, M., Amiri-Dashatan, N., Ahmadi, N. et al. (2018). Resveratrol: a miraculous natural compound for diseases treatment. *Food Science & Nutrition* 6 (8): 2473–2490. doi: 10.1002/fsn3.855.

Krishnamoorthy, A., Sevananb, M., Sugumar Mania, M.B. et al. (2019). Chrysin restores MPTP induced neuroinflammation, oxidative stress and neurotrophic factors in an acute Parkinson's disease mouse model. *Neuroscience Letters* 709: 134382. doi: 10.1016/j.neulet.2019.134382.

Kugaji, M.S., Kumbar, V.M., Peram, M.R. et al. (2019). Effect of resveratrol on biofilm formation and virulence factor gene expression of Porphyromonas gingivalis in periodontal disease. *APMIS* 127 (4): 187–195. doi: 10.1111/apm.12930.

Kumar, S. and Pandey, A.K. (2013). Chemistry and biological activities of flavonoids: an overview Shashank. *Scientific World Journal* doi: 10.1155/2013/162750.

Kwon, M., Kim, S., Park, J. et al. (2019). A caffeic acid-ferulic acid hybrid compound attenuates lipopolysaccharide-mediated inflammation in BV2 and RAW264.7 cells. *Biochemical and Biophysical Research Communications* 515 (4): 565–571. doi: 10.1016/j.bbrc.2019.06.005.

Lee, D. and Jeong, G. (2016). Butein provides neuroprotective and anti-neuroinflammatory effects through Nrf2/ARE-dependent HO-1 expression by activating the PI3K/AKT pathway. *British Journal of Pharmacology* 173 (19): 2894–2909. doi: 10.1111/bph.13569.

Lee, W. and Lee, D.G. (2017). Resveratrol induces membrane and DNA disruption via pro-oxidant activity against Salmonella typhimurium. *Biochemical and Biophysical Research Communications* 489 (2): 228–234. doi: 10.1016/j.bbrc.2017.05.138.

Lee, S., Park, Y.R., Kim, S. et al. (2016). Geraniol suppresses prostate cancer growth through down-regulation of E2F8. *Cancer Medicine* 5 (10): 2899–2908. doi: 10.1002/cam4.864.

Lee, H., Woo, E., and Lee, D.G. (2018a). Apigenin induces cell shrinkage in Candida albicans by membrane perturbation. *FEMS Yeast Research* 18 (1): foy003. doi: 10.1093/femsyr/foy003.

Lee, S., Kim, H.B., Hwang, E.S. et al. (2018b). Antidepressant-like effects of p-Coumaric Acid on LPS-induced depressive and inflammatory changes in rats. *Experimental Neurobiology* 27 (3): 189–199. doi: 10.5607/en.2018.27.3.189.

Lee, H., Ahn, J., Shin, S.S. et al. (2019). Ascorbic acid inhibits visceral obesity and nonalcoholic fatty liver disease by activating peroxisome proliferator-activated receptor α in High-Fat-Diet-Fed C57BL/6J Mice. *International Journal of Obesity* 43 (8): 1620–1630. doi: 10.1038/s41366-018-0212-0.

Li, H., Chen, Y., Zhang, B. et al. (2016a). Inhibition of sortase A by chalcone prevents Listeria monocytogenes infection. *Biochemical Pharmacology* 106: 19–29. doi: 10.1016/j.bcp.2016.01.018.

Li, J., Teng, Y., Liu, S. et al. (2016b). Cinnamaldehyde affects the biological behavior of human colorectal cancer cells and induces apoptosis via inhibition of the PI3K/Akt signaling pathway. *Oncology Reports* 35 (3): 1501–1510. doi: 10.3892/or.2015.4493.

Li, W.-L., Yu, H.-Y., Zhang, X.-J. et al. (2018a). Purple sweet potato anthocyanin exerts antitumor effect in bladder cancer. *Oncology Reports* 40 (1): 73–82. doi: 10.3892/or.2018.6421.

Li, Y., Yu, H., Han, F. et al. (2018b). Biochanin A induces S phase arrest and apoptosis in lung cancer cells. *BioMed Research International* 2018: doi: 10.1155/2018/3545376.

Li, D.A.N., Wang, G., Jin, G. et al. (2019a). Resveratrol suppresses colon cancer growth by targeting the AKT/STAT3 signaling pathway. *International Journal of Molecular Medicine* 43 (1): 630–640. doi: 10.3892/ijmm.2018.3969.

Li, G., Wang, G., Si, X. et al. (2019b). Inhibition of suilysin activity and inflammation by myricetin attenuates Streptococcus suis virulence. *Life Sciences* 223: 62–68. doi: 10.1016/j.lfs.2019.03.024.

Li, W., Xu, C., Hao, C. et al. (2020). Inhibition of herpes simplex virus by myricetin through targeting viral gD protein and cellular EGFR/PI3K/Akt pathway. *Antiviral Research* 177: 104714. doi: 10.1016/j.antiviral.2020.104714.

Liang, N., Sang, Y., Liu, W. et al. (2018). Anti-inflammatory effects of gingerol on lipopolysaccharide-stimulated RAW 264.7 Cells by inhibiting NF-κB signaling pathway. *Inflammation* 41 (3): 835–845. doi: 10.1007/s10753-018-0737-3.

Liao, C., Chen, S., Huang, H. et al. (2018). Gallic acid inhibits bladder cancer cell proliferation and migration via regulating fatty acid synthase (FAS). *Journal of Food and Drug Analysis* 26 (2): 620–627. doi: 10.1016/j.jfda.2017.06.006.

Lim, W., Ryu, S., Bazer, F.W. et al. (2018). Chrysin attenuates progression of ovarian cancer cells by regulating signaling cascades and mitochondrial dysfunction. *Journal of Cellular Physiology* 233 (4): 3129–3140. doi: 10.1002/jcp.26150.

Lin, Y., Shi, R., Wang, X. et al. (2008). Luteolin, a flavonoid with potential for cancer prevention and therapy. *Current Cancer Drug Targets* 8 (7): 634–646. doi: 10.2174/156800908786241050.

Lin, K.H., Shibu, M.A., Peramaiyan, R., and Chen, Y.F. et al. (2019). Bioactive flavone fisetin attenuates hypertension associated cardiac hypertrophy in H9c2 cells and in spontaneously hypertension rats. *Journal of Functional Foods* 52: 212–218. doi: 10.1016/j.jff.2018.10.038.

Ling, L.J., Lu, Y., Zhang, Y.-Y. et al. (2020). Flavonoids from Houttuynia cordata attenuate H1N1-induced acute lung injury in mice via inhibition of influenza virus and Toll-like receptor signalling. *Phytomedicine* 67: 153150. doi: 10.1016/j.phymed.2019.153150.

Liu, M., Wu, X., Li, J. et al. (2017). The specific anti-biofilm effect of gallic acid on Staphylococcus aureus by regulating the expression of the ica operon. *Food Control* 73 (Part B): 613–618. doi: 10.1016/j.foodcont.2016.09.015.

Liu, Q., Liang, X., Niu, C. et al. (2018). Ellagic acid promotes A549 cell apoptosis via regulating the phosphoinositide 3-kinase/protein Kinase B pathway. *Experimental and Therapeutic Medicine* 16 (1): 347–352. doi: 10.3892/etm.2018.6193.

Liu, Y., Zhang, Y., Zhou, Y. et al. (2019). Cinnamaldehyde inhibits type three secretion system in Salmonella enterica serovar Typhimurium by affecting the expression of key effector proteins. *Veterinary Microbiology* 239: 108463. doi: 10.1016/j.vetmic.2019.108463.

López, G.C. and Sánchez, C.A.C. (2017). Quercetin attenuates Staphylococcus aureus virulence by reducing alpha-toxin secretion. *Revista Argentina de Microbiología* 50 (2): 131–135. doi: 10.1016/j.ram.2017.07.002.

Lou, Z., Letsididi, K.S., Yu, F. et al. (2019). Inhibitive effect of Eugenol and its nanoemulsion on quorum sensing-mediated virulence factors and biofilm formation by Pseudomonas aeruginosa. *Journal of Food Protection* 82 (3): 379–389. doi: 10.4315/0362-028X.JFP-18-196.

Ma, X., Sun, Z., Han, X. et al. (2020). Neuroprotective effect of resveratrol via activation of Sirt1 signaling in a rat model of combined diabetes and alzheimer's disease. *Frontiers in Neuroscience* 13: 1400. doi: 10.3389/fnins.2019.01400.

Maa, F., Liu, F., Ding, L. et al. (2017). Anti-inflammatory effects of curcumin are associated with down regulating microRNA-155 in LPS-treated macrophages and mice. *Pharmaceutical Biology* 55 (1): 1263–1273. doi: 10.1080/13880209.2017.1297838.

Magalhães, C.B., Casquilho, N.V., Machado, M.N. et al. (2019). The anti-inflammatory and anti-oxidative actions of eugenol improve lipopolysaccharide-induced lung injury. *Respiratory Physiology & Neurobiology* 259: 30–36. doi: 10.1016/j.resp.2018.07.001.

Maisuria, V.B., Santos, Y.L.L., Tufenkji, N. et al. (2016). Cranberry-derived proanthocyanidins impair virulence and inhibit quorum sensing of Pseudomonas aeruginosa. *Scientific Reports* 6 (August 9): 30169. doi: 10.1038/srep30169.

Manjunatha, S., Shaik, A.H., Maruthi Prasad, E. et al. (2020). Combined cardio-protective ability of syringic acid and resveratrol against isoproterenol induced cardio-toxicity in rats via attenuating NF-kB and TNF-α pathways. *Scientific Reports* 10 (1): 3426. doi: 10.1038/s41598-020-59925-0.

Marchese, A., Erdogan, I., Daglia, M. et al. (2016). Antibacterial and antifungal activities of thymol: a brief review of the literature. *Food Chemistry* 210: 402–414. doi: 10.1016/j.foodchem.2016.04.111.

Martínez-Moreno, J., Hernandez, J.C., and Urcuqui-Inchima, S. (2020). Effect of high doses of vitamin D supplementation on dengue virus replication, Toll-like receptor expression, and cytokine profiles on dendritic cells. *Molecular and Cellular Biochemistry* 464: 169–180. doi: 10.1007/s11010-019-03658-w.

Mazokopakis, E.E., Starakis, I.K., Papadomanolaki, M.G. et al. (2014). The hypolipidaemic effects of Spirulina (Arthrospira platensis) supplementation in a Cretan population: a prospective study. *Journal of the Science of Food and Agriculture* 94 (3): 432–437. doi: 10.1002/jsfa.6261.

Ming, D., Wang, D., Cao, F. et al. (2017). Kaempferol inhibits the primary attachment phase of biofilm formation in Staphylococcus aureus. *Frontiers in Microbiology* 8: 2263. doi: 10.3389/fmicb.2017.02263.

Mir, S.M., Ravuri, H.G., Pradhan, R.K. et al. (2018). Ferulic acid protects lipopolysaccharide-induced acute kidney injury by suppressing inflammatory events and upregulating antioxidant defenses in Balb/c mice. *Biomedicine and Pharmacotherapy* 100: 304–315. doi: 10.1016/j.biopha.2018.01.169.

Mirza, Z.M., Kumar, A., Kalia, N.P. et al. (2011). Piperine as an inhibitor of the MdeA efflux pump of Staphylococcus aureus. *Journal of Medical Microbiology* 60 (10): 1472–1478. doi: 10.1099/jmm.0.033167-0.

Moghtaderi, H., Sepehri, H., Delphi, L. et al. (2018). Gallic acid and curcumin induce cytotoxicity and apoptosis in human breast cancer cell MDA-MB-231. *BioImpact* 8 (3): 185–194. doi: 10.15171/bi.2018.21.

Moreno-luna, R., Muñoz-hernandez, R., Miranda, M.L. et al. (2012). Olive oil polyphenols decrease blood pressure and improve endothelial function in young women with mild hypertension. *American Journal of Hypertension* 25 (12): 1299–1304. doi: 10.1038/ajh.2012.128.

Mori, T., Koyama, N., Tan, J. et al. (2019). Combined treatment with the phenolics (-)-epigallocatechin-3-gallate and ferulic acid improves cognition and reduces alzheimer-like pathology in mice. *Journal of Biological Chemistry* 294 (8): 2714–2731. doi: 10.1074/jbc.RA118.004280.

Morroni, F., Sita, G., Graziosi, A. et al. (2018). Neuroprotective effect of caffeic acid phenethyl ester in A mouse model of alzheimer's disease involves Nrf2/HO-1 pathway. *Aging and Disease* 9 (4): 605–622. doi: 10.14336/AD.2017.0903.

Motaghinejad, M., Motevalian, M., Fatima, S. et al. (2017). The neuroprotective effect of curcumin against nicotine-induced neurotoxicity is mediated by CREB–BDNF signaling pathway. *Neurochemical Research* 42 (10): 2921–2932. doi: 10.1007/s11064-017-2323-8.

Mousavi, S., Escher, U., Thunhorst, E. et al. (2020). Vitamin C alleviates acute enterocolitis in Campylobacter jejuni infected mice. *Scientific Reports* 10 (1): 2921. doi: 10.1038/s41598-020-59890-8.

Mun, S.H., Joung, D.K., Kim, Y.S. et al. (2013). Synergistic antibacterial effect of curcumin against methicillin-resistant Staphylococcus aureus. *Phytomedicine* 20 (8–9): 714–718. doi: 10.1016/j.phymed.2013.02.006.

Murali, K.S., Sivasubramanian, S., Vincent, S. et al. (2015). Anti-chikungunya activity of luteolin and apigenin rich fraction from Cynodon dactylon. *Asian Pacific Journal of Tropical Medicine* 8 (5): 352–358. doi: 10.1016/S1995-7645(14)60343-6.

Nagib, M.M., Tadros, M.G., Rahmo, R.M. et al. (2019). Ameliorative effects of α-Tocopherol and/or Coenzyme Q10 on phenytoin-induced cognitive impairment in rats: role of VEGF and BDNF-TrkB -CREB pathway. *Neurotoxicity Research* 35 (2): 451–462.

Naguib, M.M. and Valvano, M.A. (2018). Vitamin E increases antimicrobial sensitivity by inhibiting bacterial lipocalin antibiotic binding. *mSphere* 3: e00564–e00518. doi: 10.1128/msphere.00564-18.

Nakagawa, S., Hillebrand, G.G., and Nunez, G. (2020). Rosmarinus officinalis L. (Rosemary) extracts containing carnosic acid and carnosol are potent quorum sensing inhibitors of Staphylococcus aureus virulence. *Antibiotics* 9 (4): 149. doi: 10.3390/antibiotics9040149.

Nasri, H., Baradaran, A., Shirzad, H. et al. (2014). New concepts in nutraceuticals as alternative for pharmaceuticals. *International Journal of Preventive Medicine* 5 (12): 1487–1499.

Nguyen-Ngo, C., Willcox, J.C., and Lappas, M. (2019). Anti-diabetic, anti-inflammatory, and anti-oxidant effects of naringenin in an in vitro human model and an in vivo murine model of gestational diabetes mellitus. *Molecular Nutrition & Food Research* 63 (19): 1–12. doi: 10.1002/mnfr.201900224.

Nile, S.H., Kim, D.H., Nile, A. et al. (2020). Probing the effect of quercetin 3-glucoside from Dianthus superbus L against influenza virus infection- in vitro and in silico biochemical and toxicological screening. *Food and Chemical Toxicology* 135: 110985. doi: 10.1016/j.fct.2019.110985.

Ortea, I., Gonzalez-Fernandez, M.J., Ramos-Bueno, R.P. et al. (2018). Proteomics study reveals that docosahexaenoic and arachidonic acids exert different in vitro anticancer activities in colorectal cancer cells. *Journal of Agricultural and Food Chemistry* 66 (24): 6003–6012. doi: 10.1021/acs.jafc.8b00915.

Oskouei, B.G., Abbaspour-Ravasjani, S., Jamal Musavinejad, S. et al. (2019). In vivo evaluation of anti-hyperglycemic, anti-hyperlipidemic and anti-oxidant status of liver and kidney of thymol in STZ-induced diabetic rats. *Drug Research* 69 (1): 46–52. doi: 10.1055/a-0646-3803.

Ouyang, J., Sun, F., Feng, W. et al. (2018). Antimicrobial activity of galangin and its effects on murein hydrolases of vancomycin-intermediate Staphylococcus aureus (VISA) Strain Mu50. *Chemotherapy* 63 (1): 20–28. doi: 10.1159/000481658.

Oza, M.J. and Kulkarni, Y.A. (2018a). Biochanin A improves insulin sensitivity and controls hyperglycemia in type 2 diabetes. *Biomedicine and Pharmacotherapy* 107: 1119–1127. doi: 10.1016/j.biopha.2018.08.073.

Oza, M.J. and Kulkarni, Y.A. (2018b). Formononetin treatment in type 2 diabetic rats reduces insulin resistance and hyperglycemia. *Frontiers in Pharmacology* 9: 739. doi: 10.3389/fphar.2018.00739.

Pan, W. and Zhang, G. (2019). Linalool monoterpene exerts potent antitumor effects in OECM 1 human oral cancer cells by inducing sub-G1 cell cycle arrest, loss of mitochondrial membrane potential and inhibition of PI3K/AKT biochemical pathway. *Journal of BUON* 24 (1): 323–328.

Pan, H., Fu, C., Huang, L. et al. (2018). Anti-obesity effect of chitosan oligosaccharide capsules (COSCs) in obese rats by ameliorating leptin resistance and adipogenesis. *Marine Drugs* 16 (6): 198. doi: 10.3390/md16060198.

Panche, A.N., Diwan, A.D., and Chandra, S.R. (2016). Flavonoids: an overview. *Journal of Nutritional Science* 5: e47. doi: 10.1017/jns.2016.41.

Pandey, N., Meena, R.P., Rai, S.K. et al. (2011). Medicinal plants derived nutraceuticals: a re-emerging health aid. *International Journal of Pharma and Bio Sciences* 2 (4): 419–441.

Pandey, A.K., Kumar, P., Singh, P. et al. (2017). Essential oils: sources of antimicrobials and food preservatives. *Frontiers in Microbiology* 7: 2161. doi: 10.3389/fmicb.2016.02161.

Park, S., Bazer, F.W., Lim, W. et al. (2018). The O-methylated isoflavone, formononetin, inhibits human ovarian cancer cell proliferation by sub G0/G1 cell phase arrest through PI3K/AKT and ERK1/2 inactivation. *Journal of Cellular Biochemistry* 119 (9): 7377–7387. doi: 10.1002/jcb.27041.

Patel, J., Yin, H.B., Bauchan, G. et al. (2020). Inhibition of Escherichia coli O157:H7 and Salmonella enterica virulence factors by benzyl isothiocyanate. *Food Microbiology* 86: 103303. doi: 10.1016/j.fm.2019.103303.

Patil, S., Katolkar, U., Salve, A. et al. (2017). The neuroprotective effect of α-Tocopherol on ptz-induced epilepsy causes oxidative stress and memory impairment in rats. *Seizure* 15 (16): 17. doi: 10.20959/wjpps20176-9292.

Peng, Y., Shi, Y., Zhang, H. et al. (2017). Anti-inflammatory and anti-oxidative activities of daidzein and its sulfonic acid ester derivatives. *Journal of Functional Foods* 35: 635–640. doi: 10.1016/j.jff.2017.06.027.

Pereyra-vergara, F., Olivares-corichi, I.M., Perez-ruiz, A.G. et al. (2020). Apoptosis induced by (−)-Epicatechin in human breast cancer cells is mediated by reactive oxygen species. *Molecules* 25 (5): 1020. doi: 10.3390/molecules25051020.

Pontes, E.K.U., Melo, H.M., Nogueira, J.W.A. et al. (2019). Antibiofilm activity of the essential oil of citronella (Cymbopogon nardus) and its major component, geraniol, on the bacterial biofilms of Staphylococcus aureus. *Food Science and Biotechnology* 28 (3): 633–639. doi: 10.1007/s10068-018-0502-2.

Prakash, D., Gupta, C., and Sharma, G. (2012). Importance of phytochemicals in nutraceuticals. *Journal of Chinese Medicine Research and Development* 1 (3): 70–78.

Prakash, S., Elavarasan, N., Subashini, K. et al. (2020). Isolation of hesperetin – A flavonoid from Cordia sebestena flower extract through antioxidant assay guided method and its antibacterial, anticancer effect on cervical cancer via in vitro and in silico molecular docking studies. *Journal of Molecular Structure* 1207: 127751. doi: 10.1016/j.molstruc.2020.127751.

Qi, F., Yan, Q., Zheng, Z. et al. (2018). Geraniol and geranyl acetate induce potent anticancer effects in colon cancer Colo-205 cells by inducing apoptosis, DNA damage and cell cycle arrest. *Journal of BUON* 23 (2): 346–352.

Qi, M.Y., Wang, X.T., Xu, H.L. et al. (2020). Protective effect of ferulic acid on STZ-induced diabetic nephropathy in rats. *Food & Function* 11 (4): 3706–3718. doi: 10.1039/c9fo02398d.

Qian, W., Liu, M., Fu, Y. et al. (2020a). Antimicrobial mechanism of luteolin against Staphylococcus aureus and Listeria monocytogenes and its antibiofilm properties. *Microbial Pthogenesis* 142: 104056. doi: 10.1016/j.micpath.2020.104056.

Qian, W., Sun, Z., Wang, T. et al. (2020b). Antimicrobial activity of eugenol against carbapenem-resistant Klebsiella pneumoniae and its effect on biofilms. *Microbial Pathogenesis* 139: 103924. doi: 10.1016/j.micpath.2019.103924.

Qian, W., Wang, W., Zhang, J. et al. (2020c). Sanguinarine inhibits mono- and dual-species biofilm formation by Candida albicans and Staphylococcus aureus and Induces Mature Hypha Transition of C. albicans. *Pharmaceuticals (Basel)* 13 (1): 13. doi: 10.3390/ph13010013.

Ramírez-Espinosa, J.J., Saldaña-Ríos, J., García-Jiménez, S. et al. (2018). Chrysin induces antidiabetic, antidyslipidemic and anti-inflammatory effects in athymic nude diabetic mice. *Molecules* 23 (1): 67. doi: 10.3390/molecules23010067.

Ran, L., Zhao, W., Wang, J. et al. (2018). Extra dose of Vitamin C based on a daily supplementation shortens the common cold: a meta-analysis of 9 randomized controlled trials. *BioMed Research International* 2018: doi: 10.1155/2018/1837634.

Ranjbar-Omid, M., Arzanlou, M., Amani, M. et al. (2015). Allicin from garlic inhibits the biofilm formation and urease activity of Proteus mirabilis in vitro. *FEMS Microbiology Letters* 362 (9): fnv049. doi: 10.1093/femsle/fnv049.

Rashno, M., Ghaderi, S., Nesari, A. et al. (2020). Chrysin attenuates traumatic brain injury-induced recognition memory decline, and anxiety/depression-like behaviors in rats: insights into underlying mechanisms. *Psychopharmacology* 237 (6): 1607–1619.

Rehman, S.U., Ali, T., Alam, S.I. et al. (2019). Ferulic acid rescues LPS-induced neurotoxicity via modulation of the TLR4 receptor in the mouse hippocampus. *Molecular Neurobiology* 56 (4): 2774–2790. doi: 10.1007/s12035-018-1280-9.

Reiter, J., Levina, N., Van Der Linden, M. et al. (2017). Diallylthiosulfinate (Allicin), a volatile antimicrobial from garlic (Allium sativum), kills human lung pathogenic bacteria, including MDR strains, as a vapor. *Molecules* 22 (10): 1711. doi: 10.3390/molecules22101711.

Ren, J., Yang, M., Xu, F. et al. (2019). Acceleration of wound healing activity with syringic acid in streptozotocin induced diabetic rats. *Life Sciences* 233: 116728. doi: 10.1016/j.lfs.2019.116728.

Rizvi, S. , Raza, S.T., Ahmed, F. et al. (2014). The role of Vitamin E in human health and some diseases. *Sultan Qaboos University Medical Journal* 14 (2): e157–e165.

Rocha, G.R., Salamanca, E.J.F., de Barros, A.L. et al. (2018). Effect of tt-farnesol and myricetin on in vitro biofilm formed by Streptococcus mutans and Candida albicans. *BMC Complementary and Alternative Medicine* 18 (1): 61.

Rodenak-Kladniew, B., Castro, A., Stärkel, P. et al. (2018). Linalool induces cell cycle arrest and apoptosis in HepG2 cells through oxidative stress generation and modulation of Ras/MAPK and Akt/mTOR pathways. *Life Sciences* 199: 48–59. doi: 10.1016/j.lfs.2018.03.006.

Rodríguez-Luna, A., Ávila-Román, J., Oliveira, H. et al. (2019). Fucoxanthin and rosmarinic acid combination has anti-inflammatory effects through regulation of NLRP3 inflammasome in UVB-exposed HaCaT Keratinocytes. *Marine Drugs* 17 (8): 451.

Rúa, J., Del Valle, P., De Arriaga, D. et al. (2019). Combination of carvacrol and thymol: antimicrobial activity against Staphylococcus aureus and antioxidant activity. *Foodborne Pathogens and Disease* 16 (9): 622–629. doi: 10.1089/fpd.2018.2594.

Sabogal-Guáqueta, A.M., Osorio, E., and Cardona-Gómez, G.P. (2016). Linalool reverses neuropathological and behavioral impairments in old triple transgenic Alzheimer's mice. *Neuropharmacology* 102: 111–120. doi: 10.1016/j.neuropharm.2015.11.002.

Salem, A.M., Ragheb, A.S., Hegazy, M.G.A. et al. (2019). Caffeic acid modulates miR-636 expression in diabetic nephropathy rats. *Indian Journal of Clinical Biochemistry* 34 (3): 296–303. doi: 10.1007/s12291-018-0743-0.

Samarghandian, S., Borji, A., and Farkhondeh, T. (2017). Evaluation of antidiabetic activity of carnosol (Phenolic Diterpene in Rosemary) in streptozotocin-induced diabetic rats. *Cardiovascular & Hematological Disorders: Drug Targets* 17 (1): 11–17. doi: 10.2174/1871529x16666161229154910.

Sasso, M.D., Culici, M., Braga, P.C. et al. (2006). Thymol: inhibitory activity on escherichia coli and staphylococcus aureus adhesion to human vaginal cells. *Journal of Essential Oil Research* 18 (4): 455–461. doi: 10.1080/10412905.2006.9699140.

Sawicki, R., Golus, J., Przekora, A. et al. (2018). Antimycobacterial activity of cinnamaldehyde in a mycobacterium tuberculosis(H37Ra) model. *Molecules* 23 (9): 2381. doi: 10.3390/molecules23092381.

Seo, M., Lee, Y., Hwang, J. et al. (2015). The inhibitory effects of quercetin on obesity and obesity-induced inflammation by regulation of MAPK signaling. *The Journal of Nutritional Biochemistry* 26 (11): 1308–1316. doi: 10.1016/j.jnutbio.2015.06.005.

Sethupathy, S., Prasath, K.G., Ananthi, S. et al. (2016). Proteomic analysis reveals modulation of iron homeostasis and oxidative stress response in Pseudomonas aeruginosa PAO1 by curcumin inhibiting quorum sensing regulated virulence factors and biofilm production. *Journal of Proteomics* 145: 112–126. doi: 10.1016/j.jprot.2016.04.019.

Shafiee, G., Saidijam, M., Tavilani, H. et al. (2016). Genistein induces apoptosis and inhibits proliferation of HT29 colon cancer cells. *International Journal of Molecular and Cellular Medicine* 5 (3): 178–191.

Shahzad, S., Mateen, S., Naeem, S.S. et al. (2019). Syringic acid protects from isoproterenol induced cardiotoxicity in rats. *European Journal of Pharmacology* 849: 135–145. doi: 10.1016/j.ejphar.2019.01.056.

Shao, D. , Li, J., Li, J. et al. (2015). Inhibition of gallic acid on the growth and biofilm formation of Escherichia coli and Streptococcus mutans. *Journal of Food Science* 80 (6): M1299–M1305. doi: 10.1111/1750-3841.12902.

Sharifi-Rad, M., Varoni, E.M., Iriti, M. et al. (2018). Carvacrol and human health: a comprehensive review. *Phytotherapy Research* 32 (9): 1675–1687. doi: 10.1002/ptr.6103.

Sharma, S.H., Rajamanickam, V., and Nagarajan, S. (2018). Antiproliferative effect of p-Coumaric acid targets UPR activation by downregulating Grp78 in colon cancer. *Chemico-Biological Interactions* 291: 16–28. doi: 10.1016/j.cbi.2018.06.001.

Sheikha, B.Y., Sarker, M.M.R., Kamarudin, M.N.A. et al. (2017). Antiproliferative and apoptosis inducing effects of citral via p53 and ROS- induced mitochondrial-mediated apoptosis in human colorectal HCT116 and HT29 cell lines. *Biomedicine & Pharmacotherapy* 96: 834–846. doi: 10.1016/j.biopha.2017.10.038.

Shen, S., Zhang, T., Yuan, Y. et al. (2015). Effects of cinnamaldehyde on Escherichia coli and Staphylococcus aureus membrane. *Food Control* 47: 196–202. doi: 10.1016/j.foodcont.2014.07.003.

Shen, X.-F. , Teng, Y., Sha, K.-H. et al. (2016). Original article dietary flavonoid luteolin attenuates uropathogenic Escherichia Coli invasion of the urinary bladder. *BioFactors* 42 (6): 674–685. doi: 10.1002/biof.1314.

Shen, Y., Song, X., Li, L. et al. (2019). Protective effects of p-coumaric acid against oxidant and hyperlipidemia-an in vitro and in vivo evaluation. *Biomedicine and Pharmacotherapy* 111: 579–587. doi: 10.1016/j.biopha.2018.12.074.

Shi, C., Sun, Y., Zheng, Z. et al. (2016). Antimicrobial activity of syringic acid against Cronobacter sakazakii and its effect on cell membrane. *Food Chemistry* 197 (Pt A): 100–106. doi: 10.1016/j.foodchem.2015.10.100.

Shibata, C., Ohno, M., Otsuka, M. et al. (2014). The flavonoid apigenin inhibits hepatitis C virus replication by decreasing mature microRNA122 levels. *Virology* 462: 42–48. doi: 10.1016/j.virol.2014.05.024.

Shukla, S., Kanwal, R., and Shankar, E. (2015). Apigenin blocks IKKα activation and suppresses prostate cancer progression. *Oncotarget* 6 (31): 31216.

Si, X., Strappe, P., Blanchard, C. et al. (2017). Enhanced anti-obesity effects of complex of resistant starch and chitosan in high fat diet fed rats. *Carbohydrate Polymers* 157: 834–841. doi: 10.1016/j.carbpol.2016.10.042.

Siddhardha, B., Pandey, U., Kaviyarasu, K. et al. (2020). Chrysin-loaded chitosan nanoparticles potentiates antibiofilm activity against Staphylococcus aureus. *Pathogens* 9 (2): 115. doi: 10.3390/pathogens9020115.

Silva, R.V., Oliveira, J.T., Santos, B.L.R. et al. (2017). Long-chain Omega-3 fatty acids supplementation accelerates nerve regeneration and prevents neuropathic pain behavior in mice. *Frontiers in Pharmacology* 8: 723. doi: 10.3389/fphar.2017.00723.

Simonetto, M., Infante, M., Sacco, R.L. et al. (2019). A novel anti-inflammatory role of omega-3 PUFAs in prevention and treatment of atherosclerosis and vascular cognitive impairment and dementia. *Nutrients* 11 (10): 2279. doi: 10.3390/nu11102279.

Siriwong, S., Thumanu, K., Hengpratom, T. et al. (2015). Synergy and mode of action of Ceftazidime plus Quercetin or Luteolin on Streptococcus pyogenes. *Evidence-based Complementary and Alternative Medicine* 205.

Song, Y., Zhao, H., Liu, J. et al. (2016). Effects of citral on lipopolysaccharide-induced inflammation in human umbilical vein endothelial cells. *Inflammation* 39 (2): 663–971. doi: 10.1007/s10753-015-0292-0.

Sosnowska, B., Penson, P., and Banach, M. (2017). The role of nutraceuticals in the prevention of cardiovascular disease. *Cardiovascular Diagnosis and Therapy* 7 (Suppl 1): S21–S32. doi: 10.21037/cdt.2017.03.20.

Soulimani, R., Bouayed, J., and Joshi, R.K. (2019). Limonene: natural monoterpene volatile compounds of potential therapeutic interest. *American Journal of Essential Oils and Natural Products* 7 (4): 1–10.

Souza, A.C.A., Abreu, F.F., Diniz, L.R.L. et al. (2018). The inclusion complex of carvacrol and β-cyclodextrin reduces acute skeletal muscle inflammation and nociception in rats. *Pharmacological Reports* 70 (6): 1139–1145. doi: 10.1016/j.pharep.2018.07.002.

Srinivasan, S. and Sathish, G. (2014). Ameliorating effect of eugenol on hyperglycemia by attenuating the key enzymes of glucose metabolism in streptozotocin-induced diabetic rats. *Molecular and Cellular Biochemistry* 385 (1–2): 159–168. doi: 10.1007/s11010-013-1824-2.

Su, X., Shen, Z., Yang, Q. et al. (2019). Vitamin C kills thyroid cancer cells through ROS-dependent inhibition of MAPK/ERK and PI3K/AKT pathways via distinct mechanisms. *Theranostics* 9 (15): 4461–4473. doi: 10.7150/thno.35219.

Sun, D.W., Da Zhang, H., Mao, L. et al. (2015a). Luteolin inhibits breast cancer development and progression in vitro and in vivo by suppressing notch signaling and regulating MiRNAs. *Cellular Physiology and Biochemistry* 37 (5): 1693–1711. doi: 10.1159/000438535.

Sun, G.Y., Chen, Z., Jasmer, K.J. et al. (2015b). Quercetin attenuates inflammatory responses in BV-2 microglial cells: role of MAPKs on the Nrf2 pathway and induction of Heme Oxygenase-1. *PLoS One* 10 (10): 1–20. doi: 10.1371/journal.pone.0141509.

Sun, X. H., Zhou, T.T., Wei, C.H. et al. (2018). Antibacterial effect and mechanism of anthocyanin rich Chinese wild blueberry extract on various foodborne pathogens. *Food Control* 94: 155–161. doi: 10.1016/j.foodcont.2018.07.012.

Swaroopa, G. and Srinath, D. (2017). Nutraceuticals and their health benefits. *Indian Journal of Pure & Applied Biosciences* 5 (4): 1151–1155.

Tang, X.L., Liu, J.X., Dong, W. et al. (2014). Protective effect of Kaempferol on LPS plus ATP-induced inflammatory response in cardiac fibroblasts. *Inflammation* 38 (1): 94–101. doi: 10.1007/s10753-014-0011-2.

Tang, F., Li, L., Meng, X.M. et al. (2019a). Inhibition of alpha-hemolysin expression by resveratrol attenuates Staphylococcus aureus virulence. *Microbial Pathogenesis* 127: 85–90. doi: 10.1016/j.micpath.2018.11.027.

Tang, X.P., Guo, X.H., Geng, D. et al. (2019b). D-Limonene protects PC12 cells against corticosterone-induced neurotoxicity by activating the AMPK pathway. *Environmental Toxicology and Pharmacology* 70: 103192. doi: 10.1016/j.etap.2019.05.001.

Taylor, E.J.M., Yu, Y., Champer, J. et al. (2014). Resveratrol demonstrates antimicrobial effects against Propionibacterium acnes in vitro. *Dermatology and Therapy* 4 (2): 249–257. doi: 10.1007/s13555-014-0063-0.

Tintino, S.R., Morais-Tintino, C.D., Campina, F.F. et al. (2016). Action of cholecalciferol and alpha-tocopherol on Staphylococcus aureus efflux pumps. *EXCLI Journal* 15: 315–322.

Upadhyay, A., Upadhyaya, I., Mooyottu, S. et al. (2016). Eugenol in combination with lactic acid bacteria attenuates Listeria monocytogenes virulence in vitro and in invertebrate model Galleria mellonella. *Journal of Medical Microbiology* 65 (6): 443–455. doi: 10.1099/jmm.0.000251.

Upadhyay, A., Arsi, K., Wagle, B.R. et al. (2017). Trans-cinnamaldehyde, carvacrol, and eugenol reduce Campylobacter jejuni colonization factors and expression of virulence genes in vitro. *Frontiers in Microbiology* 8: 713. doi: 10.3389/fmicb.2017.00713.

Valdivieso-Ugarte, M., Gomez-Llorente, C., Plaza-Díaz, J. et al. (2019). Antimicrobial, antioxidant, and immunomodulatory properties of essential oils: a systematic review. *Nutrients* 11 (11): 2786. doi: 10.3390/nu11112786.

Verghese, R.J., Mathew, S.K., and David, A. (2017). Antimicrobial activity of Vitamin C demonstrated on uropathogenic Escherichia coli and Klebsiella pneumoniae. *Journal of Current Research in Scientific Medicine* 3 (2): 88–93. doi: 10.4103/jcrsm.jcrsm.

Vikram, A., Jesudhasan, P.R., Jayaprakasha, G.K. et al. (2011). Citrus flavonoid represses Salmonella pathogenicity island 1 and motility in S. Typhimurium LT2. *International Journal of Food Microbiology* 145 (1): 28–36. doi: 10.1016/j.ijfoodmicro.2010.11.013.

Vilchèze, C., Kim, J., and Jacobs, W.R. (2018). Vitamin C potentiates the killing of Mycobacterium tuberculosis by the first-line tuberculosis drugs isoniazid and rifampin in mice. *Antimicrobial Agents and Chemotherapy* 23 (3): e02165–e02117. doi: 10.1128/AAC.02165-17.

Vorilhon, P., Arpajou, B., Roussel, H.V. et al. (2019). Efficacy of vitamin C for the prevention and treatment of upper respiratory tract infection. A meta-analysis in children. *European Journal of Clinical Pharmacology* 75: 303–311.

Wang, Y. and Huang, K. (2013). In vitro anti-inflammatory effect of apigenin in the Helicobacter pylori -infected gastric adenocarcinoma cells. *Food and Chemical Toxicology* 53: 376–383. doi: 10.1016/j.fct.2012.12.018.

Wang, J., Qiu, J., Dong, J. et al. (2011). Chrysin protects mice from Staphylococcus aureus pneumonia. *Journal of Applied Microbiology* 111 (6): 1551–1558. doi: 10.1111/j.1365-2672.2011.05170.x.

Wang, B., Li, L., Jin, P. et al. (2017a). Hesperetin protects against inflammatory response and cardiac fibrosis in postmyocardial infarction mice by inhibiting nuclear factor κB signaling pathway. *Experimental and Therapeutic Medicine* 14 (3): 2255–2260. doi: 10.3892/etm.2017.4729.

Wang, L., Zhao, X., Zhu, C. et al. (2017b). Thymol kills bacteria, reduces biofilm formation, and protects mice against a fatal infection of Actinobacillus pleuropneumoniae strain L20. *Veterinary Microbiology* 203: 202–210. doi: 10.1016/j.vetmic.2017.02.021.

Wang, L.-H. , Wang, M.-S., Zeng, X.-A. et al. (2017c). Membrane and genomic DNA dual-targeting of citrus flavonoid naringenin against staphylococcus aureus. *Interactive Biology* 9 (10): 820–829. doi: 10.1039/C7IB00095B.

Wang, X., Zhao, Y., Yao, Y. et al. (2017d). Anti-inflammatory activity of di-peptides derived from ovotransferrin by simulated peptide-cut in TNF-α-induced Caco-2 cells. *Journal of Functional Foods* 37: 424–432. doi: 10.1016/j.jff.2017.07.064.

Wang, J., Song, M., Pan, J. et al. (2018a). Quercetin impairs Streptococcus pneumoniae biofilm formation by inhibiting sortase A activity. *Journal of Cellular and Molecular Medicine* 22 (11): 6228–6237. doi: 10.1111/jcmm.13910.

Wang, L., Zhang, Y., Liu, K. et al. (2018b). Carnosol suppresses patient-derived gastric tumor growth by targeting RSK2. *Oncotarget* 9 (76): 34200–34212. doi: 10.18632/oncotarget.24409.

Wang, Y., Chen, Y., Chen, Y. et al. (2018c). Eriodictyol inhibits IL-1β-induced inflammatory response in human osteoarthritis chondrocytes. *Biomedicine and Pharmacotherapy* 107 (August): 1128–1134. doi: 10.1016/j.biopha.2018.08.103.

Wang, J., Suo, Y., Zhang, J. et al. (2019a). Lycopene supplementation attenuates western diet-induced body weight gain through increasing the expressions of thermogenic/mitochondrial functional genes and improving insulin resistance in the adipose tissue of obese mice. *The Journal of Nutritional Biochemistry* 69: 63–72. doi: 10.1016/j.jnutbio.2019.03.008.

Wang, X., Wu, H., Niu, T. et al. (2019b). Downregulated expression of virulence factors induced by Benzyl Isothiocyanate in Staphylococcus Aureus: a transcriptomic analysis. *International Journal of Molecular Sciences* 20 (21): 5441. doi: 10.3390/ijms20215441.

Wang, K., Zhang, W., Wang, Z. et al. (2020). Flavokawain A inhibits prostate cancer cells by inducing cell cycle arrest and cell apoptosis and regulating the glutamine metabolism pathway. *Journal of Pharmaceutical and Biomedical Analysis* 186: 113288. doi: 10.1016/j.jpba.2020.113288.

Wei, X., Meng, X., Yuan, Y. et al. (2018). Quercetin exerts cardiovascular protective effects in LPS-induced dysfunction in vivo by regulating inflammatory cytokine expression, NF-κB phosphorylation, and caspase activity. *Molecular and Cellular Biochemistry* 446 (1–2): 43–52. doi: 10.1007/s11010-018-3271-6.

Wu, L.H., Lin, C., Lin, H.Y. et al. (2016a). Naringenin suppresses neuroinflammatory responses through inducing suppressor of Cytokine Signaling 3 expression. *Molecular Neurobiology* 53 (2): 1080–1091. doi: 10.1007/s12035-014-9042-9.

Wu, T., Jiang, Z., Yin, J. et al. (2016b). Anti-obesity effects of artificial planting blueberry (Vaccinium Ashei) Anthocyanin in high-fat diet-treated mice. *International Journal of Food Sciences and Nutrition* 67 (3): 257–264. doi: 10.3109/09637486.2016.1146235.

Wu, T., Yin, J., Zhang, G. et al. (2016c). Mulberry and cherry anthocyanin consumption prevents oxidative stress and inflammation in diet-induced obese mice. *Molecular Nutrition & Food Research* 60 (3): 687–694. doi: 10.1002/mnfr.201500734.

Wu, H., Xie, Y., Xu, Y. et al. (2020). Protective effect of Epicatechin on APAP-induced acute liver injury of mice through anti-inflammation and apoptosis inhibition. *Natural Product Research* 34 (6): 855–858. doi: 10.1080/14786419.2018.1503261.

Xiong, J.I.E., Wang, K., Yuan, C. et al. (2017). Luteolin protects mice from severe acute pancreatitis by exerting HO-1-mediated anti-inflammatory and antioxidant effects. *International Journal of Molecular Medicine* 39 (1): 113–125. doi: 10.3892/ijmm.2016.2809.

Xu, F., Yu, K., Yu, H. et al. (2017). Lycopene relieves AFB1-induced liver injury through enhancing hepatic antioxidation and detoxification potential with Nrf2 activation. *Journal of Functional Foods* 39: 215–224. doi: 10.1016/j.jff.2017.10.027.

Xu, Z., Zhang, H., Yu, H. et al. (2019). Allicin inhibits Pseudomonas aeruginosa virulence by suppressing the rhl and pqs quorum-sensing systems. *Canadian Journal of Microbiology* 65 (8): 563–574.

Xue, Z., Zhang, X., Wu, J. et al. (2016). Effect of treatment with geraniol on ovalbumin-induced allergic asthma in mice. *Annals of Allergy, Asthma & Immunology* 116 (6): 506–513. doi: 10.1016/j.anai.2016.03.029.

Xue, Y., Du, M., Zhu, M. et al. (2019). Quercetin prevents Escherichia coli O157:H7 adhesion to epithelial cells via suppressing focal adhesions. *Frontiers in Microbiology* 9: 3278. doi: 10.3389/fmicb.2018.03278.

Xuewen, H., Ping, O., Zhongwei, Y. et al. (2018). Eriodictyol protects against Staphylococcus aureus-induced lung cell injury by inhibiting alpha-hemolysin expression. *World Journal of Microbiology and Biotechnology* 34: 64. doi: 10.1007/s11274-018-2446-3.

Yan, X., Qi, M., Li, P. et al. (2017). Apigenin in cancer therapy: anti-cancer effects and mechanisms of action. *Cell & Bioscience* 7 (1): 50. doi: 10.1186/s13578-017-0179-x.

Yan, W., Ma, X., Zhao, X. et al. (2018). Baicalein induces apoptosis and autophagy of breast cancer cells via inhibiting PI3K/AKT pathway in vivo and vitro. *Drug Design, Development and Therapy* 12: 3961–3972. doi: doi:10.2147/DDDT.S181939.

Yan, H., Ma, L., Wang, H. et al. (2019). Luteolin decreases the yield of influenza A virus in vitro by interfering with the coat protein I complex expression. *Journal of Natural Medicines* 73 (3): 487–496. doi: 10.1007/s11418-019-01287-7.

Yang, P.E.I.Y.U., Hu, D.A.N.N., Kao, Y.H. et al. (2018). Butein induces apoptotic cell death of human cervical cancer cells. *Oncology Letters* 16 (5): 6615–6623. doi: 10.3892/ol.2018.9426.

Yang, W., Tian, Z.K., Yang, H.X. et al. (2019). Fisetin improves lead-induced neuroinflammation, apoptosis and synaptic dysfunction in mice associated with the AMPK/SIRT1 and autophagy pathway. *Food and Chemical Toxicology* 134: 110824. doi: 10.1016/j.fct.2019.110824.

Yao, L.H., Jiang, Y.M., Shi, J. et al. (2004). Flavonoids in food and their health benefits. *Plant Foods for Human Nutrition* 59 (3): 113–122. doi: 10.1007/s11130-004-0049-7.

Ye, Z., Liang, Z., Mi, Q. et al. (2020). Limonene terpenoid obstructs human bladder cancer cell (T24 cell line) growth by inducing cellular apoptosis, caspase activation, G2/M phase cell cycle arrest and stops cancer metastasis. *Journal of BUON* 25 (1): 280–285.

Yeo, I.J., Park, J.H., Jang, J.S. et al. (2019). Inhibitory effect of Carnosol on UVB-induced inflammation via inhibition of STAT3. *Archives of Pharmacal Research* 42 (3): 274–283. doi: 10.1007/s12272-018-1088-1.

Yeon, M.J., Lee, M.H., Kim, D.H. et al. (2019). Anti-inflammatory effects of Kaempferol on Helicobacter pylori-induced inflammation. *Bioscience, Biotechnology, and Biochemistry* 83 (1): 166–173. doi: 10.1080/09168451.2018.1528140.

Yu, J., Lin, J.J., Yu, R. et al. (2017a). Fucoxanthin prevents H2O2-induced neuronal apoptosis via concurrently activating the PI3-K/Akt cascade and inhibiting the ERK pathway. *Food & Nutrition Research* 61 (1): 1304678. doi: 10.1080/16546628.2017.1304678.

Yu, L., Yan, J., and Sun, Z. (2017b). D-limonene exhibits anti-inflammatory and antioxidant properties in an ulcerative colitis rat model via regulation of iNOS, COX-2, PGE2 and ERK signaling pathways. *Molecular Medicine Reports* 15 (4): 2339–2346. doi: 10.3892/mmr.2017.6241.

Yu, S.Y., Kwon, Y.I., Lee, C. et al. (2017c). Antidiabetic effect of chitosan oligosaccharide (GO2KA1) is mediated via inhibition of intestinal alpha-glucosidase and glucose transporters and PPARγ expression. *BioFactors* 43 (1): 90–99. doi: 10.1002/biof.1311.

Yu, R.X., Yu, R.T., and Liu, Z. (2018). Inhibition of two gastric cancer cell lines induced by fucoxanthin involves downregulation of Mcl-1 and STAT3. *Human Cell* 31 (1): 50–63. doi: 10.1007/s13577-017-0188-4.

Yuan, Z., Dai, Y., Ouyang, P. et al. (2020). Thymol inhibits biofilm formation, eliminates pre- existing biofilms, and enhances clearance of methicillin-resistant Staphylococcus aureus (MRSA) in a mouse peritoneal implant infection model. *Microorganisms* 8 (1): 99. doi: 10.3390/microorganisms8010099.

Yue, J., Yang, H., Liu, S. et al. (2018). Influence of naringenin on the biofilm formation of Streptococcus mutans. *Journal of Dentistry* 76: 24–31. doi: 10.1016/j.jdent.2018.04.013.

Yun, D.G. and Lee, D.G. (2016). Antibacterial activity of curcumin via apoptosis-like response in Escherichia coli. *Applied Microbiology and Biotechnology* 100 (12): 5505–5514. doi: 10.1007/s00253-016-7415-x.

Zeng, Y., Nikikova, A., Abdelsalam, H. et al. (2019). Activity of quercetin and kaemferol against Streptococcus mutans biofilm. *Archives of Oral Biology* 98: 9–16. doi: 10.1016/j.archoralbio.2018.11.005.

Zhang, H., Zhong, X.I.A., Zhang, X. et al. (2016a). Enhanced anticancer effect of ABT-737 in combination with naringenin on gastric cancer cells. *Experimental and Therapeutic Medicine* 11 (2): 669–673. doi: 10.3892/etm.2015.2912.

Zhang, L., Zhang, Z., Fu, Y. et al. (2016b). Trans-cinnamaldehyde improves memory impairment by blocking microglial activation through the destabilization of iNOS mRNA in mice challenged with lipopolysaccharide. *Neuropharmacology* 110: 503–518. doi: 10.1016/j.neuropharm.2016.08.013.

Zhang, R., Ai, X., Duan, Y. et al. (2017a). Kaempferol ameliorates H9N2 swine influenza virus-induced acute lung injury by inactivation of TLR4/MyD88-mediated NF-κB and MAPK signaling pathways. *Biomedicine and Pharmacotherapy* 89: 660–672. doi: 10.1016/j.biopha.2017.02.081.

Zhang, X., Du, L., Zhang, W. et al. (2017b). Therapeutic effects of baicalein on rotenone-induced Parkinson's disease through protecting mitochondrial function and biogenesis. *Scientific Reports* 7 (1): 1–14. doi: 10.1038/s41598-017-07442-y.

Zhang, M.J., Su, H., Yan, J.Y. et al. (2018a). Chemopreventive effect of Myricetin, a natural occurring compound, on colonic chronic inflammation and inflammation-driven tumorigenesis in mice. *Biomedicine and Pharmacotherapy* 97: 1131–1137. doi: 10.1016/j.biopha.2017.11.018.

Zhang, Y., Xu, W., Huang, X. et al. (2018b). Fucoxanthin ameliorates hyperglycemia, hyperlipidemia and insulin resistance in diabetic mice partially through IRS-1/PI3K/Akt and AMPK pathways. *Journal of Functional Foods* 48: 515–524. doi: 10.1016/j.jff.2018.07.048.

Zhang, Y., Liu, Y., Qiu, J. et al. (2018c). The herbal compound thymol protects mice from lethal infection by Salmonella Typhimurium. *Frontiers in Microbiology* 9: 1022. doi: 10.3389/fmicb.2018.01022.

Zhang, Y., Fan, Y., Huang, S. et al. (2018d). Thymoquinone inhibits the metastasis of renal cell cancer cells by inducing autophagy via AMPK/mTOR signaling pathway. *Cancer Science* 109 (12): 3865–3873. doi: 10.1111/cas.13808.

Zhang, W., Liu, X., Jiang, Y. et al. (2019). 6-Gingerol attenuates ischemia-reperfusion-induced cell apoptosis in Human AC16 cardiomyocytes through HMGB2-JNK1/2-NF-κB pathway. *Evidence-based Complementary and Alternative Medicine eCAM* 2019: 8798653. doi:10.1155/2019/8798653.

Zhao, M. and Du, J. (2019). Anti-inflammatory and protective effects of D-carvone on lipopolysaccharide (LPS)-induced acute lung injury in mice. *Journal of King Saud University – Science* 32 (2): 1592–1596. doi: 10.1016/j.jksus.2019.12.016.

Zhao, L., Gu, Q., Xiang, L. et al. (2017). Curcumin inhibits apoptosis by modulating Bax/Bcl-2 expression and alleviates oxidative stress in testes of streptozotocin-induced diabetic rats. *Therapeutics and Clinical Risk Management* 13: 1099–1105. doi: 10.2147/TCRM.S141738.

Zheng, J., Yuan, X., Cheng, G. et al. (2018). Chitosan oligosaccharides improve the disturbance in glucose metabolism and reverse the dysbiosis of gut microbiota in diabetic mice. *Carbohydrate Polymers* 190: 77–86. doi: 10.1016/j.carbpol.2018.02.058.

Zhu, L., Gu, P., and Shen, H. (2019). Gallic acid improved inflammation via NF-κB pathway in TNBS-induced ulcerative colitis. *International Immunopharmacology* 67: 129–137. doi: 10.1016/j.intimp.2018.11.049.

Zigangirova, N.A., Morgunova, E.Y., Fedina, E.D. et al. (2017). Lycopene inhibits propagation of chlamydia infection. *Scientifica (Cairo)* 2017: 1478625. doi: 10.1155/2017/1478625.

Zuo, J., Zhao, D., Yu, N. et al. (2017). Cinnamaldehyde ameliorates diet-induced obesity in mice by inducing browning of white adipose tissue. *Celluar Physiology and Biochemistry* 42 (4): 1514–1525. doi: 10.1159/000479268.

5

Encapsulation of Nutraceuticals in Drug Delivery System

Emmanuel Duhoranimana[1], Xiao Chen[2], and Jean Claude Dusabumuremyi[1]

[1] *Department of Biotechnologies, Faculty of Applied Fundamental Sciences, Institutes of Applied Sciences, INES-Ruhengeri, Ruhengeri, Republic of Rwanda*
[2] *School of Chemical Sciences, University of Auckland, Auckland, New Zealand*

5.1 Introduction

Nutraceuticals and functional foods have garnered increasing interest and are becoming increasingly popular worldwide. Nutraceutical is defined as a food substance or part of it that provides the body with nutritional, medical, or health benefits, including disease prevention and therapy (Khorasani et al. 2018; Maria Leena et al. 2020; Montes et al. 2019).

In recent years, a significant number of nutraceuticals and functional and medical foods have been introduced to consumers worldwide, backed by scientific research on safety and health benefits. These natural products are often less expensive, largely available and have therefore gained popularity over years (Bagchi and Nair 2017). Moreover, nutraceuticals contain appropriate amount of nourishing food components such as vitamins, proteins, carbohydrates, minerals, or essential nutrients depending on their specific needs, in addition to their pharmaceutical effects. Additionally, nutraceuticals are also referred to bioactive phytochemicals that have disease preventing, health promoting, and medicinal properties, such as the treatment of cancer, inflammation, hypertension, cardiovascular diseases, atherosclerosis, obesity, diabetes, and neurodegenerative disorders (Dubey et al. 2020; Meenambal and Srinivas Bharath 2020; Udeh et al. 2020). The utility of nutraceuticals is an attractive option owing to its natural source, biocompatibility, potential nutritional and therapeutic effects, and lower toxicity and presence of antioxidative constituents, particularly polyphenols (Meenambal and Srinivas Bharath 2020). As such, novel functional foods, including bioactive compounds such as antioxidants, minerals, vitamins, probiotics, and bioactive peptides, and so on, which may have physiological benefits and potential to reduce the risks of diseases, have been developed (Deladino et al. 2016; Nijhawan and Behl 2020).

However, utilization of these bioactive compounds in food industry is currently limited because of their poor water solubility, low bioavailability, pH sensitivity, and sensitivity to food processing and storage conditions, as well as conditions in the gastrointestinal tract (GIT) after their consumption (Montes et al. 2019; Nooshkam and Varidi 2020; Zou et al. 2015). Thus, incorporation of nutraceutical compounds into pharmaceutical and/or food matrices and their delivery to targeted

Handbook of Nutraceuticals and Natural Products: Biological, Medicinal, and Nutritional Properties and Applications,
Volume 2, First Edition. Edited by Preetha Balakrishnan and Sreerag Gopi.
© 2022 John Wiley & Sons, Inc. Published 2022 by John Wiley & Sons, Inc.

area have led to extensive research on the most appropriate technology to protect them, depending on the active ingredients and the matrix composition (Davidov-Pardo and McClements 2015; Deladino et al. 2016; Meenambal and Srinivas Bharath 2020).

Nutraceuticals are known to be practically insoluble in water; their bioaccessibility and bioavailability are very limited, and their adsorption from GIT to the blood serum is poorly controlled (Garti et al. 2016; Montes et al. 2019). It is very important to choose appropriate methods to enhance the bioaccessibility and bioavailability, and the delivery of the nutraceuticals to the targeted site with appropriate approaches and means (Garti et al. 2016; Meenambal and Srinivas Bharath 2020). Therefore, to improve the efficacy of nutraceuticals, delivery systems are required to protect nutraceuticals through GIT and ensure their delivery to the targeted site (Akbari-Alavijeh et al. 2020; Nijhawan and Behl 2020). Drug delivery systems by micro/nanotechnology using biocompatible and biodegradable polymers has improved therapeutic medicines bioavailability for preventing several health disorders. Thus, the use of nutraceuticals for managing a number of health issues by producing phytomedicine and various functional food has great potential in medicine, pharmaceutical, and food area (Nijhawan and Behl 2020; Polowsky and Janaswamy 2015).

Various technological techniques have arisen, including micro/nanoencapsulation and/or nanodelivery systems to enhance the efficacy of nutraceuticals. Therefore, encapsulation is a useful technology and technique to protect and deliver nutraceuticals, bioactive molecules, and drugs (Lakkis 2016; Montes et al. 2019). Encapsulation and controlled-release systems have been designed to rationally protect bioactive compounds from various undesirable interactions and to improve their solubility, functionality, bioaccessibility, and bioavailability (Lakkis 2016; Okagu et al. 2020; Polowsky and Janaswamy 2015), also in addition to masking the bitter taste of some nutraceuticals, ensuring adequate administration of nutraceuticals that are heat/oxidation labile and ensuring their delivery to a target site. Hence, micro/nanodelivery systems using biocompatible and biodegradable materials, such as lipids, surfactants, carbohydrates, polymers, complexes, and protein, have been designed to stabilize and enhance their biological activity (Aditya et al. 2017; Lakkis 2016).

Micro and nanotechnologies have seen widespread use in drug delivery systems with the goal of improving the efficiency of delivery systems. Some major problems in drug delivery have been solved by fabrication of micro/nanocarriers with precise control over their morphological characteristics (architecture, size, etc.) (Ahadian et al. 2020; Rabiei et al. 2020). As such, dynamic delivery systems have been fabricated using micro/nanoencapsulation technologies by which sensing, recording, and stimulating biological systems can be achieved for optimized drug delivery. Moreover, microencapsulation techniques have been used to make biomimetic GIT in vitro models in which the body's response to drugs can be recapitulated and used for better design of drugs (Ahadian et al. 2020; Rabiei et al. 2020; Tian et al. 2020). The application of micro/nanotechnology to different areas of medicine such as cancer therapy, drug delivery, biosensing, and tissue engineering has recently generated a notable impact on diagnostics and treatments (Rabiei et al. 2020).

5.2 Potential Nutraceuticals

Nutraceuticals are formulations of concentrated bioactive components present in food or derived from natural dietary products that offer preventive and/or therapeutic benefits. They are imitative of nutrition and pharmaceutical, also known as functional foods. Various substances isolated from food, such as nutrients, processed food, and dietary supplements, which are used not only for nutritional purpose but also for therapeutic and/or physiological benefits are considered as nutraceuticals (Chelluboina and Vemuganti 2020; Maria Leena et al. 2020; Nijhawan and Behl 2020).

Nutraceuticals comprises various substances such as bioactive peptides, phenolic compounds, flavonoids, carotenoids, lipids, minerals, vitamins, amino acids, antioxidants, plant metabolites, and combination of these biomolecules, dietary supplements, and processed foods. They are used in the field of healthcare and act as connection between food and production, including bioactive compounds in the form of pills, powders, capsules, and so on. Many nutraceuticals such as gallic acid, caffeine, quercetin, curcumin, and fish oils that are rich in PUFAs, essential oils, lipophilic antioxidant, coenzyme Q10 (Q10), etc. have shown health benefit properties (antiaging, antioxidant, etc.) (Davidov-Pardo and McClements 2015; Maria Leena et al. 2020; Meenambal and Srinivas Bharath 2020; Nijhawan and Behl 2020; Udeh et al. 2020).

5.2.1 Curcumin

Turmeric (*Curcuma longa*) has been used as a spice and herbal remedy in south and east Asian countries since long and has been widely used as a food-coloring agent and/or spice owing to its intense yellow color (Abbas et al. 2015; Nijhawan and Behl 2020; Zhai et al. 2020). Curcumin is the major bioactive compound in turmeric; it is a kind of native polyphenolic compound and one of the most biologically active constituents beside the other two minor curcuminoids. It exists in three major forms: curcumin, demethoxycurcumin, and bis-demethoxycurcumin (Abbas et al. 2015; Meng et al. 2021; Zou et al. 2015). Although beneficial effects of curcumin on human health are recognized by the modern medicine, its full potential is yet to be proved. Its low water solubility, poor bioavailability, and instability are the major disadvantages and limitation to this nutraceutical use. Recently, researchers have tried to use a variety of encapsulation techniques to improve its solubility, stability, and bioavailability, and also to develop functional food and pharmaceutical products (Abbas et al. 2015; Guo et al. 2018; Meng et al. 2021; Zou et al. 2015).

Moreover, curcumin has also been used for the treatment of numerous health issues, such as anemia, bacterial infections, colds, coughs, eczema, fevers, inflammation, jaundice, liver diseases, skin diseases, urinary diseases, viral infections, and wounds. The potential health benefits of curcumin have been attributed to a range of biological effects, including antibacterial, antifungal, antiaging, anti-inflammatory, antioxidant, antitumor and anticancer, and antiviral activities (Meng et al. 2021; Zou et al. 2015). Therefore, due to its potential health benefits, there has been considerable interest in incorporating curcumin into functional food products as a nutraceutical agent that may promote human health and wellness (Zou et al. 2015). However, its application is limited due to its inherent physicochemical instability, high hydrophobicity (low solubility), and inferior oral bioavailability (Meng et al. 2021). Hence, its encapsulation in micro/nanoparticles delivery systems is an effective approach to overcome the above-mentioned shortcomings.

5.2.2 Polyunsaturated Fatty Acid

Lipids rich in PUFAs. They are traditionally extracted from animals and plants but alternatively can be obtained from microbes through microbial lipid biotechnology (Ji and Ledesma-Amaro 2020).

The health benefits associated with the consumption of bioactive lipids, such as PUFAs are well known, particularly for maintaining normal brain function, reducing the risk of cancer, and preventing cardiovascular diseases (Eratte et al. 2014; Kim et al. 2016a, b; Vélez et al. 2017). They have been reported to possess diverse potent physiological functions such as anticancer, anti-inflammatory, anticarcinogenic, antiatherogenic, anti-adipogenic, antidiabetic, and antihypertensive properties (Cheng and McClements 2016; Fernandez-Avila et al. 2017; Onwulata 2012).

These functions have led to growing interest in their utilization as nutraceutical ingredients into functional food and beverage products (Kadamne et al. 2011; Nikbakht Nasrabadi et al. 2016) and have garnered renewed research interest in few past years (Fernandez-Avila et al. 2017; Jimenez et al. 2008; Kadamne et al. 2011). Omega-3 and omega-6 PUFAs present in fish oils are very important for enhancing healthiness; docosahexanoic acid (DHA) is known as an anti-inflammatory factor; however, it cannot be produced in the human body; thus, a promising way to introduce it to body is through food products or nutraceuticals capsules (Delshadi et al. 2020; Nijhawan and Behl 2020).

5.2.3 Conjugated Linoleic Acid (CLA)

CLA is a group of positional and geometric (cis or trans) isomers of linoleic acid (18:2) with a conjugated double bond that naturally occurs in dairy products (milk, cheese, etc.), ruminant tissues (beef, lamb, etc.), and also in fish and eggs. The most representative CLA isomers are 9c,11t-18:2 and 10t,12c-18:2 (Koba and Yanagita 2014; Nijhawan and Behl 2020; Nikbakht Nasrabadi et al. 2016). CLA is not to be cooked as it is temperature sensitive, so it should be consumed as medicine, as salad, or encapsulated to enhance it stability and extend its application (Duhoranimana et al. 2018; Nijhawan and Behl 2020).

CLA may be used as a nutraceutical, supplement, or pharmaceutical due to its potential health benefits (anticancer, immune modulation, atherosclerosis prevention, and cholesterol absorption and inhibitory effects). CLA has been approved as generally recognized as safe (GRAS) for certain food applications (yogurt, milk-based fruit drinks, beverages, fruit juices, etc.) (He et al. 2016; Kim et al. 2016a, b). Direct addition of free CLA aiming to supplement food products is limited by its hydrophobic nature and oxidative instability; it is very unstable in aqueous media leading to oxidative rancidity and nutritional loss (Costa et al. 2015; Nikbakht Nasrabadi et al. 2016). Hence, CLA must be encapsulated to maintain its stability and inhibit gastric digestion, while retaining its bioactivity and improving its bioaccessibility.

5.2.4 Coenzyme Q10

Q10 also known as ubiquinone is the most common form of coenzyme Q, which is one of coenzymes and naturally present in humans (Shin et al. 2020; Stratulat et al. 2013). It is a lipid-soluble benzoquinone, which is a key component of the mitochondrial respiratory chain as an intracellular antioxidant that protects mitochondrial membrane's phospholipids and protein from free radical-induced oxidative adverse consequences (Komaki et al. 2019; Shin et al. 2020). Q10 is generally known to generate energy (adenosine triphosphate [ATP]) in the mitochondria by participating in oxidative phosphorylation pathway as a coenzyme (Shin et al. 2020). It possesses interesting health benefits, such as antioxidant, antiinflammatory, anticancer, antidiabetic, cardioprotective, and neuroprotective properties (Komaki et al. 2019; Shin et al. 2020; Villanueva-Bermejo and Temelli 2020).

Q10 plays an important role in maintaining human health and vitality; as an antioxidant and anti-inflammatory bioactive, it is able to control redox balance in various physiological and pathological processes. Q10 possesses neuroprotective properties, which prevents the cascade of cell death actions by maintaining cellular association and restoring neuronal activity (Chen et al. 2020; Komaki et al. 2019; Shin et al. 2020). As such, Q10 is an active participant in many biochemical processes, including cellular respiration, ATP generation, myocardial strength maintenance, and immune system enhancement (Chen et al. 2020).

5.2.5 Essential Oils

Essential oils (Eos) are aromatic, volatile products, and/or complex mixtures of fragrant and odorless compounds characterized by a specific odor, and they are formed by aromatic plants as secondary metabolites; they are derived from plant materials through extraction (Bakry et al. 2016; Ríos 2016; Sharma et al. 2020). Essential oils are extracted from various parts of the aromatic plants such as barks, seeds, flowers, peel, fruit, roots, leaves, wood, fruits, and whole plants and are named according to the plant from which they are obtained (Ríos 2016; Sharma et al. 2020).

They possess various biological and functional properties. Their physicochemical properties may be changed due to oxidation, chemical interactions, or volatilization (Bakry et al. 2016; Sharma et al. 2020). Essential oil application is quite limited due to their physicochemical characteristics such as instability in light and oxygen, high volatility, and especially lipophilicity, which affect their solubility in aqueous medium (de Carvalho et al. 2020). In drug delivery and new drugs development, essential oils have gained great consideration, as they have a variety of compounds, which arouse interest of the researchers for presenting remarkable biological and health properties (de Carvalho et al. 2020).

To avoid and/or limit their degradation/loss during processing and storage and thus to control the delivery of the compound to the targeted site, micro/nanoencapsulation are beneficial techniques prior to their application (Bakry et al. 2016; de Carvalho et al. 2020). The protection of essential oils from the environmental factors through micro/nanoencapsulation could increase their shelf life, provide a controlled release, and improve dispersion in aqueous media (de Carvalho et al. 2020; Delshadi et al. 2020). Moreover, essential oils bioactivity can be enhanced through micro/nanoencapsulation, due to the improvement of their physicochemical stability. As such, their bioaccessibility and bioavailability can be increased, as well as their delivery to the site of action (de Carvalho et al. 2020; Shetta et al. 2019).

5.2.5.1 Peppermint oil

Peppermint oil is a complex mixture of comparatively volatile and labile components; it is a popular flavoring agent in food, perfume, and pharmaceutical industries. The most abundant component of peppermint oil is menthol; peppermint was found to have antioxidant, cytotoxic, antiallergenic, antiviral, anticancer, and strong antimicrobial activities (Abdellatief et al. 2017; Bakry et al. 2016). Peppermint oil is used as a traditional treatment for different human diseases and various pain conditions, such as headaches, postherpetic neuralgia, or mild bacterial or fungal infections of the skin. Researchers have tested the antiviral properties of peppermint oil and the findings showed that peppermint oil exhibits high levels of virucidal activity (Allahverdiyev et al. 2013; Arnal-Schnebelen et al. 2004). Furthermore, micro/nanoencapsulation has increased the stability, retention, and controlled release of peppermint oil (Dong et al. 2011; Rajkumar et al. 2020).

5.2.5.2 Cinnamaldehyde oil

Cinnamaldehyde is a yellow oily and viscous liquid with a cinnamon odor and sweet taste, which constitutes 98% of cinnamon bark essential oil (Shreaz et al. 2016; Zhu et al. 2017). It has also been considered to have medicinal properties, such as anti-inflammatory, pain relieving, and immunoregulatory, stimulant against digestive disorders, and diarrhea (Hancı et al. 2016; Hosni et al. 2017; Xie et al. 2017). It has been widely used as flavoring agents in foods, beverages, ice creams, candies and sweets, chewing gums, medical products, cosmetics and perfumes, etc., and it is an active inhibitor of bacterial growth yeast and filamentous molds (Shreaz et al. 2016; Xie et al. 2017). To retain their biological activity and at the same time to minimize the impact on the organoleptic properties of foods where incorporated, these bioactive compounds need to be encapsulated in delivery systems, which are compatible with food applications. Hence, biopolymer-based coacervates can be used for their encapsulation and stabilization.

5.2.6 Flavonoids

Flavonoids are aromatic keto-compounds found in several natural edible products, such as vegetables, fruits, legumes, and tea. They are of great therapeutic value, owing to their health properties: antioxidant, anti-inflammatory, antiviral, anticancer, and antiaging properties (Jia et al. 2020). Flavonoids are a series of compounds with C6–C3–C6 as the basic carbon model with a wide range of potentially beneficial bioactivities. They are divided into various classes: flavonols, flavanols, flavones, flavanones, isoflavones, and anthocyanidins (Kamiloglu, et al. 2020; Pu et al. 2021). They provide numerous benefits associated with health-promoting effects by reducing the risk of development of chronic diseases such as cardiovascular diseases, type 2 diabetes, and some types of cancers (Kamiloglu et al. 2020).

5.2.7 EGCG

(−)-Epigallocatechin gallate (EGCG) is the major catechin in green tea; it is the most abundant and biologically active polyphenol found in green tea and has strong health-promoting activity (He et al. 2020; Radhakrishnan et al. 2016; Shtay et al. 2019; Yu et al. 2020). They have antimicrobial, anticarcinogenic, antioxidative, anti-inflammatory, antidiabetic, antiobesity, and anticancer effects, but it can easily be degraded when exposed to light and high temperatures (He et al. 2020; Radhakrishnan et al. 2016). However, the use of EGCG is limited due to its poor bioavailability and limited stability, therefore, it has been encapsulated to better protect it against degradation during storage, digestion under simulated gastrointestinal conditions, and therapeutic application (He et al. 2020; Qin et al. 2020; Radhakrishnan et al. 2016; Shtay et al. 2019).

5.2.8 Resveratrol

Resveratrol (trans-resveratrol; trans-3,5,4'-trihydroxystilbene) is a non-flavonoid polyphenol that is found at relatively high levels in grape skins with strong antioxidant activity, but its low solubility in water leads to its underutilization, which limits its application in medicine and food (Davidov-Pardo and McClements 2015; Shao et al. 2019). It is of great interest to the food and pharmaceutical fields due to its potential beneficial effects on human health, including cardioprotective, neuroprotective, antioxidant, anti-inflammatory, anticarcinogenic, antiobesity, and chemoprevention effects (Consoli et al. 2020; Davidov-Pardo and McClements 2015). Despite the potential health benefits of resveratrol, its utilization as a nutraceutical ingredient within the food industry is currently limited due to its poor water solubility, chemical instability, and low bioavailability (Davidov-Pardo and McClements 2015). As such, due to its chemical instability and low water solubility, micro/nanoencapsulation is a good alternative as a delivery system to provide improved properties to resveratrol as a nutraceutical ingredient (Consoli et al. 2020). Hence, resveratrol has been encapsulated within emulsions and liposomes; however, the stability of liposomes is not very convenient to offer enough protection against drug leakage compared to emulsions. Polyphenols delivery to the target site can be achieved by a good choice of a delivery system to protect resveratrol from oxidation and improve its bioaccessibility and bioavailability (Fang et al. 2021; Huang et al. 2019; Shao et al. 2019).

5.3   Health Benefits of Nutraceuticals

Nutraceuticals are substances that possess nutritional and medicinal properties; they are defined as a substance that possess physiological benefit and/or provides protection against diseases. They have garnered great interest of food and pharmaceutical fields due to their potential beneficial effects on human health, including cardioprotective, neuroprotective, antioxidant, anti-inflammatory, anticarcinogenic, anticancer, antithyroid, and antiobesity effects (Davidov-Pardo and McClements 2015; Maria Leena et al. 2020; Meenambal and Srinivas Bharath 2020). Many nutraceuticals and their constituents in their natural milieu display curative effects and health properties. Nutraceuticals are either synthetic substances or chemical compounds (usually concentrated in powder, capsules [encapsulated], etc.) that can provide therapeutic or health benefits to consumers, including improved disease prevention and treatment. They possess various useful effects and are therefore used for treatment of cancer, inflammation, hypertension, cardiovascular diseases, atherosclerosis, obesity, diabetes, and neurodegenerative disorders (Maurya et al. 2021; Meenambal and Srinivas Bharath 2020; Udeh et al. 2020).

Nutraceutical consumption improves health conditions of diseased people, whereas for healthy peoples it helps in maintaining good health conditions and longevity. They can prevent stroke risk and promote stroke recovery, and also prevent oxidative, inflammatory, and cell death. Moreover, nutraceuticals improve health conditions by increasing the absorption of nutrients and supporting microflora of GIT; they can regulate blood pressure, delay neurodegeneration, and improve overall vascular health (Chelluboina and Vemuganti 2020; Diez-Gutiérrez et al. 2020; Maurya et al. 2021; Saleh et al. 2020).

They also support immune system to eliminate pathogens by increasing cytokine secretion, level of reactive oxygen, and reactive nitrogen species. Some algal nutraceuticals are immune boosters that can combat human coronavirus and other viral diseases. Moreover, nutraceuticals also help in detoxification and decrease the absorption of toxic substance in intestines. Hence, the medical benefits of nutraceuticals are due to their phytochemicals with antioxidant, anti-inflammatory, immunostimulatory, and immunomodulatory properties, which works in different ways to improve body health and even skin disease treatment (Maurya et al. 2021; Ratha et al. 2020; Raut and Wairkar 2018).

These nutraceutical phytochemicals can serve as substrate for many biochemical reactions, as cofactors for many enzymes, and can help in elimination of unwanted toxic substances, free radical scavengers, etc.; they potentially mediate these effects through their powerful antioxidant and anti-inflammatory properties (Chelluboina and Vemuganti 2020; Maurya et al. 2021). Furthermore, nutraceuticals provide multiple health benefits in addition to their nutritional benefits. They are used for alleviating hyperglycemia, lowering of cholesterol, blood pressure, and lipid; weight management; improvement of metabolism; prevention of aging; and as brain stimulant, relaxing and refreshing, and sometime for the treatment of chronic disease (Abdellatief et al. 2017; Chelluboina and Vemuganti 2020; Kim et al. 2016a, b). Additionally, being of natural origin, nutraceuticals are considered safe with have no side effects and are nontoxic. Hence, their use during serious complications such as cancer, diabetes, obesity, cardiovascular disease, neurodegenerative disorders and virus diseases has garnered increasing interest (Maurya et al. 2021; Ratha et al. 2020; Saleh et al. 2020).

Generally, nutraceutical bioavailability captures two essential features: (i) the absorption rate – how fast the bioactive agent enters the systemic circulation; and (ii) the absorption extent – how much of the bioactive agent reaches the systematic circulation (Jafari et al. 2017). As such, various external and internal factors determine the overall bioavailability rate of an ingested bioactive compound. It may be limited by various physicochemical and physiological phenomena: liberation from capsules matrices, solubility in gastrointestinal fluids, interaction with gastrointestinal components, chemical degradation or metabolism, and epithelium cell permeability. Thus, nutraceutical bioavailability can therefore be improved by designing delivery systems that control their bioaccessibility and controlled release (Gonçalves et al. 2018; McClements et al. 2015). The potential health benefits of many nutraceuticals are not fully profitable due to their physicochemical instability; they are chemically degraded during storage or within GIT. Therefore, there is a need to develop efficient delivery systems to encapsulate and protect nutraceuticals until they reach an appropriate location within the human body through the GIT (mouth, stomach, small intestine, and colon) (McClements 2017).

5.4 Nutraceutical Encapsulation

Encapsulation technology has received considerable interest in a wide range of disciplines and in numerous fields of applications such as pharmaceutical, foods, cosmetics, agricultural, electronic, and molecular diagnostic applications (Devi et al. 2017; Sobel et al. 2014). Encapsulation technologies for designing delivery systems and producing desired bioactive compound capsules have garnered increasing interest of researchers in the few past decades (Delshadi et al. 2020; Duhoranimana et al. 2017; Santos et al. 2015). Thus, encapsulation is a useful technology to protect and deliver nutraceuticals and bioactive molecules and to cope with their poor absorption, low solubility, bioaccessibility, and bioavailability (Delshadi et al. 2020; Meenambal and Srinivas Bharath 2020).

Nutraceuticals are encapsulated and therefore protected from degradation; the stability of bioactive molecules is ensured; and nutraceutical functional components are kept as fully functional (Dubey et al. 2020; Links et al. 2015; Wang et al. 2020). Therefore, for the above-mentioned purpose, numerous encapsulation techniques are available for encapsulation and protection of nutraceuticals and bioactive molecules for further delivery and controlled release of bioactive compounds.

5.4.1 Encapsulation Techniques

Nutraceuticals are nutritional substances that are used to achieve health benefits with minimal or no side effects. However, they are subject to degradation resulting from exposure to environmental factors such as humidity, oxygen, heat, light, extreme pH, and so on (Khorasani et al. 2018; Polowsky and Janaswamy 2015). Micro/nanoencapsulation techniques for improving water dispersibility, stability, and bioavailability of poorly soluble bioactive compounds and nutraceuticals have garnered increasing interest, such as emulsion, liposomes, biopolymers conjugates, coacervates, nanovehicles (or nanocarriers), especially those based on proteins and protein–polysaccharide complexes (Duhoranimana et al. 2018; Liu et al. 2020; Tang 2021; Wang et al. 2019). Moreover, as their functionality such as bioaccessibility and bioavailability greatly controls the overall efficacy, carriers and delivery systems play significant role in developing effective nutraceutical capsules (Guo et al. 2018; Polowsky and Janaswamy 2015; Zou et al. 2015).

5.4.1.1 Emulsion
Emulsion technology is widely used to create encapsulation systems for nutraceuticals, such as flavors, colors, preservatives, vitamins, and various bioactive compounds (Lv et al. 2020). Emulsion-based delivery systems are a promising encapsulation technique, when poor water-soluble drugs

are formulated, due to the fact that lipophilic bioactive components can be encapsulated within the hydrophobic core of the lipid droplets where they may be protected from degradation during storage and then released after ingestion (Davidov-Pardo and McClements 2015; Francke and Bunjes 2020). Thus, adequate stability and controlled release of nutraceuticals can be ensured through colloidal lipid emulsions. There are two most common forms of emulsion-based delivery systems: conventional emulsions (radius >100 nm) and nanoemulsions (radius ≤100 nm), which are both thermodynamically unstable systems, and they tend to breakdown during storage through a variety of instability mechanisms. However, they can be designed to have sufficient kinetic stability for many applications. Moreover, they can be used as delivery systems for lipophilic agents. Microemulsions have some characteristics similar to nanoemulsions (radius ≤25 nm), they contain very small particles and tend to be optically transparent, but they are more thermodynamically stable systems (Davidov-Pardo and McClements 2015; Piorkowski and McClements 2014).

There exist two emulsions categories: oil-in-water (O/W) or water-in-oil (W/O) emulsion, depending on the continuous phase (Bajpai 2018). Oil-in-water (O/W) emulsions and nanoemulsions are useful in designing delivery systems to encapsulate hydrophobic bioactives in the emulsion oil droplets to improve their stability and solubility in aqueous solutions. They are usually prepared by homogenizing an oil phase into an aqueous phase in the presence of water-soluble emulsifiers/stabilizers (Abbas et al. 2014; Nooshkam and Varidi 2020). Emulsions are used for parenteral nutrition and as delivery system for poorly water-soluble drugs. They are an important formulation option for many new drug developments (Francke and Bunjes 2020).

5.4.1.2 Complex Coacervation

Encapsulation techniques such as emulsion, complex coacervation, liposome, conjugates, spray drying, and extrusion have been used for the encapsulation of nutraceuticals to ensure their stability, delivery, and controlled release (Abbas et al. 2015; Dong et al. 2011; Duhoranimana et al. 2018; Geranpour et al. 2020; Liu et al. 2020; Nooshkam and Varidi 2020). Among these methods, complex coacervation has received a great deal of research interest mainly due to its high encapsulation efficiency and controlled release (Dong et al. 2011; Duhoranimana et al. 2018; Muhoza et al. 2020; Timilsena et al. 2017). Complex coacervation is a type of phase separation that occurs due to electrostatic attraction between oppositely charged polyelectrolytes and biopolymers (proteins and polysaccharides), and a neutral complex is formed when these polyelectrolytes and/or biopolymers with opposite charges are brought together (Aberkane et al. 2010; Devi et al. 2017; Kayitmazer 2017; Nooshkam and Varidi 2020). The phenomenon has received increasing research interest due to its practical application particularly in the encapsulation industry (Calderón-Oliver et al. 2017; Devi et al. 2017; Li et al. 2017). The electrostatic interactions between proteins and polysaccharides induce the formation of various supramolecular entities such as soluble complexes, insoluble complexes, and coacervates, with soluble complexes preceding coacervation (Jenkins et al. 2016; Kayitmazer 2017).

Complex coacervates structure and their stability depend on different parameters, including structure, flexibility and biopolymers charge density, molecular weight, quality of solvent, pH, ionic strength, protein–polysaccharide molar ratio, total biopolymer concentration, and so on (Devi et al. 2017; Lim et al. 2014; Yan and Zhang 2014). Researchers have reported that electrostatic interaction between protein and polysaccharide is not always the dominant driving force for coacervation; for some systems entropy gain from counterion release can overcome the enthalpic contribution of electrostatic interactions (Kayitmazer 2017; Li et al. 2012; Li et al. 2017). Hence, the effect of parameters such as pH and thermodynamic properties of protein–polysaccharide complex coacervates assessed by isothermal titration calorimetry (ITC) could provide useful information in developing complex coacervated materials for diverse applications (Dong et al. 2015a, b; Lim et al. 2014).

Additionally, the formation of protein–polysaccharide complexes can potentially lead to different functional properties to empower their uses in different industrial applications such as food, pharmaceutical, cosmetics, and agriculture (Aberkane et al. 2012; Devi et al. 2017; Kayitmazer 2017). Various application areas for complex coacervation technique have been reported, such as bioactive compounds microencapsulation, purification of proteins, and drug delivery systems (Aumiller Jr and Keating 2016; Kayitmazer 2017; Yuan et al. 2017). Hence, the design of the micro-nanoscale system for nutraceuticals and bioactive compounds encapsulation, delivery, and control release for practical applications has garnered great importance nowadays. The concept behind encapsulation by complex coacervation is the phase separation of one or many hydrocolloids from the initial solution and the subsequent deposition of the newly formed coacervate phase around bioactive compound(s) suspended or emulsified in the same reaction media (Fang and Bhandari 2010; Yan and Zhang 2014). Complex coacervation method has been used to develop effective delivery systems to encapsulate, protect, and release bioactive compounds and flavors and has several benefits such as high pay load, yield, and encapsulation efficiency (Prata and Grosso 2015; Santos et al. 2015; Sarya Aziz et al. 2014) and controlled release of encapsulated materials (Dong et al. 2011; Saravanan and Rao 2010).

Complex coacervation can be achieved in biopolymer pair of protein–polysaccharide mixtures by exact controlling of the external parameters (pH, temperature, mixing ratio, stirring rate, etc.) as shown in Figure 5.1, producing electrostatic interactions of oppositely charged macroions. Among the polymer pairs, protein–polysaccharide complex coacervation has attracted much

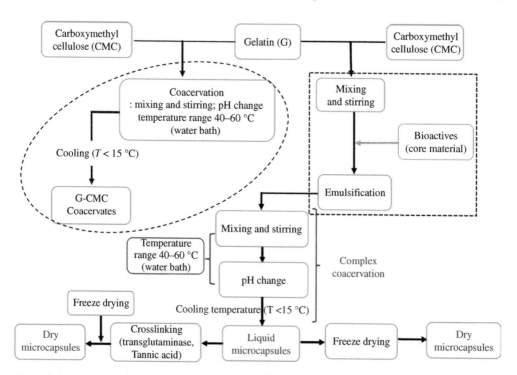

Figure 5.1 Nutraceutical encapsulation process by complex coacervation techniques with subsequent steps and potential external parameters (pH, temperature, mixing ratio, and stirring rate) influencing the encapsulation process. *Source:* Emmanuel Duhoranimana.

attention in the past few decades, particularly in the area of encapsulation of active ingredients (Devi et al. 2012, 2017; Duhoranimana et al. 2018; Muhoza et al. 2020; Timilsena et al. 2017; Zuanon et al. 2013). Proteins and polysaccharides have been extensively utilized in recent years as functional ingredients to improve texture, structure, and shelf life of most food products and for bioactive compounds coating and delivering (Anvari et al. 2015; Qiu et al. 2015; Wu and McClements 2015). Microencapsulation by complex coacervation of protein and polysaccharides, especially of gelatin and gum Arabic due to their biocompatibility, biodegradability, and safety, has been widely investigated to encapsulate nutraceuticals, and bioactive lipids, essential oils, and lipophilic bioactives (Lv et al. 2012; Piacentini et al. 2013; Qv et al. 2011). Also, other proteins (milk proteins and plant proteins) and polysaccharides (alginate, carrageenan, chitosan, pectin, CMC, gums, etc.) have been investigated and utilized (Dima et al. 2014; Dong et al. 2015a, b; Koupantsis et al. 2014; Timilsena et al. 2017).

Furthermore, encapsulating materials and core/shell interactions play a major role in design and development of nutraceutical delivery system (Maria Leena et al. 2020). Many wall materials are suitable for production of microcapsules. However, compared to other fields (pharmaceutical, cosmetic, or agrochemical industries), the selection of wall materials in the food industry to encapsulate functional ingredients via coacervation is often challenging, due to tight regulations and lower price margin (Sobel et al. 2014; Yan and Zhang 2014). Meanwhile, wall material particularly affects the capsules' stability, the process efficiency, and the degree of protection of the active core ingredients. Proteins and polysaccharides are the most widely used wall materials as their coacervates demonstrate superior new functional properties by combining advantages of both protein and polysaccharide. Therefore, wall material selection is one of the major concerns for applying coacervation technology in nutraceutical encapsulation, drug delivery, pharmaceutical, and food industry (Devi et al. 2017; Timilsena et al. 2017; Yan and Zhang 2014).

5.4.1.3 Liposomes

Liposome is a bilayer vesicle structure formed by self-assembling of phospholipids with a hydrophilic head and hydrophobic tail dispersed in aqueous solution. It can be effectively used for the selective delivery of nutraceuticals (Nandi et al. 2020; Wang et al. 2019). Liposomes are one of the most applied nanostructures for entrapping drug molecules since their membrane structures allow the encapsulation of both hydrophilic and hydrophobic drugs. Hence, liposomes can be utilized to entrap curcumin to increase curcumin solubility and prevent the degradation from hydrolysis and photo-induced reaction in the biological milieu (Laomeephol et al. 2020). Liposome delivery systems can achieve multicomponent encapsulation of hydrophilic, hydrophobic substances, and amphiphilic molecules in the interior aqueous compartment, lipid bilayers, and at the lipid/water interface (Wang et al. 2019). Moreover, liposome efficiency as a drug delivery system in pharmaceutical industry lies in their composition, which makes them biocompatible and biodegradable. Liposomes can enhance the stability and bioavailability nutraceuticals (Nandi et al. 2020; Wang et al. 2019).

5.4.1.4 Conjugates

Biopolymers Maillard conjugates based on mixtures between protein and polysaccharide using a wet heating and dry heating method, as well as their application as stabilizing agents of nutraceuticals-loaded emulsions, have garnered increasing interest of the researchers (Consoli et al. 2020). Conjugation is an effective approach for modifying the structure and functional properties of native proteins through reaction with polysaccharides via the Maillard reaction (MR) (Dai et al. 2015; Li et al. 2020). Conjugates possess improved stability against changes in pH and ionic strength compared to the native protein, which is beneficial to the wide applications of modified proteins in food processing and encapsulation technology (Dai et al. 2015). The stable nanoparticles from proteins and strong polyelectrolyte polysaccharides are a promising delivery system for hydrophobic nutrients, nutraceuticals, and drugs. Conjugates delivery systems have been extensively applied for nutraceuticals and bioactive compound encapsulation and delivery (Liu et al. 2020; Yi et al. 2018). The advantages of conjugates delivery system is that they may provide a better alternative to effectively protect and deliver hydrophobic nutraceuticals as they can improve nutraceuticals stability against environmental stress (ionic strength, heat, and pH) and thus improve their shelf life (storage stability) with enhanced antioxidant activity and bioavailability (Gu et al. 2018; Yu et al. 2020).

5.5 Application of Nutraceuticals and Nutraceuticals Capsules

Encapsulation is a very successful approach to preserve or mask flavor and aroma and to enhance thermal and oxidative stability of nutraceuticals. It allows to overcome the limitations of high volatility to control release rate and improve their poor bioavailability, thereby increasing their application in food systems. Micro/nanoencapsulation systems containing nutraceuticals can be used as a technology to produce functional foods. These encapsulation systems can provide many advantages including sustained release, antimicrobial and antioxidant activities, stability, improved bioavailability but also prevent undesirable interactions (Delshadi et al. 2020; Khorasani et al. 2021). Nutraceuticals and nutraceutical capsules have been used for various applications. Nutraceuticals and functional foods have attracted much interest as possible alternative therapies as cholesterol-lowering, reducing toxicity agent, and preventing diseases (Chen et al. 2008; Gu et al. 2018; Komaki et al. 2019; Liu et al. 2018; Radhakrishnan et al. 2016; Shin et al. 2020). Hence, nutraceutical capsules are promising entities for prophylactic and therapeutic applications.

5.6 Conclusion

Nowadays, stability and bioavailability nutraceuticals, drug, and food bioactive compounds are known as the main issues in design and development of efficient micro/nanodelivery systems. In this regard, encapsulation techniques (emulsion, complex coacervation, liposomes, conjugates, etc.) due to their applicability and materials (biopolymers, proteins, polysaccharides, lipids, etc.) due to their biocompatibility and biodegradability have garnered increased interest of the researchers for nutraceuticals and bioactive compounds encapsulation and delivery. Biopolymer-based delivery systems have shown great potential for micro/nanocapsules design and their preparation techniques, as well as their potential application in food, pharmaceutical, and medicine industries. Hence, nutraceutical encapsulation in micro/nanocarriers using above-mentioned techniques is promising for an improved stability, bioaccessibility and bioavailability, targeted delivery, and controlled release, as well as their application in functional food development, pharmaceutical, and medicine area.

Declaration of Competing Interest

All authors declare that there is no conflict of interest.

References

Abba, S., Bashari, M., Akhtar, W. et al. (2014). Process optimization of ultrasound-assisted curcumin nanoemulsions stabilized by OSA-modified starch. *Ultrasonics Sonochemistry 21* (4): 1265–1274. https://doi.org/10.1016/j.ultsonch.2013.12.017.

Abbas, S., Karangwa, E., Bashari, M. et al. (2015). Fabrication of polymeric nanocapsules from curcumin-loaded nanoemulsion templates by self-assembly. *Ultrasonics Sonochemistry 23*: 81–92. https://doi.org/10.1016/j.ultsonch.2014.10.006.

Abdellatief, S.A., Beheiry, R.R., and El-Mandrawy, S.A.M. (2017). Peppermint essential oil alleviates hyperglycemia caused by streptozotocin- nicotinamide-induced type 2 diabetes in rats. *Biomedicine & Pharmacotherapy 95*: 990–999. https://doi.org/10.1016/j.biopha.2017.09.020.

Aberkane, L., Jasniewski, J., Gaiani, C. et al. (2010). Thermodynamic characterization of acacia gum–β-lactoglobulin complex coacervation. *Langmuir 26* (15): 12523–12533. https://doi.org/10.1021/la100705d.

Aberkane, L., Jasniewski, J., Gaiani, C. et al. (2012). Structuration mechanism of β-lactoglobulin – acacia gum assemblies in presence of quercetin. *Food Hydrocolloids 29* (1): 9–20. https://doi.org/10.1016/j.foodhyd.2012.01.010.

Aditya, N.P., Espinosa, Y.G., and Norton, I.T. (2017). Encapsulation systems for the delivery of hydrophilic nutraceuticals: Food application. *Biotechnology Advances 35* (4): 450–457. https://doi.org/10.1016/j.biotechadv.2017.03.012.

Ahadian, S., Finbloom, J.A., Mofidfar, M. et al. (2020). Micro and nanoscale technologies in oral drug delivery. *Advanced Drug Delivery Reviews*. https://doi.org/10.1016/j.addr.2020.07.012 157: 37–62.

Akbari-Alavijeh, S., Shaddel, R., and Jafari, S.M. (2020). Encapsulation of food bioactives and nutraceuticals by various chitosan-based nanocarriers. *Food Hydrocolloids 105*: 105774. https://doi.org/10.1016/j.foodhyd.2020.105774.

Allahverdiyev, A.M., Bagirova, M., Yaman, S. et al. (2013). Chapter 17 – development of new antiherpetic drugs based on plant compounds. In: *Fighting Multidrug Resistance with Herbal Extracts, Essential Oils and Their Components* (ed. M.K. Rai and K.V. Kon), 245–259. San Diego: Academic Press.

Anvari, M., Pan, C.H., Yoon, W.B., and Chung, D. (2015). Characterization of fish gelatin-gum arabic complex coacervates as influenced by phase separation temperature. *International Journal of Biological Macromolecules 79*: 894–902. https://doi.org/10.1016/j.ijbiomac.2015.06.004.

Arnal-Schnebelen, B., Hadji-Minaglou, F., Peroteau, J.F. et al. (2004). Essential oils in infectious gynaecological disease: a statistical study of 658 cases. *International Journal of Aromatherapy 14* (4): 192–197. https://doi.org/10.1016/j.ijat.2004.09.003.

Aumiller, W.M. Jr. and Keating, C.D. (2016). Phosphorylation-mediated RNA/peptide complex coacervation as a model for intracellular liquid organelles. *Nature Chemistry 8* (2): 129–137. https://doi.org/10.1038/nchem.2414.

Bagchi, D. and Nair, S. (2017). Preface. In: *Developing New Functional Food and Nutraceutical Products* (ed. D. Bagchi and S. Nair), xxix–xxxi. San Diego: Academic Press.

Bajpai, P. (2018). Chapter 19 – colloid and surface chemistry. In: *Biermann's Handbook of Pulp and Paper*, 3e (ed. P. Bajpai), 381–400. Elsevier.

Bakry, A.M., Abbas, S., Ali, B. et al. (2016). Microencapsulation of oils: a comprehensive review of benefits, techniques, and applications. *Comprehensive Reviews in Food Science and Food Safety 15* (1): 143–182. https://doi.org/10.1111/1541-4337.12179.

Calderón-Oliver, M., Pedroza-Islas, R., Escalona-Buendía, H.B. et al. (2017). Comparative study of the microencapsulation by complex coacervation of nisin in combination with an avocado antioxidant extract. *Food Hydrocolloids 62*: 49–57. https://doi.org/10.1016/j.foodhyd.2016.07.028.

de Carvalho, S.Y.B., Almeida, R.R., Pinto, N.A.R. et al. (2020). Encapsulation of essential oils using cinnamic acid grafted chitosan nanogel: Preparation, characterization and antifungal activity. *International Journal of Biological Macromolecules* 166: 902–912. https://doi.org/10.1016/j.ijbiomac.2020.10.247.

Chelluboina, B. and Vemuganti, R. (2020). Therapeutic potential of nutraceuticals to protect brain after stroke. *Neurochemistry International* 142: 104908. https://doi.org/10.1016/j.neuint.2020.104908.

Chen, Z.-Y., Jiao, R., and Ma, K.Y. (2008). Cholesterol-lowering nutraceuticals and functional foods. *Journal of Agricultural and Food Chemistry* 56 (19): 8761–8773. https://doi.org/10.1021/jf801566r.

Chen, S., Zhang, Y., Qing, J. et al. (2020). Core–shell nanoparticles for co-encapsulation of coenzyme Q10 and piperine: surface engineering of hydrogel shell around protein core. *Food Hydrocolloids* 103: 105651. https://doi.org/10.1016/j.foodhyd.2020.105651.

Cheng, W. and McClements, D.J. (2016). Biopolymer-stabilized conjugated linoleic acid (CLA) oil-in-water emulsions: impact of electrostatic interactions on formation and stability of pectin-caseinate-coated lipid droplets. *Colloids and Surfaces A: Physicochemical and Engineering Aspects* 511: 172–179. https://doi.org/10.1016/j.colsurfa.2016.09.085.

Consoli, L., Hubinger, M.D., and Dragosavac, M.M. (2020). Encapsulation of resveratrol using Maillard conjugates and membrane emulsification. *Food Research International* 137: 109359. https://doi.org/10.1016/j.foodres.2020.109359.

Costa, A.M.M., Nunes, J.C., Lima, B.N.B. et al. (2015). Effective stabilization of CLA by microencapsulation in pea protein. *Food Chemistry* 168: 157–166. https://doi.org/10.1016/j.foodchem.2014.07.016.

Dai, Q., Zhu, X., Abbas, S. et al. (2015). Stable nanoparticles prepared by heating electrostatic complexes of whey protein isolate–dextran conjugate and chondroitin sulfate. *Journal of Agricultural and Food Chemistry* 63 (16): 4179–4189. https://doi.org/10.1021/acs.jafc.5b00794.

Davidov-Pardo, G. and McClements, D.J. (2015). Nutraceutical delivery systems: resveratrol encapsulation in grape seed oil nanoemulsions formed by spontaneous emulsification. *Food Chemistry* 167: 205–212. https://doi.org/10.1016/j.foodchem.2014.06.082.

Deladino, L., Teixeira, A.S., García, A.D.M., and Sofia, N.A. (2016). High-pressure-treated corn starch as an alternative carrier of molecules of nutritional interest for food systems. In: *New Polymers for Encapsulation of Nutraceutical Compounds* (ed. J.C.R. Ruiz and M.R.S. Campos), 35–58. Wiley.

Delshadi, R., Bahrami, A., Tafti, A.G. et al. (2020). Micro and nano-encapsulation of vegetable and essential oils to develop functional food products with improved nutritional profiles. *Trends in Food Science & Technology* 104: 72–83. https://doi.org/10.1016/j.tifs.2020.07.004.

Devi, N., Hazarika, D., Deka, C., and Kakati, D.K. (2012). Study of complex coacervation of gelatin A and sodium alginate for microencapsulation of olive oil. *Journal of Macromolecular Science, Part A* 49 (11): 936–945. https://doi.org/10.1080/10601325.2012.722854.

Devi, N., Sarmah, M., Khatun, B., and Maji, T.K. (2017). Encapsulation of active ingredients in polysaccharide–protein complex coacervates. *Advances in Colloid and Interface Science* 239: 136–145. https://doi.org/10.1016/j.cis.2016.05.009.

Diez-Gutiérrez, L., San Vicente, L., Barrón, R. et al. (2020). Gamma-aminobutyric acid and probiotics: multiple health benefits and their future in the global functional food and nutraceuticals market. *Journal of Functional Foods* 64: 103669. https://doi.org/10.1016/j.jff.2019.103669.

Dima, C., Cotârlet, M., Alexe, P., and Dima, S. (2014). Microencapsulation of essential oil of pimento [*Pimenta dioica* (L) Merr.] by chitosan/k–carrageenan complex coacervation method. *Innovative Food Science & Emerging Technologies* 22: 203–211. https://doi.org/10.1016/j.ifset.2013.12.020.

Dong, Z., Ma, Y., Hayat, K. et al. (2011). Morphology and release profile of microcapsules encapsulating peppermint oil by complex coacervation. *Journal of Food Engineering* 104 (3): 455–460. https://doi.org/10.1016/j.jfoodeng.2011.01.011.

Dong, D., Li, X., Hua, Y. et al. (2015a). Mutual titration of soy proteins and gum arabic and the complexing behavior studied by isothermal titration calorimetry, turbidity and ternary phase boundaries. *Food Hydrocolloids* 46: 28–36. https://doi.org/10.1016/j.foodhyd.2014.11.019.

Dong, D., Qi, Z., Hua, Y. et al. (2015b). Microencapsulation of flaxseed oil by soya proteins–gum arabic complex coacervation. *International Journal of Food Science & Technology 50* (8): 1785–1791. https://doi.org/10.1111/ijfs.12812.

Dubey, N.K., Singh, A.K., Dubey, R., and Deng, W.-P. (2020). Chapter 15 – nutraceutical encapsulation and delivery system for type 2 diabetes mellitus. In: *Biopolymer-Based Formulations* (ed. K. Pal, I. Banerjee, P. Sarkar, et al.), 353–363. Elsevier.

Duhoranimana, E., Karangwa, E., Lai, L. et al. (2017). Effect of sodium carboxymethyl cellulose on complex coacervates formation with gelatin: coacervates characterization, stabilization and formation mechanism. *Food Hydrocolloids 69*: 111–120. https://doi.org/10.1016/j.foodhyd.2017.01.035.

Duhoranimana, E., Yu, J., Mukeshimana, O. et al. (2018). Thermodynamic characterization of gelatin–sodium carboxymethyl cellulose complex coacervation encapsulating conjugated linoleic acid (CLA). *Food Hydrocolloids 80*: 149–159. https://doi.org/10.1016/j.foodhyd.2018.02.011.

Eratte, D., Wang, B., Dowling, K. et al. (2014). Complex coacervation with whey protein isolate and gum arabic for the microencapsulation of omega-3 rich tuna oil. *Food & Function 5* (11): 2743–2750. https://doi.org/10.1039/c4fo00296b.

Fang, Z. and Bhandari, B. (2010). Encapsulation of polyphenols – a review. *Trends in Food Science & Technology 21* (10): 510–523. https://doi.org/10.1016/j.tifs.2010.08.003.

Fang, Z., Cai, X., Wu, J. et al. (2021). Effect of simultaneous treatment combining ultrasonication and pH-shifting on SPI in the formation of nanoparticles and encapsulating resveratrol. *Food Hydrocolloids 111*: 106250. https://doi.org/10.1016/j.foodhyd.2020.106250.

Fernandez-Avila, C., Gutierrez-Merida, C., and Trujillo, A.J. (2017). Physicochemical and sensory characteristics of a UHT milk-based product enriched with conjugated linoleic acid emulsified by ultra-high pressure homogenization. *Innovative Food Science & Emerging Technologies 39*: 275–283. https://doi.org/10.1016/j.ifset.2017.01.001.

Francke, N.M. and Bunjes, H. (2020). Influence of drug loading on the physical stability of phospholipid-stabilised colloidal lipid emulsions. *International Journal of Pharmaceutics* X: 100060. https://doi.org/10.1016/j.ijpx.2020.100060.

Garti, N., Pinthus, E., Aserin, A., and Spernath, A. (2016). Improved solubilization and bioavailability of nutraceuticals in nanosized self-assembled liquid vehicles. In: *Encapsulation and Controlled Release Technologies in Food Systems* (ed. J.M. Lakkis), 173–203. Wiley Blackwell.

Geranpour, M., Assadpour, E., and Jafari, S.M. (2020). Recent advances in the spray drying encapsulation of essential fatty acids and functional oils. *Trends in Food Science & Technology 102*: 71–90. https://doi.org/10.1016/j.tifs.2020.05.028.

Gonçalves, R.F.S., Martins, J.T., Duarte, C.M.M. et al. (2018). Advances in nutraceutical delivery systems: from formulation design for bioavailability enhancement to efficacy and safety evaluation. *Trends in Food Science & Technology 78*: 270–291. https://doi.org/10.1016/j.tifs.2018.06.011.

Gu, L., Pan, C., Su, Y. et al. (2018). in vitro bioavailability, cellular antioxidant activity, and cytotoxicity of β-carotene-loaded emulsions stabilized by catechin–egg white protein conjugates. *Journal of Agricultural and Food Chemistry 66* (7): 1649–1657. https://doi.org/10.1021/acs.jafc.7b05909.

Guo, C., Yin, J., and Chen, D. (2018). Co-encapsulation of curcumin and resveratrol into novel nutraceutical hyalurosomes nano-food delivery system based on oligo-hyaluronic acid-curcumin polymer. *Carbohydrate Polymers 181*: 1033–1037. https://doi.org/10.1016/j.carbpol.2017.11.046.

Hancı, D., Altun, H., Çetinkaya, E.A. et al. (2016). Cinnamaldehyde is an effective anti-inflammatory agent for treatment of allergic rhinitis in a rat model. *International Journal of Pediatric Otorhinolaryngology 84*: 81–87. https://doi.org/10.1016/j.ijporl.2016.03.001.

He, H., Hong, Y., Gu, Z. et al. (2016). Improved stability and controlled release of CLA with spray-dried microcapsules of OSA-modified starch and xanthan gum. *Carbohydrate Polymers 147*: 243–250. https://doi.org/10.1016/j.carbpol.2016.03.078.

He, A., Guan, X., Song, H. et al. (2020). Encapsulation of (−)-epigallocatechin-gallate (EGCG) in hordein nanoparticles. *Food Bioscience 37*: 100727. https://doi.org/10.1016/j.fbio.2020.100727.

Hosni, A.A., Abdel-Moneim, A.A., Abdel-Reheim, E.S. et al. (2017). Cinnamaldehyde potentially attenuates gestational hyperglycemia in rats through modulation of PPARγ, proinflammatory cytokines and oxidative stress. *Biomedicine & Pharmacotherapy 88*: 52–60. https://doi.org/10.1016/j.biopha.2017.01.054.

Huang, X., Liu, Y., Zou, Y. et al. (2019). Encapsulation of resveratrol in zein/pectin core-shell nanoparticles: stability, bioaccessibility, and antioxidant capacity after simulated gastrointestinal digestion. *Food Hydrocolloids 93*: 261–269. https://doi.org/10.1016/j.foodhyd.2019.02.039.

Jafari, S.M., Katouzian, I., Rajabi, H., and Ganje, M. (2017). 13 – Bioavailability and release of bioactive components from nanocapsules. In: *Nanoencapsulation Technologies for the Food and Nutraceutical Industries* (ed. S.M. Jafari), 494–523. Academic Press/Elsevier.

Jenkins, S.I., Collins, C.M., and Khaledi, M.G. (2016). Perfluorinated alcohols induce complex coacervation in mixed surfactants. *Langmuir 32* (10): 2321–2330. https://doi.org/10.1021/acs.langmuir.5b04701.

Ji, X.-J. and Ledesma-Amaro, R. (2020). Microbial lipid biotechnology to produce polyunsaturated fatty acids. *Trends in Biotechnology 38* (8): 832–834. https://doi.org/10.1016/j.tibtech.2020.02.003.

Jia, J.-Y., Zang, E.-H., Lv, L.-J. et al. (2020). Flavonoids in myocardial ischemia-reperfusion injury: therapeutic effects and mechanisms. *Chinese Herbal Medicines* https://doi.org/10.1016/j.chmed.2020.09.002.

Jimenez, M., Garcia, H.S., and Beristain, C.I. (2008). Sensory evaluation of dairy products supplemented with microencapsulated conjugated linoleic acid (CLA). *LWT – Food Science and Technology 41* (6): 1047–1052. https://doi.org/10.1016/j.lwt.2007.07.008.

Kadamne, J.V., Castrodale, C.L., and Proctor, A. (2011). Measurement of conjugated linoleic acid (CLA) in CLA-rich potato chips by ATR-FTIR spectroscopy. *Journal of Agricultural and Food Chemistry 59* (6): 2190–2196. https://doi.org/10.1021/jf104204e.

Kamiloglu, S., Tomas, M., Ozdal, T., and Capanoglu, E. (2020). Effect of food matrix on the content and bioavailability of flavonoids. *Trends in Food Science & Technology 117*: 15–33. https://doi.org/10.1016/j.tifs.2020.10.030.

Kayitmazer, A.B. (2017). Thermodynamics of complex coacervation. *Advances in Colloid and Interface Science 239*: 169–177. https://doi.org/10.1016/j.cis.2016.07.006.

Khorasani, S., Danaei, M., and Mozafari, M.R. (2018). Nanoliposome technology for the food and nutraceutical industries. *Trends in Food Science & Technology 79*: 106–115. https://doi.org/10.1016/j.tifs.2018.07.009.

Khorasani, S., Ghandehari Yazdi, A.P., Taghavi, E. et al. (2021). 3.32 – recent trends in the nanoencapsulation processes for food and nutraceutical applications. In: *Innovative Food Processing Technologies* (ed. K. Knoerzer and K. Muthukumarappan), 532–545. Oxford: Elsevier.

Kim, B., Lim, H.R., Lee, H. et al. (2016a). The effects of conjugated linoleic acid (CLA) on metabolic syndrome patients: a systematic review and meta-analysis. *Journal of Functional Foods 25*: 588–598. https://doi.org/10.1016/j.jff.2016.07.010.

Kim, Y., Kim, D., and Park, Y. (2016b). Conjugated linoleic acid (CLA) promotes endurance capacity via peroxisome proliferator-activated receptor δ-mediated mechanism in mice. *The Journal of Nutritional Biochemistry* 38: 125–133. https://doi.org/10.1016/j.jnutbio.2016.08.005.

Koba, K. and Yanagita, T. (2014). Health benefits of conjugated linoleic acid (CLA). *Obesity Research & Clinical Practice* 8 (6): e525–e532. https://doi.org/10.1016/j.orcp.2013.10.001.

Komaki, H., Faraji, N., Komaki, A. et al. (2019). Investigation of protective effects of coenzyme Q10 on impaired synaptic plasticity in a male rat model of Alzheimer's disease. *Brain Research Bulletin 147*: 14–21. https://doi.org/10.1016/j.brainresbull.2019.01.025.

Koupantsis, T., Pavlidou, E., and Paraskevopoulou, A. (2014). Flavour encapsulation in milk proteins – CMC coacervate-type complexes. *Food Hydrocolloids* 37: 134–142. https://doi.org/10.1016/j.foodhyd.2013.10.031.

Lakkis, J.M. (2016). Introduction. In: *Encapsulation and Controlled Release Technologies in Food Systems* (ed. J.M. Lakkis), 1–15. Wiley Blackwell.

Laomeephol, C., Ferreira, H., Kanokpanont, S. et al. (2020). Dual-functional liposomes for curcumin delivery and accelerating silk fibroin hydrogel formation. *International Journal of Pharmaceutics 589*: 119844. https://doi.org/10.1016/j.ijpharm.2020.119844.

Li, D., Kelkar, M.S., and Wagner, N.J. (2012). Phase behavior and molecular thermodynamics of coacervation in oppositely charged polyelectrolyte/surfactant systems: a cationic polymer JR 400 and anionic surfactant SDS mixture. *Langmuir 28* (28): 10348–10362. https://doi.org/10.1021/la301475s.

Li, X., Hua, Y., Chen, Y. et al. (2017). Two-step complex behavior between Bowman–Birk protease inhibitor and ι-carrageenan: Effect of protein concentration, ionic strength and temperature. *Food Hydrocolloids* 62: 1–9. https://doi.org/10.1016/j.foodhyd.2016.07.029.

Li, L., Wang, C., Li, K. et al. (2020). Influence of soybean protein isolate-dextran conjugates on the characteristics of glucono-δ-lactone-induced tofu. *LWT* 139: 110588. https://doi.org/10.1016/j.lwt.2020.110588.

Lim, S., Moon, D., Kim, H.J. et al. (2014). Interfacial tension of complex coacervated mussel adhesive protein according to the hofmeister series. *Langmuir 30* (4): 1108–1115. https://doi.org/10.1021/la403680z.

Links, M.R., Taylor, J., Kruger, M.C., and Taylor, J.R.N. (2015). Sorghum condensed tannins encapsulated in kafirin microparticles as a nutraceutical for inhibition of amylases during digestion to attenuate hyperglycaemia. *Journal of Functional Foods 12*: 55–63. https://doi.org/10.1016/j.jff.2014.11.003.

Liu, F., Wang, L.-Y., Li, Y.-T. et al. (2018). Protective effects of quercetin against pyrazinamide induced hepatotoxicity via a cocrystallization strategy of complementary advantages. *Crystal Growth & Design 18* (7): 3729–3733. https://doi.org/10.1021/acs.cgd.8b00576.

Liu, Q., Cui, H., Muhoza, B. et al. (2020). Fabrication of low environment-sensitive nanoparticles for cinnamaldehyde encapsulation by heat-induced gelation method. *Food Hydrocolloids 105*: 105789. https://doi.org/10.1016/j.foodhyd.2020.105789.

Lv, Y., Zhang, X., Abbas, S., and Karangwa, E. (2012). Simplified optimization for microcapsule preparation by complex coacervation based on the correlation between coacervates and the corresponding microcapsule. *Journal of Food Engineering* 111 (2): 225–233. https://doi.org/10.1016/j.jfoodeng.2012.02.030.

Lv, S., Zhou, H., Bai, L. et al. (2020). Development of food-grade Pickering emulsions stabilized by a mixture of cellulose nanofibrils and nanochitin. *Food Hydrocolloids* 113: 106451. https://doi.org/10.1016/j.foodhyd.2020.106451.

Maria Leena, M., Mahalakshmi, L., Moses, J.A., and Anandharamakrishnan, C. (2020). Chapter 14 – nanoencapsulation of nutraceutical ingredients. In: *Biopolymer-Based Formulations* (ed. K. Pal, I. Banerjee, P. Sarkar, et al.), 311–352. Elsevier.

Maurya, A.P., Chauhan, J., Yadav, D.K. et al. (2021). Chapter 11 – nutraceuticals and their impact on human health. In: *Preparation of Phytopharmaceuticals for the Management of Disorders* (ed. C. Egbuna, A.P. Mishra and M.R. Goyal), 229–254. Academic Press.

McClements, D.J. (2017). Recent progress in hydrogel delivery systems for improving nutraceutical bioavailability. *Food Hydrocolloids 68*: 238–245. https://doi.org/10.1016/j.foodhyd.2016.05.037.

McClements, D.J., Li, F., and Xiao, H. (2015). The nutraceutical bioavailability classification scheme: classifying nutraceuticals according to factors limiting their oral bioavailability. *Annual Review of Food Science and Technology 6* (1): 299–327. https://doi.org/10.1146/annurev-food-032814-014043.

Meenambal, R. and Srinivas Bharath, M.M. (2020). Nanocarriers for effective nutraceutical delivery to the brain. *Neurochemistry International 140*: 104851. https://doi.org/10.1016/j.neuint.2020.104851.

Meng, R., Wu, Z., Xie, Q.-T. et al. (2021). Preparation and characterization of zein/carboxymethyl dextrin nanoparticles to encapsulate curcumin: physicochemical stability, antioxidant activity and controlled release properties. *Food Chemistry 340*: 127893. https://doi.org/10.1016/j.foodchem.2020.127893.

Montes, C., Villaseñor, M.J., and Ríos, Á. (2019). Analytical control of nanodelivery lipid-based systems for encapsulation of nutraceuticals: achievements and challenges. *Trends in Food Science & Technology 90*: 47–62. https://doi.org/10.1016/j.tifs.2019.06.001.

Muhoza, B., Xia, S., Wang, X., and Zhang, X. (2020). The protection effect of trehalose on the multinuclear microcapsules based on gelatin and high methyl pectin coacervate during freeze-drying. *Food Hydrocolloids 105*: 105807. https://doi.org/10.1016/j.foodhyd.2020.105807.

Nandi, U., Onyesom, I., and Douroumis, D. (2020). Anti-cancer activity of sirolimus loaded liposomes in prostate cancer cell lines. *Journal of Drug Delivery Science and Technology 23*: 102200. https://doi.org/10.1016/j.jddst.2020.102200.

Nijhawan, P. and Behl, T. (2020). Nutraceuticals in the management of obesity. *Obesity Medicine 17*: 100168. https://doi.org/10.1016/j.obmed.2019.100168.

Nikbakht Nasrabadi, M., Goli, S.A.H., and Nasirpour, A. (2016). Stability assessment of conjugated linoleic acid (CLA) oil-in-water beverage emulsion formulated with acacia and xanthan gums. *Food Chemistry 199*: 258–264. https://doi.org/10.1016/j.foodchem.2015.12.001.

Nooshkam, M. and Varidi, M. (2020). Maillard conjugate-based delivery systems for the encapsulation, protection, and controlled release of nutraceuticals and food bioactive ingredients: a review. *Food Hydrocolloids 100*: 105389. https://doi.org/10.1016/j.foodhyd.2019.105389.

Okagu, O.D., Verma, O., McClements, D.J., and Udenigwe, C.C. (2020). Utilization of insect proteins to formulate nutraceutical delivery systems: Encapsulation and release of curcumin using mealworm protein-chitosan nano-complexes. *International Journal of Biological Macromolecules 151*: 333–343. https://doi.org/10.1016/j.ijbiomac.2020.02.198.

Onwulata, C.I. (2012). Encapsulation of new active ingredients. *Annual Review of Food Science and Technology 3* (1): 183–202. https://doi.org/10.1146/annurev-food-022811-101140.

Piacentini, E., Giorno, L., Dragosavac, M.M. et al. (2013). Microencapsulation of oil droplets using cold water fish gelatine/gum arabic complex coacervation by membrane emulsification. *Food Research International 53* (1): 362–372. https://doi.org/10.1016/j.foodres.2013.04.012.

Piorkowski, D.T. and McClements, D.J. (2014). Beverage emulsions: recent developments in formulation, production, and applications. *Food Hydrocolloids 42*: 5–41. https://doi.org/10.1016/j.foodhyd.2013.07.009.

Polowsky, P.J. and Janaswamy, S. (2015). Hydrocolloid-based nutraceutical delivery systems: Effect of counter-ions on the encapsulation and release. *Food Hydrocolloids 43*: 658–663. https://doi.org/10.1016/j.foodhyd.2014.07.033.

Prata, A.S. and Grosso, C.R.F. (2015). Production of microparticles with gelatin and chitosan. *Carbohydrate Polymers* 116 (0): 292–299. https://doi.org/10.1016/j.carbpol.2014.03.056.

Pu, P., Zheng, X., Jiao, L. et al. (2021). Six flavonoids inhibit the antigenicity of β-lactoglobulin by noncovalent interactions: a spectroscopic and molecular docking study. *Food Chemistry 339*: 128106. https://doi.org/10.1016/j.foodchem.2020.128106.

Qin, X.-S., Luo, Z.-G., and Li, X.-L. (2020). An enhanced pH-sensitive carrier based on alginate-Ca-EDTA in a set-type W1/O/W2 double emulsion model stabilized with WPI-EGCG covalent conjugates for probiotics colon-targeted release. *Food Hydrocolloids* 106460. https://doi.org/10.1016/j.foodhyd.2020.106460.

Qiu, C., Zhao, M., and McClements, D.J. (2015). Improving the stability of wheat protein-stabilized emulsions: Effect of pectin and xanthan gum addition. *Food Hydrocolloids* 43: 377–387. https://doi.org/10.1016/j.foodhyd.2014.06.013.

Qv, X.-Y., Zeng, Z.-P., and Jiang, J.-G. (2011). Preparation of lutein microencapsulation by complex coacervation method and its physicochemical properties and stability. *Food Hydrocolloids* 25 (6): 1596–1603. https://doi.org/10.1016/j.foodhyd.2011.01.006.

Rabiei, M., Kashanian, S., Samavati, S.S. et al. (2020). Nanotechnology application in drug delivery to osteoarthritis (OA), rheumatoid arthritis (RA), and osteoporosis (OSP). *Journal of Drug Delivery Science and Technology* 61: 102011. https://doi.org/10.1016/j.jddst.2020.102011.

Radhakrishnan, R., Kulhari, H., Pooja, D. et al. (2016). Encapsulation of biophenolic phytochemical EGCG within lipid nanoparticles enhances its stability and cytotoxicity against cancer. *Chemistry and Physics of Lipids 198*: 51–60. https://doi.org/10.1016/j.chemphyslip.2016.05.006.

Rajkumar, V., Gunasekaran, C., Paul, C.A., and Dharmaraj, J. (2020). Development of encapsulated peppermint essential oil in chitosan nanoparticles: characterization and biological efficacy against stored-grain pest control. *Pesticide Biochemistry and Physiology 170*: 104679. https://doi.org/10.1016/j.pestbp.2020.104679.

Ratha, S.K., Renuka, N., Rawat, I., and Bux, F. (2020). Prospectives of algae derived nutraceuticals as supplements for combating COVID-19 and human coronavirus diseases. *Nutrition* 83: 111089. https://doi.org/10.1016/j.nut.2020.111089.

Raut, G. and Wairkar, S. (2018). Management of psoriasis with nutraceuticals: an update. *Complementary Therapies in Clinical Practice 31*: 25–30. https://doi.org/10.1016/j.ctcp.2018.01.007.

Ríos, J.-L. (2016). Chapter 1 – essential oils: what they are and how the terms are used and defined. In: *Essential Oils in Food Preservation, Flavor and Safety* (ed. V.R. Preedy), 3–10. San Diego: Academic Press.

Saleh, S.R., Abdelhady, S.A., Khattab, A.R., and El-Hadidy, W.F. (2020). Dual prophylactic/therapeutic potential of date seed, and nigella and olive oils-based nutraceutical formulation in rats with experimentally-induced Alzheimer's disease: A mechanistic insight. *Journal of Chemical Neuroanatomy 110*: 101878. https://doi.org/10.1016/j.jchemneu.2020.101878.

Santos, M.G., Bozza, F.T., Thomazini, M., and Favaro-Trindade, C.S. (2015). Microencapsulation of xylitol by double emulsion followed by complex coacervation. *Food Chemistry* 171 (0): 32–39. https://doi.org/10.1016/j.foodchem.2014.08.093.

Saravanan, M. and Rao, K.P. (2010). Pectin–gelatin and alginate–gelatin complex coacervation for controlled drug delivery: Influence of anionic polysaccharides and drugs being encapsulated on physicochemical properties of microcapsules. *Carbohydrate Polymers 80* (3): 808–816. https://doi.org/10.1016/j.carbpol.2009.12.036.

Sarya Aziz, J.G., Dutilleul, P., Neufeld, R., and Kermasha, S. (2014). Microencapsulation of krill oil using complex coacervation. *Journal of Microencapsulation 31* (8): 774–784.

Shao, P., Feng, J., Sun, P., and Ritzoulis, C. (2019). Improved emulsion stability and resveratrol encapsulation by whey protein/gum arabic interaction at oil-water interface. *International Journal of Biological Macromolecules 133*: 466–472. https://doi.org/10.1016/j.ijbiomac.2019.04.126.

Sharma, S., Barkauskaite, S., Jaiswal, A.K., and Jaiswal, S. (2020). Essential oils as additives in active food packaging. *Food Chemistry 343*: 128403. https://doi.org/10.1016/j.foodchem.2020.128403.

Shetta, A., Kegere, J., and Mamdouh, W. (2019). Comparative study of encapsulated peppermint and green tea essential oils in chitosan nanoparticles: Encapsulation, thermal stability, in-vitro release, antioxidant and antibacterial activities. *International Journal of Biological Macromolecules 126*: 731–742. https://doi.org/10.1016/j.ijbiomac.2018.12.161.

Shin, J.Y., Choi, J.-W., Kim, D.-G. et al. (2020). Protective effects of coenzyme Q10 against acute pancreatitis. *International Immunopharmacology 88*: 106900. https://doi.org/10.1016/j.intimp.2020.106900.

Shreaz, S., Wani, W.A., Behbehani, J.M. et al. (2016). Cinnamaldehyde and its derivatives, a novel class of antifungal agents. *Fitoterapia 112*: 116–131. https://doi.org/10.1016/j.fitote.2016.05.016.

Shtay, R., Keppler, J.K., Schrader, K., and Schwarz, K. (2019). Encapsulation of (−)-epigallocatechin-3-gallate (EGCG) in solid lipid nanoparticles for food applications. *Journal of Food Engineering 244*: 91–100. https://doi.org/10.1016/j.jfoodeng.2018.09.008.

Sobel, R., Versic, R., and Gaonkar, A.G. (2014). Chapter 1 – introduction to microencapsulation and controlled delivery in foods. In: *Microencapsulation in the Food Industry* (ed. A.G. Gaonkar, N. Vasisht, A.R. Khare and R. Sobel), 3–12. San Diego: Academic Press/Elsevier.

Stratulat, I., Britten, M., Salmieri, S. et al. (2013). Encapsulation of coenzyme Q10 in a simple emulsion-based nutraceutical formulation and application in cheese manufacturing. *Food Chemistry 141* (3): 2707–2712. https://doi.org/10.1016/j.foodchem.2013.05.057.

Tang, C.-H. (2021). Strategies to utilize naturally occurring protein architectures as nanovehicles for hydrophobic nutraceuticals. *Food Hydrocolloids 112*: 106344. https://doi.org/10.1016/j.foodhyd.2020.106344.

Tian, B., Liu, Y., and Liu, J. (2020). Smart stimuli-responsive drug delivery systems based on cyclodextrin: a review. *Carbohydrate Polymers 251*: 116871. https://doi.org/10.1016/j.carbpol.2020.116871.

Timilsena, Y.P., Wang, B., Adhikari, R., and Adhikari, B. (2017). Advances in microencapsulation of polyunsaturated fatty acids (PUFAs)-rich plant oils using complex coacervation: a review. *Food Hydrocolloids 69*: 369–381. https://doi.org/10.1016/j.foodhyd.2017.03.007.

Udeh, E.L., Nyila, M.A., and Kanu, S.A. (2020). Nutraceutical and antimicrobial potentials of Bambara groundnut (*Vigna subterranean*): a review. *Heliyon 6* (10): e05205. https://doi.org/10.1016/j.heliyon.2020.e05205.

Vélez, M.A., Perotti, M.C., Zanel, P. et al. (2017). Soy PC liposomes as CLA carriers for food applications: preparation and physicochemical characterization. *Journal of Food Engineering* https://doi.org/10.1016/j.jfoodeng.2017.06.001.

Villanueva-Bermejo, D. and Temelli, F. (2020). Optimization of coenzyme Q10 encapsulation in liposomes using supercritical carbon dioxide. *Journal of CO2 Utilization 38*: 68–76. https://doi.org/10.1016/j.jcou.2020.01.011.

Wang, X., Liu, L., Xia, S. et al. (2019). Sodium carboxymethyl cellulose modulates the stability of cinnamaldehyde-loaded liposomes at high ionic strength. *Food Hydrocolloids 93*: 10–18. https://doi.org/10.1016/j.foodhyd.2019.02.004.

Wang, C., Pei, X., Tan, J. et al. (2020). Thermoresponsive starch-based particle-stabilized Pickering high internal phase emulsions as nutraceutical containers for controlled release. *International Journal of Biological Macromolecules 146*: 171–178. https://doi.org/10.1016/j.ijbiomac.2019.12.269.

Wu, B.-C. and McClements, D.J. (2015). Microgels formed by electrostatic complexation of gelatin and OSA starch: Potential fat or starch mimetics. *Food Hydrocolloids 47*: 87–93. https://doi.org/10.1016/j.foodhyd.2015.01.021.

Xie, Y., Huang, Q., Wang, Z. et al. (2017). Structure-activity relationships of cinnamaldehyde and eugenol derivatives against plant pathogenic fungi. *Industrial Crops and Products 97*: 388–394. https://doi.org/10.1016/j.indcrop.2016.12.043.

Yan, C. and Zhang, W. (2014). Coacervation processes. In: *Microencapsulation in the Food Industry* (ed. N. Vasisht, A.R. Khare and R. Sobel), 125–137. San Diego: Academic Press.

Yi, J., Liu, Y., Zhang, Y., and Gao, L. (2018). Fabrication of resveratrol-loaded whey protein–dextran colloidal complex for the stabilization and delivery of β-carotene emulsions. *Journal of Agricultural and Food Chemistry 66* (36): 9481–9489. https://doi.org/10.1021/acs.jafc.8b02973.

Yu, J., Cui, H., Zhang, Q. et al. (2020). Adducts derived from (−)-epigallocatechin gallate-amadori rearrangement products in aqueous reaction systems: characterization, formation, and thermolysis. *Journal of Agricultural and Food Chemistry 68* (39): 10902–10911. https://doi.org/10.1021/acs.jafc.0c5098.

Yuan, Y., Kong, Z.-Y., Sun, Y.-E. et al. (2017). Complex coacervation of soy protein with chitosan: Constructing antioxidant microcapsule for algal oil delivery. *LWT – Food Science and Technology 75*: 171–179. https://doi.org/10.1016/j.lwt.2016.08.045.

Zhai, X., Wang, X., Zhang, J. et al. (2020). Extruded low density polyethylene-curcumin film: a hydrophobic ammonia sensor for intelligent food packaging. *Food Packaging and Shelf Life* 100595. https://doi.org/10.1016/j.fpsl.2020.100595.

Zhu, R., Liu, H., Liu, C. et al. (2017). Cinnamaldehyde in diabetes: a review of pharmacology, pharmacokinetics and safety. *Pharmacological Research 122*: 78–89. https://doi.org/10.1016/j.phrs.2017.05.019.

Zou, L., Zheng, B., Liu, W. et al. (2015). Enhancing nutraceutical bioavailability using excipient emulsions: influence of lipid droplet size on solubility and bioaccessibility of powdered curcumin. *Journal of Functional Foods 15*: 72–83. https://doi.org/10.1016/j.jff.2015.02.044.

Zuanon, L.A.C., Malacrida, C.R., and Telis, V.R.N. (2013). Production of turmeric oleoresin microcapsules by complex coacervation with gelatin–gum arabic. *Journal of Food Process Engineering 36* (3): 364–373. https://doi.org/10.1111/jfpe.12003.

6

Extraction and Purification of Bioactive Ingredients from Natural Products

Swetha Sunkar[1], G. Ranimol[2], Jayshree Nellore[3], C. Valli Nachiyar[3], S. Karthick Raja Namasivayam[3], and K. Renugadevi[3]

[1] Department of Bioinformatics, Sathyabama Institute of Science and Technology, Chennai, Tamil Nadu, India
[2] Department of Biotechnology Engineering, Sahrdaya College of Engineering and Technology, Thrissur, Kerala, India
[3] Department of Biotechnology, Sathyabama Institute of Science and Technology, Chennai, Tamil Nadu, India

6.1 Introduction

Natural medicine in daily life of ancient people has taken the main seat as defense against disease, and this, during the course of civilization, has been infused into the minds of people and their lifestyle. With the advancement in technology, these were explored by the research community, and today, this natural medicine caters to basic health needs of people. These compounds that are known to have medicinal benefits are called as active ingredients or active principles of natural medicines that offer more drug-like features to molecules from combinatorial chemistry in terms of functional groups, chirality, and structural complexity (Atanasov et al. 2015). The benefits of natural sources such as prebiotic, microbial, plants, and animals sources result from the combination of these active compounds (Tonthubthimthong et al. 2011).

Medicinal plants are the richest bio-resource of drugs of traditional systems of medicine, nutraceuticals, food supplements, and pharmaceutical intermediates; and chemical entities for crude and synthetic drugs (Pandey and Tripathi 2001). Various extracts of different parts of plants have been widely used in folk medicines and perfumes as well as in food flavor and preservatives and are more commonly utilized in chronic as well as common diseases. Plants contain several active compounds such as alkaloids, steroids, tannins, glycosides, volatile oils, fixed oils, resins, phenols, and flavonoids that are deposited in their different parts.

Bioactive natural products (NPs) more commonly utilized in chronic as well as infectious diseases (Duraipandiyan et al. 2006) such as cancer, diabetes and asthma, anti-inflammatory, analgesic, antipyretic solutions and as alternatives for hormone replacement therapy (Burman 2003; Li and Yu 2006; Liao et al. 1995). It also uses as a remedy for the treatment of gastropathy, hepatitis, nephritis, edema, chest pain, fever and cough of pneumonia, bronchitis, and arthritis (Ahmad et al. 2009). Today, natural medicines not only provide the primary healthcare needs for the majority of the population in developing countries but also have attracted more and more attention in the developed countries due to the high healthcare cost and low or no side effect.

Handbook of Nutraceuticals and Natural Products: Biological, Medicinal, and Nutritional Properties and Applications,
Volume 2, First Edition. Edited by Preetha Balakrishnan and Sreerag Gopi.
© 2022 John Wiley & Sons, Inc. Published 2022 by John Wiley & Sons, Inc.

Despite their widespread existence and importance, the bioactive NPs are not sufficient. The amounts of bioactive potential compounds in natural medicines are always fairly low. The main hindrance in the extraction of these compounds is that it is time consuming and lab intensive and has been the main issue in the application of NPs in drug development. Therefore, there is need to develop effective methods to selectively purify the desired NPs.

6.2 Extraction Methods

Extraction is the crucial first step in the analysis of medicinal plants using selective and standard procedures as it is necessary to extract the desired chemical components from the plant materials for further separation and characterization (Bulugahapitiya 2013). There are several extractions methods and can be called conventional (long been used) and modern (developed more recently). Conventional techniques are the one that use organic solvents or water and are carried out generally at atmospheric pressure while modern techniques use pressure and/or elevated temperatures (Njila et al. 2017).

The main stages in the extraction process are:

1) The solvent penetrates into the solid matrix;
2) The solute dissolves in the solvents;
3) The solute is diffused out of the solid matrix;
4) The extracted solutes are collected (Zhang et al. 2018).

Diffusivity and solubility are two factors that facilitate extraction process along with the solvent employed. Selectivity, solubility, cost and safety should be considered in selection of solvents. Based on the law of similarity and intermiscibility (like dissolves like), solvents with a polarity value near to the polarity of the solute, are likely to perform better and vice versa. Alcohols (mainly ethyl alcohol and methyl alcohol) are universal solvents for phytochemical examination. Also, solvents such as chloroform, water, hexane, dichloromethane, ethyl acetate (EtOAc), etc. are most commonly used. The conventional extraction methods generally use organic solvents and require a large volume of solvents and long extraction time (Rathi et al. 2006). The modern extraction methods have also been applied in NPs extraction and they offer some advantages such as lower organic solvent consumption, shorter extraction time and improve extraction yield (Brusotti et al. 2014).

When a non-soluble matrix is used, stability and polarity of the extract, volatility, toxicity, viscosity, and purity of the extraction solvent, probability of artifact formation and the amount of material used for extraction are matters of concern. The particle size of the raw materials, properties of the extraction solvent, the solvent-to-solid ration, the extraction duration and the extraction temperature will affect the extraction efficiency (Du et al. 2011; Li et al. 2008; Yi et al. 2012; Zhou et al. 2012). Generally, the finer the particle size, the better result the extraction achieves. Small particle size enables better penetration of solvent and diffusion of solute thereby increasing extraction efficiency. Too fine particle size will lead to excessive absorption of solute in solid and difficulty in subsequent filtration.

High temperatures increase the solubility and diffusion while very high temperatures lead to loss of thermolabile compounds and undesirable impurities. Increased extraction time facilitates better extraction until equilibrium of the solute is reached inside and outside the solid material. The greater the solvent-to-solid ratio is, the higher the extraction yield is; however, too high ratio will cause excessive extraction solvent and requires a long time for concentration.

The various methods of extraction are given below.

6.2.1 Maceration

This is a simple method where in solid plants parts are placed in a stoppered container with the whole of the solvent and allowed to stand for a period of at least three days (upto one week) with frequent agitation, until soluble matter is dissolved. The mixture is then strained (through sieves/nets), the marc pressed and the combined liquids clarified, cleaned by filtration or by decantation, after standing. When the solvent is water and the period of maceration is long, a small quantity of alcohol may be added to prevent microbial growth (Handa et al. 2008). It could be used for the extraction of thermolabile components. Though simple, it has disadvantages like long extraction time and low extraction efficiency. Compounds like phenols and anthocyanins were effectively extracted from chokeberry fruit using maceration technique (Ćujić et al. 2016). Likewise catechin was also extracted from *Arbutus unedo* L. fruits using maceration which was effective in low temperatures with yield similar to microwave-assisted extraction (MAE) and therefore could be translated into economic benefits (Albuquerque et al. 2017). Various methods like maceration, heat assisted extraction and ultrasonic extraction (UAE) were used to extract polyphenols from *Serpylli herba* and it was observed that not much variation for these methods (Jovanović et al. 2017).

6.2.2 Percolation

This method is mostly used to extract compounds for preparing tinctures and fluid extracts. The plant material is taken in a percolation tube plugged with cotton or fitted with a filter and a stopcock and solvent is added into the plant material and allowed to stand for approximately four hours in a well closed container. This is followed by packing the mass and top of percolator closed. The system is kept at room temperature for 24 hours after which the solvent along with the extracted material is collected and mixed liquid is clarified (Handa et al. 2008). Percolation is more efficient than maceration because it is a continuous process in which the saturated solvent is constantly being replaced by fresh solvent. A study by Zhang et al. (2014) reported that percolation was much efficient than reflux method to extract fucoxanthin from *Undaria pinnatifida*.

6.2.3 Digestion

This is a kind of maceration in which mild heat (40–60 °C) is applied. It is used when moderately elevated temperature is not objectionable (Bimakr et al. 2011). Modifications can be done where in solvent mixing can be done using mechanical stirrer, magnetic stirrer, or by shaking occasionally by hand. After 8–12 hours, the extract is filtered and fresh solvent is added and the process repeated till all the desired products are extracted.

6.2.4 Infusion

In this process, the plant material is macerated for a short period of time with either cold or boiling water (Vidyadhar et al. 2010). It is a dilute solution of the readily soluble components of the crude drugs.

6.2.5 Decoction

This process is generally employed in Ayurvedic extracts called –quath or –kawath where in, the powdered plant materials is boiled in a specified volume of water for a defined time, then cooled and strained or filtered. This procedure is mainly used for extracting water-soluble, heat-stable constituents. The starting ratio of crude drug to water is fixed (e.g. 1:4 or 1:16) and the volume is then brought down to one-fourth to its original volume by boiling during the extraction. Then, the concentrated extract is filtered that can be used as such or processed further (Vidyadhar et al. 2010). This process contains a large amount of water-soluble impurities and cannot be used for the extraction of thermolabile or volatile components.

6.2.6 Reflux

This is a hot extraction process wherein the material is treated with boiling solvent and the solvent vapor is recycled by a condenser. It cannot be used for the extraction of thermolabile NPs (Zhang et al. 2018). A study showed that this process is more efficient than percolation or maceration and requires less extraction time and solvent. The reflux method was found to be better than the decoction method which was shown in a report where highest yields of baicalin and puerarin were obtained from the reflux method with 60% ethanol as the extraction solvent (Zhang 2013).

6.2.7 Tincture

It is the extract of plant material in alcohol with the ratio of 1:5. Because of the alcohol content, the tinctures can be stored at room temperatures without being decomposed.

6.2.8 Pressurized Liquid Extraction (PLE)

Also known as accelerated solvent extraction system (ASE) or enhanced solvent extraction system (ESE), this method uses elevated pressure and temperature. Increased temperature increases the diffusivity of the solvent and increased pressure keeps the organic solvent in liquid state without boiling and also forces the solvent to penetrate the matrix pores (Lv et al. 2010).

6.2.9 Soxhlet Extraction

The Soxhlet extraction method integrates the advantages of the reflux extraction and percolation, which utilizes the principle of reflux and siphoning to continuously extract the herb with fresh solvent. Named after Franz Ritter von Soxhlet, a German agricultural chemist, it is the best method for the continuous extraction of a solid by a hot solvent (Grigonis et al. 2005). Soxhlet apparatus is a specialized glass refluxing unit and is mainly used for organic solvent extractions. The powdered solid material is placed in a thimble made up of filter paper and is placed inside the Soxhlet apparatus. The apparatus is fitted to a round bottomed flask containing the solvent and to a reflex condenser. The solvent in the flask is boiled gently, the vapor passes up through the side tube, condensed by the condenser and falls into the thimble containing the material and slowly fills the Soxhlet. When the solvent reaches the top of the attached tube it siphons over into the flask, thus removes the portion of the substance, which it has extracted. This method is an automatic continuous extraction method with high extraction efficiency and requires less time and solvent. But high temperature and long extraction time will increase the possibilities of thermal degradation.

6.2.10 Distillation

Volatile compounds especially oils are mainly obtained by distillation techniques, although working at elevated temperatures can lead to chemical changes or decomposition. Hydro distillation (HD) and steam distillation (SD) are two commonly used methods. Recent developments include microwave SD which applies microwaves to increase disruption of glands and cells while steam is passing through the plant material and carrying the essential oil.

6.2.10.1 Steam Distillation

It is the standard process for the isolation of volatile oils from crude plant material. It is simple vaporization achieved by passing steam directly through the material and the volatile oil is recovered by condensation, where oil separates out from water. This can be used for the extraction of acyclic olefins, phenols, ketones, esters, alcohols and carboxylic acids (Okonkwo and Ohaeri 2020)

6.2.10.2 Hydro Distillation

This is the extensively used process for isolation of essential oils where the plant material is soaked in water and boiled using a heating mantle. The presence of hot water makes the essential oil free from the oil glands in the plant tissues and passes along with the steam. Using Clevenger apparatus, the steam oil mixture is condensed and oil is separated from water and the condensed water is recycled (Alupului et al. 2012). There can be a decrease or increase in the contents of some components as extraction time increases (Yahya and Yunus 2013).

6.2.11 Expression

Expression or cold pressing is a method of extraction specific to citrus essential oils. In the past, sponge pressing was carried out by hand. The released oil is absorbed by sponge and it was recovered by squeezing the sponge. It is reported that oil produced through this method contains more of the fruit odor character than oil produced by any other method (Bulugahapitiya 2013).

6.2.12 Enfluerage

Delicate fragrances from flowers are extracted using this method. The flower petals are spread over a layer of refined fat that picks up the odor of the flowers and the saturated fat is treated with a solvent, usually alcohol in which the fragrant components are soluble. The residual fat dissolved in alcohol may be removed by cooling the alcohol extract to 20 °C, when fat separates out. The alcohol is evaporated under reduced pressure and pure oils are obtained.

6.2.13 Supercritical Fluid Extraction (SFE)

This extraction system is the most technologically advanced. It involves the use of gases, usually CO_2, and compressing them into a dense liquid which is then pumped through a cylinder containing the material to be extracted. From there, the extract-laden liquid is pumped into a separation chamber where the extract is separated from the gas and the gas is recovered for re-use. Varying the pressure and temperature would affect the solvent properties of CO_2. The main advantages of SFE is that no solvent residues are left in it as CO_2 evaporates completely (Patil and Shettigar 2010). Also, organic solvents used in extraction technologies which are detrimental to environment are replaced by supercritical CO_2 and hence and finds increasing application in extraction.

It uses supercritical fluid (SF) as the extraction solvent can dissolve a wide variety of NPs and has similar solubility to liquid and similar diffusivity to gas. Their solvating properties dramatically changed near their critical points due to small pressure and temperature changes. Supercritical carbon dioxide (S-CO_2) was chosen in SFE because it has low critical temperature (31 °C), inertness, selectivity, non-toxicity, low cost, and capability to extract thermally labile compounds. S-CO_2 having low polarity makes it perfect for the extraction of nonpolar NPs such as lipid and volatile oils.

An addition of modifier can enhance the solvating properties of S-CO$_2$ significantly. Several studies showed a very keen interest in polyphenols extraction using SFE. Pure S-CO$_2$ is a safe solvent generally used for this purpose. Nevertheless, the extraction efficiency may be enhanced significantly with the use of ethanol.

6.2.14 Ultrasonic Extraction

Also called as UAE or sonication, high frequency sound/ ultrasonic wave energy is used to release natural compounds from the plant tissues by damaging the cell wall. UAE can be used with mixtures of immiscible solvents such as hexane with methanol (MeOH)/water. The process creates heat so that heat labile compounds may decompose (Chemat et al. 2017) and therefore the extraction container is placed in ice bath to reduce the temperature. In UAE the plant material is covered by the extraction solvent and put into an ultrasonic bath. This process has become popular because it decreases extraction time and improves extraction yields due to mechanical stress which induces cavitations and cellular breakdown. Ultrasound produces cavitation and accelerates the dissolution and diffusion of the solute as well as the heat transfer and therefore improves the extraction efficiency. Low solvent and energy consumption, reduction of extraction temperature and time are the main advantages of UAE and therefore appropriate for the extraction of thermolabile and unstable compounds.

Certain bioactive compounds like bixin and catechin, chrysin, chlorogenic acid, licochalcone A, butein, hypoletin, and xanthohumol were successfully isolated from annatto seeds using ultrasound-assisted extraction (Quiroz et al. 2019) and their antioxidant activity was also analyzed.

6.2.15 Microwave-Assisted Extraction

It is also termed as microwave extraction and is a combination of microwave and traditional solvent extraction. This method heats solvents in contact with a sample for separating compounds of interest using electromagnetic radiation within a frequency ranging from 300 MHz to 300 MHz (Riss et al. 2016). Revolution in organic compound synthesis has been promoted by microwave-assisted organic syntheses (MAOS) by which small molecules are built up into large polymers in a fraction of time (Jacob 2012). Microwave-assisted heating the solvents and plant tissue augments the kinetics of extraction that assists partition of analytes from the sample matrix into the solvent (Trusheva et al. 2007). The heat induced by microwave directly affects the polar materials. Microwave radiation interacts with dipoles of polar and polarizable materials causes heating near the surface of the materials and heat is transferred by conduction. Dipole rotation of the molecules disrupts hydrogen bonding; enhancing the migration of dissolved ions and promotes solvent penetration into the matrix (Altemimi et al. 2015). In nonpolar solvents, poor heating occurs as the energy is transferred by dielectric absorption only (Popova et al. 2008).

MAE offers many advantages, such as decreasing the thermal degradation, selective heating of vegetal material and increasing the extract yield. MAE is also considered as a green technology as it reduces the usage of organic solvent. MAE methods can be solvent-free extraction (normally for volatile compounds) and solvent extraction (usually for nonvolatile compounds) (Chemat and Cravotto 2013). Though MAE may degrade bioactive carbohydrates because of high temperature, it is still considered to be an effective method to extract marine bioactive compounds. Studies have suggested the use of MAE in the extraction of compounds from fish, oysters, shrimps (Bhattacharya et al. 2015; Reyes et al. 2009; Tsiaka et al. 2015) etc. Also, this is found to be suitable for degrading algal cell walls rich in carbohydrates, extracting sulfated polysaccharides from Brown Seaweed (Yuan and Macquarrie 2015).

A study successfully isolated various compounds using MAE from the edible wild fruit *Gordonia axillaris* that possessed strong antioxidant activity. The compounds were further characterized using UPLC-MS/MS and were identified as gallic acid, rutin, epicatechin, protocatechuic acid, gallate, p-coumaric acid, 2-hydrocinnamic acid, chlorogenic acid, quercetin and ferulic acid (Li et al. 2017).

6.2.16 Solid Phase Extraction (SPE)

This is a sensitive, rapid and economical technique which uses different types of cartridges and disks and variety of sorbents. Here the solute molecules are preferentially attached over the stationary phase. Sample preparation and concentration can be achieved in a single step (Żwir-Ferenc and Biziuk 2006). Normal phase, reverse phase and ion exchange SPE units are available. A study reported the isolation of different volatile water-soluble compounds of rose aromatic water samples using SPE. Liquid–liquid extraction and head space technique. It was observed that SPE was quick compared to other methods and also SPE showed good recoveries and high repeatability (Canbay 2017).

This method was suggested to be a reliable technique for routine analysis of phloridzin from NPs namely apples and plums along with Amberlite XAD4 followed by HPLC analysis (Marchev et al. 2013). Another study employed SPE to fractionate marine organic extracts containing high concentration of salt that hampers the recovery of secondary metabolites. They suggested that this technique was found to be particularly effective in the extraction and fractionation of sarains, the complex alkaloids of the Mediterranean sponge *R. sarai.* (Cutignano et al. 2015).

6.2.17 Pressurized Liquid Extraction

PLE is also called as ESE, accelerated solvent extraction, accelerated fluid extraction, pressurized fluid extraction and high-pressure solvent extraction by different research groups. PLE applies high pressure in extraction which keeps solvents in a liquid state above their boiling point resulting in a high solubility and high diffusion rate of lipid solutes in the solvent, and a high penetration of the solvent in the matrix. PLE dramatically decreased the consumption of extraction time and solvent and had better repeatability compared to other methods. This technique needs solvents in low quantities because of the combination of high pressure and temperatures that provides faster extraction. The elevated extraction temperature can support higher analyte solubility by increasing both solubility and mass transfer rate and, also decrease the viscosity and surface tension of solvents, thus improving extraction rate (Ibañez et al. 2012).

Experimental evidences suggested that PLE was effective in significantly decreasing the time consumption and solvent use (Richter et al. 1996) when compared with Soxhlet extraction. PLE is considered as an potential alternative for the extraction of polar compounds in contrast to SFE (Kaufmann and Christen 2002). This was also found to be useful to isolate compounds from marine sponges (Ibañez et al. 2012).

6.2.18 Pulsed Electric Field (PEF) Extraction

PEF extraction significantly increases the extraction yield and decreases the extraction time as it can increase mass transfer during extraction by destroying membrane structures. Electric potential passes through the membrane of a cell when cell suspension is subjected to electrical field. The electric potential separates molecules according to their charge in the cell membrane which is mainly based on dipole nature of membrane molecules. When potential of approximately 1 V of transmembrane potential exceeds, repulsion occurs between the charge carried by the molecules resulting in the formation of pores in the weak areas of the membrane thereby increasing permeability (Bryant and Wolfe 1987). Generally, for plant materials, PEF is done using a simple circuit with exponential decay pulses which has a treatment chamber with two electrodes where the plant materials are placed. The PEF process can work in either continuous or batch mode depending on the design of treatment chamber (Puértolas et al. 2010).

The efficiency of PEF treatment depends on several factors that include field strength, pulse number, specific energy input, treatment temperature and properties of the materials to be treated. This is a non-thermal method and minimizes the degradation of the thermolabile compounds. The yield of water-soluble phenolic compounds and flavonoid compounds from onion was enormously increased after PEF treatments according to studies which showed noteworthy antioxidant activity (Liu et al. 2018). PEF is known to be used in the isolation of various compounds like lipids, carbohydrates, amino acids, pigments from different classes of microbes like bacteria, yeast and microalgae (Martínez et al. 2020).

6.2.19 Enzyme-Assisted Extraction (EAE)

The main barriers to the extraction of NPs are the structure of the cell membrane and cell wall, the coagulation and denaturation of proteins at high temperatures during extraction micelles formed by macromolecules such polysaccharides and protein. EAE would enhance extraction efficiency due to the hydrolytic action of the enzymes on the components of the cell wall and membrane and the macromolecules inside the cell. This facilitates the release of the NPs. Cellulose, α-amylase and pectinase are generally employed in EAE.

Enzyme-assisted aqueous extraction (EAAE) and enzyme-assisted cold pressing (EACP) are the two approaches in EAE (Latif and Anwar 2009). The extractions of the oils from various seeds are done using EAAE method (Hanmoungjai et al. 2001; Rosenthal et al. 2001; Sharma et al. 2002). In EAAE system polysaccharide-protein colloid is available but in EACP technique this protein is not available therefore the former is used to hydrolyze the seed cell wall with the help of enzymes (Concha et al. 2004). The vital factors for extraction are particle size of plant materials, enzyme composition and concentration, solid to water ratio and hydrolysis time (Niranjan and Hanmoungjai 2004). The EAE uses water as solvent instead of organic chemicals and therefore it is considered an ecofriendly technology for extraction of bioactive compounds and oils (Puri et al. 2012). Saad et al. (2019) suggested that this was an ecofriendly process for the effective recovery of lipophilic compounds and polyphenols from promace press cake. Another report revealed that EAE was successful in augmenting the extraction yield of phenolic compounds from pistachio green hull. Also a combination of enzymes was more effective in increasing the extraction yield than using enzymes separately thereby recommending the use of multiple enzymes for extraction (Yazdi et al. 2019).

Summary of the various extraction methods with their advantages and disadvantages are provided in Table 6.1.

6.3 Purification of Bioactive Compounds

The extracts obtained contain mixture of compounds with different polarities, belonging to different categories based on their chemical structure and characteristics. Pure compounds or the active ingredients have to be separated further based on the physical and chemical differences between the compounds. Some of the methods used for separation of compounds are given below:

Table 6.1 Summary of the various extraction methods with their advantages and disadvantages.

Method	Solvent	Volume of organic solvent consumed	Temperature	Pressure	Time	Polarity of natural products extracted	Advantage	Disadvantage
Maceration	Water, aqueous and nonaqueous solvents	Large	Room temperature	Atmospheric	Long	Dependent on extracting solvent	• Maceration is a simple method using non-complicated utensil and equipment. Skilled operator not required. • Energy saving process. • For certain substances which are very less soluble in solvent and requires only prolonged contact with solvent is ideal. • Suitable method for less potent and cheap drugs.	• Unfortunately, the duration of extraction time is long and sometimes takes up to weeks. • Not exhaustively extract the drug. • It is very slow process and time consuming. • Solvent required is more.
Percolation	Water, aqueous and nonaqueous solvents	Large	Room temperature occasionally under heat	Atmospheric	Long	Dependent on extracting solvent	• Requires less time than maceration. Extraction of thermolabile constituents can be possible. Suitable method for potent and costly drugs. • Short time and more complete extraction	• Requires more time than Soxhalation. • More solvent is required. • Skilled person is required. • Special attention should be paid on particle size of material and throughout process
Decoction	Water	None	Under heat	Atmospheric	Moderate	Polar compounds	• Suitable for extracting heat-stable compounds. • This method does not required more and expensive equipment. • It is easy to perform. • No need trained operator.	• Unfortunately, it is not advised for the extraction of heat sensitive constituents.

(Continued)

Table 6.1 (Continued)

Method	Solvent	Volume of organic solvent consumed	Temperature	Pressure	Time	Polarity of natural products extracted	Advantage	Disadvantage
Reflux extraction	Aqueous and nonaqueous solvents	Moderate	Under heat	Atmospheric	Moderate	Dependent on extracting solvent	• Less extraction time • Less amount of solvent required	• It cannot be used for the extraction of thermolabile compounds
Soxhlet extraction	Organic solvents	Moderate	Under heat	Atmospheric	Long	Dependent on extracting solvent	• Large amount of plants materials can be extracted at a time. • Repeatedly can use solvent • This method does not require filtration after extraction • This method does not depend upon the type of matrix. • It is a very simple technique. • The displacement of transfer equilibrium by repeatedly bringing fresh solvent into contact with the solid matrix.	• The samples are heated to a high temperature for a relatively long period thus the risk of thermal destruction of some compounds cannot be overlooked if the plant material contains heat labile compounds. • The extraction time is lengthy and the process is labor intensive • The process allows manipulations of limited variables. • The time and the requirement of a large amount of solvent result in wide criticism of Soxhlet extraction technique [14]
Pressurized liquid extraction	Water, aqueous and nonaqueous solvents	Small	Under heat	High	short	Dependent on extracting solvent	• Less solvent • Less time of extraction	• Not suitable for thermolabile compounds

Method	Solvent		Temperature	Pressure	Time	Polarity	Advantages	Disadvantages
Supercritical fluid extraction	Supercritical fluid (usually S-CO$_2$), sometimes with modifier	None or small	Near room temperature	High	short	Nonpolar to moderate polar compounds	• Ecofriendly • Suitable for thermolabile compounds	• High capital investment • Requirement of high pressure
Ultrasound-assisted extraction	Water, aqueous and nonaqueous solvents	Moderate	Room temperature, or under heat	Atmospheric	short	Dependent on extracting solvent	• Ecofriendly • Can replace the solvents with generally recognized as safe (GRAS) solvents • High extraction efficiency • Reduced extraction time • Good for thermolabile compounds	• Lack of uniformity in the distribution of ultra sound energy • Decline of power with time
Microwave-assisted extraction	Water, aqueous and nonaqueous solvents	None or moderate	Room temperature	Atmospheric	short	Dependent on extracting solvent	• Reduced solvent usage • Higher extraction rate • Improved extraction yield	• High capital cost
Pulsed electric field extraction	Water, aqueous and nonaqueous solvents	Moderate	Room temperature, or under heat	Atmospheric	short	Dependent on extracting solvent	• Increases extraction yield • Lower extraction time	• High capital cost
Enzyme-assisted extraction	Water, aqueous and nonaqueous solvents	Moderate	Room temperature, or heated after enzyme treatment	Atmospheric	Moderate	Dependent on extracting solvent	• extraction efficiency will be enhanced	• The structure of the cell membrane and cell wall, micelles formed by macromolecules such polysaccharides and protein, and the coagulation and denaturation of proteins at high temperatures during extraction, are the main barriers

(Continued)

Table 6.1 (Continued)

Method	Solvent	Volume of organic solvent consumed	Temperature	Pressure	Time	Polarity of natural products extracted	Advantage	Disadvantage
Hydro distillation and steam distillation	Water	None	Under heat	Atmospheric	Long	Essential oil (usually nonpolar)	• Higher oil yield. • Components of the volatile oil are less susceptible to hydrolysis and polymerization (the control of wetness on the bottom of the still affects hydrolysis, whereas the thermal conductivity of the still walls affects. polymerization). • If refluxing is controlled, then the loss of polar compounds is minimized. • Oil quality produced by steam and water distillation is more reproducible. • No organic solvent needed so this process is cheap and environment friendly.	• Complete extraction is not possible. • As the plant material near the bottom of the still comes in direct contact with the fire from the furnace, it may char and thus impart an objectionable odor to the essential oil. • The prolonged action of hot water can cause hydrolysis of some constituents of the essential oil, such as esters. • Heat control is difficult, which may lead to variable rates of distillation. • It requires a greater number of stills, more space and more fuel. Thus, the process becomes uneconomical.

6.3.1 Solvent Method

6.3.1.1 Acid and Basic Solvent Method

The compounds in the extract possess different acidity and alkalinity based on which purification is carried out. Alkaline organic compounds that are water insoluble (e.g. alkaloids) can form salts with inorganic acids and can be separated. Components that are acidic in nature such as phenolic hydroxyl groups or carboxyl groups can be salted out by using bases and can be dissolved in water. Lactone or lactum-containing compounds can be saponified and dissolved in water which can be later separated from other components. Extracts can be divided into acidic, basic, and neutral parts by completely dissolving in lipophilic organic solvents and extracting them separately using acid water and alkali water. Varying the pH value can also facilitate the extraction when organic solvents are used for extracts dissolved in water. The alkalinity or acidity of the fractions are different and can be separated further by pH gradient extraction. In this process, strength of acidity or alkalinity, heating temperature, the contact time with the separated components, and time are important parameters that should be catered to as they lead to structural changes of some compounds under extreme conditions which sometimes may be irreversible.

6.3.1.2 Polarity Gradient Extraction Method

This method utilizes the different polarities and different partition coefficients of the components of the extracts. Usually two-phase solvent systems are used according to the polarities. For strong polarity compounds, n-butanol-water system is used, while for medium polarity compounds, ethyl acetate-water system is used and for weak polarity compounds, chloroform (or ether)-water system is used. The sequence of steps involved in this process is provided in Figure 6.1.

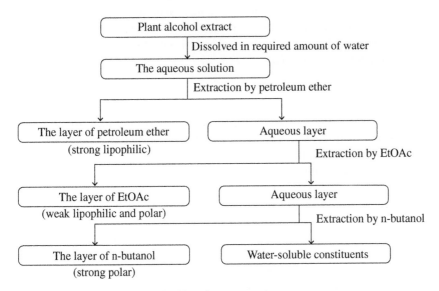

Figure 6.1 General steps involved in solvent extraction.

The success of solvent extraction depends on selecting the right solvent with an appropriate polarity based on the law of "like dissolves like". Therefore, hydrophilic constituents dissolve in hydrophilic solvents and vice versa which could be predicted by polarity. Terpenoids and steroids can be dissolved in lipophilic solvents such as ether and chloroform as they possess low polarity unlike carbohydrates and amino acids that prefer water and ethanol as they are highly polar. The solvents based on their order of polarity from weak to strong are petroleum ether < carbon tetrachloride < benzene < dichloromethane < chloroform < ether < ethyl acetate < n-butanol < acetone < ethanol < methanol < water (Feng et al. 2019).

6.3.2 Precipitation Method

Certain phytochemicals form precipitate with specific reagents and reduce their solubility. This is a reversible reaction as the target compounds have to form precipitates, and if the nontarget compounds forms precipitates, it has to be removed. Artemisinin is extracted by using ionic liquids and pure compound is obtained after simple precipitation (Lapkin et al. 2006).

6.3.3 Solvent Precipitation Method

The solubility of components in a mixture can be altered by adding a particular solvent that is also soluble in the solution and hence can be precipitated from the solution. Fractional precipitation is the gradual precipitation that happens when the polarity or amount of solvent is changed. For instance, for an aqueous extract, ethanol is added to increase its alcohol content to more than 80% and then other compounds such as proteins, polysaccharides, gum, and starch will be precipitated and removed after filtration. This is referred to as water extraction followed by ethanol precipitation (Koh et al. 2009).

6.3.3.1 Exclusive Reagent Precipitation Method

Certain reagents selectively react with certain chemicals to produce reversible precipitation and this is called as exclusive reagent precipitation method. For instance, Reynolds ammonium salt is used to precipitate alkaloids from non-alkaloids and water-soluble alkaloids. Likewise cholesterol and sterol saponins can be separated from triterpene saponins, and tannins are precipitated using gelatins. The selection of the right kind of reagent based on the properties of target components is the key to an ideal separation of molecules.

Extraction by precipitation was experimented with *Eurycoma longifolia* where solvent fractionation followed by acetone precipitation was performed to obtain saponins which showed higher anti-proliferative activity than the crude extract (Chua et al. 2019). Likewise, methanol was found to be an ideal solvent for the extraction of various phytochemical constituents that displayed several biological activities from *Severinia buxifolia*.

6.3.4 Salting Out Method

The principle is based on the electrolyte–nonelectrolyte interaction where the nonelectrolyte could be less soluble at high salt concentrations. It is generally used for purification of proteins and also for preventing protein denaturation due to excessive dilution of samples (Garrett 2013). The salt concentration required for protein precipitation differs from protein to protein. This method is also used to concentrate dilute solutions of proteins.

Solubility of certain components in water extract of plants can be reduced by adding certain inorganic salts at a particular concentration or saturation condition. This helps in the separation of water-soluble compounds. The commonly used inorganic salts for salting out are sodium sulfate, sodium chloride, ferric sulfate, magnesium sulfate, etc. For example, extractions of berberine from *Berberis poiretii and* tetrandrine from *Daemonorops margaritae* could be achieved by salting out with sodium chloride or ammonium sulfate. Some water-soluble substances, such as ephedrine, protoanemonin, and matrine, are often extracted with organic solvents after adding a certain amount of salt to the water extract.

6.3.5 Dialysis Method

It is the process of selective penetration of certain substances through semipermeable membranes (ex dialysis bags) which can be natural or synthetic under the influence of concentration difference, potential difference, and pressure difference to ensure separation, purification, classification, or concentration. During the process of separation and purification of various plant compounds, dialysis enables the removal of inorganic salts, monosaccharides, and other impurities. Also, the semipermeable membrane can be used to separate small molecular substances into the outside solution while the large molecules can be left in semipermeable membrane (Tahara et al. 2017). Vanillin, which is one of the most important elements in food industry for its aroma, is isolated from ferulic acid which is a product from agricultural waste using pervaporation and dialysis. Dialysis worked even at low temperatures and can be used to restore the consumed substrate (Camera-Roda et al. 2019).

6.4 Fractional Distillation Method

This method is based on separating liquid components based on their different boiling points. It can be classified as atmospheric distillation, vacuum distillation, molecular distillation (MD), etc. and is mainly used to separate volatile oils and certain liquid alkaloids in plants. If the difference in boiling point of two compounds is above 100 °C, then repeated distillation can efficiently separate the compounds. For instance, two alkaloids coniine and conhydrine of *Cicuta virosa* have boiling points of 166–167 and 226 °C, respectively, and can be effectively separated by fractional distillation. If the difference is less than 25 °C, fractionation column is required to purify. The smaller the boiling point difference is, the finer the fractionation device is essential (Hanif et al. 2017). Fractional distillation was used to obtain organic liquid products from palm oil under laboratory scale. Along this process, other components such as kerosene, diesel, and gasoline were also obtained and characterized (Fereira et al. 2017).

6.5 Crystallization Method

This is a process wherein the solute precipitates from mother liquor with complex components which is an effective method for preparing pure substances. Crystallization is not a single-step process as initial crystallization often contains impurities and therefore has to be crystallized again and is called as recrystallization. This method separates compounds from the mixture based on the difference of solubility of each component in the solvent. Crystallization is one of the significant technologies for plant chemists to prepare pure compounds. If the extract contains high amount of a certain phytochemical, then crystals can be obtained by cooling or slightly concentrating the extract with a suitable solvent. Selection of solvent is the key for effective crystallization. The criteria for choosing a solvent are low solubility at low temperature, high solubility for the components to be purified at high temperature, insoluble for the impurities at high and low temperatures or soluble for the impurities at high and low temperatures, no chemical reaction with the components to be crystallized, moderate boiling point, safe, low cost, easy to obtain, etc.

Commonly used solvents are ethanol, methanol, ethyl acetate, acetone, pyridine, acetic acid, etc. Sometimes, combination of solvents can be used for crystallization when one solvent is not sufficient to form crystals. The two solvents used are generally miscible with one having high solubility for the component to be crystallized while the other solvent has low solubility. This is a stepwise process where the sample to be crystallized is heated first and dissolved in few solvents with high solubility. This is followed by using second solvent that has low solubility in the hot solution to make it turbid. The first solvent is added again to dissolve the sample. When the solution reaches the saturation point, crystals are formed when cooled. Crystal color, form, melting point, melting range, thin-layer chromatography (TLC), and paper chromatography are preliminary techniques to identify the purity of the crystal formed.

A plant compound called rutin from *Sophora japonica* was isolated using crystallization whose structure was analyzed using experimental techniques that included X-ray powder diffraction and thermogravimetric analysis coupled with differential scanning calorimetry. The solvents used were methanol, ethanol, and 2-propanol. 99% purity was obtained for crystalline rutin trihydrate (Horosanskaia et al. 2017).

Another study successfully crystallized vitamin D3 in continuous flow using an in-line continuous filtration step where in just 1 min of cooling time ~50% (w/w) crystals of vitamin D_3 were directly obtained (Escriba-Gelonch et al. 2018). An overview of conventional separation techniques are provided in Table 6.2.

6.5.1 Chromatographic Methods

6.5.1.1 Classical Methods

The most common method of separation of chemical constituents from NPs is chromatography. Chromatography is used because of high separation efficiency, simplicity, and rapidity. Phytochemicals can be purified by choosing the appropriate separation principles, different chromatographic packings, different operation modes, or applying various chromatographic methods jointly.

Table 6.2 Comparison of conventional separation techniques.

Method	Principle	Advantages	Disadvantages
Crystallization	Crystallization is based on the principles of solubility. The principle behind the crystallization is that the amount of solute that can be dissolved by a solvent increases with temperature and the fact that the solubility decreases with temperature. This causes the precipitation of the solute. If the cooling is slow enough, the solvent forms crystals (some hydrated) on any surface. The crystals thus formed have highly regular internal structure, the basis of which is called the crystal lattice.	• High purification can be obtained in a single step. • Produces a solid phase which may be suitable for direct packaging and sale. • Operates at a lower temperature and with lower energy requirements than corresponding distillation separations.	• Generally purifies only one component • Yield is limited by phase equilibria • Process kinetics are complex.
Fractional distillation	The process involves repeated distillations and condensations, and the mixture is usually separated into component parts. The separation happens when the mixture is heated at a certain temperature where fractions of the mixture start to vaporize. Different liquids boil and evaporate at different temperatures. Therefore, when the mixture is heated, the substance with lower boiling point starts to boil first and convert into vapors.	• Easy to implement • Highly effective and efficient	Can be expensive Operational hazards Cause pollution

Table 6.2 (Continued)

Method	Principle	Advantages	Disadvantages
Salting out	It is based on the electrolyte–nonelectrolyte interaction, in which the nonelectrolyte could be less soluble at high salt concentrations.	It is used as a method of purification for proteins, as well as preventing protein denaturation due to excessively diluted samples during experiments.	Salting out proteins requires prior knowledge of the protein's solubility Any contaminants present in the initial sample may still be present in the fraction containing the protein of interest It may be necessary to remove the salt from the protein sample and so further processing in the form of either dialysis or chromatography will be required.
Dialysis	Dialysis works on the principles of the diffusion of solutes and ultrafiltration of fluid across a semipermeable membrane. Diffusion is a property of substances in water; substances in water tend to move from an area of high concentration to an area of low concentration.	Low energy consumption Membrane technique operates under normal pressure and has not a state change Less operating cost Low installation cost Easy operation High stability and reliability of the process.	Low processing capability Slow compared with pressure-driven processes
Solvent precipitation method	The organic solvents decrease the dielectric constant of organic compound resulting in a loss of solubility and therefore precipitation. Organic solvents, such as acetone, are also used for protein precipitation, often in conjunction with TCA.	Very simple equipment and easy handling Precipitation, phase separation, and isolation at constant temperature Good control of precipitated mass of polymer via volume of precipitant when precipitation behavior of the system is known.	It is difficult to obtain narrow fractions of high MW Increase in the fractionation volume with each fractionation step A gradient of precipitant concentration occurs near the precipitant inlet.
Acid-base solvent extraction	Acid-base extraction is typically used to separate organic compounds from each other based on their acid-base properties. It is a type of liquid–liquid extraction. It typically involves different solubility levels in water and organic solvents. The organic solvent may be any carbon-based liquid that does not dissolve very well in water; common ones are ether, ethyl acetate, or dichloromethane.	Solubilities of these acidic and basic components can be manipulated to our advantage by applying simple acid-base reactions Can be used directly to isolate a desired acidic or basic compound or to remove acidic or basic impurities	Procedure works only for acids and bases with a large difference in solubility between their charged and their uncharged form Does not work for zwitter ions, very lipophilic amines, very lipophilic acids, lower amines like ammonia, and hydrophilic acids

6.5.1.1.1 Adsorption Chromatography In this technique, separation is carried out based on the difference of adsorptive capacity of adsorbents to different compounds. Adsorbents such as alumina, activated carbon, silica, and polyamide are commonly used. Out of these, silica gel adsorption chromatography is extensively used in the separation of most of the plant chemical constituents. Alkaline or neutral lipophilic components, such as steroids, alkaloids, and terpenoids, are mainly separated using the method of alumina adsorption chromatography. Water-soluble substances, such as amino acids, carbohydrates, and some kinds of glycosides, are mainly separated by activated carbon. Separation of phenols, anthraquinones, quinones, flavonoids, tannins, etc. can be carried using polyamide. This process is based on the formation of hydrogen bonds (Poole 2018)

Plant alkaloids belonging to the methyl chanofruticosinate group including six new alkaloids, prunifolines A–F, were obtained from the leaf of *Kopsia arborea* by initial silica gel column chromatography using gradient MeOH–trichloromethane (CHCl₃) as the mobile phase followed by centrifugal TLC using ammonia saturated diethyl ether (Et2O)–hexane or EtOAc/hexane systems as the eluent (Lim and Kam 2008).

6.5.1.1.2 Gel Chromatography (Exclusion Chromatography, Molecular Sieve Chromatography) The main principle of gel chromatography is molecular sieve which separates the mixture based on the pore size of the gel and molecular size of the compounds. The gel used in this technique is a solid with a porous network structure. The ability of the separated substances to enter the gel is different because the molecules of the separated substances are different in sizes. The molecules can enter the gel interior freely if the molecules are smaller than the gel pores, and if the molecules are larger than the gel pores, the molecules cannot enter the gel but can pass through gel particle gaps. Different movement speeds therefore emerged. The retention time of the molecules of larger sizes is shorter. The retention time of the molecules with smaller sizes is longer because of its diffusion into the pores. Commercial gel, hydroxypropyl dextran gel, and dextran gel are the many kinds of commonly used gels (Porath 1997).

6.5.1.1.3 Ion Exchange Chromatography This method separates the components of the given mixture based on the dissociation degree. In this method the mobile phase used is water or solvent mixed with water and the stationary phase used is ion exchange resin. The ion exchange resin absorbs the ionic components existing in the mobile phase. The method which is most suitable for the separation of ionic compounds such as peptides, organic acids, alkaloids, flavonoids and amino acids is ion exchange chromatography. The reaction between the ion exchange resins and compounds in this method is majorly influenced by the compound's dissociation degree and the amount of electrical charges. The exchange of compounds is facilitated if the dissociation degree of a compound is high, that is acidic or alkaline but difficult to elute. Hence, in a mixture of given compounds those with lower degree of dissociation are quicker to elute than those with higher degree of dissociation (Gerberding and Byers 1998).

The media used in this technique have charged functional groups to which molecules with opposite charges bind to. The bound molecules are eluted by displacement by applying an increased concentration of similarly charged molecules. Since this is also based on adsorption, it can be used to separate positively and negatively molecules. Based on pH and conductivity of the sample, the target will be adsorbed and the other molecules or contaminants are unretained, which is known as positive chromatography and in reverse it is known as negative chromatography. Media generally used are Sepharose, MiniBeads, MonoBeads, MacroCap, Capto, Sephadex, and SOURCE.

Studies have reported the use of CM Sephadex C-25 for the separation of chitooligomers (Li et al. 2012), SP-Sephadex C-25 cation exchanger for the separation of antioxidant peptide from Blue Mussel *(Mytilus edulis)* hydrolysate (Park et al. 2016).

6.5.1.1.4 Macroporous Adsorption Resin Chromatography   This method is based on the principle of adsorption and molecular sieve. This method's behavior has reversed-phase properties. An example of a macroporous material is a macroporous resin, a solid macro molecular material, with no dissociable group, insoluble in water and porous in structure. Natural compounds are majorly enriched and separated using this process due to high stability of their physical and chemical properties. Water-containing alcohol with low to high concentration is usually used to separate water solution of the mixture. This mixture can be separated into several components. The regeneration of the adsorbent resin is suitable. Generally, 1 mol/l hydrochloric acid and 1 mol/l sodium hydroxide solution is used to wash the mixture followed by washing with distilled water to make it neutral, and is stored in ethanol or methanol. But before using, the alcohol should be removed with distilled water.

20(S)-Protopanaxatriol saponins (PTS) and 20(S)-protopanaxadiol saponins (PDS), two major bioactive components in the root of Panax notoginseng, were successfully separated with macroporous resin column (Comeskey et al. 2009; Feng and Zhao 2010). Lately, Meng et al. (2017) demonstrated the isolation of saponins from *Panacis Japonici Rhizoma* (PJRS) using D101 macroporous resin (Meng et al. 2017).

6.5.1.1.5 Partition Chromatography   This method is used to separate components by using different partition coefficients between two immiscible liquids that form the mobile phase and stationary phase. This type of chromatography can be categorized into reverse phase chromatography and normal phase chromatography. The stationary phase has more polarity than that of the mobile phase in normal partition chromatography and mainly used to separate moderately polar and polar molecules. Carriers such as silica gel, cellulose powder, and diatomite are usually used in normal phase distribution chromatography. Carriers such as silica gel, which is most commonly used for partition chromatography with water content more than 17%, is used for partition chromatography due to its loss of adsorption. The mobile phase has more polarity than that of the stationary phase in reverse phase partition chromatography. Octadecylsilylated silica (ODS) is the most commonly used stationary phase. Acetonitrile water system or methanol water, which is mainly used for the separation of nonpolar and moderately polar molecular compounds, is generally used as mobile phase.

6.5.1.2 New Technologies and Methods

6.5.1.2.1 High-Performance Liquid Chromatography (HPLC)   HPLC is a rapid separation and analysis technology developed on the foundation of conventional column chromatography. The principle of HPLC is the same as regular column chromatography, including gel chromatography, adsorption chromatography, ion exchange chromatography, partition chromatography, and other methods. HPLC columns are produced with particle fillers where the particle diameter is around 5–20 μm and high-pressure homogenate column loading technology. High-pressure infusion pump is used to press the eluents into the column. It is equipped with high-sensitive detectors and automatic recording and collection devices. Therefore, it is far advanced to that of conventional column chromatography in terms of separation speed and efficiency. Its characteristics include high speed, high efficiency, and automation.

Preparative HPLC can be used to obtain a large amount of samples with high purity. When it comes to plant compounds separation, qualitative and quantitative analysis HPLC has played a very enormously increasing role. Constant concentration eluents are mostly used in preparative HPLC while in certain samples gradient elution is also used. Furthermore, HPLC maintains the advantage of liquid chromatography (LC) such as mobile phase change flexibility and wide range of applications. It can be used for chemical components of difficult gasification, thermal stability, or high molecular weight. The most commonly used detectors in HPLC are differential refractive index detectors and ultraviolet (UV) detectors but with limitations. UV detectors cannot detect samples without UV absorption while differential refractive index detectors are sensitive to temperature change, the detection of small amount of substances is often not absolute, and gradient elution cannot be used. In recent times, evaporative light scattering detector (ELSD), a kind of mass detector, has been used in HPLC. Overcoming the issues, this detector can detect samples without UV absorption and also use gradient elution, thereby making this the most suitable technique for nonvolatile compounds (Ji et al. 2018).

Currently HPLC is generally combined with qualitative equipment such as mass spectrometry (MS) and LC followed by tandem mass spectrometric detection (LC–MS/MS) to characterize peptide sequences, thereby foraying into the structural elucidation of protein and peptides. Besides to overcome the disadvantages of the existing methods, HPLC with evaporative light scattering detection (HPLC-ELSD) for purification and quantification, ultra-high-performance liquid chromatography-tandem mass spectrometry (UHPLC-MS/MS) analysis, and rapid resolution liquid chromatography-tandem mass spectrometry (RRLC–MS) were developed (Rizzetti et al. 2017; Tenon et al. 2017).

6.5.1.2.2 Droplet Counter-Current Chromatography (DCCC)

DCCC is a superior liquid–liquid partition chromatography based on the counter-current partition method. When the mobile phase passes through a liquid stationary phase column, droplets are formed. These droplets contact the stationary phase effectively and form new surfaces in thin partition extraction tubes constantly, which support the partition of solutes in two-phase solvents. The chemical components of mixtures are isolated in immiscible two-phase droplets due to different partition coefficients. This method is appropriate for the separation of phytochemicals with very high polarity. The separation effect is usually better than counter-current partition chromatography, and there is no emulsification phenomenon.

Additionally, nitrogen is used to steer the mobile phase to ensure that the separated substance will not be oxidized by oxygen in the atmosphere. Selection of solvent system, which can generate droplets, is important as the amount of sample treated is small and special equipment is needed. DCCC can handle crude extract samples of milligram to gram grade and possesses good reproducibility. It can be used in either basic or acidic conditions. Since no solid separation carriers are used, band broadening of chromatographic peaks and irreversible adsorption can be avoided. DCCC consumes less solvent when compared with preparative HPLC, but the separation time is longer and the resolution is lower.

A study reported the separation of the indole alkaloids from the root barks of *Tabernaemontana hilariana* (Apocynaceae) benzene extracts. The crude alkaloid fraction initially obtained was fractionated by DCCC using a low polarity mixture (hexane:ethyl acetate:ethanol:water). Nine indole alkaloids were identified using TLC, gas chromatography (GC) coupled with MS, and nuclear magnetic resonance spectroscopy (NMR). There was no decomposition seen both during and after the separation process. High amount of time and the volume of solvents were needed, which are limitations of this technique. Also, cheap solvents are used, and no buffer time and no complex gradient of mobile phase were required, and it is carried out on its own. This method allows the fractionation of a highly sensitive plant extract but has very minor disadvantages compared to the advantages. Moreover, it was noticed that the extract showed no decomposition during or after the separation process. The main issues that need attention are, first, it is time consuming, and second, it needs high amounts of solvents. However, the solvents used are cheap, buffer is not required, no complex gradient of mobile phase, and the process can be carried out automatically. In comparison to the limitations, the advantages are promising for the fractionation of highly sensitive plant extract (Cardoso and Wilegas 1999).

6.5.1.2.3 *High-speed counter-current chromatography (HSCCC)*

HSCCC is a liquid–liquid partition chromatography with no solid support, hence avoiding the loss of substrate by binding to the column. The only media in contact with the sample is the solvent. The chemical components with higher partition coefficient in mobile phase are eluted first while those with higher partition coefficient in stationary phase are eluted later. This chromatography can overcome the inadequacies of irreversible adsorption and abnormal tailing of chromatographic peaks that are generally caused by solid carriers in LC because it does not require solid carriers. The recovery of the sample is near 100%. It also possesses other advantages such as high purity of separated compounds, good reproducibility, and swiftness. It is apt for the isolation and purification of wide range of phytochemicals, such as alkaloids, saponins, anthraquinoids, flavonoids, lignans, proteins, carbohydrates, and triterpenes.

HSCCC was successful in fingerprinting the active constituents of Chinese traditional medicine which are impacted by soil, climate, and growth stages. The extract of Salvia miltiorrhiza Bunge obtained from different locations was subjected to HSCCC, and twelve components were separated with high precision that met the national standards in the fingerprint development, thereby making HSCCC a viable method for the development of fingerprints (Gu et al. 2004).

6.5.1.2.4 *High-performance capillary electrophoresis (HPCE)*

Developed in the late 1980s, this method combines classical electrophoresis with modern microcolumn separation strategies. In pharmaceutical context, the generally used separation modes are micellar electrokinetic capillary chromatography, capillary zone electrophoresis, and capillary gel electrophoresis. It is a competent separation method for large and small molecules which uses a hollow, thin capillary with an inner diameter of 10–200 μm. The two ends of the capillary are immersed in a buffer solution and electrodes connected with a high voltage power supply are inserted separately. The voltage makes samples migrate along the capillary. Under high voltage, different molecules are separated based on their charge and volume. In zone capillary electrophoresis, separation will be attained by the movement of electrophoresis and electroosmotic flow. The strength of electroosmotic flow depends on the pH value of electrolyte, the strength of electric field, ionic strength, composition of buffer solution, internal friction, and so on. Sample injection could be accomplished by atmospheric pressure or voltage. HPCE displays certain advantages such as high efficiency, economy, microamount, high automation, and wide applications but poses issues such as low sensitivity, poor preparation ability, and poor separation reproducibility which have to be taken care of.

Advancement in HPLC and HPCE methods has facilitated the analysis of low-molecular weight compounds such as catechins which are poly phenols, purine alkaloids in tea. These techniques enable to determine the variations of the chemical components with respect to taste, place of production, character of the cultivars, quality, manufacturing styles, and cultivation methods (Horie and Kohata 2000).

6.5.1.2.5   *Affinity Chromatography (AC)*   This is a special type of chromatography method which is based on the principle of reversible combination of high affinity and specificity between molecules. Based on the concept of specific and reversible interactions between biomolecules, this technique uses adsorption medium together with affinity ligands in the stationary phase to adsorb target compounds. This is an advancement of adsorption chromatography. This technique can selectively separate and analyze specific chemical components from complex samples. The chromatographic column is made of ligands that can specifically bind to target fixed on the filler. The mixture comprising the target compounds is then passed through the column.

The target compounds that specifically show affinity with the ligands will bind to the ligands and remain in the column. Finally, the adsorbed target compounds are eluted by changing the composition of the mobile phase and are thus separated from other chemical constituents. Air conditioning is mainly used for the separation and purification of proteins, especially antigens, enzymes, and antibodies. Its application range has been increasing along with the constant development of technology in recent years. Experimental evidence suggests the positive role of this method in isolating certain plant-based compounds. A study demonstrated the isolation of structurally variant flavonoids – with hydroxyl rings and without hydroxyl rings using high-performance AC based on their affinity or binding to human serum albumin. (Cao et al. 2019). An overview of the chromatographic techniques is provided in Table 6.3.

6.5.2   Other Separation Techniques

6.5.2.1   Molecular Distillation

This method separates molecules through distillation under vacuum at a temperature far below its boiling point. It is an appropriate method for thermosensitive and high-molecular weight compounds. Borgarello et al. (2015) extracted thymol which showed antioxidant properties from oregano essential oil through this method modeled by artificial neural networks. Another study isolated three kinds of phthalates from sweet orange oil through this method under ideal conditions (Xiong et al. 2013).

6.5.2.2   Preparative Gas Chromatography (pGC)

GC is the most common technique used for separating and analyzing compounds that can be vaporized without decomposition. Since its invention in 1941, much technological advancement in this technique led to its integration with computer. Preparative GC (pGC) generally uses large-diameter columns to purify relatively large quantities of materials by using a sample collection system at the column outlet.

Essentially, pGC seems to be a practical alternative to other preparative techniques such as preparative HPLC, especially for volatile compounds. pGC can be applied in the field of synthetic chemistry, the fine chemical industry, the preparation of flavors and fragrances, or odoriferous constituents which are chiefly used in cosmetic industry, environmental chemistry, biology, pharmaceuticals, toxicology, and compound-specific radio carbon analysis. The main components of pGC system are carrier gas system, an injection system, a separation column, splitter and detector, and a trap used to collect the effluents, which were not included in the analytical equipment. Today, most of the pGC systems reported in the literature for preparative purposes have been modified from the analytical systems (Zuo et al. 2012a).

A study by Yang et al. (2011) reported the successful separation of five volatile compounds, namely curzerene, β-elemene, curzerenone, curcumenol, and curcumenone, from the methanol extract of

Table 6.3 Comparison of different chromatography-based separation techniques.

Method	Principle involved	Mobile phase examples	Stationary phase examples	Components separated	Advantages	Disadvantages
Affinity chromatography (solid–liquid separation)	Components are separated according to differences in their binding affinity.	Buffer containing a variety of biomolecules from DNA to proteins (depending on the purification experiment)	Agarose, cellulose, acrylamide, polystyrene, polymethyl acrylate, silica, glass	Antibody, proteins, carbohydrate residues, DNA, hormones, alkaloids, etc.	• Highly specific • High purity product can be obtained • Process is reproducible • Remove specific contaminants	• Expensive ligands • Degradation of solid support • Limited lifetime
High-performance capillary electrophoresis (solution in capillary)	Analytical technique that separates ions based on their electrophoretic mobility with the use of an applied voltage.	Organic solvents and aqueous buffer mixtures	Organic polymer-based monoliths, inorganic silica-based reversed-phase packing	Proteins, enzymes, sugars, nucleic acids, peptides, amino acids, and phospholipids	• Rapid analysis times • Automation • Minute sample volume requirements • Number of detection methods	• High concentration limit of detection
High-speed counter-current chromatography (liquid–liquid separation)	Technique is based on the effects of gravitational and centrifugal force on the solvent flow behavior in a helical-shaped tubing.	For polar compounds: 1-butanol/acetic acid/water. For moderately hydrophobic compounds – hexane/ethyl acetate/methanol/0.1 M HCl. For hydrophobic compounds – hexane/ethanol/water or hexane/acetonitrile.	Two immiscible solvent systems	Kavain and demethoxyyangonin, flavonoids, indole auxins, tetracycline derivatives, DNP amino acid, sulforaphane, bioactive lignans and its acetate	• No sample loss • High recovery rates • Low solvent usage • High resolution and separation speed • Enhances the repeatability • Versatility of the experiment	• Unreliable • Range of equipment available is poor and typically only available at the preparative scale, requiring gram-size sample injections. Hence it is a problem for small molecule research and development.

(Continued)

Table 6.3 (Continued)

Method	Principle involved	Mobile phase examples	Stationary phase examples	Components separated	Advantages	Disadvantages
Droplet counter-current chromatography (liquid–liquid separation)	Based on the partitioning of solute between a steady stream of droplets of moving phase and a column of surrounding stationary liquid phase. The principle of separation involves the partition of a solute between two immiscible solvents (mobile phase and stationary phase). The relative proportion of solute passing into each of the two solvents determined by partition coefficient.	Chloroform: water. Chloroform:acetic acid: aqueous 0.1 M HCl. Chloroform: methanol: water "n"-butanol-water: modifier such as acetic acid, pyridine or n-propanol	n-hexane (or heptane), ethyl acetate, methanol, and water in different proportions.	Saponins, alkaloids, Senna glycosides, monosaccharides, triterpene glycosides, flavone glycosides, xanthones, iridoid glycosides, vitamin B_{12} lignans, imbricatolic acid, gallic acid, carotenoids, and triterpenoids.	Adsorptive sample loss and denaturation is less Tailing of solute peaks and contamination is less High recovery rate and ease of scale up	Poor stabilization of stationary phase Poor mixing
High-performance liquid chromatography (solid–liquid separation)	It relies on pumps to pass a pressurized liquid solvent containing the sample mixture through a column filled with a solid adsorbent material. Each component in the sample interacts slightly differently with the adsorbent material, causing different flow rates for the different components and leading to the separation of the components as they flow out of the column.	Hexane ethyl acetate n-butanol methanol	Silica and polymers	Flavonoids, phenolic acids, dihydrochalcones, pro anthocyanidins, ellagitannins, soyasaponins, sugars, amino acids, phytosterols, lignan	Higher resolution and speed of analysis Columns are reusable Easy automation Greater reproducibility Adaptability to large scale	Tedious to detect co-elution High cost Complex to operate

Technique	Principle	Mobile phase	Stationary phase	Applications	Advantages	Disadvantages
Partition chromatography (liquid–liquid separation)	Partition chromatography exploits the fact that a solute in contact with two immiscible liquids (or phases) will distribute itself between them according to its distribution coefficient, K. The separation depends on different partition coefficient.	Water: chloroform:n-butanol solvent mixture. Acetate/methanol/water Ethyl acetate/methanol/water	Silica gel, diatomaceous earth, cellulose, polytetrafluoroethylene (PTFE), polystyrene	Coumarins, saponins, chlorophyll, carotenoids, anthocyanins, phenolic compounds, alkaloids, tannins, lignans	Simple to operate inexpensive, high efficiency Can separate small organic and inorganic compounds Accurate results	Data cannot be stored long Automation made complication expensive, solvent requirement is more.
Macroporous adsorption resin chromatography (resin-based separation)	The principle of adsorption is based on electrostatic force, hydrogen-bonding interaction, and size sieving action between macroporous resins and different molecular from the solution	Ethanolic extract containing solute	Macroporous resin	Proteins, carbohydrates, saponins, flavonoids, anthocyanins, glycosides	Convenient with low operational cost Lower solvent consumption Absence of chemical residues in the product Good stability, high adsorption capacity, and selectivity Fast adsorption and desorption, and easy regeneration	• Time consuming for both adsorption and desorption processes to reach the equilibrium
Ion exchange chromatography (resin-based liquid separation)	The molecules are separated on the basis of their charge and are eluted using a solution of varying ionic strength. By passing such a solution through the column, highly selective separation of molecules according to their different charges takes place.	Sample followed by either of these buffers (acetate buffer, pyridine, tris-buffer buffer, phosphate buffer, and citrate buffers)	Cellulose/polystyrene/agarose/polyacrylamide resins	Polypeptides, proteins, polynucleotides, enzymes, growth factors, and nucleic acids	Most powerful way to separate charged particles Used for both analytical and preparative reasons Inorganic ions can also be isolated	Buffer requirement Only charged molecules can be isolated High operating cost Stability and reproducibility become questionable after repeated use

(Continued)

Table 6.3 (Continued)

Method	Principle involved	Mobile phase examples	Stationary phase examples	Components separated	Advantages	Disadvantages
Gel permeation chromatography (gel-based liquid separation)	Separation of components is based on the difference in molecular weight or size.	Liquid used to dissolve the biomolecules	Porouspolymer gel beads (e.g. dextran, agarose, acrylamide, sephadex, and sepharose)	Polypeptides, proteins, polynucleotides, enzymes	Short analysis time, well-defined separation Narrow band and good sensitivity Less sample loss Flow rate can be set. Small amount of mobile phase can be used.	Limited number of peaks that can be resolved within the short time scale of the run Filtrations must be performed
Adsorption chromatography (solid–liquid/gas separation)	Chemicals are retained based on their adsorption and desorption at the surface of the support, which also acts as the stationary phase through electrostatic interactions, hydrogen bonding, dipole–dipole interactions, and dispersive interactions (i.e., van der Waals forces)	Solvent mixture	Silica, alumina, and charcoal	Carotenoids, porphyrins, natural oil and flavor extracts, and cannabinol.	Used for separating many molecules that cannot be distinguished from other methods Uses a broad range of mobile phases Very few types of equipment are used	Automation is making it more complicated and expensive Some solutes have longer retention times Can cause catalytic variations in the sample Some results are difficult to reproduce

Curcuma Rhizome by pGC. Similarly, natural isomers cis-asarone and trans-asarone were separated from the oil of Acorus tatarinowii (Zuo et al. 2012b). pGC has become a major separation method for natural volatile compounds; however, a large-diameter preparative column and a heavier sample load were found to decrease the efficiency (Ozek and Demirci 2012). Certain disadvantages of pGC such as lack of commercial pGC equipment, the decomposition of thermolabile compounds under high operation temperature, consumption of a large volume of carrier gas, low production, and the difficulties of fraction collection need to be addressed which can augment its use further.

6.5.2.3 Supercritical Fluid Chromatography (SFC)

SF is a fluid which has low viscosity, high diffusivity, and high dissolving capacity as the mobile phase and hence allows fast and efficient separation. SFC is helpful in separating thermally labile compounds or nonvolatile compounds. This facilitates the separation of thermally liable and nonvolatile compounds for which GC is not compatible. Additionally this set up is compatible with a wide range of detectors. Elution strength can be enhanced by using certain modifiers such as acetonitrile and methanol which seems to be a reliable option for the separation of polar natural compounds (Hartmann and Ganzera 2015; Speybrouck and Lipka 2016). A study by Zhao et al. (2013) demonstrated the separation of three pairs of 25 R/S diastereomeric spirostanol saponins from Trigonellae Semen on two CHIRALPAK IC columns coupled in tandem. Likewise, another study reported the use of this technique for separating two pairs of 7-epimeric spirooxindole alkaloids from stems of Uncaria macrophylla (Yang et al. 2017). This technique is also used in separating natural enantiomers (R, S)-goitrin using acetonitrile as modifier (Nie et al. 2016).

6.5.2.4 Molecular Imprinted Technology

This technique has become a promising option for the separation of compounds because of its unique features such as low cost, high selectivity, and easy preparation.

Molecularly imprinted polymers (MIP) are the cross-linked polymeric materials that can resist chemical and physical stress such as heat, organic solvents, acid, bases, and others (Haupt et al. 1998). The thought of polymer that can specifically and selectively distinguish desired molecules has grabbed the attention of research community in the recent past. This kind of identification of polymers is analogous to the biological recognition systems in the body such as enzymes, antibodies, and DNA. The imprinted polymers created from the polymerization process possess cavities that are complementary to the shape of the desired molecules.

The binding between the polymer and the selected compounds can be through covalent method, non-covalent method, and semi-covalent method. The most prevalent method is the non-covalent approach in which the templates bond to monomers with a non-covalent intermolecular bonding which can be destroyed and created easily. Weak metal coordination, hydrogen bonds, electrostatic interactions, and hydrophobic interactions comprises non-covalent forces used by both molecules which are chemically and geometrically complementing each other (Yusof et al. 2010).

Once polymerized, the templates can be removed via simple diffusion using a polar or acidic solvent which can destroy the non-covalent interaction between template and polymer (Bergmann and Peppas 2008). Non-covalent approach is cost effective and hence preferred compared to covalent approach.

A study reported the preparation of multi-template MIP for the separation of denichine using DL-tyrosine and phenylpyruvic acid as the template from the water extract of *Panax notoginseng*. The templates possess amino group, carboxylic group, and α-keto acid which are also found in denichine (Ji et al. 2016). Likewise, solanesol was separated from tobacco leaves by flash chromatography based on MIP which was methyl methacrylate with the monomer solanesol as the template molecule and ethylene glycol dimethacrylate as the crosslinker (Ma et al. 2016).

You et al. (2014) used thermo-responsive magnetic MIP for the separation of three major curcuminoids, which were curcumin, demethoxycurcumin, and bisdemethoxycurcumin, from the TCM *Curcumae Longae Rhizoma*. This MIP was found to display good imprinting factor for curcuminoids.

6.5.2.5 Simulated Moving Bed Chromatography (SMBC)

This technique uses multiple smaller columns with solid adsorbent (beds) instead of one large column, and the beds move in the opposite direction of the fluid for obtaining a concurrent flow rather than flowing fluids through one static bed. This simulated movement is performed throughout the multiport valves interspersed between columns so that the input (feed and eluent) and output (extract and raffinate) can be switched from time to time from column to column depending on the direction of flow of the fluid. Instead of working with one column, all fluid streams can be applied simultaneously and can be withdrawn at appropriate times between these columns. When running at a steady state, the various stages of separation are carried out simultaneously by different columns in a continuous cycle.

The SMBC process made LC economically practical on an industrial scale due to its high productivity relative to single-column methods. This improved productivity (up to 20-fold) is achieved through much more proficient consumption of the solid and liquid phases required for separation. In simplest terms, SMBC does more with less. A more recent variation of SMBC adapts the multicolumn approach to higher separation factor applications, such as AC.

Reports suggest the use of SMBC in the extraction of various NPs. A study demonstrated the separation of two cyclopeptides, namely cyclolinopeptides C and E, from flax seed oil using SMBC along with HPLC (Okinyo-Owiti et al. 2014). Similarly, paclitaxel, 13-dehydroxybaccatin III, and 10-deacetylpaclitaxel were obtained using SMBC (Kang et al. 2010). Studies showed that SFs can also be used as the desorbent in SMBC chromatography. Liang et al. (2013) successfully separated resveratrol and emodin by applying $S-CO_2$ with ethanol as the desorbent for a three-zone SMBC from a crude extract of the TCM Polygoni Cuspidati Rhizoma Radix.

6.5.2.6 Multidimensional Chromatographic Separation

Generally, the components in a mixture are huge in number and pose a real problem for their separation qualitatively and quantitatively. Separating them unidimensionally is possible to a certain extent. Therefore, multidimensional separation is preferred, wherein SPE with multiple columns and different stationary phases are used, that is found to greatly enhance the separation efficiency. With the advent of multidimensional separation more of NPs are separated rapidly, efficiently with adequate automation. Multidimensional separation can be attained using the same type separation equipment (LC or GC) or different types of equipment (GC and LC). Several studies reported the use of this approach to separate compounds from a mixture.

Sciarrone et al. (2013) demonstrated the use of three-dimensional pGC to isolate a novel volatile compound (2E, 6E)-2-methyl-6-(4-methylcyclohex-3-enylidene) hept-2-enal from wampee essential oil. Also they separated sesquiterpenes in patchouli essential oil by three-dimensional pGC (Sciarrone et al. 2016). Likewise, five antioxidant compounds which included two alkaloids (glusodichotomine AK and glusodichotomine B) and three flavonoids (tricin, luteolin, and homoeriodictyol) were separated using a two-dimensional HPLC method from *Arenaria kansuensis* (Cui et al. 2017).

Pantò et al. (2015) applied two three-dimensional approaches (LC–GC–GC and GC–GC–GC) to separate the sesquiterpene alcohols from the sandalwood essential oil. They found that the first-dimensional separation using LC reduced the sample complexity and increased the productivity of low-concentration components.

6.6 Structural Identification of Natural Compounds

NP is a chemical compound or substance that is produced by living organisms and can be classified based on many criteria and characteristics, such as source, biosynthetic pathway, biological function, and physical and chemical properties. In recent times, NPs find a broad range of applications related to human life including medicine.

Of late, NPs have been the starting point for drug discovery process as potential drug hits and leads. This necessitates the identification of structures of these NPs which instigate various in silico approaches in drug discovery. These structures form the basis for studies on bioactivities, structure activity relationships, in vivo metabolism studies, structural modifications, analogue studies, and synthesis of active biomolecules. The natural produces obtained generally are of less quantity that makes their structural analysis difficult. Therefore, spectral analysis is preferred.

After the purification of bioactive molecules, the structure of the molecule is characterized by various spectroscopic techniques. The basic principle of spectroscopy is based on measuring the amount of radiation absorbed by any organic molecule when electromagnetic radiation is passed through it. The amount of radiation is measured and a spectrum is produced, which is specific to certain bonds in a molecule. Based on these spectra, the structure of the molecule can be identified. The spectra produced from either three or four regions – UV, visible, infrared (IR), radio frequency, and electron beam (Popova et al. 2009) – are of major interest for the research group for structural clarification. The techniques generally used are explained below.

6.6.1 UV-Visible Spectroscopy

UV-visible spectroscopy can be carried out for qualitative analysis and for identification of some class of compounds in both pure and biological mixtures. This method is well preferred for aromatic molecules as they are powerful chromophores. Many natural compounds can be resolved by using UV-visible spectroscopy for phenolic compounds including tannins, anthocyanins, phenols, and polymer dyes (Kemp 1991). This technique is quick and cost effective compared to other techniques (Urbano et al. 2006).

6.6.2 Infrared Spectroscopy

When IR light is passed through a sample, some of the frequencies are absorbed by the compound while some are transmitted. This leads to vibrational changes in the molecule due to bonds which can be observed in the IR spectrum (Urbano et al. 2006). Fourier transform infrared spectroscopy (FTIR) is a high-resolution analytical tool to identify the chemical constituents and elucidate the structural compounds and this offers a rapid and nondestructive investigation to fingerprint herbal extracts or powders.

6.6.3 Nuclear Magnetic Resonance Spectroscopy

NMR is mainly related to the magnetic properties of certain atomic nuclei, notably the nucleus of the hydrogen atom, the proton, the carbon, and an isotope of carbon. NMR spectroscopy enabled the study molecules by recording the differences between the various magnetic nuclei and thereby giving a clear picture of the positions of these nuclei in the molecule. Also, it demonstrates which atoms are present in neighboring groups. Therefore, it can conclude how many atoms are present in each of these environments (Kemp 1991).

6.6.4 Mass Spectroscopy

MS displays the capability ranging from small-molecule analysis to protein characterization. MS is a potent analytical technique that is used to identify unknown compounds, to quantify known compounds, and to elucidate the structure and chemical properties of molecules. The molecular weight of sample can be determined from MS spectrum. Structural information can also be generated from certain types of mass spectrometers. This procedure is useful for the structural elucidation of organic compounds, for peptide or oligonucleotide sequencing, and for monitoring the existence of previously characterized compounds in complex mixtures with a high specificity by defining both the molecular weight and a diagnostic fragment of the molecule simultaneously.

6.6.5 X-Ray Crystallography

This experimental technique is based on the fact that X-rays are diffracted by crystals. X-rays have the proper wavelength to be scattered by the electron cloud of an atom of comparable size. Based on the diffraction pattern obtained from X-ray scattering off the periodic assembly of molecules or atoms in the crystal, the electron density can be reconstructed. Additional phase information can be extracted either from the diffraction data or from supplementing diffraction experiment to complete the reconstruction. A model is then progressively built into the experimental electron density, refined against the data, and the result is a quite accurate molecular structure.

6.7 Summary

The use of NPs in the field of medicine in recent times has increased enormously. The extraction of these compounds is lab intensive and time consuming and hence posed difficulty in the application of these products in medicine. With the advancement in technology and automation, several methods or combination of methods have been suggested for efficient extraction of these natural compounds, which could meet the requirement of high throughput screening. The selection of the right extraction methods depends on the selectivity, extraction yield, stability of extracts, and process safety. Isolating the compounds depends on the packaging material that would enhance the efficiency. Isolation and purification of natural compounds is always challenging owing to their use in drug design, and hence the right approach would ensure proper extraction and purification of compounds.

References

Ahmad, A., Alkarkhi, A.F.M., Henaand, S., and Lima, L.H. (2009). Extraction, separation and identification of chemical ingredients of Elephantopus Scaber L using factorial design of experiment. *International Journal of Chemistry* 1 (1): 36–49.

Albuquerque, B.R., Prieto, M.A., Barreiro, M.F. et al. (2017). Catechin-based extract optimization obtained from Arbutus unedo L. fruits using maceration/microwave/ultrasound extraction techniques. *Industrial Crops and Products* 95: 404–415.

Altemimi, D.A. Lightfoot, M. Kinsel, and D.G. Watson. (2015). Employing response surface methodology for the optimization of ultrasound assisted extraction of lutein and β-carotene from spinach. *Molecules* 20 (4): 6611–6625, https://doi.org/10.3390/molecules20046611.

Alupului, A., Calinecu, I., and Lavric, V. (2012). Microwave extraction of active principles from medicinal plants, *U.P.B. Science Bulletin, Series B* 74 (2): 129–142.

Atanasov, A.G., Waltenberger, B., Pferschy-Wenzig, E.M. et al. (2015). Discovery and resupply of pharmacologically active plant-derived natural products: a review. *Biotechnology Advances* 33 (8): 1582–1614.

Bergmann, N.M. and Peppas, N.A. (2008). Molecularly imprinted polymers with specific recognition for macromolecules and proteins. *Progress in Polymer Science* 33: 271–288.

Bhattacharya, M., Srivastav, P.P., and Mishra, H.N. (2015). Thin-layer modeling of convective and microwave-convective drying of oyster mushroom (Pleurotus ostreatus). *Journal of Food Science and Technology* 52 (4): 2013–2022.

Bimakr, M., Rahman, R.A., Taip, F.S. et al. (2011). Comparison of different extraction methods for the extraction of major bioactive flavonoid compounds from spearmint (Mentha spicata L.) leaves. *Food and Bioproducts Processing* 89: 67–72. https://doi.org/10.1016/j.fbp.2010.03.002.

Borgarello, A.V., Mezza, G.N., Pramparo, M.C., and Gayol, M.F. (2015). Thymol enrichment from oregano essential oil by molecular distillation. *Separation and Purification Technology* 153: 60–66.

Brusotti, G., Cesari, I., Dentaaro, A. et al. (2014). Isolation and characterization of bioactive compounds from plant resources: the role of analysis in the ethno pharmacological approach. *Journal of Pharmaceutical and Biomedical Analysis* 87: 218–22 https://doi. org/10.1016/j.jpba.2013.03.007.

Bryant, G. and Wolfe, J. (1987). Electromechanical stress produced in the plasma membranes of suspended cells by applied electrical fields. *Journal of Membrane Biology* 96 (2): 129–139.

Bulugahapitiya, V. (2013). Plant based natural products extraction and phytochemical analysis. *Self.* https://www.researchgate.net/publication/324136585.

Burman, J.J.R. (2003). *Tribal Medicine*, 1e, vol. 12. A Mittal Publication.

Camera-Roda, G., Loddo, V., Palmisano, L., Parrino, F. (2019). Green synthesis of Vanillin: pervaporation and dialysis for process intensification in a membrane reactor. *Chemical Engineering Transactions* 75. https://doi.org/10.3303/CET1975001.

Canbay, H.S. (2017). Effectiveness of liquid-liquid extraction, solid phase extraction, and headspace technique for determination of some volatile water-soluble compounds of rose aromatic water. *International Journal of Analytical Chemistry.* https://doi.org/10.1155/2017/4870671.

Cao, H., Liu, X.J., Ulrihc, N.P. et al. (2019). Plasma protein binding of dietary polyphenols to human serum albumin: a high performance affinity chromatography approach. *Food Chemistry* 270: 257–263. https://doi.org/10.1016/j.foodchem.2018.07.111.

Cardoso, C.A.L. and Wilegas, W. (1999). Droplet counter-current chromatography of indole alkaloids from Tabernaemontana hilariana. *Phytochemical Analasis* 10: 60–63.

Chemat, F. and Cravotto, G. (2013). *Microwave-Assisted Extraction for Bioactive Compounds*. Boston, MA: Springer.

Chemat, F., Rombaut, N., Sicaire, A.G. et al. (2017). Ultrasound assisted extraction of food and natural products. Mechanisms, techniques, combinations, protocols and applications. *Ultrasonics Sonochemistry* 34: 540–560. https:// doi.org/10.1016/j.ultsonch.2016.06.035.

Chua, L.S., Lau, C.H., Chew, C.Y., and Dawood, D.A.S. (2019). Solvent fractionation and acetone precipitation for Crude Saponins from Eurycoma longifolia extract. *Molecules* 24: 1416. https://doi.org/10.3390/molecules24071416.

Comeskey, D.J., Montefiori, M., Edwards, P.J.B., and McGhie, T.K. (2009). Isolation and structural identification of the anthocyanin components of red kiwifruit. *Journal of Agricultural and Food Chemistry* 57 (5): 2035–2039.

Concha, J., Soto, C., Chamy, R., and Zuniga, M.E. (2004). Enzymatic pretreatment on Rose-Hip oil extraction: hydrolysis and pressing conditions. *Journal of American Oil Chemist's Society* 81 (6): 549–552.

Cui, Y., Shen, N., Yuan, X. et al. (2017). Two-dimensional chromatography based on on-line HPLCDPPH bioactivity-guided assay for the preparative isolation of analogue antioxidant compound from Arenaria kansuensis. *Journal of Chromatography B* 1046: 81–86.

Ćujić, N., Šavikin, K., Janković, T. et al. (2016). Optimization of polyphenols extraction from dried chokeberry using maceration as traditional technique. *Food Chemistry* 194: 135–142.

Cutignano, A., Nuzzo, G., Ianora, A. et al. (2015). Development and application of a Novel SPE-method for bioassay-guided fractionation of marine extracts. *Marine Drugs* 13: 5736–5749. https://doi.org/10.3390/md13095736.

Du, G., Zhao, H.Y., Song, Y.L. et al. (2011). Rapid simultaneous determination of isoflavones in Radix puerariae using high-performance liquid chromatography-triple quadrupole mass spectrometry with novel shell-type column. *Journal of Separation Science* 34 (19): 2576–2585.

Duraipandiyan, V., Ayyanarand, M., and Ignacimuthu, S. (2006). Antimicrobial activity of some ethnomedicinal plants used by Paliyar tribe from Tamil Nadu, *India. BMC Complementary and Alternative Medicine* 6 (35): 35–41. https://doi.org/10.1186/1472-6882-6-35.

Escriba-Gelonch, M., Hessel, V., Maier, M.C. et al. (2018). Continuous-flow in-line solvent-swap crystallization of vitamin D3. *Organic Process Research and Development* 22: 178–189. https://doi.org/10.1021/acs.oprd.7b00351.

Feng, L. and Zhao, F. (2010). Separation of polyphenols in tea on weakly acidic cation-exchange gels. *Chromatographia* 71 (9): 775–782.

Feng, W., Li, M., Hao, Z., and Zhang, J. (2019). Analytical methods of isolation and identification. *IntechOpen.* https://doi.org/10.5772/intechopen.88122.

Fereira, C.C., Costa, E.C., de Castro, D.A.R. et al. (2017). Fractional distillation of organic liquid compounds produced by catalytic cracking of fats, oils, and grease, distillation – innovative applications and modeling, *Marisa Fernandes Mendes. IntechOpen* . https://doi.org/10.5772/66759.

Garrett, R.H. (2013). *Reginald Biochemistry*. Belmont: Brooks/Cole, Cengage Learning.

Gerberding, S.J. and Byers, C.H. (1998). Preparative ion-exchange chromatography of proteins from dairy whey. *Journal of Chromatography A* 808: 141–151.

Grigonis, D., Sivik, P., Sandahl, M., and Eskilsson, C. (2005). Comparison of different extraction techniques for isolation of antioxidants from sweet grass (Hierochloeodorata). *Journal of Supercritical Fluids* 33 (15): 223–233. https://doi.org/10.1016/j.foodchem.2004.08.006.

Gu, M., Ouyang, F., and Su, Z.G. (2004). Comparison of high-speed countercurrent chromatography and highperformance liquid chromatography on fingerprinting of Chinese traditional medicine. *Journal of Chromatography A* 1022: 139–144. https://doi.org/10.1016/j.chroma.2003. 09.038.

Handa, S.S., Khanuja, S.P.S., Longo, G., and Rakesh, D.D. (2008). *Extraction Technologies for Medicinal and Aromatic Plants*, 1e, no. 66. Italy: United Nations Industrial Development Organization and the International Centre for Science and High Technology.

Hanif, M.A., Nawaz, H., Naz, S., et al. (2017). Raman spectroscopy for the characterization of different fractions of hemp essential oil extracted at 130°C using steam distillation method. *Spectrochimica Acta Part A: Molecular and Biomolecular Spectroscopy* 182: 168–174. https://doi.org/10.1016/j.saa.2017.03.072.

Hanmoungjai, P., Pyle, D.L., and Niranjan, K. (2001). Enzymatic process for extracting oil and protein from rice bran. *Journal of the American Oil Chemists Society* 78 (8): 817–821.

Hartmann, A. and Ganzera, M. (2015). Supercritical fluid chromatography – theoretical background and applications on natural products. *Planta Medica* 81 (17): 1570–1581.

Haupt, K., Dzgoev, A., and Mosbach, K. (1998). Assay system for the herbicide 2,4-dichlorophenoxyacetic acid using a molecularly imprinted polymer as an artificial recognition element. *Analytical Chemistry* 70: 628–631.

Horie, H. and Kohata, K. (2000) Analysis of tea components by high-performance liquid chromatography and highperformance capillary electrophoresis. *Journal of Chromatography A*. 881 (1–2): 425–438. https://doi.org/10.1016/S0021-9673(99)01345-X.

Horosanskaia, E., Tan, N.M., Tien, V.D. et al. (2017). Crystallization-based isolation of pure Rutin from herbal extract of Sophora Japonica L. *Organic Process Research & Development* 21 (11): 1769–1778.

Ibañez, E., Herrero, M., Mendiola, J.A., and Castro-Puyana, M. (2012). Extraction and characterization of bioactive compounds with health benefits from marine resources: macro and micro algae, cyanobacteria, and invertebrates. In: *Marine Bioactive Compounds: Sources, Characterization and Applications* (ed. M. Hayes), 55–98. Springer.

Jacob, J. (2012). Microwave assisted reactions in organic chemistry: a review of recent advances. *International Journal of Chemistry* 4 (6): 29–43. https://doi.org/10.5539/ijc.v4n6p29.

Ji, S., Wang, S., Xu, H. et al. (2018). The application of on-line two-dimensional liquid chromatography (2DLC) in the chemical analysis of herbal medicines. *Journal of Pharmaceutical and Biomedical Analysis* 160: 301–331. https://doi.org/10.1016/j.jpba.2018.08.014.

Ji, W., Xie, H., Zhou, J. et al. (2016). Water-compatible molecularly imprinted polymers for selective solid phase extraction of denchine from the aqueous extract of Panax notoginseng. *Journal of Chromatography B* 1008: 225–233.

Jovanović, A.A., Đorđević, V.B., Zdunić, G.M. et al. (2017). Optimization of the extraction process of polyphenols from Thymus serpyllum L. herb using maceration, heat- and ultrasound-assisted techniques. *Separation and Purification Technology* 179: 369–380.

Kang, S.H., Kim, J.H., and Mun, S. (2010). Optimal design of a tandem simulated moving bed process for separation of paclitaxel, 13-dehydroxybaccatin III, and 10-deacetylpaclitaxel. *Process Biochemistry* 45 (9): 1468–1476.

Kaufmann, B. and Christen, P. (2002). Recent extraction techniques for natural products: microwaveassisted extraction and pressurized solvent extraction. *Phytochemical Analysis* 13 (2): 105–113.

Kemp, W. (1991). Infrared spectroscopy. In: *Organic Spectroscopy*, 19–56. London, UK: Macmillan Press Ltd.

Koh, G.Y., Chou, G., and Liu, Z.P. (2009). Purification of a water extract of Chinese sweet tea plant (Rubus suavissimus S. lee) by alcohol precipitation. *Journal of Agricultural and Food Chemistry* 57: 5000–5006. https://doi.org/10.1021/jf900269r.

Lapkin, A., Plucinski, P.K., and Cutler, M. (2006). Comparative assessment of technologies for extraction of artemisinin. *Journal of Natural Products* 69: 1653–1664.

Latif, S. and Anwar, F. (2009). Physicochemical studies of hemp (Cannabis sativa) seed oil using enzyme-assisted cold-pressing. *European Journal of Lipid Science and Technology* 111 (10): 1042–1048.

Li, J., Mao, C., Li, L. et al. (2014b). Pharmacokinetics and liver distribution study of unbound curdione and curcumol in rats by microdialysis coupled with rapid resolution liquid chromatography (RRLC) and tandem mass spectrometry. *Journal of Pharmaceutical and Biomedical Analysis* 95: 146–150.

Li, J.X. and Yu, Z.Y. (2006). Cimicifugaerhizoma: from origins, bioactive constituents to clinical outcomes. *Current Medicinal Chemistry* 13 (27): 2927–2951.

Li, K., Xing, R., Liu, S. et al. (2012). Separation of chito-oligomers with several degrees of polymerization and study of their antioxidant activity. *Carbohydrate Polymers* 88 (3): 896–903. https://doi. org/10.1016/j.carbpol.2012.01.033.

Li, P., Xu, G., Li, S.P. et al. (2008). Optimizing ultra performance liquid chromatographic analysis of 10 diterpenoid compounds in Salvia miltiorrhiza using central composite design. *Journal of Agricultural and Food Chemistry* 56 (4): 1164–1171.

Li, P., Yin, Z.Q., Li, S.L. et al. (2014a). Simultaneous determination of eight flavonoids and pogostone in Pogostemon cablin by high performance liquid chromatography. *Journal of Liquid Chromatography & Related Technologies* 37 (12): 1771–1784.

Li, Y., Li, S., Lin, S.-J. et al. (2017). Microwave-assisted extraction of natural antioxidants from the Exotic Gordonia axillaris fruit: optimization and identification of phenolic compounds. *Molecules* 22: 1481. https://doi.org/10.3390/ molecules22091481.

Liang, M.T., Liang, R.C., Yu, S.Q., and Yan, R.A. (2013). Separation of resveratrol and emodin by supercritical fluid-simulated moving bed chromatography. *Journal of Chromatography and Separation Techniques* 4 (3): 1000175.

Liao, J.F., Jan, Y.M., Huang, S.Y. et al. (1995). Evaluation with receptor binding assay on the water extracts of ten CNS-active Chinese herbal drugs. *Proceedings of the National Science Council, Republic of China* 19 (3): 151–158.

Lim, K.H. and Kam, T.S. (2008). Methyl chanofruticosinate alkaloids from Kopsia arborea. *Phytochemistry* 69 (2): 558–561.

Liu, Z.-W., Zeng, X.-A., and Ngadi, M. (2018). Enhanced extraction of phenolic compounds from onion by pulsed electric field (PEF). *Journal of Food Processing and Preservation* 42 (9): e13755.

Lv, G.P., Huang, W.H., Yang, F.Q. et al. (2010). Pressurized liquid extraction and GC–MS analysis for simultaneous determination of seven components in Cinnamomum cassia and the effect of sample preparation. *Journal of Separation Science* 33 (15): 2341–2348. https://doi.org/10.1002/ jssc.201000208.

Ma, X., Meng, Z., Qiu, L. et al. (2016). Solanesol extraction from tobacco leaves by Flash chromatography based on molecularly imprinted polymers. *Journal of Chromatography B* 1020: 1–5.

Marchev, A., Ivanov, I., Vrancheva, R., and Pavlov, A. (2013). Solid phase extraction and HPLC determination of phloridzin in natural products. *Bulgarian Journal of Agricultural Science Supplement* 19 (2): 201–203.

Martínez, J.M., Delso, C., Álvarez, I., and Raso, J. (2020). Pulsed electric field-assisted extraction of valuable compounds from microorganisms. *Comprehensive Reviews in Food Science and Food Safety* 19 (2): 530–552. https://doi.org/10.1111/1541-4337.12512.

Meng, F.C., Wu, Q.S., Wang, R. et al. (2017). A novel strategy for quantitative analysis of major ginsenosides in Panacis Japonici Rhizoma with a standardized reference fraction. *Molecules* 22 (12): 2067.

Nie, L., Dai, Z., and Ma, S. (2016). Improved chiral separation of (R, S)-goitrin by SFC: an application in traditional Chinese medicine. *Journal of Analytical Methods in Chemistry* 5: 2016.

Niranjan, K. and Hanmoungjai, P. (2004). Enzyme-aided aquous extraction. In: *Nutritionally Enhanced Edible Oil Processing* (ed. N.T. Dunford and H.B. Dunford). AOCS Publishing.

Njila, N.I.M., Mahdi, E., and Lembe, M.D. et al. (2017). Review on extraction and isolation of plant secondary metabolites. *7th Int'l Conference on Agricultural, Chemical, Biological and Environmental Sciences*, pp. 67–72. doi: 10.15242/IIE.C051720.

Okinyo-Owiti, D.P., Burnett, P.G.G., and Reaney, M.J.T. (2014). Simulated moving bed purification of flaxseed oil orbitides: unprecedented separation of cyclolinopeptides C and E. *Journal of Chromatography B* 965: 231–237.

Okonkwo, C.O. and Ohaeri, O.C. (2020). Comparative study of steam distillation and soxhlet for the extraction of botanical oils. *Asian Journal of Biological Sciences* 13: 62–69.

Ozek, T. and Demirci, F. (2012). Isolation of natural products by preparative gas chromatography. *Methods in Molecular Biology* 864: 275–300.

Pandey, A. and Tripathi, S. (2001). Concept of standardization, extraction and pre phytochemical screening strategies for herbal drug. *Journal of Pharmacognosy and Phytochemistry* 2 (5): 115–119.

Panto, S., Sciarrone, D., Maimone, M. et al. (2015). Performance evaluation of a versatile multidimensional chromatographic preparative system based on three-dimensional gas chromatography and liquid chromatography-two-dimensional gas chromatography for the collection of volatile constituents. *Journal of Chromatography A* 1417: 96–103.

Park, S.Y., Kim, Y.S., Ahn, C.B., and Je, J.Y. (2016). Partial purification and identification of three antioxidant peptides with hepatoprotective effects from blue mussel (Mytilus edulis) hydrolysate by peptic hydrolysis. *Journal of Functional Foods* 20: 88–95. https://doi.org/10.1016/j.jff.2015.10.023.

Patil, P.S. and Shettigar, R. (2010). An advancement of analytical techniques in herbal research. *Journal of Advanced Scientific Research* 1 (1): 8–14.

Poole, C.F. (2018). Chromatographic test methods for characterizing alkylsiloxane-bonded silica columns for reversed-phase liquid chromatography. *Journal of Chromatography B* 1092: 207–219. https://doi.org/10.1016/j.jchromb.2018.06.011.

Popova, I.E., Hall, C., and Kubátová, A. (2008). Determination of lignans in flaxseed using liquid chromatography with time-of-flight mass spectrometry. *Journal of Chromatography A* 1216 (2): 217–229. https://doi.org/10.1016/j.chroma.11.063.

Popova, I.E., Hall, C., and Kubátová, A. (2009). Determination of lignans in flaxseed using liquid chromatography with time-of-flight mass spectrometry. *Journal of Chromatography A* 1216 (2): 217–229.

Porath, J. (1997). From gel filtration to adsorptive size exclusion. *Journal of Protein Chemistry* 16: 463–468.

Puértolas, E., López, N., Saldaňa, G. et al. (2010). Evaluation of phenolic extraction during fermentation of red grapes treated by a continuous pulsed electric fields process at pilot-plant scale. *Journal of Food Engineering* 119 (3): 1063–1070.

Puri, M., Sharma, D., and Barrow, C.J. (2012). Enzyme-assisted extraction of bioactives from plants. *Trends in Biotechnology* 30 (1): 37–44.

Quiroz, J.Q., Duran, A.M.N., Garcia, M.S. et al. (2019). Ultrasound-assisted extraction of bioactive compounds from annatto seeds, evaluation of their antimicrobial and antioxidant activity, and identification of main compounds by LC/ESI-MS. *Analysis International Journal of Food Science.* https://doi.org/10.1155/2019/3721828.

Rathi, B.S., Bodhankar, S.L., and Baheti, A.M. (2006). Evaluation of aqueousleaves extract of Moringaoleifera Linn for wound healing in albino rats. *Indian Journal of Experimental Biology* 44: 898–901.

Reyes, L.H., Mar, J.L., Rahman, G.M. et al. (2009). Simultaneous determination of arsenic and selenium species in fish tissues using microwave-assisted enzymatic extraction and ion chromatography-inductively coupled plasma mass spectrometry. *Talanta* 78 (3): 983–990.

Richter, B.E., Jones, B.A., Ezzell, J.L. et al. (1996). Accelerated solvent extraction: a technology for sample preparation. *Analytical Chemistry* 68 (6): 1033–1039.

Riss, T.L., Moravec, R.A., Niles, A.L. et al. (2016). Cell viability assays. In: *Assay Guidance Manual* (ed. S. Markossian, G.S. Sittampalam, A. Grossman, et al.). Bethesda, MD: Eli Lilly & Company and the National Center for Advancing Translational Sciences.

Rizzetti, T.M., de Souza, M.P., Prestes, O.D. et al. (2017). A simple and fast method for the determination of 20 veterinary drug residues in bovine kidney and liver by ultra-highperformance liquid chromatography tandem mass spectrometry. *Food Analytical Methods* 10 (4): 854–864. https://doi.org/10.1007/s12161-016-0649-5.

Rosenthal, A., Pyle, D.L., Niranjan, K. et al. (2001). Combined effect of operational variables and enzyme activity on aqueous enzymatic extraction of oil and protein from soybean. *Enzyme and Microbial Technology* 28 (6): 499–509.

Saad, N., Louvet, F., Tarrade, S., et al. (2019). Enzyme-assisted extraction of bioactive compounds from Raspberry (Rubus idaeus L.) Pomace. *Journal of Food Science* 84 (6): 1371–1381. https://doi.org/10.1111/ 1750-3841.14625.

Sciarrone, D., Panto, S., Donato, P., and Mondello, L. (2016). Improving the productivity of a multidimensional chromatographic preparative system by collecting pure chemicals after each of three chromatographic dimensions. *Journal of Chromatography A* 1475: 80–85.

Sciarrone, D., Panto, S., Rotondo, A. et al. (2013). Rapid collection and identification of a novel component from Clausena lansium Skeels leaves by means of three-dimensional preparative gas chromatography and nuclear magnetic resonance/infrared/mass spectrometric analysis. *Analytica Chimica Acta* 785: 119–125.

Sharma, A., Khare, S.K., and Gupta, M.N. (2002). Enzyme-assisted aqueous extraction of peanut oil. *Journal of American Oil Chemist's Society* 79 (3): 215–218.

Speybrouck, D. and Lipka, E. (2016). Preparative supercritical fluid chromatography: a powerful tool for chiral separations. *Journal of Chromatography A* 1467: 33–55.

Tahara, S., Yamamoto, S., Yamajima, Y. et al. (2017). A rapid dialysis method for analysis of artificial sweeteners in foods (2nd report). *Shokuhin Eiseigaku Zasshi* 58 (3): 124–131. https://doi.org/10.3358/shokueishi.58.124.

Tenon, M., Feuillère, N., Roller, M., and Birtić, S. (2017). Rapid, cost-effective and accurate quantification of Yucca schidigera Roezl. steroidal saponins using HPLC-ELSD method. *Food Chemistry* 221: 1245–1252.

Tonthubthimthong, P., Chuaprasert, S., Douglas, P., and Luewisutthichat, W. (2011). Supercritical CO_2 extraction of nimbin from neem seeds an experimental study. *Journal of Food Engineering* 47 (4): 289–293. https://doi.org/10.1016/S0260-8774(00)00131-X.

Trusheva, B., Trunkova, D., and Bankova, V. (2007). Different extraction methods of biologically active components from propolis: a preliminary study. *Chemistry Central Journal* 1 (13). https://doi.org/10.1186/1752-153X-1-13.

Tsiaka, T., Zoumpoulakis, P., Sinanoglou, V.J. et al. (2015). Response surface methodology toward the optimization of high-energy carotenoid extraction from Aristeus antennatus shrimp. *Analytica Chimica Acta* 877: 100–110.

Urbano, M., Luque de Castro, M.D., Pérez, P.M. et al. (2006). Ultraviolet–visible spectroscopy and pattern recognition methods for differentiation and classification of wines. *Food Chemistry* 97: 166–175. https://doi.org/10.1016/j.foodchem.2005.05.001.

Vidyadhar, S., Saidulu, M., Gopal, T.K. et al. (2010). in vitro anthelmintic activity of the whole plant of Enicostemmalittorale by using various extracts. *International Journal of Applied Biology and Pharmaceutical Technology* 1 (3): 1119–1125.

Xiong, Y., Zhao, Z., Zhu, L. et al. (2013). Removal of three kinds of phthalates from sweet orange oil by molecular distillation. *LWT –Food Science and Technology* 53 (2): 487–491.

Yahya, A. and Yunus, R.M. (2013). Influence of sample preparation and extraction time on chemical composition of steam distillation derived patchouli oil. *Procedia Engineering* 53: 1–6.

Yang, F.Q., Wang, H.K., Chen, H. et al. (2011). Fractionation of volatile constituents from Curcuma rhizome by preparative gas chromatography. *Journal of Automated Methods & Management in Chemistry* 2011: 942467.

Yang, W., Zhang, Y., Pan, H. et al. (2017). Supercritical fluid chromatography for separation and preparation of tautomeric 7-epimeric spiro oxindole alkaloids from Uncaria macrophylla. *Journal of Pharmaceutical and Biomedical Analysis* 134: 352–360.

Yazdi, A.P.G., Barzegar, M., Sahari, M.A., and Gavlighi, H.A. (2019). Optimization of the enzymeassisted aqueous extraction of phenolic compounds from pistachio green hull. *Food Science & Nutrition* 7 (1): 356–366. https://doi.org/10.1002/fsn3.900.

Yi, Y., Zhang, Q.W., Li, S.L. et al. (2012). Simultaneous quantification of major flavonoids in "Bawanghua", the edible flower of Hylocereus undatus using pressurised liquid extraction and high performance liquid chromatography. *Food Chemistry* 135 (2): 528–533.

You, Q., Zhang, Y., Zhang, Q. et al. (2014). High-capacity thermo-responsive magnetic molecularly imprinted polymers for selective extraction of curcuminoids. *Journal of Chromatography A* 1354: 1–8.

Yuan, Y. and Macquarrie, D. (2015). Microwave assisted extraction of sulfated polysaccharides (fucoidan) from Ascophyllum nodosum and its antioxidant activity. *Carbohydrate Polymers* 129: 101–107.

Yusof, N.A., Beyan, A., Haron, J., and Ibrahim, N.A. (2010). Synthesis and characterisation of a molecularly imprinted polymer for Pb2+ uptake using 2-vinylpyridine as the complexing monomer. *Sains Malaysiana* 39 (5): 829–835.

Zhang, H., Wang, W., Fu, Z.M. et al. (2014). Study on comparison of extracting fucoxanthin from Undaria pinnatifida with percolation extraction and refluxing methods. *Zhongguo Shipin Tianjiaji* 9: 91–95.

Zhang, L. (2013). Comparison of extraction effect of active ingredients in traditional Chinese medicine compound preparation with two different method. *Heilongjiang Xumu Shouyi* 9: 132–133.

Zhang, W.Q., Lin, G.L., and Ye, C.W. (2018). Techniques for extraction and isolation of natural products: a comprehensive review. *Chinese Medicine* 13 (20): 1–26. https://doi.org/10.1186/s13020-018-0177-x.

Zhao, Y., McCauley, J., Pang, X. et al. (2013). Analytical and semipreparative separation of 25 (R/S)-spirostanol saponin diastereomers using supercritical fluid chromatography. *Journal of Separation Science* 36 (19): 3270–3276.

Zhou, Y.Q., Zhang, Q.W., Li, S.L. et al. (2012). Quality evaluation of semen oroxyli through simultaneous quantification of 13 components by high performance liquid chromatography. *Current Pharmaceutical Analysis* 8 (2): 206–213.

Zuo, H.-L., Yang, F.-Q., Huang, W.-H., and Xia, Z.-N. (2012a). Preparative gas chromatography and its applications. *Journal of Chromatographic Science* 1–12. https://doi.org/10.1093/ chromsci/bmt040.

Zuo, H.L., Yang, F.Q., Zhang, X.M., and Xia, Z.N. (2012b). Separation of cis- and trans-Asarone from Acorus tatarinowii by preparative gas chromatography. *Journal of Analytical Methods in Chemistry* 5. https://doi.org/10.1155/2012/402081.

Żwir-Ferenc, A. and Biziuk, M. (2006). Solid phase extraction technique – trends, opportunities and applications. *Polish Journal of Environmental Studies* 15 (5): 677–690.

7

Health Benefits of Turmeric and Ginger

Jean Claude Dusabumuremyi[1], Emmanuel Duhoranimana[1], and Xiao Chen[2]

[1] Department of Biotechnologies, Faculty of Applied Fundamental Sciences, Institutes of Applied Sciences, INES-Ruhengeri, Ruhengeri, Republic of Rwanda
[2] School of Chemical Sciences, University of Auckland, Auckland, New Zealand

7.1   Introduction

Ginger (*Zingiber officinale* Rosc.) is a spicy plant that belongs to the same family (Zingiberaceae) as turmeric and cardamom. Ginger is one of most important spices all over the world and cultivated in almost tropical and subtropical countries, where its majority is produced in India (Sangwan et al. 2012; Tanaka et al. 2015). Even if ginger grows in those countries, it grows well in medium temperate regions in the world. Many countries in the world especially in Asia such as India, China, and Japan, people hugely utilize ginger as both food and medical substances for many diseases.

Concerning its health benefits, ginger is used as drug for colds, cough, vomiting, dizziness, hypertension, impaired vision problems, fever, and stomach diseases, and it is used to remove mucus in the body for a long time and helps to protect human health, among others (Lete and Allué 2016; Shaban et al. 2017). The consumption of ginger is high in many parts of the world, and this is attributed to its high phytochemical compositions that are considered potential antioxidants that allow it to play a big importance in human life (Shukla and Singh 2007). These phytochemical compositions are divided into two categories those of which are volatiles and nonvolatiles, which separately play different roles in human life.

The volatiles include sesquiterpene and monoterpenoid hydrocarbon categories and are responsible for distinct aroma and taste of ginger, while nonvolatile include gingerols, shogaols, paradols, and zingerone, which are accountable for the warm and pungent sensation in the human mouth (Jolad et al. 2004).

Ginger can be processed into many products that are used in many forms of foods and that many people get used because of many reasons including its therapeutic effect in human body. These products include the fresh ginger that can be taken to cure the nausea and vomiting (Lete and Allué 2016), dried ginger powder that is used as spices for curing throat inflammation, and reduce gastritis (Nikkhah Bodagh et al. 2019), while its extracted oil and extracts are used in ginger wine, ginger nonalcoholic beverage beer, juice, tea, among others (Sci et al. 2014; Ade-Omowaye et al. 2015; Jangra et al. 2018). In many countries all over the world, ginger is used as one of the ingredients in the production of biscuits, cakes, soup, and pickle (Adebayo-oyetoro et al. 2016).

Turmeric (*Curcuma longa*) is a rhizomatous herbaceous perennial plant that belongs to Zingiberaceae family. Turmeric provides a bright yellow to orange spice that is produced from its dried and ground underground rhizome and responsible for flavor and color (Benzie and Wachtel-Galor 2011; Rajkumari and Sanatombi 2018). It is also used as aroma and flavor enhancers due to its curcuma, with slightly peppery and bitter and with a subtle ginger taste. In addition, it has natural phytochemical compositions called curcuminoids, which is mostly in the form of curcumin as active ingredient in turmeric.

The health benefits induced by antioxidants, antimicrobial, and anti-inflammatory activity of turmeric are due to its phytochemical compositions such as curcumin, alkaloid, saponin, tannin, sterol, phytic acid, flavonoid, and phenols (Ikpeama et al. 2014; Mughal 2019). Turmeric can be processed into important ingredients that have significant role in human body and food products. It is with concerns that it can be transformed into powder that is used as spice and contributed as food preservatives, flavoring agent, and household remedy for treatment of many diseases (Al-Reza et al. 2010; Xiang et al. 2011).

Basing on the turmeric phytochemicals, it is traditionally used to cure the following diseases: gastrointestinal diseases, especially for biliary and hepatic disorder, diabetic wounds, rheumatism, inflammation, sinusitis, anorexia, coryza, and cough. Based on traditional medicinal uses of turmeric, it acts as anticancer, antidiabetic, antioxidant, hypolipidemic, anti-inflammatory, antimicrobial, antifertility, antivenom, hepatoprotective, nephroprotective, anticoagulant, among others (Akram et al. 2010; Chanda and Ramachandra 2019).

Apart from its traditional medicinal uses, it is nutritionally rich in starch, carbohydrates, proteins, fats, vitamins, and minerals (Suphrom et al. 2012; Rajkumari and Sanatombi 2018). Therefore, turmeric can be produced into a range of products that can nutritionally support human health. This chapter is aimed at exploring health benefit of ginger and turmeric in human body and in food products.

7.2 Nutritional Content of Ginger

Ginger plant is made of different parts that are used depending on its nutritional content. The main part that is used as spice on the plant itself is called the rhizomes or ginger root. This root is processed in different forms and used in food products. For instance, in western countries cuisine, ginger is processed into ginger cake, ginger snaps, gingerbread, ginger biscuits, and ginger ale, among others. Ginger rhizome is also produced into powder, which can also be added in different products in order to increase the flavor, color, antioxidant properties, antimicrobial properties, and nutritional content of desired food products. In terms of nutritional compositions, ginger rhizome contains different minerals in different proportions such as vitamins (β-carotene, vitamin C), carbohydrates, fats, proteins, and water. On basis of mineral content, ginger root powder was reported to have the following predominant mineral elements: zinc, manganese, copper, calcium, iron, sodium, phosphorus, and potassium; it contains also crude fibers (10.36%), ash (6.57%), ether extract (6.48%), nitrogen-free extract (64.82%), and crude proteins (5.45%) (Ogbuewu et al. 2014).

The nutrition composition may vary depending on the processing method used. For instance, if the ginger root is dried under different drying conditions such as shade, solar, oven, and microwave. Several research studies showed the ranges of ginger nutrients under drying conditions.

These include proteins, crude fibers, fats, and ash contents ranged from 5.02 to 5.82, 4.97 to 5.61, 0.76 to 0.90, and 3.38 to 3.66%, respectively (Broad et al. 2004). In terms of vitamin content, ginger is highly rich in β-carotene and ascorbic acid content in the following proportions 0.81 mg/100 g and 3.83 mg/100 g, respectively (Sangwan et al. 2014). The nutritional content indicate that ginger can be used as functional food and dietary supplements so that it can be used to prevent some micronutrient deficiency diseases.

7.3 Antioxidant Properties of Ginger

Antioxidant are very important for human body as they help it to prevent oxidative stress that normally led the imbalanced formation of reactive oxygen species as one source of several diseases such as cancer, heart diseases, neurodegenerative diseases, among others, and prolonged antioxidant defense system (Malaysiana et al. 2015). This imbalanced condition results in the formation of free radicals such as superoxide radicals and hydrogen peroxide, which are destructive to human body cells, especially in a hepatoma cell line (Line et al. 2005). Consumption of food with antioxidant prevent and reduce the destruction of cells in different ways and enhance the normal function of the cells.

Ginger root is reported to possess high level of antioxidants that are used to protect the formation of different kind of free radicals and protect cell membrane lipids from oxidation activity (Pangastuti and Maret 2018). Several studies showed that ginger antioxidants reduce the formation of lipid peroxidation in human and rat (Pangastuti and Maret 2018). It has been revealed that ginger antioxidant capacity to be comparable to ascorbic acid capacity. To play such role in human body, ginger root contains active compound called 6-gingerol as one type of gingerols that are responsible for pungency characteristics. This active compound of ginger has strong antioxidant capacity to prevent and treat different diseases (Ali et al. 2008).

It has been revealed that ginger antioxidant properties have the potential to increase antioxidant enzyme blood levels such as CuZn-superoxide dismutase and catalase activity, and levels of glutathione peroxidase and total glutathione and decrease oxidative stress blood levels such as malondialdehyde and NO_2-/NO_3 that are capable of providing high levels of reactive oxygen species (Kuhad et al. 2006; Danwilai et al. 2017). Besides, the animal studies was conducted to explore the power of ginger and revealed that ginger 6-gingerol active compound has the capacity to protect kidney against harmful effects and cisplatin-induced oxidative stress in Wistar rats (Kuhad et al. 2006). The extracted ginger ethanol indicated its capacity to protect acute renal damage and cisplatin induced in mice (Danwilai et al. 2017).

The study conducted by Jolad et al. (2004) on antioxidant activity of ginger revealed that ginger has antioxidant activity in cancer patients receiving chemotherapy. Several studies explored the antioxidant power of ginger and showed that it can be used to alleviate nausea and vomiting, especially in patients receiving adjuvant chemotherapy (Thamlikitkul et al. 2017), and found to strongly prevent postoperative nausea and vomiting during pregnancy (Chaiyakunapruk et al. 2006; Thomson et al. 2014). Ginger supplementation also was found to effectively reduce severity of acute chemotherapy-induced nausea (Konmun et al. 2017).

As ginger has the capacity to reduce the level of oxidative stress, it can also prevent inflammation using two active compounds, 6-gingerol and 6-shogaol. It is known that the oxidative stress and inflammation are the main factors that lead to aging and the development of degenerative diseases; the ginger active compounds are able to counteract these processes (Fatin et al. 2019). As most of pathogenesis of different aging related and degenerative diseases such as arthritis and rheumatism, Alzheimer's disease, Parkinson's disease, atherosclerosis, cardiovascular disease, hypertension, and type 2 diabetes mellitus are caused by oxidative stress and inflammation, the use of antioxidant, and anti-inflammation-rich ingredients like ginger, can significantly lead to prevention and treatment of these diseases (Campisi et al. 2011; Shidfar et al. 2015; Tosukhowong et al. 2016; Stambler 2017). In addition, ginger also is used to treat many diseases including migraine (Maghbooli et al. 2014).

The study conducted by Mahluji et al. (2013) reported that ginger antioxidant effect reduces insulin resistance in diabetes by improving glucose transport activity and enhance glucose tolerance. In animal study, antioxidant properties of ginger were proven to decreasing cholesterol, serum glucose, and triacylglycerol, urine protein levels and to cause hypoglycemia, hypocholesterolemia, and hypolipidemia (Al-amin et al. 2006).

Thus, ginger is a good source of potential antioxidants that can be used to prevent and cure different human diseases.

7.4 Antimicrobial Properties of Ginger

Ginger antibacterial activity is different depending on the used extraction method and part of ginger that has been used. For instance, alcohol extract of ginger root exhibits higher antimicrobial effect than alcohol extract of its leaves and water extract of ginger root (Sebiomo et al. 2011). Several studies have proven the ginger extracts to have antimicrobial activity against fungal, and both gram-negative and gram-positive bacteria. The study conducted by Zainal-abidin et al. (2017) on in vitro antibacterial activity of ginger and *Orthosiphon stamineus* showed a great effect against gram-positive Enterococcus. Another study conducted by Sebiomo et al. (2011) also proven the ginger extracts to inhibit and eliminate the gram-positive bacteria *Staphylococcus aureus* and *Streptococcus pyogenes*. In addition, the ginger has antibacterial activities to effectively kill *Pseudomans aeruginosa* in human body and inhibiting the biofilm formation (Chakotiya et al. 2017). The ginger extracts showed also its potential to kill microorganism that can spoil foods and lead to food-borne illness. Therefore, ginger ingredients can be used to preserve food products.

7.4.1 Anti-inflammatory Activities of Ginger

As the inflammation is one of the sources of some pathogenesis of various diseases, ginger has the antioxidant properties and anti-inflammatory activity that inhibit the cyclooxygenase-2 and reduce the inflammatory signals such as nuclear factor TNF-α and IL-β (Mozaffari-khosravi et al. 2016).

7.4.2 Neuroprotective Activity of Ginger

Several studies were conducted on potential of ginger polyphenol compounds in reducing neurotoxic effect. The study carried out by El-akabawy and El-kholy (2014), showed the beneficial effects of ginger active compounds in reducing the oxidative stress as one of the causes of neuronal damage, inflammation, and apoptosis in human brain of people with diabetes. These antioxidants of ginger were also confirmed by the study conduct by Baluchnejadmojarad and Roghani (2011). In addition to this study, it showed the antioxidant activity of this spicy plant capable of protecting neurons against a variety of experimental neurodegenerative conditions.

7.5 Nutritional Content of *Curcumin Longa*

Like ginger, turmeric is a medicinal plant that botanically belongs to Zingiberacea family and exhibits the differences among other spicy plants in the same family (Chattopadhyay et al. 2004). It is highly known as spice, color enhancer due to its curcuminoids and much known because of its medicinal properties for curing different diseases (Luthra et al. 2001). Turmeric is consumed in both tropical and subtropical countries, especially in Africa because turmeric is highly nutritious and have different active compounds, which play a big role in treating different diseases. Turmeric like other medicinal plants, it is rich in vitamins, minerals, water, carbohydrates, proteins, and fats. The studies conducted by Ikpeama et al. (2014) and Mughal (2019) revealed that turmeric possess beta-carotene, provitamin C, and contains some polyphenols that are highly connected with fatty acid and essential oil. Another study reported that turmeric is highly rich in carbohydrates, proteins, and minerals, which can increase its chance to be used as one of food supplement (Sánchez-andica and Cauca-colombia 2020). The rhizome of turmeric was found to have new carbohydrates such as stigmasterole, β-sitosterole, cholesterol, and 2-hydroxymethyl anthraquinone (Kapoor 2001).

Furthermore, the fiber content of turmeric is very important in human body as it contributes to the removal of carcinogens from digestive tract, prevention of excess intake of cholesterol. Importantly, turmeric dietary fiber contributes to addition of bulk of the food and prevents the intake of excessive starchy foods as result of preventing hypercholesterolemia and diabetes mellitus, among others (Okwu and Josiah 2006). In addition, turmeric contains minerals such as 0.20% calcium, 0.63% phosphorus, 0.46% potassium, and 0.05% iron (Sánchez-andica and Cauca-colombia 2020).

Regular consumption of turmeric is very important as its mineral content helps in strengthening the bones, allows muscle contraction and relaxation, reduction in blood pressure, and maintenance of hemoglobin formation due to its iron content. Therefore, turmeric can be used to treat anemia (Peschel et al. 2007). Due to the nutritional content of turmeric plant, it can be used as functional food and dietary supplements, which can reduce the main human diseases and enhance consumer healthy.

7.6 Antioxidant Properties of Turmeric

Some health-related diseases are cured by the presence of biologically active compounds such as carotenoids, polyphenols, and dietary supplements, among others. Different herbs and spices can be used to treat different human diseases due to their specific contained active compounds. Turmeric (*C. longa*) contains curcuminoids that are phenolic compounds, whose main characteristic is curcumin, and different phytochemical compounds in different proportions such as 0.76% alkaloid, 0.45% saponin, 1.08% tannin 0.03% sterol, 0.82% phytic acid, 0.40% flavonoid, and 0.08% phenols (Ikpeama et al. 2014; Mughal 2019). These curcuminoids and phytochemical compositions of turmeric provide different antioxidant properties against different human diseases.

The curcuminoid content of turmeric is mostly present in rhizomes and considered biological active compound of plant (Mesa et al. 2000; Ali et al. 2014), of which curcumin is represented as a combination of three main components such as curcumin (1,7-bis(4-hydroxy-3-methoxyphenyl)-1,6-heptadiene-3,5-dione), dimethoxy-curcumin, and bis-dimethoxy-curcumin. The antioxidant properties of turmeric are due to the contained curcumin component. Curcumin is a polyphenolic component of curcuminoid, which is characterized by the keto and enol groups that it owns (Sánchez-andica and Cauca-colombia 2020). This curcumin is very powerful and is found to be stable at high temperature range and acidic state, but is volatile in alkaline environments, as well as in the presence of heat. Besides, curcumin is soluble in oil and alkali, and at acid and neutral pH, it is virtually insoluble in water (Iniaghe et al. 2009).

Several studies were conducted to explore the antioxidant properties of turmeric plant. It was found that turmeric alkaloids are more effective to treat different diseases such as hypertension-related headaches, colds, and treat chronic migraine while the rest of turmeric phytochemicals such as saponins, flavonoids, and tannins were reported to reduce cholesterol, prevent harmful cytotoxins, enhance sex hormones, and reduce inflammation due to antioxidant properties (Ikpeama et al. 2014). Other studies reported the antioxidant properties of tannins of turmeric to cure some intestinal diseases such as dysentery and diarrhea (Okwu and Josiah 2006; Hewlings & Kalman 2017).

The flavonoid content of turmeric was found to be more powerful in improving human health through absorption of the biological radicals and superoxide anions radicals. Moreover, flavonoids were also reported to show anti-inflammatory, antiangionic, antiallergic effects, analgesic, and antioxidant properties (Bisht et al. 2010; Heeba et al. 2014). The saponins is one of the turmeric phytochemicals. This phytochemical was found to be more helpful in lowering cholesterol and to have a deleterious cytotoxic property like permeabilization of the intestine (Ikpeama et al. 2014). The study conducted on polyphenol content of turmeric explored and revealed that turmeric has capacity to both reduce low-density lipoprotein cholesterol level and increase high-density lipoprotein cholesterol level while also increasing antihypertensive effects (Dinelli et al. 2009; Mughal 2019).

Many studies reported the curcumin of turmeric to be used as an inhibitor as superoxide dismutase to prevent auto-oxidation of epinephrine while producing free antiradical activity (Restrepo-Osorio et al. 2020) and prevent lipid peroxidation and oxidation of food products. This curcumin is also effective in protecting the organism from aging and cell death by oxidative damage while enhancing the repairing and maintenance of biological body structure. It has been reported in many studies that curcumin is able to prevent and reduce the free radical (anions, superoxide, and hydroxyl) formation, which always result in cell damage and influence enzymatic activity due to its antioxidant capacity (Gülçin 2006).

As antioxidant power is attributed to curcumin content in turmeric, this herbaceous and spicy plant is found to be very important in preventing and treating different associated human diseases such as cardiovascular, inflammation suppression, antimicrobial, obesity, tumorigenesis, chronic tiredness, antidepressant and neurological function, anxiety, muscle and bone loss, and neuropathic pain, among others (Stambler 2017).

7.7 Antimicrobial Effect of Turmeric Extract

Antimicrobial activity of turmeric plant was studied by many researchers. This activity is attributed to turmeric polyphenol content and other phytochemical compositions. The polyphenol compounds of this plant are found to be an excellent antioxidant and venotonics, antibacterial, and antifungal tannins that act as natural antibiotics (Mughal 2019). The antimicrobial properties of turmeric extracts were used as antimicrobial agents to inhibit the growth of fungi and bacteria. The study conducted on antimicrobial activity of turmeric indicated that its extracts have inhibitory effects against both gram-negative and gram-positive such as *Bacillus subtilis, P. aeruginosa, S. aureus, Escherichia coli, Aspergillus niger, Penicillium citrinum, Micrococcus,* and *Streptococcus faecalis* (Ikpeama et al. 2014). As the turmeric has the potential of killing different spoilage bacteria and pathogens, its antimicrobial properties can be therefore used to preserve food products.

7.8 Conclusion

Ginger and turmeric are rhizomatous perennial herbs of Zingiberaceae family. These are used as spices and in food applications. Ginger is nutritionally rich in β-carotene, vitamin C, carbohydrates, fats, proteins, crude fibers, and minerals such as zinc, manganese, copper, calcium, iron, sodium, phosphorus, and potassium, while turmeric contains vitamins, minerals, and highly rich in carbohydrates and proteins. In addition, both ginger and turmeric have separate health benefits where they are all used as antioxidants, antimicrobial against fungal infections and both gram-positive and gram-negative bacteria, anti-inflammatory, among others. These antioxidant properties of ginger were found to be attributed to its active compound called 6-gingerol as one type of gingerols, while turmeric antioxidant power comes from curcuminoids to prevent and treat different human diseases. Therefore, ginger and turmeric can be used as functional food, dietary supplements, and for therapeutic purposes.

References

Adebayo-Oyetoro, A.O., Ogundipe, O.O., Azoro, C.G., and Adeyeye, S.A.O. (2016). Production and evaluation of ginger spiced cookies from wheat-plantain composite flour. *Pacific Journal of Science and Technology* 17 (1): 280–287.

Ade-Omowaye, B.I.O., Adedeji, T.O., and Oluwalana, I.B. (2015). The effect of ginger extract on the acceptability and storability of a non-alcoholic beverage (sorghum stem sheath drink) in Nigeria. *Journal of Scientific Research and Reports* 30: 178–184.

Akram, M., Shahab-Uddin, A.A., Usmanghani, K.H.A.N. et al. (2010). Curcuma longa and curcumin: a review article. *Romanian Journal of Biology – Plant Biology* 55 (2): 65–70.

Al-Amin, Z.M., Thomson, M., Al-Qattan, K.K. et al. (2006). Anti-diabetic and hypolipidaemic properties of ginger (*Zingiber officinale*) in streptozotocin-induced diabetic rats. *British Journal of Nutrition* 96 (4): 660–666.

Ali, B.H., Blunden, G., Tanira, M.O., and Nemmar, A. (2008). Some phytochemical, pharmacological and toxicological properties of ginger (*Zingiber officinale Roscoe*): a review of recent research. *Food and Chemical Toxicology* 46 (2): 409–420.

Ali, S., Sagheer, M., Hassan, M. et al. (2014). Insecticidal activity of turmeric (*Curcuma longa*) and garlic (*Allium sativum*) extracts against red flour beetle, *Tribolium castaneum*: a safe alternative to insecticides in stored commodities. *Journal of Entomology and Zoology Studies* 2 (3): 201–205.

Al-Reza, S.M., Rahman, A., Sattar, M.A. et al. (2010). Essential oil composition and antioxidant activities of *Curcuma aromatica* Salisb. *Food and Chemical Toxicology* 48 (6): 1757–1760.

Baluchnejadmojarad, T. and Roghani, M. (2011). Chronic epigallocatechin-3-gallate ameliorates learning and memory deficits in diabetic rats via modulation of nitric oxide and oxidative stress. *Behavioural Brain Research* 224 (2): 305–310.

Benzie, I.F. and Wachtel-Galor, S. (ed.) (2011). *Herbal Medicine: Biomolecular and Clinical Aspects.* CRC Press.

Bisht, K., Wagner, K.H., and Bulmer, A.C. (2010). Curcumin, resveratrol and flavonoids as anti-inflammatory, cyto-and DNA-protective dietary compounds. *Toxicology* 278 (1): 88–100.

Broad, B., Cho-cho, C., Double, C. et al. (2004). *Nutritive Value of Indian Foods*, vol. 2004, 1–2. Hyderabad: National Institute of Nutrition, ICMR.

Campisi, J., Andersen, J.K., Kapahi, P., and Melov, S. (2011). Cellular senescence: a link between cancer and age-related degenerative disease? *Seminars in Cancer Biology* 21 (6): 354–359.

Chaiyakunapruk, N., Kitikannakorn, N., Nathisuwan, S. et al. (2006). The efficacy of ginger for the prevention of postoperative nausea and vomiting: a meta-analysis. *American Journal of Obstetrics and Gynecology* 194 (1): 95–99.

Chakotiya, A.S., Tanwar, A., Narula, A., and Sharma, R.K. (2017). *Zingiber officinale*: its antibacterial activity on Pseudomonas aeruginosa and mode of action evaluated by flow cytometry. *Microbial Pathogenesis* 107: 254–260.

Chanda, S. and Ramachandra, T.V. (2019). Phytochemical and pharmacological importance of turmeric (*Curcuma longa*): a review. *Research & Reviews: A Journal of Pharmacology* 9 (1): 16–23.

Chattopadhyay, I., Biswas, K., Bandyopadhyay, U., and Banerjee, R.K. (2004). Turmeric and curcumin: biological actions and medicinal applications. *Current Science* 87 (1): 44–53.

Danwilai, K., Konmun, J., Sripanidkulchai, B.O., and Subongkot, S. (2017). Antioxidant activity of ginger extract as a daily supplement in cancer patients receiving adjuvant chemotherapy: a pilot study. *Cancer Management and Research* 9: 11–18.

Dinelli, G., Marotti, I., Bosi, S. et al. (2009). Physiologically bioactive compounds of functional foods, herbs, and dietary supplements. *Advances in Food Biochemistry* 1–52.

El-Akabawy, G. and El-Kholy, W. (2014). Neuroprotective effect of ginger in the brain of streptozotocin-induced diabetic rats. *Annals of Anatomy-Anatomischer Anzeiger* 196 (2-3): 119–128.

Fatin, N., Mohd, N., and Makpol, S. (2019). Ginger (*Zingiber officinale Roscoe*) in the prevention of ageing and degenerative diseases: evidence based complement. *Alternative Medicine* 2019: 5054395.

Gülçin, İ. (2006). Antioxidant and antiradical activities of L-carnitine. *Life Sciences* 78 (8): 803–811.

Heeba, G.H., Mahmoud, M.E., and Hanafy, A.A.E. (2014). Anti-inflammatory potential of curcumin and quercetin in rats: role of oxidative stress, heme oxygenase-1 and TNF-α. *Toxicology and Industrial Health* 30 (6): 551–560.

Hewlings, S.J. and Kalman, D.S. (2017). Curcumin: a review of its effects on human health. *Foods* 6 (10): 92.

Ikpeama, A., Onwuka, G.I., and Nwankwo, C. (2014). Nutritional composition of turmeric (*Curcuma longa*) and its antimicrobial properties. *International Journal of Scientific and Engineering Research* 5 (10): 1085–1089.

Iniaghe, O.M., Malomo, S.O., and Adebayo, J.O. (2009). Proximate composition and phytochemical constituents of leaves of some Acalypha species. *Pakistan Journal of Nutrition* 8 (3): 256–258.

Jangra, M., Jangra, S., and Jain, A. (2018). Production and characterization of wine from ginger, honey and production and characterization of wine from ginger, honey and sugar blends. *Global Journal of Bioscience and Biotechnology* 7 (1): 74–80.

Jolad, S.D., Lantz, R.C., Solyom, A.M. et al. (2004). Fresh organically grown ginger (*Zingiber officinale*): composition and effects on LPS-induced PGE2 production. *Phytochemistry* 65 (13): 1937–1954.

Kapoor, L.D. (2001). *Handbook of Ayurvedic Medicinal Plants*. CRC Press.

Konmun, J., Danwilai, K., Ngamphaiboon, N. et al. (2017). A phase II randomized double-blind placebo-controlled study of 6-gingerol as an anti-emetic in solid tumor patients receiving moderately to highly emetogenic chemotherapy. *Medical Oncology* 34 (4): 1–10.

Kuhad, A., Tirkey, N., Pilkhwal, S., and Chopra, K. (2006). 6-Gingerol prevents cisplatin-induced acute renal failure in rats. *Biofactors* 26 (3): 189–200.

Lete, I. and Allué, J. (2016). The effectiveness of ginger in the prevention of nausea and vomiting during pregnancy and chemotherapy. *Integrative Medicine Insights* 11–17.

Line, H.C., Hanif, H.A., Murad, N.A. et al. (2005). Effects of *Zingiber officinale* on superoxide dismutase, glutathione peroxidase, catalase, glutathione and malondialdehyde content in HepG2 cell line. *Malaysian Journal of Biochemistry and Molecular Biology* 11: 36–41.

Luthra, P.M., Singh, R., and Chandra, R. (2001). Therapeutic uses of *Curcuma longa* (turmeric). *Indian Journal of Clinical Biochemistry* 16 (2): 153–160.

Maghbooli, M., Golipour, F., Moghimi Esfandabadi, A., and Yousefi, M. (2014). Comparison between the efficacy of ginger and sumatriptan in the ablative treatment of the common migraine. *Phytotherapy Research* 28 (3): 412–415.

Mahluji, S., Ostadrahimi, A., Mobasseri, M. et al. (2013). Anti-inflammatory effects of *Zingiber officinale* in type 2 diabetic patients. *Advanced Pharmaceutical Bulletin* 3 (2): 273–276.

Malaysiana, S., Oksidatif, T., and Kajian, S. (2015). Oxidative stress-associated pathology: a review. *Sains Malaysiana* 44 (10): 1441–1451.

Mesa, M.D., Ramírez Tortosa, M.C., Aguilera García, C.M. et al. (2000). Efectos farmacológicos y nutricionales de los extractos de *Curcuma longa* L. y de los cucuminoides. *Ars Pharmaceutica* 41 (3): 307–321.

Mozaffari-Khosravi, H., Naderi, Z., Dehghan, A. et al. (2016). Effect of ginger supplementation on proinflammatory cytokines in older patients with osteoarthritis: outcomes of a randomized controlled clinical trial. *Journal of Nutrition in Gerontology and Geriatrics* 35 (3): 209–218.

Mughal, M.H. (2019). Turmeric polyphenols: a comprehensive review. *Integrative Food, Nutrition and Metabolism* 6: 1–6.

Nikkhah Bodagh, M., Maleki, I., and Hekmatdoost, A. (2019). Ginger in gastrointestinal disorders: a systematic review of clinical trials. *Food Science & Nutrition* 7 (1): 96–108.

Ogbuewu, I.P., Jiwuba, P.D., Ezeokeke, C.T. et al. (2014). Evaluation of phytochemical and nutritional composition of ginger rhizome powder. *International Journal of Agriculture and Rural Development* 17 (1): 1663–1670.

Okwu, D.E. and Josiah, C. (2006). Evaluation of the chemical composition of two Nigerian medicinal plants. *African Journal of Biotechnology.* 5 (4): 357–361.

Pangastuti, A. and Maret, U.S. (2018). Total phenolic content and antioxidant activity of ginger extract and SNEDDS with eel fish bone oil (*Anguilla* spp.). *Nusantara Bioscience* 10: 164–169.

Peschel, D., Koerting, R., and Nass, N. (2007). Curcumin induces changes in expression of genes involved in cholesterol homeostasis. *The Journal of Nutritional Biochemistry* 18 (2): 113–119.

Rajkumari, S. and Sanatombi, K. (2018). Nutritional value, phytochemical composition, and biological activities of edible Curcuma species: a review. *International Journal of Food Properties* 20 (3): S2668–S2687.

Restrepo-Osorio, J., Nobile-Correa, D.P., Zuñiga, O., and Sánchez-Andica, R.A. (2020). Determination of nutritional value of turmeric flour and the antioxidant activity of *Curcuma longa* rhizome extracts from agroecological and conventional crops of Valle del Cauca-Colombia. *Revista Colombiana de Quimica* 49 (1): 26–32.

Sánchez-andica, R.A. and Cauca-colombia, V. (2020). Applied and analytical chemistry determination of nutritional value of turmeric flour and the antioxidant activity of *Curcuma longa* rhizome extracts from agroecological and conventional crops of de cúrcuma y la actividad antioxidante de extractos de culti. *Revista Colombiana de Quimica* 49 (1): 26–32.

Sangwan, A., Kawatra, A., & Sehgal, S. (2014). Nutritional composition of ginger powder prepared using various drying methods. *Journal of Food Science and Technology*, 51(9), 2260–2262. https://doi.org/10.1007/s13197-012-0703-2.

Sangwan, A., Kawatra, A., and Sehgal, S. (2014). Nutritional composition of ginger powder prepared using various drying methods. *Journal of Food Science and Technology* 51 (9): 2260–2262.

Sci, J.E., Resources, N., Ahammed, S. et al. (2014). Processing and preservation of ginger juice. *Journal of Environmental Science and Natural Resources* 7 (1): 117–120.

Sebiomo, A., Awofodu, A.D., Awosanya, A.O. et al. (2011). Comparative studies of antibacterial effect of some antibiotics and ginger (*Zingiber officinale*) on two pathogenic bacteria. *Journal of Microbiology and Antimicrobials* 3 (1): 18–22.

Shaban, M.I., NF, E.L.-G., El-said, A., and El-sol, H. (2017). Ginger: it's effect on blood pressure among hypertensive patients. *IOSR—Journal of Nursing and Health Sciences (IOSR-JNHS)* 6 (5): 79–86.

Shidfar, F., Rajab, A., Rahideh, T. et al. (2015). The effect of ginger (*Zingiber officinale*) on glycemic markers in patients with type 2 diabetes. *Journal of Complementary and Integrative Medicine* 12 (2): 165–170.

Shukla, Y. and Singh, M. (2007). Cancer preventive properties of ginger: a brief review. *Food and Chemical Toxicology* 45 (5): 683–690.

Stambler, I. (2017). Recognizing degenerative aging as a treatable medical condition: methodology and policy. *Aging and Disease* 8 (5): 583–589.

Suphrom, N., Pumthong, G., Khorana, N. et al. (2012). Anti-androgenic effect of sesquiterpenes isolated from the rhizomes of *Curcuma aeruginosa* Roxb. *Fitoterapia* 83 (5): 864–871.

Tanaka, K., Arita, M., Sakurai, H. et al. (2015). Analysis of chemical properties of edible and medicinal ginger by metabolomics approach. *BioMed Research International* 2015: 671058.

Thamlikitkul, L., Srimuninnimit, V., Akewanlop, C. et al. (2017). Efficacy of ginger for prophylaxis of chemotherapy-induced nausea and vomiting in breast cancer patients receiving adriamycin-cyclophosphamide regimen: a randomized, double-blind placebo-controlled, crossover study. *Supportive Care in Cancer* 25 (2): 459–464. https://doi.org/10.1007/s00520-016-3423-8.

Thomson, M., Corbin, R., and Leung, L. (2014). Effects of ginger for nausea and vomiting in early pregnancy: a meta-analysis. *The Journal of the American Board of Family Medicine* 27 (1): 115–122.

Tosukhowong, P., Boonla, C., Dissayabutra, T. et al. (2016). Biochemical and clinical effects of Whey protein supplementation in Parkinson's disease: a pilot study. *Journal of the Neurological Sciences* 367: 162–170. https://doi.org/10.1016/j.jns.2016.05.056.

Xiang, Z., Wang, X.Q., Cai, X.J., and Zeng, S. (2011). Metabolomics study on quality control and discrimination of three *Curcuma* species based on gas chromatograph–mass spectrometry. *Phytochemical Analysis* 22 (5): 411–418.

Zainal-Abidin, Z., Abdul-Wahab, N.A., Ghazi-Ahmad, M.K., and Mohd-Said, S. (2017). In vitro antibacterial activity of *Zingiber officinale* and *Orthosiphon stamineus* on *Enterococcus faecalis*. *Journal of Agricultural Science* 9 (13): 112–121.

8

Carbohydrates, Proteins, and Amino Acids

As Natural Products and Nutraceuticals

S. Sudha, L. Inbathamizh, and D. Prabavathy

Department of Biotechnology, School of Bio and Chemical Engineering, Sathyabama Institute of Science and Technology, Chennai, Tamil Nadu, India

8.1 Introduction

Natural products are compounds produced by living organisms for their own intrinsic function and survival. The evolutionary processes and natural selection have shaped the structural diversity of the natural products with unique biological or pharmacological activities that were used over hundreds of thousands of years. Nutraceuticals are substances that have physiological benefits and provide protection against chronic diseases (Nasri et al. 2014). The broad and diverse range of products within nutraceuticals comprises individual nutrients and biologically active phytochemicals, supplements, functional foods, and herbal products (Gupta et al. 2010). Hasler and Brown (2009) stated that nutraceuticals are products isolated or purified from food, generally sold in medicinal forms not usually associated with food. The success of treatment using natural products is due to the art of balancing the effect of one variety of product with other so that all complement each other. A report stated that 70% of patients normally consult a medical physician before or during traditional therapy, which shows condemnation toward natural therapy (Kessler et al. 2001). However, people are aware about the side effects, contraindications caused by the chemical agents used for short- and long-term therapy. Thus, the interest to prevent any kind of disease with the help of nutritional approaches came into trend and consequently that leads to new research on alternative therapy using nutraceuticals.

8.2 Significance of Carbohydrates in Human

Carbohydrate is the major macronutrient with no established minimum requirement. It is the product of photosynthesis and produces chemical energy such as adenosine triphosphate and nicotinamide adenine dinucleotide phosphate by catabolism. This chemical energy is utilized by the cells to synthesize proteins, lipids, and other compounds (Lia Noemi Gerschenson et al. 2017). Most of the population have thrived with carbohydrates for survival; it is needed for optimal health, longevity, and sustainability.

Carbohydrates are the main source of energy for all body functions, mostly for brain functions, and are essential for the metabolism of other nutrients. Other important effects of carbohydrates on human physiology are satiety and gastric emptying, control of blood glucose, insulin metabolism and serum cholesterol, and enhancement of colonic microflora and gastrointestinal processes such as laxation and fermentation (Muir et al. 2009).

8.3 Classification of Carbohydrates

The dietary carbohydrates are classified based on the character of individual monomers, degree of polymerization (DP), and kind of linkage (α or β) (Cummings and Stephen 2007) (Table 8.1)

8.4 Natural Carbohydrates

8.4.1 Monosaccharide

Monosaccharides include D-glucose, D-fructose, D-galactose, L-xylose, D-mannose, and L-arabinose. The monosaccharides consist of a single unit of 5, 6, or 7 carbon-atom skeleton (aldoses or ketoses). Monosaccharides require no digestion and can be absorbed directly into the bloodstream. All monosaccharides can be synthesized by the body (Hounsome et al. 2008).

Glucose is a simple sugar and an important energy source for our brain and body (Kearns et al. 2017). All other carbohydrates (including other sugars) are converted into glucose during the digestion of food (MedlinePlus on Blood Sugar). Glucose is naturally found in some fruits, vegetables, and nectar or sap (U.S. Agricultural Research Service Food Data Central). Glucose provides energy required to support daily activities, to enhance endurance, to boost cognition (Clemens et al. 2016), to recover energy, for physiological processes, to regulate temperature, to build muscle, and as a natural preservative (https://drhealthbenefits.com/vitamin-supplement/glucose/

Table 8.1 Classification of carbohydrates.

Class (DP[a])	Subgroup	Principal components
Sugars (1–2)	Monosaccharides	Glucose, fructose, and galactose
	Disaccharides	Sucrose, lactose, maltose, and trehalose
	Polyols (sugar alcohols)	Sorbitol, mannitol, lactitol, xylitol, erythritol, isomalt, and maltitol
Oligosaccharides (3–9) (short-chain carbohydrates)	Maltooligosaccharides (α-glucans)	Maltodextrins
	Non-α-glucan oligosaccharides	Raffinose, stachyose, fructo- and galactooligosaccharides, polydextrose, and inulin
Polysaccharides (≥10)	Starch (α-glucans)	Amylose, amylopectin, and modified starches
	Non-starch polysaccharides (NSPs)	Cellulose, hemicellulose, pectin, arabinoxylans, β-glucan, glucomannans, plant gums and mucilages, and hydrocolloids

[a] Degree of polymerization or number of monomeric (single sugar) units.
Source: Based on Food and Agriculture Organization/World Health organization "Carbohydrates in Human Nutrition" report (1998), and Cummings and Stephen (2007).

health-benefits-of-glucose). Fructose is a major component of fruits, fruit juices, honey, and corn syrup (Park and Yetley 1993). Galactose is mostly found in milk and yogurt, lactose-free milk, instant coffee granules, ground black pepper, and on digestion of lactose. Recent reports stated that diseases affecting brain function have been associated with galactose (Coelhoa et al. 2015). In hepatic encephalopathy or Alzheimer's patients, galactose removes the neurotoxic compound ammonia and uses it as a substrate for its conversion to amino acids (Waisbren et al. 2012). Dysfunction of the insulin receptor system is associated with dementia, followed by reduction in glucose transport to and subsequent metabolism in brain cells. As galactose is transported to the brain, it can act as an alternative source of energy owing to its metabolism into glucose (Berry et al. 1995). Daily oral galactose administration is a new promising nontoxic therapy for the treatment of resistant nephrotic syndrome (Berry et al. 2004).

8.4.2 Disaccharides

The commonly known disaccharides are sucrose, a dimer of glucose and fructose; lactose, dimer of glucose and galactose; and maltose, a dimer of two glucose units (Muir et al. 2009). Sucrose is a nonreducing sugar extracted and refined from sugarcane or sugar beet root. Lactose is a reducing sugar present abundantly in most mammalian milk. Maltose, the malt sugar, is found in germinating grains such as barley, malted wheat, breads, bagels, breakfast cereals, energy bars, sweet potatoes, peaches, pears, as well as in malt or malted foods and beverages.

Trehalose the disaccharide made up of two molecules of glucose, obtained from mushrooms and edible fungi, some seaweeds, lobsters, shrimp, Honey, Wine & beers. Recent studies suggest that the trehalose is an important component of Kyoto solution, which is used for the preservation of pancreatic tissue enhance clinical outcomes in transplantation surgery (Matsumoto et al. 2010). Trehalose has been more effective in improving objective signs of dry eye in patients with moderate or severe dry eye (Matsuo 2004; Matsuo et al. 2002).

Isomaltulose is another disaccharide composed of glucose and fructose linked by an ($\alpha1\rightarrow6$)-glycosidic linkage. It contains 42% of the sweetness of sucrose and is found naturally at low levels in honey and sugarcane extract (Siddiqui and Furgala 1967; Takazoe 1985). The consumption of isomaltulose does not cause tooth decay (Lina et al. 2002), and it has a glycemic index (GI) = 32–37 with low insulinemic response. Hence it is considered to be more suitable for diabetics than sucrose (Mitchell 2006). In a study, replacement of sucrose with isolactulose for 12 weeks in individuals with type 2 diabetes resulted in lower blood triglyceride levels but not lower HbA1c levels (Brunner et al. 2012).

8.4.3 Polyols

Sugar alcohols or sugar polyols are produced by the reduction of the corresponding aldoses and ketoses. Sorbitol and mannitol are the natural polyols found in a wide range of fruits and vegetables. Mannitol is present in several vegetables such as celery, carrot, parsley, pumpkin, onion, endive, and asparagus (Hounsome et al. 2008) while sorbitol is found in many fruits. Some researchers have reported that mannitol and sorbitol are applied as indicators of the authenticity or adulteration of foods (Martínez-Montero et al. 2004; Ruiz-Matute et al. 2007). Man-made polyols can also be sneaked into processed food items such as hard candies, toffees, ice cream, jams and preserves, chewing gum, chocolates, protein powders, baked goods, nutritional supplements, diabetic supplements, cough drops, and throat lozenges (Archived by WebCite® at http://www.webcitation.org/6bry3HwOU, Archived by WebCite® at http://www.webcitation.org/6YbYCAip1).

8.4.4 Oligosaccharides

The oligosaccharides have the property of enhancing the quality of food. They have been exhibiting numerous health-promoting activities which were recorded from many clinical studies, including improving *Bifidobacterium* growth in the human intestine, neutralizing intestinal bacteria, modulating the immune response, suppressing cancers and tumors as well as encouraging mineral absorption (Benito-Román et al. 2013). Most of the oligosaccharides are prebiotics, the nondigestible food ingredients that beneficially affect the host by selectively stimulating the growth and/or activity of one or a limited number of bacteria in the colon, thus improving host health (Gibson and Roberfroid 1995), and all the prebiotics are called as dietary fiber. The oligosaccharides (DP 3-9), including arabinoxylanoligosaccharide (AXOS), are classified as dietary fiber (De Menezes et al. 2013).

Isomaltooligosaccharide (IMO) is a mixture of glucose oligomers such as isomaltose, panose, isomaltotriose, isomaltotetrose, isomaltopentose, isomaltohexose, and isomaltoheptose. IMOs are branched oligosaccharides containing a series of α-(1,6) bonds in its structure. IMOs are found naturally in various fermented foods such as miso, sake or soy sauce, and also in honey (Playne and Crittenden 2004). IMOs are the nondigestible carbohydrates with prebiotic properties to enhance human microbiome (Goffin et al. 2011; Rycroft et al. 2001). Panesar et al. (2011) documented the principal hypotriglyceridemic mechanism of action for IMO use to decrease liver lipogenesis through increased production of short-chain fatty acids (SCFAs) by intestinal microbiota in the colon. SCFA production from IMOs leads to increased portal vein concentrations of the ratio between propionate and acetate, which inhibits lipogenesis in hepatocytes (Panesar et al. 2011)

Fructants and fructooligosaccharides (FOS, e.g. nystose and kestose) and galactooligosaccharides (GOS, e.g. raffinose and stachyose) are considered FODMAPs (the fermentable short-chain carbohydrates such as oligo-, di-, and monosaccharides and polyols that can be poorly absorbed by the small intestine) and prebiotic carbohydrates (Muir et al. 2009). About 15% of flowering plant species store fructans in any of their organs during their lifecycle. Fructan polysaccharide is a general term used for any carbohydrates in which fructosylfructose links constitute the majority of the glycosidic bonds. High amount of fructants are found in garlic and Jerusalem artichokes (Muir et al. 2007). The cultured plants of Jerusalem artichoke have the highest concentration of FOS. The prebiotic effect of FOS made it popular and has been used as dietary supplements in Japan since the 90s and now in Western cultures. FOS improve the overall gastrointestinal tract (GIT) health by serving as a substrate for microflora in the large intestine. Many studies have found that FOS and the polysaccharide inulin enhance calcium absorption in both animal and human gut.

Inulin, a polymer of fructose monomers naturally present in onions, garlic, and asparagus (Bosscher et al. 2009), enhances the growth of bifidobacteria, whereas, it suppresses the growth of potential pathogenic bacteria such as *Escherichia coli, Salmonella*, and *Listeria* (Bosscher et al. 2009; Chong 2014). When inulin and oligofructose were added to a controlled diet, significant increase in the concentration of bifidobacterial populations was noted in colon, and it has been stated that these changes improve both colonic and systemic health through modification of the intestinal microflora (Jenkins et al. 1999). Inulin can reduce triglyceride and/or cholesterol concentration, reduce serum urea levels in renal disease, and reduce NH_3 levels in hepatic encephalopathy (Reddy et al. 1994).

The GOS include raffinose, stachyose, and verbascose and are found in legumes. They consist of a terminal sucrose to which one (raffinose), two (stachyose), or three (verbascose) galactose monomers are linked. Raffinose is a trisaccharide containing a galactose-linked α-(1,6), whereas the bond between galactose and the glucose unit of the terminal sucrose is α-1,3. Stachyose is a tetrasaccharide containing a galactose-linked α-(1,6) to the terminal galactose unit of raffinose (Middlebos and Fahey 2008).

These GOS are also considered as dietary fibers, and humans cannot digest these oligosaccharides because they do not have α-galactosidase, which is needed for their hydrolysis. These oligosaccharides have been found to provide beneficial effects in the GIT of humans not only by stimulating growth of selected members of the intestinal microflora but also through their anti-adhesive activity. GOS specifically were found to inhibit infections by enteric pathogens (Ho et al. 2003).

Transgalactooligosaccharides (TGOS) are nondigestible carbohydrates that consist of chains of galactose molecules ending mainly with glucose molecule, varying with chain length (DP 2-8) and linkage type. They are α-D-Glcp-(1-4)-[β-D-Galp-(1-6)]n with $n = 2$–5 produced from lactose with the aid of transgalactosylase (Hammes 2004). Like other nondigestible oligosaccharides, TGOS escape digestion in the human stomach and small intestine, consequently arriving quantitatively to the colon (Van Den Heuvel et al. 2000).

Xylooligosaccharides (XOS) are unusual oligosaccharides whose main constituent is xylose linked by β(1-4)-linkages having a DP of 26. XOS are naturally present in minimal concentrations in honey, fruits, vegetables, bamboo shoots, etc. The prebiotic activity of XOS includes improvement of bowel and immune functions with antimicrobial and other health benefits (Azevedo Carvalho et al. 2013). The consumption of XOS has shown to be of significant importance in maintaining the gut health and functionality of human beings. XOS selectively stimulate growth or activity of specific group of bacteria (Immerzeel et al. 2014), which is associated with improved health, reduced gut infection, and suppression of colon cancer (Macfarlane et al. 2006).

8.4.5 Polysaccharides

Starch is synthesized by plants during photosynthesis as a major energy source for all organisms. Starch is stored in cereal grains (wheat, oats, rye, barley, buckwheat, rice, etc.) potatoes, and legumes (beans, peas, and lentils). It is made up of long chains of glucose called α-glucan. The amylose and amylopectin are the two types of α-glucans, which represent approximately 98–99% of the dry weight. The ratio of the two polysaccharides varies according to the botanical origin of the starch (Tester et al. 2004). Amylose is a linear molecule of (1-4)-linked α-D-glucopyranosyl units, but some molecules are slightly branched by (1-6)-α-linkages. The linear macromolecules are degraded by pure β-amylase and completely converted into maltose, whereas branched chains also give one β-limit dextrin consisting of the remaining inner core polysaccharide structure with its outer chains recessed. Amylopectin is the highly branched component of starch: it is made up of long chains of α-D-glucopyranosyl residues linked together mainly by (1-4)-linkages but with 56% of (1-6) bonds at the branch points. Amylopectin is a branched polysaccharide comprised of hundreds of short (1-4)-α-glucan chains, which are interlinked by (1-6)-α-linkages (Buléon et al. 1998).

The starches from the brewing industries are used as thickening agents in baked goods and confectionery products (Tester et al. 2004). Starch is a safe, cheap, natural, biocompatible, biodegradable, and a multifunctional material with many pharmaceutical applications (Builders and Arhewoh 2016). The oat grain contains starch as the major component of about 60% of the total dry weight. The amylopectin:amylose ratio is about 3:1. The digestibility of oat starch is about 100% but it digests slowly, partly due to the presence of high amounts of fiber and the high oil content in whole grain oat, which retards stomach emptying and improves digestion. Finally, it gradually supplies glucose to the intestine, which maintains a long feeling of satiety. As a result, whole grain oat foods have a low GI, which is advantageous in diabetes and obesity (Mathews 2011; White 2011).

Cellulose is the non-starch polysaccharide and the most abundant carbohydrate polymer found in nature. The cell walls of plants, algae, and bacteria are predominantly made up of cellulose (Akeem and Olatunde 2018; Cao et al. 2009). Cellulose is a homopolymer made up of chains of glucose unit ranging from 700 to 25 000 joined together by β-1,4 glycosidic linkages (Akeem and Olatunde 2018). Cellulose possesses good thermal and chemical stability, high hydrophilicity, and excellent biocompatibility making it an ideal biomaterial for drug delivery systems (Dai and Si 2017). The hemicellulose is the second most abundant natural carbohydrate polymer in the biosphere next to cellulose. In plant cell wall, the hemicellulose is thick in primary and secondary layers associated with cellulose and lignin (Ghose and Bisaria 1987). They can diverge greatly in different cell types and in different species (Waldron et al. 2003).

Pectin is an abundant, multifunctional component of the cell wall of all land plants (Willats et al. 2006). The best grade of pectins in foods are found in citrus fruits such as lime, lemon, grapefruit, and orange. Pectic polysaccharides made up of more linear polymers of galacturonic acid (GalA) are called homogalacturonans (HG; α-1,4-linked GalA monomers). The rhamnogalacturonan-I (RG-I) areas comprised significant amounts of rhamnose, arabinose, and galactose, as well as the RG-II and the xylogalacturonan domains of pectins constituted 13 different monosaccharides (Vincken et al. 2003). Pectin is considered a soluble dietary fiber with several beneficial gastrointestinal physiological effects including delaying gastrointestinal emptying (Flourie et al. 1985), slowing down gut transit time (Spiller et al. 1980), reducing glucose absorption (Jenkins et al. 1977), increasing fecal bulk, and lowering cholesterol (Kay and Truswell 1977). As with other dietary fibers, pectin reaches the large intestine intact where it is fermented by the gut microflora (McBurney and Thompson 1989).

Xylans are a diverse group of polysaccharides belonging to the hemicellulose group of the cell wall polymers of vegetables with the common feature of a β-(1-4)-linked L-xylose backbone. Xylans obtained from bamboo along with xylose, XOSD, and water-soluble lignin have been significantly inhibiting the viability of leukemia cells that were derived from acute lumphoblastic leukemia (ALL) in a dose-dependent manner. But the xylans did not inhibit the viability of leukemia cells that were derived from myelogenous leukemia (ML-2) or lymphoma (SupT-1) and also the viability of normal lymphocytes (Ando et al. 2004). This report stated that the cytotoxic effect of these isolated xylans might be specific for ALL-derived cells.

β-glucans are polysaccharides of D-glucose monomers linked through β-glycosidic bonds, naturally present in common cereals (barley, oats, wheat, and rye). The largest (seed) amounts of β-glucans are found in barley (3–11%) and oats (3–7%) (Patterson 2008). β-Glucans from cereals help to lower cholesterol and blood glucose levels (Zhu et al. 2016). It is a soluble fiber that has been shown to have effects on the glycemic level, insulin, and cholesterol responses to foods (Tiwari and Cummings 2009). Xin-Zhong et al. (2015) reported that the inclusion of 5% oat beta-glucans in a high-fat diet resulted in significantly reduced body weight, and epididymal and subcutaneous adipose tissue weight compared with human flora-associated mice fed with high-fat diet ($p < 0.01$). Oat-specific beta-glucans are soluble food fibers. In addition, oat fibers increase the fecal bulk, which contributes to normal stool and have a positive impact on the functioning of the microbiome (Mathews 2011). Beta-glucans with immunostimulatory properties were also shown to be beneficial in preventing infectious diseases and gastrointestinal cancer, particularly colorectal cancer (Jurczyńska et al. 2012).

Chitin and Chitosan are the polysaccharides obtained from animal sources includes exoskeleton of arthropods like shrimps, insects, lobsters, crabs, and the cell walls of certain fungi (Aravamudhan et al. 2014). Chitin polysaccharide made up of 2-acetamido-2-deoxy-β-d-glucose monomers that are connected via β-(1 → 4)-linkages (Akeem and Olatunde 2018; Rathore and Gupta 2015). The N-deacetylation of chitin develop a crystalline, cationic, and hydrophilic polymer with excellent gelation and film-forming chitosan (Panos et al. 2008). Chitosan is a linear polysaccharide made up of D-glucosamine monomers with randomly located N-acetylglucosamine substituents that are β-(1 → 4) linked (Akeem and Olatunde 2018). The biopharmaceutical and medical includes drug/gene delivery, wound dressings, implants, contact lenses, tissue engineering, and cell encapsulation (Shariatinia 2019).

Alginates are produced by marine algae and also certain strains of bacteria, e.g. *Pseudomonas aeruginosa* (Rinaudo 2014). Alginates are linear polymers composed of $(1 \rightarrow 4)$-α-L-guluronic acid units (GG) and $(1 \rightarrow 4)$-β-D-mannuronic acid units (MM), along with some heteropolymeric sequences of M and G units (MG blocks) (Pawar 2011). Both M/G ratio and the distribution of M and G units along the chain influence the biological and physical properties of alginates in aqueous media (Aarstad et al. 2012; Rinaudo 2014). Monosodium salts of alginates are soluble in water and form a viscous solution, which has valuable applications (Rinaudo 2014), whereas divalent and multivalent cations of alginates (except Mg2+) form gels or precipitates (Anademanantina and Rinaudo 2010). Alginic acid or alginates also form gels in acidic pH through formation of intermolecular hydrogen bonds (Anademanantina and Rinaudo 2010). Alginates are widely used in biomedical field for controlled drug release (Fundueanu et al. 1998), cells encapsulation (Yi et al. 2005), tissue engineering (Kong and Mooney 2005), and for preparation of dental molds (Draget and Taylor 2011; Lee and Mooney 2012; Rinaudo 2014).

Carrageenan (CRG) is a natural anionic sulfated linear polysaccharide obtained from red seaweeds belonging to the rhodophyceae family (*Chondrus, Eucheuma, Gigartina*, and *Hypnea* species) (Prajapati et al. 2014). CRG is made up of long linear chains of repeating D-galactose units and D-anhydrogalactose copolymer by alternating α-(1–4) and β-(1–3)-linkages with ester sulfates (15–40%) as substitutes (Jiao et al. 2011). CRG has numerous pharmaceutical applications including drug delivery, formulations, and also for making pH- and temperature-sensitive delivery systems (Campo et al. 2009; Desbrieres et al. 2018). Additionally, CRG is a biocompatible, biodegradable polymer with water-retention and gel-forming properties, which allow use in buccal, ophthalmic, and vaginal drug delivery systems, and other biomedical applications, e.g. wound healing and tissue engineering (Desbrieres et al. 2018; Liu et al. 2015).

8.5 Carbohydrate Components as Nutraceuticals

8.5.1 Disaccharide Components as Nutraceuticals

Lactulose is a nondigestible, non-absorbable synthetically produced disaccharide derived from lactose, consisting of D-galactose and D-fructose (4-*O*-β-D-galactopyranosyl-β-D-fructofuranose) (Figure 8.1). Lactulose is available in trade names such as Cholac, Generlac, Consulose, Duphalac, and 4-*O*-β-D-Galactosyl-D-fructose. It is mainly used medicinally as an oral osmotic laxative to treat constipation, orally or as a rectum suppository in portosystemic encephalopathy (ASHSP 2015).

Ballongue et al. (1997) observed that the gut microorganisms ferment the lactulose easily and produce high concentrations of SCFAs that lead to a reduction in the pH of the gut. This acidic pH altered gut microbiota by increasing *Bifidobacterium*, Lactobacillus, and Streptococcus while

Figure 8.1 Lactulose.

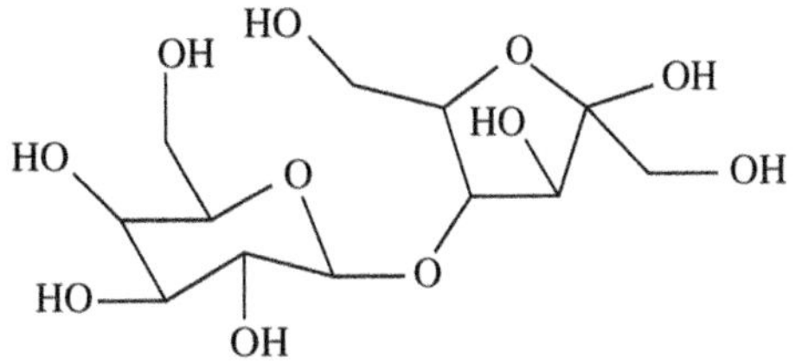

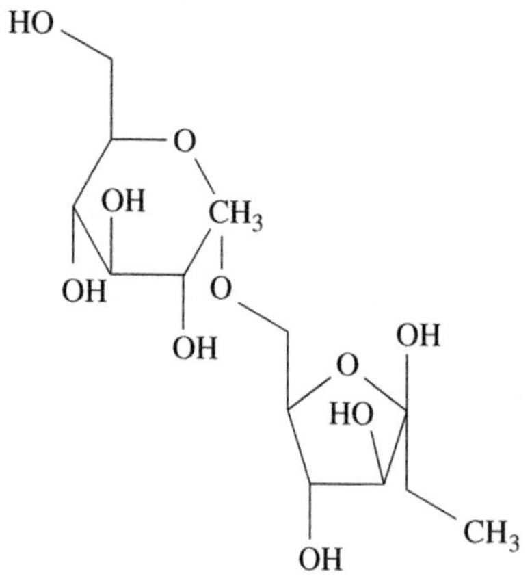

Figure 8.2 Isomaltulose.

reducing the number of Bacteroides, Clostridium, Coliforms, and Eubacterium. Simultaneously, the concentrations of acetic and lactic acids were increased in the fecal matter, while there is a reduction in the concentrations of butyric, propionic, and valeric acid. Tuohy et al. (2002) also demonstrated that lactulose increased the concentration of bifidobacteria significantly in the gut. Lactulose helps in protonating ammonia (NH_3) to ammonium ion (NH_4) that stopped the diffusion of ammonia across the gut epithelium into the portal vein and be carried to the liver (Shukla et al. 2011).

Isomaltulose was synthesized by controlled hydrolysis of dextran by following the previously described procedure (Mountzouris et al. 2002). It was also produced by the enzymatic rearrangement of sucrose (glucose-[α1→2]-β-fructose) using a sucrose mutase found in bacteria, e.g. *Protaminobacter rubrum* (Pelzer et al. 2012). Commercial isolmaltulose syrup is a mixture of glucosyl saccharides with both α-(1→6)-linkages and α-(1→4)-linkages (Yun et al. 1994). But in recent years, the enzymatic preparation of isolmaltulose syrup is made with the mixture of glucooligosaccharides linked by α-(1→6)-linkage with lower proportion of α-(1→3) (nigerooligosaccharides) or α-(1→2) (kojioligosaccharides) glucosidic linkages (Yamamoto et al. 2004) (Figure 8.2). It is generally used as a non-cariogenic sucrose replacer. The digestibility properties of isomaltulose was studied in vitro with mammalian intestinal α-glucosidases (including human) indicating that the rate of hydrolysis of this sugar is significantly slower than that of sucrose and maltose (Tsuji et al. 1986). Animal studies have shown that isomaltulose is completely digested and absorbed in the small intestine, but the postprandial glycemic and insulinemic responses rise at a slow rate, with maximum concentrations of glucose and insulin being lower than for sucrose (Van Can et al. 2012). The slowly digestible property of isolmaltulaose products makes it a suitable ingredient for consumers with diabetic and pre-diabetic dispositions.

8.5.2 Polyol Components as Nutraceuticals

Mannitol is an isomer of sorbitol (Figure 8.3) commercially used as a sweetener and medication. Mannitol in the consumed food is absorbed very slowly in the intestine; because of this property it is widely used in diabetic food as a sweetener. As a medication, it is used to reduce pressure in the eyes, in glaucoma, and to suppress the increased intracranial pressure (Varzakas et al. 2012; Wakai et al. 2013). Medically, it is given in the form of injection with the trade name Osmitrol and other names such as D-mannitol, mannite, and manna sugar. In industrial level, production of mannitol involves high pressure hydrogenation of fructose/glucose mixtures in aqueous solution at high temperature (120–160 °C) with Raney nickel as a catalyst and hydrogen gas. Mannitol is produced from

Figure 8.3 Mannitol.

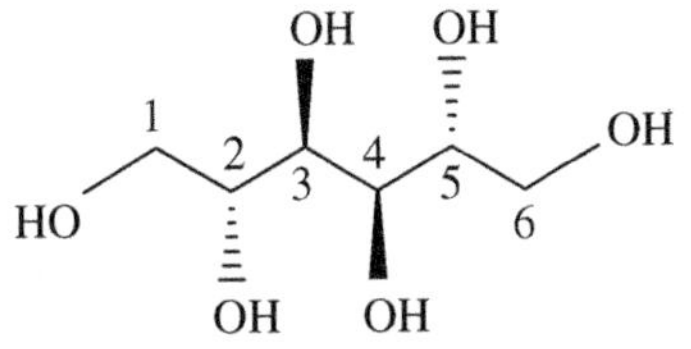

Figure 8.4 Xylitol.

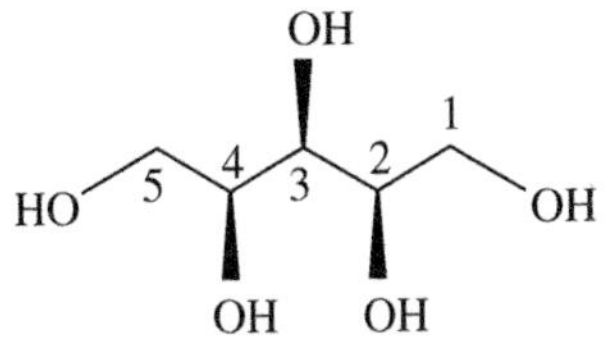

α-fructose and sorbitol is from β-fructose. The glucose is hydrogenated exclusively to sorbitol. Due to poor selectivity of the nickel catalyst, the hydrogenation of a 50:50 fructose/glucose mixture results in an approximately 25:75 mixture of mannitol and sorbitol. It is comparatively tough to separate sorbitol and mannitol. Mannitol is used as a powerful osmotic diuretic medicine (to enhance the formation of urine to prevent and treat acute renal failure and also to discard the toxic substances from the body) and in different types of operation for the prevention of kidney failure (to alter the osmolarity of the glomerular filtrate) and to reduce dye and brain edema (increased brain water content). Hypertonic mannitol can enhance the transport of drugs across the blood–brain barrier for the treatment of life-threatening brain diseases (Rapoport 2000). In cystic fibrosis patients the inhaled mannitol improves the hydration and surface properties of sputum (Daviskas et al. 2010).

Xylitol is a sugar alcohol with the chemical formula of $C_5H_{12}O_5$, or $HO(CH_2)(CHOH)_3(CH_2)OH$ (Figure 8.4). It is naturally present in the fibers of many fruits and vegetables in low concentration and can be extracted from different berries, oats, and mushrooms, as well as a fibrous material such as corn husks and sugarcane bagasse. However, industrial production starts from xylan (a hemicellulose) extracted from hardwoods or corncobs, which is hydrolyzed into xylose and catalytically hydrogenated into xylitol. It is available in the market by different names such as Birch Sugar, E967, Meso-Xylitol, Meso-Xylitol, Pentane-1,2,3,4,5-pentol, Sucre de Bouleau, Xilitol, Xylit, Xylite, and Xylo-pentane-1,2,3,4,5-pentol. Xylitol chewing gum appears to decrease rates of acute otitis (inflammation of the ear) media in children going to day care by 25%. Xylitol nasal sprays decrease the incidence of acute otitis media as well as being a very effective way of both assisting and stimulating the body's own natural nasopharyngeal washing and reducing both bacterial colonization and allergenic pollution, with their accompanying problems. Consumption of xylitol as a food increased the bone volume in rats in studies conducted in 2001 and 2011, and these results have generated interest in the sugar that would be examined to determine whether it could be used for treatment of osteoporosis in humans. (https://www.webmd.com/vitamins/ai/ingredientmono-996/xylitol)

8.5.3 Oligosaccaharide Components as Nutraceuticals

FOS consist of a fructose unit polymerized to different extent. Oligomers with two fructose units are known as 1-kestose, three fructose units are 1-nystose, and four fructose units are 1-fructofuranosyl-nystose. The sugars are linked by β-2,1 position of sucrose (Sangeetha et al. 2005). FOS are enzymatically synthesized from the sugar syrup and molasses are from beet containing 620 and 570 mg/ml sucrose, respectively (Ghazi et al. 2006). The production of FOS was increased by lowering the early pH value of syrup (7.5) and molasses (8.9) to 5.5. The fructose unit, 1-kestose,

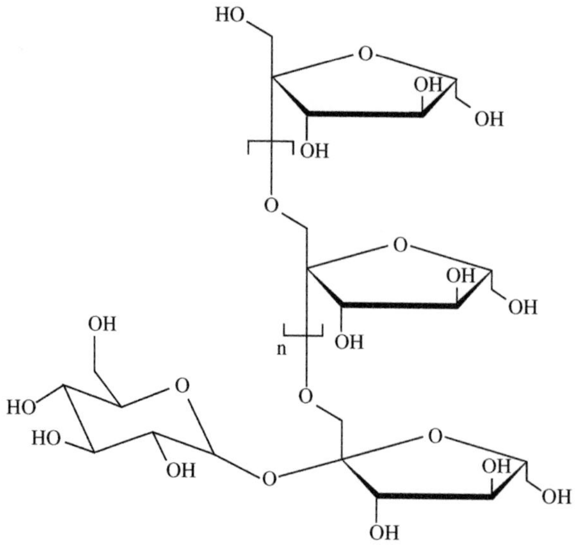

Figure 8.5 Inulin.

has enhanced therapeutic properties than those with a high polymeric degree (GFn. 4). There are four fructan-type oligosaccharides available in nutraceutical market:

1) Inulin (Sigma)
2) Raftiline HP (an inulin-containing product produced by Orafti Active Food Ingredients, Tienen, Belgium)
3) Nutraflora (FOS; GTC Nutrition Company, Westminster, CO)
4) Raftilose P95 (Orafti)

The inulin (Figure 8.5) obtained from Sigma (Inu-S) and from Orafti (Inu-O) are both extracted from chicory root and vary in the DP only slightly, with both averaging more than 23 fructose monomers per molecule. But, raftilose P95 is obtained by fractional hydrolysis of inulin, yielding an FOS product containing ca. 75% of fructose-only chains (FFn) with degrees of polymerization ranging from 2 to 7. The balance (ca. 25%) is of the GFn form. Nutraflora is manufactured enzymatically to produce FOS species consisting of a glucose (G) monomer linked to two, three, or four fructose (F) molecules. This product is denoted as the GFn type of FOS. FOS can also be obtained by inulin hydrolysis caused by endoinulinase produced by several microorganisms, mainly fungi and some bacteria (Guio et al. 2009). Addition of XOS and FOS at 5.4% in the diet reduced the occurrence of colonic aberrant crypt foci, which are considered as early markers for tumors, by 76 and 48%, respectively (Hsu et al. 2004) (Table 8.2).

GOS are the complex mixtures of oligosaccharides ranging from two to eight moieties and different glycosidic linkages: β-(1,1), β-(1,2), β-(1,3), β-(1,4), and β-(1,6) (Figure 8.6) (Playne and Crittenden 2009). It is synthesized by enzymatic catalysis of lactose using glycosidase hydrolases (de Roode et al. 2003). The conversion of lactose into GOS by β-galactosidases is performed in a kinetically controlled reaction, by means of competition between hydrolysis and transgalactosylation. GOS play an inhibitory role in colon cancer by reducing risk factors for colon cancer development, such as reducing bacterial reductase enzymes, secondary bile acids, ammonia, and indole (Sako et al. 1999). Animal studies have also shown a decrease in the induction of colorectal tumors after consuming GOS (Wijnands et al. 2001).

Table 8.2 Structure and composition of some commercial prebiotic oligosaccharides.

Oligosaccharide	Chemical structure	Composition (%)[a]
Inulin (Inu-S)	α-Glu-(1→2)-[β-Fru-(1→2)]$_{>20}$	95
Raftiline HP (Inu-O)	α-Glu-(1→2)-[β-Fru-(1→2)]$_{>20}$	100
Nutraflora (GFn)	α-Glu-(1→2)-[β-Fru-(1→2)]$_{2-4}$	97
Raftilose P95 (FFn)	β-Fru-(1→2)-[β-Fru-(1→2)]$_{1-10}$ and α-Glu-(1→2)-[β-Fru-(1→2)]$_{2-10}$	75 and 25
Lactulose	β-Gal-(1→4)-β-Fru	95
Raffinose	α-Gal-(1→6)-α-Glu-(1→2)-β-Fru	98
Oligomate (GOS)	α-Glu-(1→4)-[β-Gal-(1→6)]$_{2-4}$	100[b]

[a] From the manufacturer.
[b] After purification.
Source: Infection and Immunity, December 2006, pp. 6920–6928, Vol. 74, No. 12 0019-9567/06/$08.000 doi:10.1128/IAI.01030-06

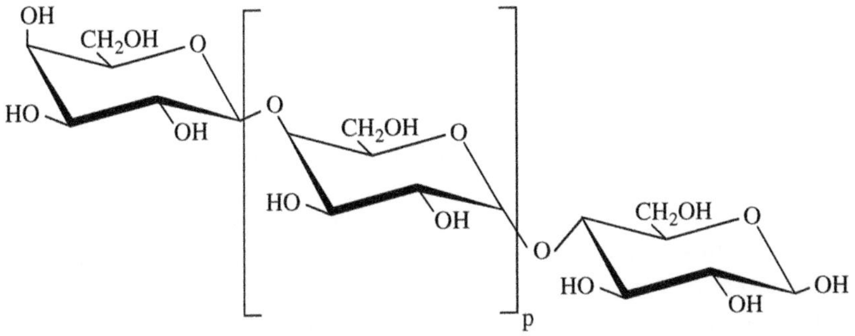

Figure 8.6 Galactooligosaccharide.

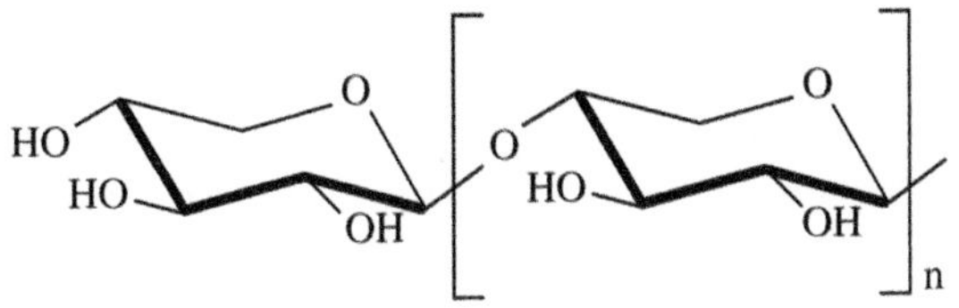

Figure 8.7 Xylooligosaccharide.

Xylooligosaccharides or feruloyl oligosaccharides are oligosaccharides consisting of many xylose moieties linked by β-(1,4) bonds, with a polymerization degree ranging from 2 to 10 monosaccharides (Figure 8.7). It is naturally present in plant sources such as Bengal gram husk, wheat bran and straw, spent wood, barley hulls, brewery spent grains, almond shells, bamboo, and corn cob. It is also produced by the microorganisms such as *Aspergillus*, *Trichoderma*, *Penicillium*, *Bacillus*, and *Streptomyces*. The consumption of XOS mainly provides prebiotic effect in consumers. It offers beneficial effect in diabetes, in treatment of arteriosclerosis, in reducing total cholesterol and LDL in patients with type 2 diabetes mellitus (DM), and in colon cancer (Chung et al. 2007; Madhukumar and Muralikrishna 2010).

AXOS is an arabinan polysaccharide exhibiting linkage of 1,3- and 1,5-α-L-arabinofuranosyl residues (Vogel 1991). Arabinose occurs naturally in arabinans, arabinogalactans, or arabinoxylans present in plant cell wall components. It is commercially manufactured from flaxseed mucilage using pectinase, followed by mild acid thermal hydrolysis and then xylanase (Guilloux et al. 2012); from wheat bran and psyllium seed husk using xylanase hydrolysis or mechanical ball milling (Van Creaeyveld et al. 2008), rye AX is initially heated to improve xylanase-catalyzed hydrolysis from two glycoside hydrolase families (RmXyn10A from GH10 and Pentopan Mono BG from GH11) and to provide AXOS mixtures of greater than 60% with xylobiose a major product (Falck et al. 2014); or from switch grass biomass using mechanical ball milling (Mazumder and York 2010). AXOS intake induced cecal and colon enlargement associated with an important bifidogenic effect, as it increased the level of circulating satietogenic peptides produced by the colon (peptide YY and glucagon-like peptide-1) and coherently counteracted high-fat diet-induced body weight gain and fat mass development. In addition, high-fat-induced hyperinsulinemia and the homestasis model assessment of insulin resistance were decreased due to AXOS consumption. AXOS consumption also reduced high-fat-induced metabolic endotoxemia, macrophage infiltration (mRNA of F4/80) in the adipose tissue, and the pro-inflammatory cytokine, interleukin-6 (IL6), in the plasma (Poesen et al. 2016).

Pectin oligosaccharides POS I and POS II are isolated from the agricultural by-products such as sugar beet, apple, olive, and citrus. POS are obtained through partial hydrolysis of pectin polymers. POS I and POS II preparations induced apoptosis in HT29 colon cancer cells (Olano-Martin et al. 2003). Cell growth was inhibited in the presence of POS and their parent pectins (10 mg/ml). This decrease in cell yield was not due to necrosis nor differentiation, and DNA laddering was observed following agarose gel electrophoresis. These effects were also observed in the presence of butyrate and D-GalA. Caspase-3 activity, but no alkaline phosphatase activity, was also present. These potentially anticancer effects of pectic oligosaccharides lends further support to other reports of pectin fragments with anticancer activity. A pectin fragment was observed to compete with the galectin binding involved in tumor cell metastasis (Pienta et al. 1995; Platt and Raz 1992). Pectin-derived acidic oligosaccharides (pAOS) from higher plant products such as fruits and vegetables have wide applications in infant formulas to subside diarrhea and increase in absorption of minerals and calcium ions, and these also have antioxidant effects (Liu et al. 2010).

Chitosan is a natural nontoxic biopolymer produced by the deacetylation of chitin, a major component of the shells of crustaceans such as crab, shrimp, and crawfish. Chitosan has amino/acetamido group as well as both primary and secondary hydroxyl groups at the C-2, C-3, and C-6 positions as the reactive functional groups. Chitooligosaccharides (COS) is the degraded product of chitosan or chitin. The COS have been produced by several methods, such as enzymatic and acidic, and their derivatives have been proved for their best implications as nutraceutical and pharmacological moieties to play major role against some important health complications (Kim 2017; Xia et al. 2011). The properties and new modification reactions of chitin, chitosan, COS, and their derivatives are completely studied for applying these macromolecules in the promising fields of medicine, pharmacy, cosmetics, toiletries, food processing, agriculture, etc. (Kim 2010). COS has been used as an antioxidative agent, antitumor agent, and antimicrobial agent. Chitosan oligosaccharides have been verified to protect normal cells from apoptosis (Liu et al. 2010).

Alginate oligosaccharides (AOS) comprises 2–25 alginate monomers formed from depolymerization of alginate by different methods, including physical, chemical, and enzymatic methods such as fermentation, organic synthesis, and biosynthesis. AOS are reported to have unique bioactivities and impart health benefits acting as immunomodulatory, antimicrobial, antioxidant, prebiotic, antihypertensive, antidiabetic, antitumor, and anticoagulant agents (Fang et al. 2017;

Hu et al. 2019). They have been successfully utilized as novel feed supplements that improve aquaculture, poultry, and swine production. Enzymatically depolymerized AOS can cause cytotoxic cytokine production in human mononuclear cells. Commercially the low-molecular-weight alginate derivatives such as propylene glycol alginate sodium sulfate and propylene glycol mannuronate sulfate have shown antioxidation benefits and prevention of cardiovascular and cerebrovascular diseases. Khan et al. (2012) previously found that AOS especially reach in GG acid monomers and were also able to kill multidrug-resistant bacteria by modulating biofilm formation and persistence reducing the resistance to antibiotic treatment.

8.5.4 Polysaccharide Components as Nutraceuticals

Polydextrose (PDX) is a polysaccharide rather than an oligosaccharide. It is a polymer of glucose with sorbitol and traces of citric acid catalyst attached to the polymer through mono- and di-ester bonds. PDX is produced by vacuum thermal polymerization of glucose, using sorbitol and an approved food acid as a catalyst. Random polymerization and branching yield various types of glycosidic bonds in the structure, which is comprised of α- and β-linked $1\rightarrow2$, $1\rightarrow3$, $1\rightarrow4$, and $1\rightarrow6$ glycosidic linkages, although the α- and β-$(1\rightarrow6)$-linkages predominate (Lahtinen et al. 2010) (Figure 8.8). PDX, unlike other lower molecular weight (MW) nondigestible oligosaccharides, is slowly and only partially fermented by gut microbiota, remaining as an energy substrate for the microbiota throughout the length of the large intestine, including the distal portion where much of proteolytic fermentation usually takes place. Much of the more fermentable carbohydrate substrate is utilized in the proximal and traverse colonic regions (Mäkeläinen et al. 2010).

Tiihonen et al. (2011) evaluated PDX at 1 and 2% v/v concentrations in vitro for their effects on total SCFA production, as compared with baseline fermentations. The researchers observed a positive dose-response by indicating that the number of genes differentially regulated by the lower PDX dose doubled, from 307–710 genes, when the dose was doubled to 2% v/v. PDX was demonstrated to regulate key cancer-causing genes by PDX fermentation metabolites, which influenced the number of active cells by inducing apoptosis of colon cancer cells.

Resistant starch: The isolated and extracted resistant starch has been used to fortify foods to increase their dietary fiber content (Fuentes-Zaragoza et al. 2010; Sayago-Ayerdi et al. 2011). The RS2 resistant starch is from high amylose corn, RS3 resistant starch from cassava, and RS4 resistant starch from wheat and potato are widely used in food fortification. The resistant starch content is not getting lost in these sources, because they can survive varying degrees of food processing (Sajilata et al. 2006). These types of resistant starch (RS1, RS2, and RS3) are fermented by the large intestinal microbiota, conferring benefits to human health through the production of SCFAs, increased bacterial mass, and promotion of butyrate-producing bacteria (Brouns et al. 2002).

Figure 8.8 Polydextrose.

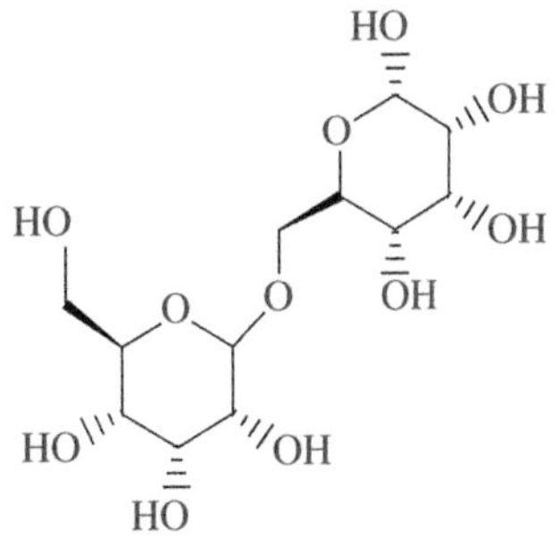

In healthy individuals, the RS does not get absorbed in the small intestine but later in the colon, and the RS is fermented by natural microflora and produce SCFAs.

Dextrins are the partial degradation product of starch and are promising source of prebiotics (Slizewska 2013). It is produced by acid or enzymatic hydrolysis of starch or by a combination of both. Dextrin is a group of low-molecular-weight carbohydrates, mixtures of polymers of D-glucose units linked with α(1-4) or α(1-6) glycosidic bonds (Figure 8.9). The molecular distribution and oligosaccharide profiles determine the physicochemical properties. Dextrins are widely used for their functional properties, whereas their physicochemical properties are dependent on their molecular distribution and oligosaccharide profiles (Sun et al. 2010). **Nutriose** (FB06) is a soluble dextrin produced from wheat or maize starch by a highly controlled process of dextrinization followed by a chromatographic fractionation step (Fouache et al. 2003). Specific glycosidic bonds are added to the typical starch α-1,4- and α-1,6-linkages during the dextrinization, which involves repolymerization. Lefranc-Millot et al. (2012) confirmed the prebiotic activity of the soluble fiber Nutrioset, which can provide a beneficial effect on colonic microbial population. The upgrading consequence of therapeutic compounds in the developed insulin resistance and inflammation response is a basic strategy in the management of type 2 diabetes. Through a randomized controlled clinical trial, Aliasgharzadeh et al. (2015) determined that supplementation with prebiotic-resistant dextrin (Nutriose FB06) effectively ameliorates insulin resistance and can modulate inflammation in women with type 2 diabetes.

Maltodextrins: The products of starch hydrolysis with DE values below 20 are called maltodextrins (Sun et al. 2010) (Figure 8.10). Maltodextrins with different DE can produce different yields of prebiotic glucooligosacarides by fermentation with gluconobacter oxydans NCIMB 4943 (Wichienchot et al. 2009). Slavin (2013) described the use of maltodextrins as placebo in studies of prebiotic effect and of weight loss.

Resistant maltodextrins are short-chain polymers of glucose that are hardly resistant to digestion in the human digestive system produced by dextrinization. Most of the resistant maltodextrins in food products are manufactured from starch by treating with heat and/or acid and/or enzymes (Barczynska et al. 2010). **Fibersol-2** is a familiar soluble and nondigestible starch-derived resistant

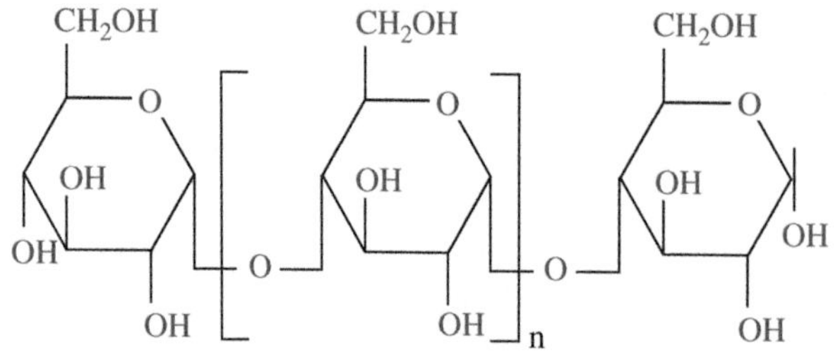

Figure 8.9   Dextrin.

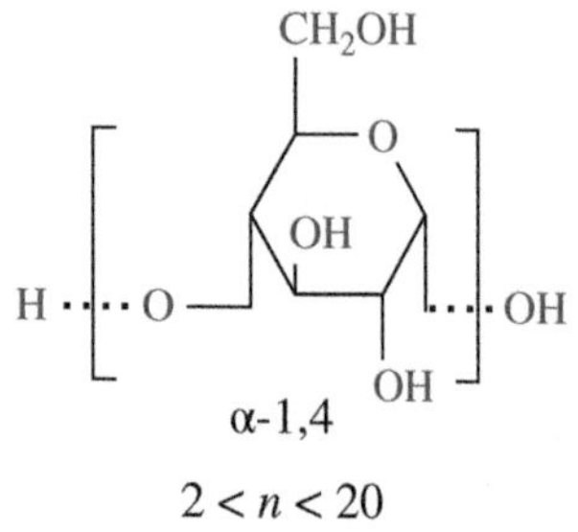

Figure 8.10   Maltodextrin.

Figure 8.11   Beta-Glucan.

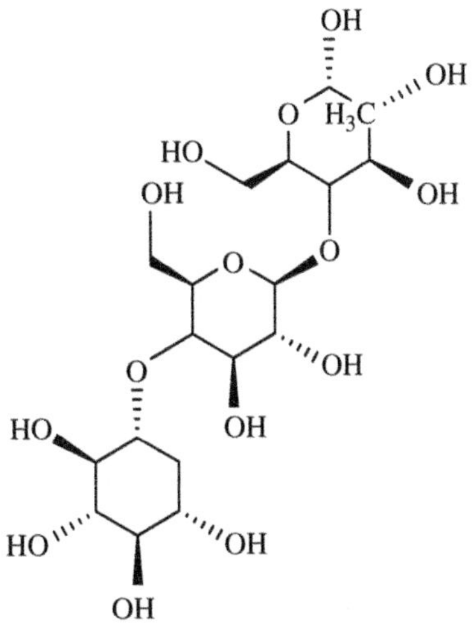

maltodextrin (Barczynska et al. 2010). It is synthesized from corn starch by following pyrolysis and subsequent enzymatic treatment to convert a portion of the normal α-1,4 glucose linkages to random 1,2-, 1,3-, and 1,4-α-or β-linkages. Fibersol-2 can efficiently decrease postprandial levels of blood glucose and insulin, the blood levels of triacylglycerols and serum cholesterol, and can also promote beneficial bacteria growth in the colon.

Citric acid-resistant dextrin (Ca-Dextrin) is the resistant starch synthesized from native potato starch (Slizewska 2013). The enzyme-resistant dextrin was synthesized by heating potato starch in the presence of hydrochloric (0.1% dry starch basis) and citric (0.1% dry starch basis) acids at 130 °C for 3 hours, obtaining CA-dextrin for enzyme hydrolysis in colon. Later its prebiotic activity was determined.

β-glucans are polysaccharides with a MW of 30–50 kDa (Figure 8.11) and have been extracted from Agaricus blazei Murill mushrooms using hot water (Kim et al. 2005). The soluble form of β-glucans is obtained from the sources such as yeast and cereals by fractionation method. The β-glucans dissolved in water, alkali, and other bases will be used for the preparation of drugs and cosmetics. In the digestive tract, the soluble fibers easily dissolve in water and are transported in gelatinous form, eliminating cholesterol from the body and balancing the blood glucose simultaneously. The increasing demand of the product in pharmaceutical formulations is increasing the production of soluble β-glucans over the forecast period. The insoluble β-glucan powder is well-matched with numerous ingredients and is used in the manufacture of cosmetics. In the cosmetics industry, the insoluble form of β-glucan products are used for manufacturing antifungal cream, antimicrobial cream, deodorants, and other oral care products that are likely to drive the industry growth. The consumption of the β-glucan products provide many health benefits including cardiovascular health improvement, cognitive improvement, and cancer prevention (Beta-glucan Market Size, Share, Global Industry Report, 2018–2025).

8.5.5   Microbial Polysaccharides Components as Nutraceuticals

Dextran is a bacterial polysaccharide obtained from certain lactic acid bacteria (genera *Lactobacillus*, *Leuconostoc*, and *Streptococcus*) during sucrose fermentation (Varshosaz 2012). The large class of dextran (Figure 8.12) is a branched α-D-glucans with repeating anhydro-D-glucopyranose units as their main molecular chain. Dextrans contain more α-1,6-linkages with regular α(1–3) branching.

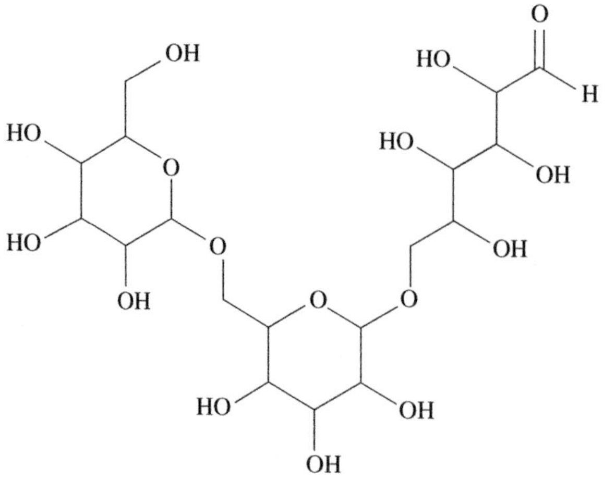

Figure 8.12   Dextran.

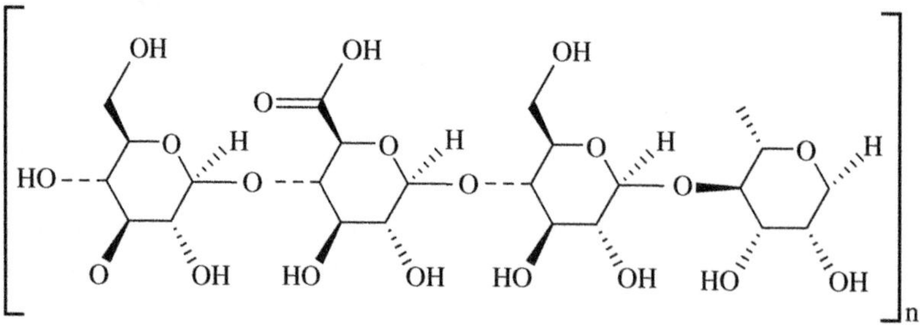

Figure 8.13   Gellan gum.

The pharmaceutically significant dextrans contain 95% α-1,6-glucopyranosidic linkages and 5% α-1,3-linkages (Dhaneshwar et al. 2006).

Gellan gum is an extracellular anionic polysaccharide produced by *Sphingomonas elodea bacterium* as a fermentation product. Gellan gum is a linear polysaccharide made up of repeating units of a β-l-rhamnose, β-D-glucose, and β-D-glucuronate in the molar ratios 1:2:1 (BeMiller 2019). Natural gellan contains two ester groups of the same glucosyl unit, namely, L-glyceryl and acetyl groups. By alkaline hydrolysis, these ester groups can be removed form a de-esterified gellan, which is also known as low-acetyl or low-acyl gellan (Figure 8.13). In a temperature-dependent process with the addition of mono-, di-, and trivalent cations, hydrogels are generated from native and low-acyl gellan. Native gellan forms soft, easily deformable gels in the presence of positively charged ions, whereas the low-acyl gellan forms rigid and brittle gels under similar conditions. The gelation property, coupled with biodegradability and nontoxicity, led to extensive use of gellan gum as a multifunctional excipient in many pharmaceutical dosage forms (Osmałek et al. 2014).

Pullulan is an exopolysaccharide produced by a fungi *Aureobasidium pullulans* by starch fermentation (Rekha and Sharma 2007). Pullulan is a water-soluble, neutral linear polysaccharide composed of regularly repeating α-(1 → 4)-maltotriosyl units (3-D-glucopyranosyl) joined through α-(1 → 6)-linkages (Figure 8.14). Based on the fermentation condition, the MW of this exopolysaccharide varied between 4.5×10^4 and 6×10^5 Da (Grigoras 2019). Pullulan is biodegradable,

Figure 8.14 Pullulan.

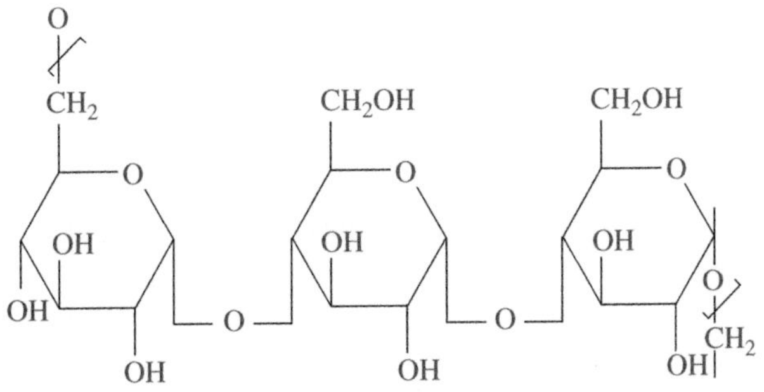

impermeable to oxygen, nonhygroscopic, and nonreducing polymer. Also, pullulan dissolves easily in water to form clear and viscous solution with high adhesion and film-forming abilities (LeDuy et al. 2002). Additionally, pullulan is responsive to chemical modifications, which yields derivatives with low or no water solubility (Grigoras 2019). Furthermore, pullulan is not nontoxic and nonimmunogenic. Owing to this, pullulan and its derivatives are being explored for various applications in biomedical field, especially for targeted drug/gene delivery and imaging (Rekha and Sharma 2007).

Xanthan gum is an extracellular branched polysaccharide produced by bacterial fermentation (*Xanthomonas campestris*). The backbone of xanthan gum consists of repeating units of cellobiose and the side chains consists of a trisaccharide-containing D-mannose (β-1,4), D-glucuronic acid (β-1,2), and D-mannose, which are linked to backbone (alternate glucose residues) through α-1,3-linkages as shown in Figure 8.15 (Petri 2015). Aqueous solutions of

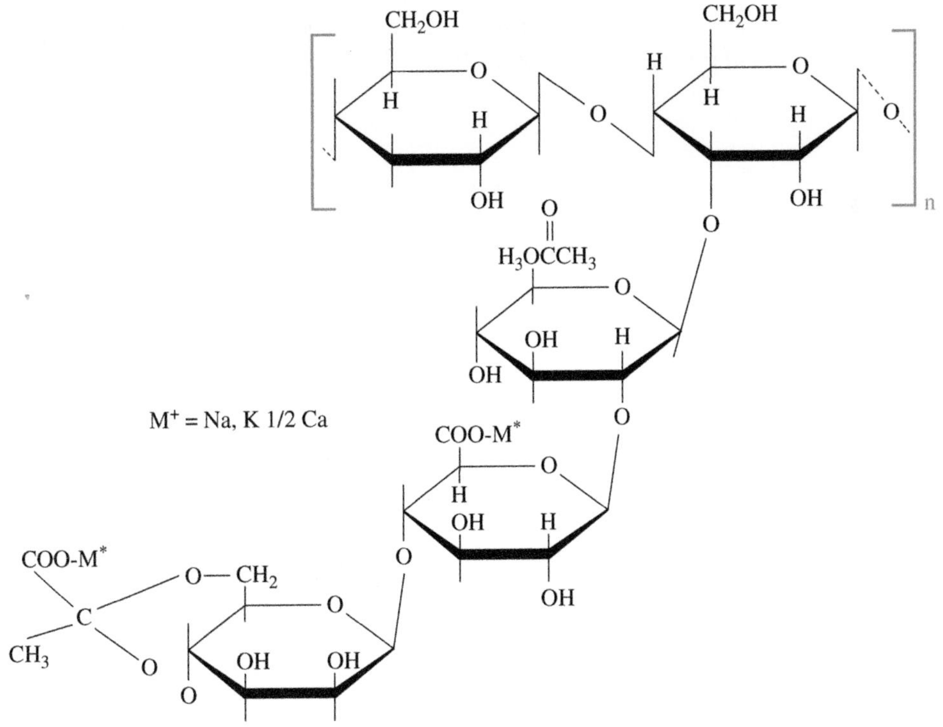

Figure 8.15 Xanthan.

xanthan gum show pseudoplastic behavior, pH stability, and thermal stability. The structural properties of xanthan in solution can be manipulated by varying temperature and ionic strength. For example, xanthan chains exist in helical conformation under high ionic strength or low temperature, whereas they are coiled under low ionic strength or high temperature. Furthermore, the high MW of xanthan gums favors the formation of physical and chemical networks, making them suitable for development of carriers for drugs and proteins (Petri 2015). Therefore, xanthan gum has been expansively used in combination with other polymers as excipient in tablet formulations or as supporting hydrogels for drug-release applications (Jansson et al. 1983).

8.5.6 Conjugated Carbohydrate Components as Nutraceuticals

Glucosamine ($C_6H_{13}NO_5$) is an amino sugar and a prominent precursor in the biochemical synthesis of glycosylated proteins and lipids (Figure 8.16). Glucosamine is part of the structure of the polysaccharides, chitosan, and chitin. Produced commercially by the hydrolysis of shellfish exoskeletons or, less commonly, by fermentation of a grain such as corn or wheat, glucosamine has many names depending on country (Glucosamine. Drugs.com 2019). Although **glucosamine** is a common dietary supplement, there is little evidence that it is effective for relief of arthritis or pain and is not an approved prescription drug (Robert 2016).

Chondroitin sulfate is a sulfated glycosaminoglycan (GAG) composed of a chain of alternating sugars (N-acetylgalactosamine and glucuronic acid) (Figure 8.17). It is usually found attached to proteins as part of a proteoglycan. A chondroitin chain can have over 100 individual sugars, each of which can be sulfated in variable positions and quantities. Chondroitin sulfate is an important structural component of cartilage and provides much of its resistance to compression (Baeurle et al. 2009). Along with glucosamine, chondroitin sulfate has become a widely used dietary supplement for treatment of osteoarthritis (Robert 2016).

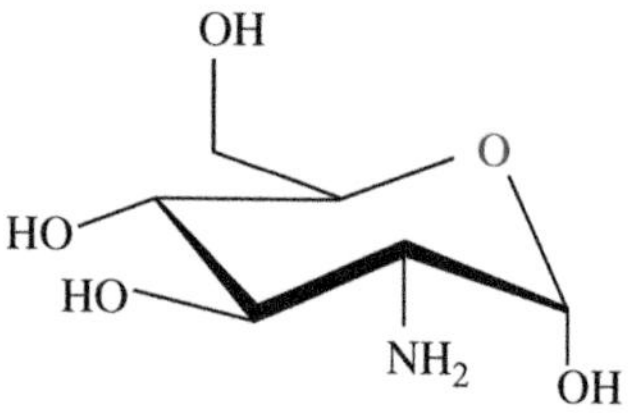

Figure 8.16 Glucosamine.

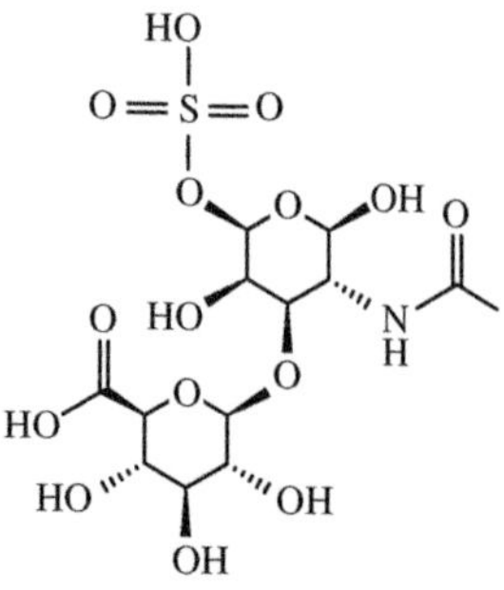

Figure 8.17 Chondroitin sulfate.

8.6   Protein and Amino Acids

Protein and amino acids are produced by a huge number of plant and animal species. Animal protein has a balanced level of all amino acids; hence, it is called complete protein. The rich sources of animal proteins are meat, milk, milk products, egg, poultry, and fishes. In contrast, plant (vegetable) protein is incomplete protein; soybean protein is an exception to this. Plant proteins are abundantly found in legumes, vegetables, greens, and nuts. Animal protein is largely connected with high fat content, so high consumption of animal protein leads to high risks of diseases such as high blood pressure and heart diseases (Nehete et al. 2013). Animal proteins contain essential amino acids needed for an adult's diet. This section describes the importance of some natural proteins, amino acids from plant and animal sources, also the purified form of protein, and amino acids with nutraceutical potentials.

8.7   Significance of Protein and Amino Acids in Human

Proteins are essential for growth and maintenance of tissues and organs of all living organisms. Proteins as enzymes carry out thousands of biochemical reactions including digestion, energy production, blood clotting, muscle contraction, etc. (Martínez-Cuesta et al. 2015). Amino acid chains of various lengths form protein and peptides which make up several hormones that are involved in cell signaling between cells, tissues, and organs. A group of fibrous proteins including keratin, collagen, and elastin provide various parts of your body with structure, strength, and elasticity. Proteins act as a buffer system (Hamm et al. 2015). Antibodies are formed by proteins that protect the body from foreign disease-causing organisms such as bacteria and viruses. Albumin and globulin are proteins found in blood that maintain the body's fluid balance by attracting and retaining water (Hankins 2006). Some proteins are involved in nutrient transport throughout the entire body while others store them. Protein can serve as a valuable energy source but only in situations of fasting, exhaustive exercise, or inadequate calorie intake (Carbone et al. 2014).

8.8   Natural Proteins

8.8.1   Milk Proteins

Casein and whey protein are the major milk proteins. Casein is found in about 80% (29.5 g/l) of the total protein in bovine milk, and whey protein accounts for about 20% (6.3 g/l) (Parodi 2007). It contains high concentration of cysteine, glutamine, lysine, phenylalanine, and branched-chain amino acids (BCAA), including leucine, isoleucine, and valine. It is a heterogeneous family of four major components including alpha- (α_{s1}- and α_{s2}-casein), beta-, gamma-, and kappa-casein (k-casein) (McLachlan 2001; Pihlanto 2011). α_{s1}-casein (23.6 kDa, 4.94 a pI, net charge − 21.9 at a pH of 6.6), α_{s2}-casein (net charge − 13.8, 5.37 pI, hydrophilic due to high-charge density), β-casein (polar N-terminal amphipathic protein with large hydrophobic domain, Ca 2 + sensitive, at 4 °C solubility increases), and casein (not Ca 2 + sensitive) which make up 38, 10, 36, and 13% of the casein composition, respectively, have a unique property to form films (Audic et al. 2003).

Caseins are heat stable and have little secondary or tertiary structure because of high proline content. Its open structure imparted proteolytic cleavage and the characteristic acid-soluble calcium–phosphate linking makes an excellent target-activated release mechanism for delivering drug to the stomach (Livney 2010). Evidence point out that casein might protect the body against some cancers by preventing the fecal beta-glucuronidase, an enzyme produced by intestinal bacteria and deconjugates procarcinogenic glucuronides to carcinogens (Parodi 2007). Casein also defends against colon cancer through its influence on the immune system, specifically by stimulating phagocytic activities and increasing lymphocytes (Parodi 1998).

Some reports suggested that casein might contribute to the beneficial effects of milk on oral health (Johansson and Lif Holgerson 2011). k-casein may fight against dental caries by decreasing the activity of glucosyltransferase, a plaque-promoting enzyme produced by *Streptococcus mutans*, and the ability of this enzyme to adhere to dental surfaces (Vacca-Smith et al. 1994). Casein has also been revealed to reduce the adherence of *S. mutans* to the S-HA surfaces of teeth (Johansson 2002). In hypercholesterolemic persons, who consumed 2 doses of casein (30 or 50 g) in the form of beverage, total cholesterol concentrations were reduced during 16 weeks (Tonstad et al. 2002).

Whey protein is a collection of globular proteins containing high level of α-helix structure with the acidic-basic and hydrophobic-hydrophilic amino acids distributed in a fairly balanced form (Madureira et al. 2007). It contains high concentration of BCAA, including leucine, isoleucine, and valine. Other amino acids include glutamine, proline, aspartic acid, serine, tyrosine, and histidine. Alpha-lactalbumin (α-LA) and beta-lactoglobulin (β-LG) are the predominant whey proteins and comprise about 70–80% of the total whey proteins. The biological components of whey, including lactoferrin, beta-lactoglobulin, α-LA, glycomacropeptide (GMP), and immunoglobulins, demonstrate a range of immune-enhancing properties. In addition, whey has the ability to act as an antioxidant, antihypertensive, antitumor, hypolipidemic, antiviral, antibacterial, and chelating agent (Keri Marshall 2004). In animal studies where colon cancer was induced, whey demonstrated significantly lower incidence of tumors, as well as fewer aberrant crypts (Kuhara et al. 2000).

8.8.2 Egg Protein

Eggs consist of ovalbumin (54%), ovotransferrin (12%), ovomucoid (11%), lysozyme (3.5%), and ovomucin (3.5%) which are considered as the main proteins and avidin (0.05%), cystatin (0.05%), ovomacroglobulin (0.5%), ovoflavoprotein (0.8%), ovoglycoprotein (1.0%), and ovoinhibitor (1.5%) are the minor proteins (Kovacs-Nolan et al. 2005).

Ovalbumin comprises 54% of the total egg white proteins and is synthesized in the hen's oviduct (Stadelman and Cotterill 2001). The ovalbumin is made up of 386 amino acids with the MW of 45 kDa. Ovalbumin a has unique amino acid composition compared with other proteins (Nisbet et al. 1981); the C-terminal amino acid is proline and the N-terminal amino acid is acetylated glycine. It is also called as a glycoprotein and has a carbohydrate group attached to the N-terminal. Ovalbumin is made of three components, A1, A2, and A3, that contain 2, 1, and no phosphate group, respectively. The relative proportion of the subcomponents is 85:12:3 (Stadelman and Cotterill 2001). Like the human blood albumin, the egg ovalbumin also has potential to be used as a drug carrier (Kratz 2008). Ovalbumin has tumor necrosis releasing factors, which can be used for tumor suppression (Kovacs-Nolan et al. 2000).

Ovotransferrin is a monomeric glycoprotein containing a MW of 76 kDa and 686 amino acids (Stadelman and Cotterill 2001). The amino acid sequence of ovotransferrin is similar to the transferrin found in human serum and has 15 disulfide bonds (Oe et al. 1988). It was also called conalbumin but later renamed as ovotransferrin after its finding property with iron (Williams 1968). It transports iron in the body by binding with two iron molecules folded into two lobes and four domains with each lobe composed of two distinct α- and β-domains. These two domains are linked with antiparallel β strands that open and close by a hinge (Huopalahti et al. 2007). At pH > 7.0, iron (Fe^{3+}) can be easily attached to ovotransferrin but is removed at pH < 4.5 (Ko and Ahn 2008). The two iron-binding sites are situated within the inter-domain cleft of each lobe. Ovotransferrin releases the bound iron at pH < 4.5 effortlessly (Ko and Ahn 2008). Ibrahim and Kiyono (2009) reported that ovotransferrin underwent thiol-linked auto-cleavage after reduction, and produced partially hydrolyzed products with very strong anticancer effects against colon and breast cancer cells.

Another significant protein found in egg white is lysozyme. In nature, there are various forms of lysozyme found, but the egg owns the most soluble and stable lysozyme among them. It is a universal enzyme that can degrade the β-linkage between *N*-acetylneuraminic acid and *N*-acetylglucosamine in the bacterial cell wall (Huopalahti et al. 2007); so it is also called *N*-acetyl-muramic-hydrolase and consists of leucine and lysine in the C- and N-terminal, respectively. Lysozyme consists of a single polypeptide chain made up of 129 amino acids with a MW of 4400 Da. This protein occasionally present as a dimer with more thermal stability but exists as a monomer in nature. It is measured as a strong basic protein present in egg white (Huopalahti et al. 2007). Lysozyme contains four disulfide bridges making the thermal stability high, and its isoelectric point is 10.7. It has an affinity of binding to negatively charged proteins such as ovomucin in egg white (Wan et al. 2006). Lysozyme acts as an immune-modulating and immune-stimulating agent and has the capability of suppressing tumor cells (Kovacs-Nolan et al. 2005). Therefore, lysozyme can be used as an anticancer agent.

Ovomucin is another main egg white protein, which constitutes 3.5% of the total egg white protein. Ovomucin is made up of soluble and insoluble components: the soluble component consists of 8300 Da and insoluble component ranges from 220 to 270 kDa (Omana et al. 2010). Earlier reports have revealed that four types of carbohydrate chains are present in ovomucin, which include galalctose, galacrosamine, sialic acid, and sulfate with a molecular ratio of 1:1:1:1. On average, 33% of ovomucin is carbohydrates (Mine 2008). Ovomucin primarily contains two types of subunits and they are called α and β; α-ovomucin is homogeneous, whereas β-ovomucin is heterogeneous. α-Ovomucin has two subunits called α1 and α2, which have less carbohydrate group than β-ovomucin, which is rich in carbohydrates. Ovomucin has more coiled regions at its edges, like the structure of human mucin. Because of the long-coiled areas, a randomly coiled structure is observed. β-Ovomucin is made up of the amino acids like serine and threonine and the α-ovomucin consist of the acidic amino acids such as aspartic acid and glutamic acid, but there is no difference in the ovomucin found in thick egg white and thin egg white (Omana et al. 2010). Ovomucin is also reported to have antitumor activity and antiviral effects (Oguro et al. 2000; Omana et al. 2010). Therefore, not only ovotransferrin but also ovomucin can be used to control tumor growth.

Ovomucoid is the highly glycosylated protein found in egg white (Kovacs-Nolan et al. 2000). The MW of ovomucoid is 28 kDa, but the band in SDS-PAGE appears at 30–40 kDa. It is also called as trypsin inhibitor and it is considered as the main food allergen present in egg white. Each ovomucoid molecule binds with one molecule of trypsin, and its three-dimensional structure is held with the three disulfide bonds in it (Oliveira et al. 2009). Nagata and Yoshida (1984) documented that ovomucoid can be used to prevent the *Streptomyces erythraeus*. Though the protein has the property of trypsin inhibition, which is a negative property of the protein, it has the ability of controlling microorganisms (Kovacs-Nolan et al. 2005) and it has been reported that the biospecific ligand of ovomucoid can be used as a drug delivery agent. It is also enhancing the surface migration of primordial germ cells, which helped the expression of PGCs from E3 to E7 in male embryo cells (Halfter et al. 1996).

8.8.3 Meat Proteins

Sarcoplasmic, stromal, and myofibrillar proteins are the three major proteins obtained from fish and animal meat. Sarcoplasmic proteins represent 20–40% of the total muscle proteins. These proteins are globular and exhibit solubility in water and diluted salt solutions and are constituted mainly by enzymes involved in cellular metabolism (Nakagawa et al. 1998). They are found in the sarcoplasm or fluid surrounding the myofibrils. They are made up of mostly oxidative enzymes, heme pigments (myoglobin), the mitochondrial oxidative enzymes (Glyceraldehyde phosphate dehydrogenase, aldolase, enolase, creatine kinase, lactate dehydrogenase, pyruvate kinase, phosphorylase). Lysosomal enzymes, and nucleoproteins. There are around 90 different proteins that belong to the group of sarcoplasmic proteins among which myoglobin and hemoglobin are the main sarcoplasmic proteins.

The watery substance of connective tissue is dispersed with matrix of stromal-protein fibrils. Stromal proteins are used for making edible films and coatings, which are soluble in salt solutions. The main types of stromal proteins include collagen and elastin. Collagen is a fibrous stromal protein extracted from the connective tissue, tendons, skin, bones, and the vascular system and is a waste product of meat processing. Collagen formed a super helical structure by the combination of three parallel alfa-chains and forms gelatin (Haug et al. 2004). Collagen exposed to mild heat treatment under acidic or alkaline conditions forms gelatin (Badii and Howell 2006). Several reports suggested that the consumption of collagen may have a variety of health benefits, from relieving joint pain to improving skin health (Asserin et al. 2015; Bello and Oesser 2006).

Elastin is existing in the walls of the circulatory system as well as in connective tissues throughout the animal body and provides elasticity to those tissues. Elastin is yellow in color, so it is referred to as "yellow" connective tissue. The elastin-derived peptides have been shown to play an important role in the physiological maintenance of arteries (Qin 2015). The experiment reports supported that BEP may prevent and regulate photo aging of the skin by decreasing the elastase activities, inhibiting fibroblast apoptosis, and by increasing the hydroxyproline and water content (Liu et al. 2018).

The myofibrillar proteins include contractile, structural, and regulatory proteins (Hopkins 2014). The contractile proteins are myosin and actin, which are thin and thick filaments that are involved in the skeletal muscle contraction and relaxation. The regulatory proteins comprise of troponin and tropomyosin. The structural proteins include titin, nebulin, α-actinin, β-actinin, tropomodulin, desmin, filamin, C-protein, H-protein, and myomesin.

8.8.3.1 Contractile Proteins

Myosin is a filamentous protein with the MW of 520 kD that forms the thick filaments of muscle cells and is the principal protein of the A-band (Strasburg et al. 2008). The quaternary structure of myosin has six subunits, which include two myosin heavy chains (MHC), two essential myosin light chains (MLC1), and two regulatory myosin light chains (MLC2) with MWs of approximately 220, 23, and 20 kDa, respectively (Swartz et al. 2009).

Actin is the building block of thin filaments with the MW of 42 kDa and is found in two forms, namely globular actin (G-actin) and filamentous actin (F-actin) (Strasburg et al. 2008). F-actin is formed by the polymerization of G-actin into double-stranded coiled filaments. During muscle contraction, actin binds myosin to form actomyosin cross-bridges, which activate the myosin ATPase, leading to the pulling of thin filaments by myosin toward the M-line, resulting in shortening of the sarcomere (Lawrie 2006).

8.8.3.2 Regulatory Proteins

Tropomyosin and troponin are two main proteins that regulate muscle contraction and relaxation (Choi and Kim 2009). They prevent the activation of actomyosin ATPase in the absence of calcium ions by interacting with actin filaments to block the myosin-binding site. Tropomyosin is a long, coiled protein (MW 65 kDa) that comprises two a-helix polypeptide subunits: α- and β-tropomyosin. Tropomyosin molecules bind head-to-tail along the F-actin filament. Each tropomyosin molecule is attached to a troponin complex (MW 80 kDa) which is made up of troponin C (MW 18 kDa), troponin I (MW 21 kDa), and troponin T (MW 31 kDa).

Troponin C acts as the calcium binding site; troponin T connects troponin complex to tropomyosin while troponin I inhibits actomyosin ATPase activity when it is bound to actin (Lehman and Craig 2008). At high calcium ion concentration, calcium ions bind to troponin C, which initiates a conformation change in the tropomyosin–troponin complex, dislocating troponin I and allowing the action of actomyosin ATPase for muscle contraction.

8.8.3.3 Structural Proteins

The structural proteins control the filamentous structure and integrity of myofibrils (Obinata et al. 1981). Titin, also known as connectin, with a MW of 4200 kDa, serves as the backbone of thick filaments in the A-band. It also acts as a molecular spring in the I-band, which provides elasticity to the sarcomere during muscle contraction (Labeit and Kolmerer 1995). The structural protein nebulin (MW 800 kDa) is involved in regulation of the length of thin filaments (Strasburg et al. 2008). α-Actinin (MW 95 kDa) is the major component of the Z-disk; β-actinin is a heterodimer made up of α- and β-subunits (MW 37 and 34 kDa, respectively), which is also called as CapZ protein. β-Actinin binds the α-actinin in the Z-disk and stops network development between the actin filaments (Swartz et al. 2009). Tropomodulin (MW 40 kDa) combines tropomyosin and actin and also controls the length of thin filaments by preserving the number of G-actin monomers (Clark et al. 2002).

Desmin (MW 55 kDa) and filamin (MW 300 kDa) are involved in the linking of myofibrils to the sarcolemma and also in stabilizing muscle structure (Strasburg et al. 2008). The A-band of thick filaments contain the myosin-binding proteins called C-protein (MW 140 kDa) and H-protein (MW 58 kDa) (Xiong 1997). These proteins are assumed to contribute to the arrangement and stabilization of the thick filaments. In the M-line, the major protein is myomesin (MW 185 kDa). It is involved for the binding of titin and myosin and for maintaining the structure of the thick filaments.

8.8.4 Silk Protein

The cocoon of the silkworm *Bombyx mori* provided silk to weave. The silk is made up of the protein fibroin and sericin with good biocompatibility, slow biodegradability, self-assembly, excellent mechanical properties, controllable structure, and morphology that make it a favorable material for drug delivery and tissue engineering (Numata and Kaplan 2010). Fibroin is a glycoprotein and constitutes of two protein subunits that are covalently linked by disulfide bonds. The fibroin filament is composed of both crystalline and amorphous domains. The amorphous domains are characterized by the presence of amino acids, whereas the crystalline domains are characterized by high percentage of alanine, glycine, and serine (Lesile et al. 2003). The γ-irradiated silk fibroin shows higher proliferative effect in the mouse peritoneal macrophages in a concentration-dependent manner, and this shows the antitumor activity of γ-irradiated silk fibroin (Byun et al. 2010).

The protein sericin can be classified into three fractions based on its solubility: A, B, and C. Sericin A is comprised of 17.2% of nitrogen and amino acids. It is the outmost layer and insoluble in hot water. The middle layer is sericin B and is hydrolyzed by acid; it yields amino acids of sericin A in addition to tryptophan. It contains 16.8% of nitrogen. Sericin C is the innermost layer that is adjacent to fibroin (Sprange 1975).

8.9 Plant Proteins

8.9.1 Oats Protein

Oats (100 g) contain 16.9 grams of protein, namely avenalin and avenin. Oats proteins are similar to the protein of soy beans, which is recognized as being almost equal in quality to the protein in meat, milk, and eggs. The hull-less oat kernel (groat) has a protein content of 12–24%, which is the highest among cereals. The main protein (80%) in oats is globulin protein, called avenalin, which is found only in oats and not in other grains. The water-soluble property of globulins helps to make oats milk but not bread (Lasztity 1999). The remaining 20% of oat protein is a prolamine, called avenin, which is related to wheat gluten (Chatuevedi et al. 2011).

People with celiac disease may experience adverse reactions when they eat foods containing prolamine proteins, especially gluten. Oats lack many of the prolamines found in wheat; however, oats do contain avenin. Though the minor protein in oats is prolamine protein, a number of scientific studies found that people with celiac disease can tolerate most varieties of gluten-free oats (Tapsas et al. 2014). About 90% of oat protein is highly digestible, which is similar to the protein digestibility of rice and corn. The oat proteins composition suits well to fulfill the human needs of essential amino acids; the amounts of lysine and threonine in whole grain oats almost meet the dietary requirements (80%) for both amino acids (Peterson 2011).

8.9.2 Soyabean (*Glycine max*) Protein

The soyabean seeds contain approximately 90% of storage proteins. The major globulins found in soybean are glycinin and β-conglycinin that account for about 70–80% of the total seed globulin fraction (Krishnan et al. 2009). The total soybean protein content and the quality is higher than that of other plant proteins and is equal to animal protein (Hughes et al. 2011). The protein digestibility corrected amino acid scores (PDCAAS) for soy protein range from 0.9 to 1.0 depending on the specific soy food (Hughes et al. 2011; Rutherfurd et al. 2015). In the meta-analysis conducted among 743 subjects, 38 separate studies showed that consumption of soy protein resulted in significant reduction in total cholesterol (9.3%), LDL cholesterol (12.9%), and triglycerides (10.5%); HDL cholesterol showed small but insignificant increase (2.4%) (Anderson et al. 1995).

8.9.3 Pea (*Pisum sativum*) Protein

During the development, the pea seeds accumulated large amounts of protein in the seed cotyledons. Protein content varies from 18 to 30% depending on environment factors and the cultivar. Unlike animal proteins, pea proteins contain essential amino acids in essential proportions, whereby methionine is the limiting amino acid in peas. Pea proteins have five protein fractions which are albumins (water soluble), globulins (soluble in dilute salt solution), prolamins (soluble in 70% ethanol solution), glutelins (soluble in dilute alkaline solution), and residue protein (left over protein) based on the Osborne classification (Osborne 1924). The most dominant class of proteins in peas is globulins, which consists of 7S (vicilin) and 11S (legumin) globulin proteins.

8.9.4 Peanuts (*Arachis hypogaea*) Protein

The protein content ranges from 22 to 30% of its total calories, making peanuts a great source of plant-based protein (Pancholy et al. 1978). Pea protein contains all nine essential amino acids – histidine, isoleucine, leucine, lysine, methionine, phenylalanine, threonine, tryptophan, and valine – that your body cannot create and must get from food. However, it is relatively low in methionine (Tömösközi et al. 2010) It is also a great source of BCAA. Peanut proteins have been customarily classified as albumins (water soluble) or globulins (saline soluble). Most of the storage proteins are globulins, which make up 87% of the total protein. Peanut protein provides many health benefits, especially arginine, which promotes healthy blood flow and heart health and leucine, isoleucine, and valine, which promote muscle growth (Latif et al. 2013).

8.9.5 Rice (*Oryza sativa*) Protein

Rice grain contains albumin (4–22%), globulin (5–13%), prolamin (1–5%), and predominantly glutelin (60–80% of total protein) (Kim et al. 2013) Glutelin of rice is a protein of high MW (6×10^4 B 6×10^5), also soluble in dilute acid and composed of subunits bound by disulfide linkages (Tecson et al. 1971), while rice globulin is composed of low-molecular-weight ($12-20 \times 10^3$) protein components (Cagampang et al. 1976). The rice protein prolamin stimulated cytokine release from normal peripheral blood mononuclear cells (PBMC) to inhibit growth and induce differentiation of human leukemic U937 cells. The gastrointestinal enzymes digest the prolamin, avoiding its contact with leukocytes (Chen et al. 2010).

8.9.6 Spinach Amino Acids

Fresh leaves of spinach contained 2.36 g of total amino acids in 100 g of edible parts. Essential amino acids constituted 49% of total amino acids. The dominant amino acids were glutamic acid (12% of the total content of amino acids) and aspartic acid (11%) (Lisiewska et al. 2011).

8.9.7 ʟ-Arginine

ʟ-Arginine is essential for children and nonessential for adults; hence it is known as semi-essential or conditionally essential amino acid. The endogenous synthesis of ʟ-arginine takes place mainly by the tissues of the kidney, from citrulline, which is released mainly by the small intestine (Dhanakoti et al. 1990). The amount of ʟ-arginine synthesized by the liver will be completely reutilized in the urea cycle so that the liver contributes little or not at all to plasma arginine flux (Watford 1991). In a healthy adult diet, 5–7% of the amino acid content is ʟ-arginine only. It is estimated that the average intake of ʟ-arginine is 2.5–5 g/day, which only meets the body's minimal requirement for tissue repair, protein synthesis, and immune cell maintenance. In the GIT, ʟ-arginine is absorbed in the jejunum and ileum of the small intestine. The absorbed arginine (60%) is metabolized by the GIT and only 40% reaches the systemic circulation intact. Most dietary proteins have a relatively balanced mixture of amino acids, and thus the only way to selectively deliver more ʟ-arginine to an individual would be to supplement with the individual amino acid itself. ʟ-Arginine is naturally present in various animal and plants sources, the concentration of ʟ-arginine in different sources is listed in Table 8.3.

ʟ-Arginine has been demonstrated to improve peripheral circulation (2004), renal function (Klahr 1999), and immune function (Park et al. 1991). It also possesses antistress and adaptogenic

Table 8.3 Sources of L-arginine.

Source	Grams/cup of L-arginine
Nuts and seeds	
Pumpkin seeds	6.905 g
Watermelon seeds	5.289
Sesame seeds	4.875
Dried walnut	4.522
Almonds	3.525
Pine nuts	3.258
Meat products	
Turkey breast	16.207
Chicken	2.790
Pork loin	2.661
Beef	4.131
Legumes	
Soybeans	5.865
Raw peanuts	4.567
Chickpeas	3.878
Seaweed	4.645

Source: Medical New today, by Jenna Fletcher on 4 October 2018. Medically reviewed by Katherine Marengo LDN.R.D

capabilities (Gupta et al. 2005). L-Arginine stimulates the release of growth hormone as well as the release of pancreatic insulin and glucagon and pituitary prolactin (Boger and Bode Boger 2001).

8.10 Protein Isolates as Nutraceuticals

8.10.1 Collagen Peptide (Bovine Origin)

Bovine collagen is a protein product mainly derived from cows. It is prescribed for several health benefits, including relief from arthritis, improved skin health, and prevention of bone loss. Collagen is an abundant protein found in humans and numerous animals. It is the major building blocks in skin, bones, tendons, ligaments, muscles, and blood vessels (Avila Rodríguez et al. 2018; Vollmer et al. 2018). This protein is also widely used as a food additive and supplement. Nowadays, it is popular in cosmetic industry as a potential remedy to reduce the effects of skin aging.

Majority of the collagen supplements are derived from a variety of animal and plant sources including the bovine animals such as pigs and marine species such as fish, jellyfish, and sponges. Less common sources include genetically modified yeast and bacteria (Silva et al. 2014; Vollmer et al. 2018). Bovine collagen obtained from the bovine species include yak, antelope, bison, water buffalo, and cows, but primarily cows. It is prepared by boiling the cow bones or other cattle by-products in water and then the collagen is extracted and dried to form powdered supplement.

Bovine collagen has been found to increase types I and III collagen, whereas marine collagen boosts types I and II (Silva et al. 2014; Song et al. 2018).

The human skin is primarily made up of types I and III collagen; so bovine collagen is mainly useful for reducing wrinkles, promoting elasticity, and increasing skin moisture (Song et al. 2018). Bovine collagen is used to reduce the symptoms of osteoarthritis, a common type of arthritis caused by the disintegration of the protective cartilage at the ends of bones. It can lead to pain and stiffness in your hands, knees, and hips, among other body parts (Guo and Dou 2020). In in-vitro studies in mouse cells, bovine collagen increased bone formation and mineralization, which may support osteoarthritis (Liu et al. 2014). Additionally, in a 13-week study in 30 people with osteoarthritis affecting their knees, those given 5 grams of bovine collagen twice daily experienced improvements in symptoms (Kumar et al. 2015).

8.10.2 Soy Protein Hydrolysates (SPHs)

Soy bean hydrolysates are produced from soy proteins by following different protein processing technologies such as hydrolysis and thermal treatments, or through biological processes including enzymatic digestion, gastrointestinal digestion, and microbial fermentation (Ashaolu 2020). Soy protein contains the entire essential amino acids, including its peptic hydrolysates (Ashaolu and Yupanqui 2017) similar to animal proteins. The PDCAAS of casein, egg, and soy protein are same. This confirms that the nutritional and biological values of SPHs are equivalent to animal protein (Singh et al. 2014). On the other hand, soy protein is free from cholesterol, gluten, and lactose, and its enzymatically hydrolyzed forms are hypoallergenic, which makes it a suitable food for lactose-intolerant consumers, vegetarians, and milk-allergy patients (Ashaolu and Yupanqui 2017, 2018). Soy proteins comprises 65–80% of glycinin and β-conglycinin in its total protein content, often acting as the precursor of soy peptides isolation.

The hydrolysates or biopeptides prepared from soy protein confer numerous biological functions, which have preventive or therapeutic applications such as treating obesity, cancer, and CVDs (Ashaolu et al. 2019). Numerous biologically potential peptides are isolated from animal and plant sources such as milk, meat, egg, fish, oyster, cereals (rice, wheat, soybean, buckwheat, barley, and corn), soybean, and radish seeds (Lafarga and Hayes 2014) including marine macroalgae (seaweeds or sea vegetables) and microalgae (Ko et al. 2012). The size of the bioactive peptides are from 2 to 30 amino acids in length (with a few exceptions such as lunasin, which has 43 amino acids) and are usually less than 6 kDa in size (Sarmadi and Ismail 2010). Soy biopeptides may influence cardiovascular, digestive, nervous, and immune systems of the body, based on their amino acids sequence. The biopeptides have been identified with antimicrobial (Andavan and Lemmens-Gruber 2010), immunomodulatory (Ashaolu et al. 2019), angiotensin converting enzyme (ACE)-inhibitory (Wijesekara and Kim 2010), antioxidant (Lule et al. 2015), and anticoagulant (Kim and Wijesekara 2010) properties.

8.10.3 Egg White Protein Hydrolysate

Chiang et al. (2006) produced bioactive peptides by hydrolyzing the egg white by thermolysin that can inhibit the activity of ACE. Miguel and Aleixandre (2006) also produced peptides by hydrolyzing egg white with pepsin. The amino acid sequences of the peptides with Tyr-Arg-Glu-Glu-Arg-Tyr-Pro-Ile-Leu, Arg-Ala-Asp-His-Pro-Phe-Leu, and Ile-Val-Phe exhibited strong ACE-inhibitory activities. Feeding these peptides to spontaneously hypertensive rats reduced the blood pressure in rats.

Fujita et al. (2000) produced seven ACE-inhibitory peptides –LKA, LKP, LAP, IKW, FQKPKR, FKGRYYP, and IVGRPRHQG – by hydrolyzing ovalbumin with pepsin, trypsin, and α-chymotrypsin.

Some of the peptides produced from ovalbumin showed strong ACE-inhibitory effects and also lowered blood lipid content (Manso et al. 2008; Miguel et al. 2007) due to the vasodilation effect of the peptides derived from egg white as well as from ovalbumin. Yu et al. (2012) reported that ovokinins 2 to 7 showed the most prominent ACE-inhibitory activities among the peptides produced.

Bioactive peptides of ovotransferrin showed strong antimicrobial activity (Ibrahim et al. 2000). But ovotransferrin lost its ability to bind with iron after hydrolysis (Wu and Acero-Lopez 2012). Peptides of ovotransferrin also exhibited strong antioxidant activity. The hydrolysis of ovotransferrin with the enzymes such as protamex, alkalse, trypsin, and α-chymotrypsin showed protective effects against oxidative stress including DNA damage in human leukocytes (Moon et al. 2013). Also, the hydrolysates of ovotransferrin having the peptide sequence of Lys-Val-Arg-Glu-Gly-Thr had strong ACE-inhibitory activity as well as vasodilatory activity (Wu and Acero-Lopez 2012). Peptides derived from ovomucoid and ovomucin showed immunomodulating activity against T-cells and macrophage-stimulating activities in vitro, respectively (Kovacs-Nolan et al. 2005), indicating that they can also be good candidates for pharmaceutical use in humans.

8.10.4 Casein Protein Hydrolysate

Casein from milk or any dairy foods is the main source of casein-derived bioactive peptides. Milk-derived peptides are commonly ingested in both functional foods and drugs. Biologically active peptides hidden within the intact milk proteins are released and activated by gastrointestinal digestion of milk, fermentation of milk by proteolysis starter cultures, or hydrolysis by proteolytic enzymes. Peptides from casein protein and whey proteins such as opioid peptides, antihypertensive peptides, casein phosphopeptides (CPPs), GMP, and lactorphins exhibit numerous physiological roles, such as opioid-like features, immunostimulating activities, antihypertensive activities, antibacterial and antiviral impacts, and also improving the calcium absorption (Jauhiainen and Korpela 2007). Kampa et al. (1997) described that many casomorphin peptides belonging to opioid peptide groups derived from α- and β-casein suppressed the proliferation of some prostatic cancer cell lines, including LNCaP, PC3, and DU145, through the involvement of opioid receptors. Many experiments have been done to observe the effect of casein-derived bioactive peptides on immune function. It was found that in-vitro digests of casein produced by peptidases of *Lactobacillus rhamnosus* inhibited protein kinase C translocation and downregulated IL-2 mRNA expression. These findings demonstrated in-vitro suppression of T-cell activation by casein digests (Pessi et al. 2001). Caseicidin, a defense peptide purified by chymosin hydrolysis of casein at neutral pH, showed inhibitory activity against *Staphylococci*, *Sarcina spp*, *B. subtilis*, *Diplococcus pneumoniae*, and *Streptococcus pyogenes* (Lahov and Regelson 1996).

8.10.5 Whey Protein Hydrolysate

Whey protein products are derived from the protein fraction of whey. There are three major whey protein powders: concentrate (WPC), isolate (WPI), and hydrolysate (WPH). These products are the source of high-quality complete protein comprised of all types of essential amino acids. These are also easily digestible, absorbed from the gut easily, when compared to all other types of proteins. Among the three types of products, whey protein concentrate is the most common type and also very cheap. As a dietary supplement, whey protein is widely popular among bodybuilders, athletes, and others who want additional protein in their diet. Whey protein is effective for the prevention of age-related muscle loss, as well as for improved strength and a better-looking body (Paddon-Jones and Rasmussen 2009). Whey protein consumption promotes muscle growth due to the presence of high concentration of leucine, the growth-promoting branched amino acid of whey protein. For muscle growth, whey protein has been shown to be slightly better compared to other types of protein, such as casein or soy (Hartman et al. 2007; Pennings et al. 2011).

Whey protein consumption has been found to be effective at moderating blood sugar by increasing both the levels of insulin and the sensitivity to its effects. These properties of whey protein may even be comparable to those of diabetic drugs, such as sulfonylurea (Ma et al. 2009; Pal and Ellis 2010). Taking a whey protein supplement before or with a high-carb meal has been shown to moderate blood sugar in both healthy people and type 2 diabetics (Frid et al. 2005). A huge review study shows that the high doses of whey protein supplements significantly reduced C-reactive protein (CRP), a key marker of inflammation in the body (Zhou et al. 2015). Whey proteins contain high cysteine which boost the body's natural antioxidant defenses (Kimball and Jefferson 2006). A number of studies in both humans and rodents have found that whey proteins may reduce oxidative stress and increase levels of glutathione (de Aguilar-Nascimento et al. 2011).

Many animal studies have scrutinized the effects of whey and its immune-enhancing components, including lactoferrin and beta-lactoglobulin. When whey-based protein powders were compared to soy-based protein powders, similar effects were also observed. Hakkak et al. (2009) demonstrated that lactoferrin has the ability to inhibit metastasis of primary tumors in mice with cancer. Bovine serum albumin (10–15% of total whey protein) has demonstrated inhibition of growth in human breast cancer cells in vitro (Yoo et al. 1998). A hamster study confirmed that fractionated whey has the ability to prevent and treat 5-fluorouracil chemotherapy-induced oral mucositis (Laursen et al. 1990). This protection is thought to occur via induction of tumor growth factor-beta (TGF-β), which reduces basal epithelial cell proliferation (Clarke et al. 2002)

8.10.6 L-Arginine

L-Arginine is a conditionally essential amino acid found in the diet. It is mostly used by athletic people as a dietary supplement because it directly produces nitric oxide using *nitric oxide synthase* enzymes. It is usually used as drug for the periods of illness and chronic conditions such as hypertension and type II diabetes, because these states increase the enzyme arginase that degrades L-arginine, resulting in a transient deficiency of L-arginine. This leads to an increase in blood pressure in these states and can be partially remedied by an increase in L-arginine intake or resolution of the illness/disease state (http://examine.com/supplements/arginine/).

A summary of some of the positive results for L-arginine in the prevention and improvement of CVD include: 6.6 g/day oral in hypercholesterolemic patients with peripheral arterial disease (Heartbar) – at two weeks increased pain-free period, increased total walking distance (by 66 and 23%), and increased quality of life (Maxwell et al. 2000); and 15 g/day oral in patients with congestive heart failure – at five days improved glomerular filtration rate, natriuresis, and plasma endothelin levels (Watanabe et al. 2000).

Oral administration of 500 mg arginine–HCl per day to infertile men for six to eight weeks markedly increased sperm counts and motility in a majority of patients and resulted in successful pregnancies (Tanimura 1967).

Dietary L-arginine has been shown to improve collagen deposition and wound strength in both humans (Kirk et al. 1993) and animals (Arbss et al. 2000). The healing effect of L-arginine is also extended to cover burn injuries. Oral dietary L-arginine supplementation of 100–400 mg/kg/day shortened re-epithelization times, increased amounts of hydroxyproline, and accelerated the synthesis of reparative collagen in burned rats (Chen et al. 1999). Evidence suggests that arginine supplementation may be an effective way to improve endothelial function in individuals with DM (Giugliano et al. 1997).

Administration of L-arginine (1.6 g/day) in 16 elderly patients with senile dementia has been found to be effective in reducing lipid peroxidation and increasing cognitive function (Ohtsuka and Nakaya 2000). In their recent report, Yi et al. (2009) explored the possible role of L-arginine in Alzheimer's disease (AD), taking into consideration known functions for L-arginine in atherosclerosis, redox stress and the inflammatory process, regulation of synaptic plasticity and neurogenesis, and modulation of glucose metabolism and insulin activity

8.10.7 Mineral Amino Acid Chelate

Calcium glycinate, calcium proteinate, chromium proteinate, polysaccharide chromium complex, copper proteinate, and magnesium aspartate are the feed-grade mineral amino acids chelates. These mineral amino acid chelates are the combinations of inorganic micro-minerals (Zn, Cu, Mn, Fe, and Co) or macro-minerals (Mg, Ca) with an amino acid in a 1:1 molar ratio. The chelates help the metals from being tied up by antagonisms (Fe, Mo, and S) during digestion and allows the metal to remain part of this organic molecule as it is absorbed primarily in the jejunal area of the small intestine. These amino-chelated minerals are thought to be more digestible than nonchelated forms. The organic ligand molecule consists of amino acids, hydrolyzed protein chains (usually from soy), sugars, or other compounds that may or may not offer absorptive value to the human body. The nutritive value of the ligands is not needed to improve the function of mineral rather the ligand's mechanism of making the mineral more biologically effective than its inorganic counterpart (Keith 2013).

Glucose and hydrolyzed soy proteins are very cheap ligands, and hydrolyzed proteins are available in an assortment of unidentified protein chains. The large-sized ligands are not stable in the digestive process. General medical research and laboratory studies have shown that the amino acid glycine is the ideal size and type of ligand (Ferrari et al. 2012). The amino acid glycine is produced by the human body naturally as a building block for larger protein chains. By comparison, glycine is a very small and precise amino acid molecule that makes a very stable chelate. These factors make a glycine chelate superior. Unfortunately, the cost of this single amino acid is quite high because of the level of sophistication required to manufacture it. A small ligand like glycine bonds to the mineral and creates a complete chelated molecule small enough to be picked by protein receptors in the digestive process – a key factor for increased mineral bioavailability (Keith 2013).

8.11 Conclusion

Carbohydrates, proteins, and amino acids are the distinct group of chemically defined components with a range of physical and physiological properties and health benefits for consumers. The major role of these components is to provide energy, build structure and functions of cells, tissues, and organs. Many forms of these components are found in natural sources with potential properties. Recently, the consumption of natural products was improved among the population for getting better health, to improve body building, and to treat various diseases. Knowledge from various sources help the people to design their diet with prebiotics, dietary fiber, meat, milk, egg, vegetables, and fruits for obtaining natural carbohydrates, protein, and amino acids. The natural sources are the chief supplier of potential carbohydrates, protein, and amino acids without any major side effects. The development in the technology separates the compounds from the natural sources in a purified form and made them available as a nutraceutical to treat many diseases. This chapter describes the common types of carbohydrate, protein, and amino acid nutraceuticals possessing anticancer, antitumor, immunomodulatory, antimicrobial, antioxidant, anti-hypertensive, antidiabetic, anticoagulant, and prebiotic potential. These types of nutraceuticals are also prescribed for treating brain diseases, nephrotic syndrome, osteoporosis, and colon cancer.

References

Aarstad, O.A., Tondervik, A., Sletta, H., and Skjak-Brak, G. (2012). Alginate sequencing: an analysis of block distribution in alginates using specific alginate degrading enzymes. *Biomacromolecules* 13 (1): 106–116.

de Aguilar-Nascimento, J.E., Prado Silveira, B.R., and Dock-Nascimento, D.B. (2011). Early enteral nutrition with whey protein or casein in elderly patients with acute ischemic stroke: a double-blind randomized trial. *Nutrition 27* (4): 440–444. https://doi.org/10.1016/j.nut.2010.02.013.

Akeem, M.A. and Olatunde, O.C. (2018). Recent developments on the application of carbohydrate polymers. IOSR. *J. Appl. Chem.* 11 (7): 68–80.

Aliasgharzadeh, A., Dehghan, P., Gargari, B.P., Asghari-Jafarabadi, M. (2015). Resistant dextrin, as a prebiotic, improves insulin resistance and inflammation in women with type 2 diabetes: a randomised controlled clinical trial. *Br. J. Nutr.*, 113(2):321–330. doi:https://doi.org/10.1017/S0007114514003675.

Anademanantina, H. and Rinaudo, M. (2010). Relationship between the molecular structure of alginates and their gelation in acidic conditions. *Polym. Int.* 59 (11): 1531–1541.

Andavan, G.S.B. and Lemmens-Gruber, R. (2010). Cyclodepsipeptides from marine sponges: natural agents for drug research. *Marine Drugs* 8 (3): 810–834.

Anderson, J.J.W., Johnstone, B.M., and Cook-newell, M.E. (1995). Meta-analysis of the effects of soy protein intake on serum lipids. *New Engl. J. Med.* 333: 276–282.

Ando, H., Ohba, H., Sakaki, T. et al. (2004). Hot-compressed-water decomposed products from bamboo manifest a selective cytotoxicity against acute lymphoblastic leukemia cells. *Toxicol. in vitro* 18: 763–771.

Aravamudhan, A., Ramos, D.M., Nada, A.A., and Kumbar, S.G. (2014). Natural polymers: polysaccharides and their derivatives for biomedical applications. In: *Natural and synthetic biomedical polymers* (ed. S.G. Kumbar, C.T. Laurencin and M. Deng), 67–89. Oxford: Elsevier.

Arbss, M.A., Ferrando, J.M., Vidal, J. et al. (2000). Early effects of exogenous arginine after the implantation of prosthetic material into the rat abdominal wall. *Life Sci.* 67 (20): 2493–2512.

TJ Ashaolu. (2020). Health applications of soy protein hydrolysates. *International Journal of Peptide Research and Therapeutics* doi:https://doi.org/10.1007/s10989-020-10018-6

Ashaolu, T.J. and Yupanqui, C.T. (2017). Suppressive activity of enzymatically-euced soy protein hydrolysates on degranulation in IgEantigen complex-stimulated RBL-2H3 cells. *Funct. Foods Health Dis.* 7 (7): 545–561.

Ashaolu, T.J. and Yupanqui, C.T. (2018). Hypoallergenic and immunomodulatory prospects of pepsin-educed soy protein hydrolysates. *Croat. J. Food Sci. Technol.* 10 (2): 270–278.

Ashaolu, T.J., Saibandith, B., Yupanqui, C.T., and Wichienchot, S. (2019). Human colonic microbiota modulation and branched chain fatty acids production affected by soy protein hydrolysate. *Int. J. Food Sci. Technol.* 54 (1): 141–148.

Asserin, J., Lati, E., Shioya, T., and Prawitt, J. (2015). The effect of oral collagen peptide supplementation on skin moisture and the dermal collagen network: evidence from an ex vivo model and randomized, placebo-controlled clinical trials. *J. Cosmet. Dermatol.* 14 (4): 291–301.

Audic, J.L., Chaufer, B., and Daufin, G. (2003). Non-food applications of milk components and dairy co-products: a review. *Lair* 83: 417–438.

Avila Rodríguez, M.I., Rodríguez Barroso, L.G., and Sánchez, M.L. (2018). Collagen: a review on its sources and potential cosmetic applications. *J. Cosmet. Dermatol.* 17 (1): 20–26. https://doi.org/10.1111/jocd.12450.

Azevedo Carvalho, A.F., De Oliva Neto, P., Fernandes Da Silva, D., and Pastore, G.M. (2013). Review. Xylooligosaccharides from lignocellulosic materials: chemical structure, health benefits and production by chemical and enzymatic hydrolysis. *Food Res. Int.* 51: 75–85.

Badii, F. and Howell, N.K. (2006). Fish gelatine: structure, gelling properties and interaction with egg albumen proteins. *Food Hydrocoll.* 20: 630–640.

Baeurle, S.A., Kiselev, M.G., Makarova, E.S., Nogovitsin, E.A. (2009). Effect of the counterion behavior on the frictional–compressive properties of chondroitin sulfate solutions. *Polymer*, 50 (7), 1805–1813. doi:https://doi.org/10.1016/j.polymer.2009.01.066.

Ballongue, J., Schuman, C., and Quignon, P. (1997). Effects of lactulose and lactitol on colonic microflora and enzymatic activity. *Scand. J. Gastroenterol.* 222: 41–44.

Barczynska, R., Jochym, K., Śliżewska, K. et al. (2010). The effect of citric acidmodified enzyme-resistant dextrin on growth and metabolism of selected strains of probiotic and other intestinal bacteria. *J. Funct. Foods* 2: 126–133.

Bello, A.E. and Oesser, S. (2006). Collagen hydrolysate for the treatment of osteoarthritis and other joint disorders: a review of the literature. *Curr. Med. Res. Opin.* 22 (11): 2221–2232. https://doi.org/10.1185/030079906X148373.

BeMiller, J.N. (2019). Gellans, curdlan, dextrans, levans, and pullulan. In: *Carbohydrate Chemistry for Food Scientists*, 3e (ed. J.N. BeMiller), 271–278. AACC International Press.

Benito-Román, O., Alonso, E., and Cocero, M.J. (2013). Ultrasound-assisted extraction of β-glucans from barley. *LWT* 50: 57–63.

Berry, G.T., Nissim, I., Lin, Z. et al. (1995). Endogenous synthesis of galactose in normal men and patients with hereditary galactosaemia. *Lancet 346* (8982): 1073–1074. https://doi.org/10.1016/s0140-6736(95)91745-.

Berry, G.T., Moate, P.J., Reynolds, R.A. et al. (2004). The rate of de novo galactose synthesis in patients with galactose-1-phosphate uridyltransferase deficiency. *Mol. Genet. Metab. 81* (1): 22–30. https://doi.org/10.1016/j.ymgme.2003.08.026.

Boger, R.H. and Bode Boger, S.M. (2001). The clinical pharmacology of l-arginine. *Annu. Rev. Pharmacol. Toxicol.* 41: 79–99.

Bosscher, D., Breynaert, A., Pieters, L., and Hermans, N. (2009). Food-based strategies to modulate the composition of the intestinal microbiota and their associated health effects. *J. Physiol. Pharmacol.* 60 (Suppl 6): 5–11.

Brouns, Fred., Kettitz, Bernd., Arrigoni, Eva. (2002). Resistant starch and the butyrate revolution. *Trends Food Sci. Technol.,* 13 (8), 251–261. doi:https://doi.org/10.1016/S0924-2244(02)00131-0.4.

Brunner, S., Holub, I., Theis, S. et al. (2012). Metabolic effects of replacing sucrose by isomaltulose in subjects with type 2 diabetes: a randomized double-blind trial. *Diabetes Care 35* (6): 1249–1251. https://doi.org/10.2337/dc11-1485.

Builders, P.F. and Arhewoh, M.I. (2016). Pharmaceutical applications of native starch in conventional drug delivery. *Starch—Stärke* 68 (9–10): 864–873.

Buléon, A., Colonna, P., Planchot, V., and Ball, S. (1998). Mini review Starch granules: structure and biosynthesis. *Int. J. Biol. Macromol.* 23: 85–112.

Byun, E.B., Sung, N.Y., Kim, J.H. et al. (2010). Enhancement of anti-tumor activity of gammairradiated silk fibroin via immunomodulatory effects. *Chem. Biol. Interact.* 186 (1): 90–95.

Cagampang, G.B., Perdon, A.A., and Juliano, B.O. (1976). Changes in salt-soluble proteins of rice during rain development. *Biochemist* 15 (10): 1425–1429.

Campo, V.L., Kawano, D.F., da Silva, D.B., and Carvalho, I. (2009). Carrageenans: biological properties, chemical modifications and structural analysis – a review. *Carbohydr. Polym.* 77 (2): 167–180.

van Can, J. G., van Loon, L. J., Brouns, F, and Blaak, E. E. (2012). Reduced glycaemic and insulinaemic responses following trehalose and isomaltulose ingestion: Implications for postprandial substrate use in impaired glucose-tolerant subjects. *Br. J. Nutr.*, 108 (07),1210–7. doi: https://doi.org/10.1017/S0007114511006714.

Cao, Y., Wu, J., Zhang, J. et al. (2009). Room temperature ionic liquids (RTILs): a new and versatile platform for cellulose processing and derivatization. *Chem. Eng. J.* 47 (1): 13–21.

Carbone, J.W., Pasiakos, S.M., Vislocky, L.M. et al. (2014). Effects of short-term energy deficit on muscle protein breakdown and intramuscular proteolysis in normal-weight young adults. *Appl. Physiol. Nutr. Metab. 39* (8): 960–968. https://doi.org/10.1139/apnm-2013-0433.

Chatuevedi, N., Yadav, S., and Shukla, K. (2011). Diversified therapeutic potential of Avena sativa: an exhaustive review. *Asian J. Plant Sci. Res.* 1 (3): 103–114.

Chen, X., Li, Y., Cai, X. et al. (1999). Dose–effect of dietary larginine supplementation on burn wound healing in rats. *Chin. Med. J.* 112 (9): 828–831.

Chen, Y.-J., Chen, Y.-Y., Wu, C.-T. et al. (2010). Prolamin, a rice protein, augments anti-leukaemia immune response. *J. Cereal Sci.* 51 (2): 189–197.

Chiang, W., Lee, M., Guo, W., and Tsai, T. (2006). Protein hydrolysates batch production with angiotensin I–Converting enzyme inhibitory activity from egg whites. *J. Food Drug Anal.* 14: 385–390.

Choi, Y.M. and Kim, B.C. (2009). Muscle fiber characteristics, myofibrillar proteinisoforms and meatquality. *Livest. Sci.* 122: 105–118.

Chong, E.S. (2014). A potential role of probiotics in colorectal cancer prevention: review of possible mechanisms of action. *World J. Microbiol. Biotechnol. 30* (2): 351–374. https://doi.org/10.1007/s11274-013-1499-6.

Chung, Y., Hsu, C., and Ko, C. (2007). Dietary intake of xylooligosaccharides improves the intestinal microbiota, fecal moisture, and pH Value in the elderly. *Nutr. Res.* 27: 756–761.

Clark, K.A., McElhinny, A.S., Beckerle, M.C., and Gregorio, C.C. (2002). Striated muscle cyto architect ure:anintricatewebofformandfunction. *Annu. Rev. Cell Dev. Biol* 18: 637–706.

Clarke, J., Butler, R., and Howarth, G. (2002). Exposure of oral mucosa to bioactive milk factors reduces severity of chemotherapy-induced mucositis in the hamster. *Oral Oncol.* 38: 478–485.

Clemens, R.A., Jones, J.M., Kern, M. et al. (2016). Functionality of sugars in foods and health. *Compr. Rev. Food Sci. Food Saf.* 15: 433–470.

Coelhoa, A.I., Berryb, G.T., and Rubio-Gozalboa, M.E. (2015). Galactose metabolism and health. *Opin. Clin. Nutr. Metab. Care* 18: 422–427.

Cop©MedlinePlus on Blood Sugar

Cummings, J.H. and Stephen, A.M. (2007). Carbohydrate terminology and classification. *Eur. J. Clin. Nutr.* 61 (Suppl. 1): S5–S18.

Dai, L. and Si, C. (2017). Recent advances on cellulose-based nano-drug delivery systems: design of prodrugs and nanoparticles. *Curr. Med. Chem.* 24: 1–19.

Daviskas, E., Anderson, S.D., Jaques, A., and Charlton, B. (2010). Inhaled mannitol improves the hydration and surface properties of sputum in patients with cystic fibrosis. *Chest 137* (4): 861–868. https://doi.org/10.1378/chest.09-2017.

De Menezes, E.W., Giuntini, E.B., Dan, M.C.T. et al. (2013). Codex dietary fiber definition. Justification for inclusion of carbohydrates from 3 to 9 degrees of polymerisation. *Food Chem.* 140: 581–585.

De Roode, B.M., Franssen, A.C.R., van der Padt, A., and Boom, R.M. (2003). Perspectives for the industrial enzymatic production of glycosides. *Biotechnol. Prog.* 19 (5): 1391–1402.

Desbrieres, J., Peptu, C.A., Savin, C.L., and Popa, M. (2018). Chemically modified polysaccharides with applications in nanomedicine. In: *Biomass as Renewable Raw Material to Obtain Bioproducts of High-Tech Value* (ed. V. Popa and I. Volf), 351–399. Elsevier.

Dhanakoti, S.N., Brosnan, J.T., Herzberg, G.R., and Brosnan, M.E. (1990). Renal arginine synthesis: studies in vitro and in vivo. *Am. J. Phys.* 259 (3 Pt 1): E437–E442.

Dhaneshwar, S.S., Mini, K., Gairola, N., and Kadam, S. (2006). Dextran: a promising macromolecular drug carrier. *Indian J. Pharm. Sci.* 68 (6): 705.

Draget, K.I. and Taylor, C. (2011). Chemical, physical and biological properties of alginates and their biomedical implications. *Food Hydrocoll.* 25 (2): 251–256.

Falck, P., Aronsson, A., Grey, C. et al. (2014). Production of arabinoxylan-oligosaccharide mixtures of varying composition from rye bran by combination of process conditions and type of xylanase. *Bioresour. Technol.* 174: 118–125.

Fang, W.S., Bi, D.C., Zheng, R.J. et al. (2017). Identification and activation of TLR4-mediated signalling pathways by alginate-derived guluronate oligosaccharide in RAW264.7 macrophages. *Sci. Rep.* 7: 1663.

Ferrari, P., Nicolini, A., Manca, M.L. et al. (2012). Treatment of mild non-chemotherapy-induced iron deficiency anemia in cancer patients: comparison between oral ferrous bisglycinate chelate and ferrous sulfate. *Biomed. Pharmacother.* 66 (6): 414–418. https://doi.org/10.1016/j.biopha.2012.06.003.

Flourie, B., Vidon, N., Chayvialle, J.A. et al. (1985). Effect of increased amounts of pectin on a solid-liquid meal digestion in healthy man. *Am. J. Clin. Nutr.* 42 (3): 495–503. https://doi.org/10.1093/ajcn/42.3.495.

Fouache, C., Duflot, P., Looten, P. (2003). Branched maltodextrins and method of preparing them. U.S. Patent 6,630,586 B1

Frid, A.H., Nilsson, M., Holst, J.J., and Björck, I.M. (2005). Effect of whey on blood glucose and insulin responses to composite breakfast and lunch meals in type 2 diabetic subjects. *Am. J. Clin. Nutr.* 82 (1): 69–75. https://doi.org/10.1093/ajcn.82.1.69.

Fuentes-Zaragoza, E., Riquelme-Navarrete, M. J., Sánchez-Zapata, E., Pérez-Álvarez, J. A. (2010). Resistant starch as functional ingredient: a review. *Food Res. Int.*, 43 (4), 931–942. doi:https://doi.org/10.1016/j.foodres.2010.02.004.

Fujita, H., Yokoyama, K., and Yoshikawa, M. (2000). Classification and antihypertensive activity of Angiotensin I–converting enzyme inhibitory peptides derived from food proteins. *Food Chem. Toxicol.* 65: 564–569.

Fundueanu, G., Esposito, E., Mihai, D. et al. (1998). Preparation and characterization of Ca-alginate microspheres by a new emulsification method. *Int. J. Pharm.* 170 (1): 11–21.

Gerschenson, L.N., Rojas, A.M., and Fissore, E.N. (2017). Carbohydrates. In: *Nutraceutical and Functional Food Components Effects of Innovative Processing Techniques* (ed. C.M. Galanakis), 39–101. Amsterdam: Elsevier Academic Press.

Ghazi, I., Fernandez-Arrojo, L., Gomez De Segura, A. et al. (2006). Beet sugar syrup and molasses as low-cost feedstock for the enzymatic production of fructo-oligosaccharides. *J. Agric. Food Chem.* 54 (8): 2964–2968.

Ghose, T.K. and Bisaria, V.S. (1987). Measurement of hemicellulase activities. Part 1: Xylanases. *Pure Appl. Chem.* 59 (12): 1739–1752.

Gibson, G.R. and Roberfroid, M.B. (1995). Dietary modulation of the human colonic microbiota: introducing the concept of prebiotics. *J. Nutr.* 125 (6): 1401–1412. https://doi.org/10.1093/jn/125.6.1401.

Giugliano, D., Marfella, R., Verrazzo, G. et al. (1997). l-Arginine for testing endothelium-dependent vascular functions in health and disease. *Am. J. Phys.* 273 (3 Pt 1): E606–E612.

Glucosamine. Drugs.com. 31 July 2019. Retrieved 14 September 2019

Goffin, D., Delzenne, N., Blecker, C. et al. (2011). Wll isomaltooligosaccharides, a well-established functional food in Asia, break through the European and American market? The status of knowledge on these prebiotics. *Crit. Rev. Food Sci. Nutr.* 51: 394–409.

Grigoras, A.G. (2019). Drug delivery systems based on pullulan polysaccharides and their derivatives. In: *Pharmaceuticals from Microbes*, Environmental Chemistry for a Sustainable World, vol. 26 (ed. D. Arora, C. Sharma, S. Jaglan and E. Lichtfouse), 99–141. Cham: Springer.

Guilloux, K., Gaillard, I., Courtois, J. et al. (2012). Production of arabinoxylan-oligosaccharides from flaxseed (*Linum usitatissimum*). *J. Agric. Food Chem.* 57 (23): 1130–11313.

Guio, F., Rodriguez, M.A., Almeciga-Diaz, C.J., and Sanchez, O.F. (2009). Recent trends in fructooligosaccharides production. *Recent Pat. Food Nutr. Agric.* 1: 221–230.

Guo, J. and Dou, D. (2020). Influence of prior hip arthroscopy on outcomes after hip arthroplasty: a meta-analysis of matched control studies. *Medicine* 99 (29): e21246. https://doi.org/10.1097/MD.0000000000021246.

Gupta, V., Gupta, A., Saggu, S. et al. (2005). Antistress and adaptogenic activity of l-arginine supplementation. *Evid. Based Complement. Alternat. Med.* 2 (1): 93–97.

Gupta, S., Chauhan, D., Mehla, K. et al. (2010). An overview of nutraceuticals: current scenario. *J. Basic Clin. Pharmacol.* 1 (2): 55–62.

Hakkak, R., Korourian, S., and Shelnutt, S.R. (2009). Diets containing whey proteins or soy protein isolate protect against 7,12- dimethylbenz(a)anthracene-induced mammary tumors in female rats. *Cancer Epidemiol. Biomark. Prev.* 9: 113–117.

Halfter, W., Schurer, B., Hasselhorn, H.M. et al. (1996). An ovomucin-like protein on the surface of migrating primordial germ cells of the chick and rat. *Development* 122: 915–923.

Hamm, L.L., Nakhoul, N., and Hering-Smith, K.S. (2015). Acid-base homeostasis. *Clin. J. Am. Soc. Nephrol.* 10 (12): 2232–2242. https://doi.org/10.2215/CJN.07400715.

Hammes, W.P. (2004). How selective are the prebiotics? In: *Functional Food: Safety Aspects* (ed. Senate Commission on Food Safety). Weinheim, Germany: Wiley VCH Verlag GmbH & Co. KGaA.

Hankins, J.(2006). The role of albumin in fluid and electrolyte balance. *J. Infus. Nurs.*, 29(5):260–265. doi:https://doi.org/10.1097/00129804-200609000-00004

Hartman, J.W., Tang, J.E., Wilkinson, S.B. et al. (2007). Consumption of fat-free fluid milk after resistance exercise promotes greater lean mass accretion than does consumption of soy or carbohydrate in young, novice, male weightlifters. *Am. J. Clin. Nutr.* 86 (2): 373–381. https://doi.org/10.1093/ajcn/86.2.373.

Hasler, C.M., Brown, A.C., and American Dietetic Association (2009). Position of the American Dietetic Association: functional foods. *J. Am. Diet. Assoc.* 109 (4): 735–746. https://doi.org/10.1016/j.jada.2009.02.023.

Haug, I.J., Draget, K.I., and Smidsrod, O. (2004). Physical and rheologicalproperties of fish gelatin compared to mammalian gelatin. *Food Hydrocoll.* 18: 203–213.

Ho, S.C., Liu, J.H., and Wu, R.Y. (2003). Establishment of the mimetic aging effect in mice caused by D-galactose. *Biogerontology* 4 (1): 15–18. https://doi.org/10.1023/a:1022417102206.

Hopkins, L. (2014). Tenderizingmechanisms. Mechanical. In: *Encyclopedia of Meat Sciences*, 2e (ed. C. Devine and M. Dikeman), 443–451. London: Academic Press.

Hounsome, N., Hounsome, B., Tomos, D., and Edwards-Jones, G. (2008). Plant metabolites and nutritional quality of vegetables. *J. Agric. Food Chem.* 57: 554–565.

Hsu, C.-K., Liao, J.-W., Chung, Y.-C. et al. (2004). Xylooligosaccharides and fructooligosaccharides affect the intestinal microbiota and precancerous colonic lesion development in rats. *J. Nutr.* 134: 1523–1528.

Hu, Y., Feng, Z., Feng, W.J. et al. (2019). AOS ameliorates monocrotaline-induced pulmonary hypertension by restraining the activation of P-selectin/p38MAPK/NF-kappa B pathway in rats. *Biomed. Pharmacother.* 109: 1319–1326.

Hughes, G.J., Ryan, D.J., Mukherjea, R., and Schasteen, C.S. (2011). Protein digestibility-corrected amino acid scores (PDCAAS) for soy protein isolates and concentrate: Criteria for evaluation. *J. Agric. Food Chem.* 59: 12707–12712.

Huopalahti, R., Fandino, R.L., Anton, M., and Schade, R. (2007). *Bioactive Egg Compounds.* New York, NY: Springer.

Ibrahim, H.R. and Kiyono, T. (2009). Novel anticancer activity of the autocleaved ovotransferrin against human colon and breast cancer cells. *J. Agric. Food Chem.* 57: 11383–11390.

Ibrahim, H.R., Sugmito, Y., and Akoi, T. (2000). Ovotransferrin antimicrobial peptide (OTAP-92) kills bacteria through a membrane damage mechanism. *Boichim. Biophys. Acta* 1523: 196–205.

Immerzeel, P., Falc, P., Galbe, M. et al. (2014). Extraction of water-soluble xylan from wheat bran and utilization of enzymatically produced xylooligosaccharides by Lactobacillus, Bifidobacterium and Weissella spp. *LWT Food Sci. Technol.* 56: 321–327.

Jansson, P.E., Lindberg, B., and Sandford, P.A. (1983). Structural studies of gellan gum, an extracellular polysaccharide elaborated by Pseudomonas elodea. *Carbohydr. Res.* 124 (1): 135–139.

Jauhiainen, T. and Korpela, R. (2007). Milk peptides and blood pressure. *J. Nutr.* 137: 825S–829S.

Jenkins, D.J., Gassull, M.A., Leeds, A.R. et al. (1977). Effect of dietary fiber on complications of gastric surgery: prevention of postprandial hypoglycemia by pectin. *Gastroenterology 73* (2): 215–217.

Jenkins, D.J., Kendall, C.W., and Vuksan, V. (1999). Inulin, oligofructose and intestinal function. *J. Nutr. 129* (7 Suppl): 1431S–1433S. https://doi.org/10.1093/jn/129.7.1431S.

Jiao, G., Yu, G., Zhang, J., and Ewart, S.H. (2011). Chemical structures and bioactivities of sulfated polysaccharides from marine algae. *Mar. Drugs* 9 (2): 196–223.

Johansson, I. (2002). Milk and dairy products: possible effects on dental health. *Food Nutr. Res.* 46: 119–122.

Johansson, I. and Lif Holgerson, P. (2011). Milk and oral health. *Nestle Nutr. Workshop Ser. Pediatr. Program* 67: 55–66.

Jurczyńska, E., Saczko, J., Kulbacka, J. et al. (2012). Beta-glukan, jako naturalny antykarcynogen. *Pol. Merkur. Lekarski* 196: 217–220. (in Polish).

Kampa, M., Bakogeorgou, E., Hatzoglou, A. et al. (1997). Opioid alkaloids and casomorphin peptides decrease the proliferation of prostatic cancer cell lines (LNCaP, PC3 and DU145) through a partial interaction with opioid receptors. *Eur. J. Pharmacol.* 335 (2–3): 255–265.

Kay, R.M. and Truswell, A.S. (1977). Effect of citrus pectin on blood lipids and fecal steroid excretion in man. *Am. J. Clin. Nutr. 30* (2): 171–175. https://doi.org/10.1093/ajcn/30.2.171.

Kearns, C.E., Apollonio, D., and Glantz, S.A. (2017). Sugar industry sponsorship of germ-free rodent studies linking sucrose to hyperlipidemia and cancer: an historical analysis of internal documents. *PLoS Biol. 15* (11): e2003460. https://doi.org/10.1371/journal.pbio.2003460.

Keith, G. (2013). *Understanding Chelated Minerals.* Nutritional Outlook.

Keri Marshall, K. (2004). Therapeutic applications of whey protein. *Altern. Med. Rev. 9* (2): 136–156.

Kessler, R.C., Davis, R.B., Foster, D.F. et al. (2001). Long-term trends in the use of complementary and alternative medical therapies in the United States. *Ann. Intern. Med. 135* (4): 262–268.

Khan, S., Tøndervik, A., Sletta, H. et al. (2012). Overcoming drug resistance with alginate oligosaccharides able to potentiate the action of selected antibiotics. *Antimicrob. Agents Chemother.* 56 (10): 5134_5141.

Kim, S.K. (2010). *Chitin, Chitosan, Oligosaccharides and Their Derivatives: Biological Activities and Applications*, 643. Boca Raton, Florida, USA: CRC Press.

Kim, S.K. (2017). Seaweed polysaccharides. *Crit. Rev. Biotechnol.* 111–155. https://doi.org/10.1016/B978-0-12-809816-5.00001-3.

Kim, S.K. and Wijesekara, I. (2010). Development and biological activities of marine-derived bioactive peptides: a review. *J. Funct. Foods* 2 (1): 1–9.

Kim, Y.W., Kim, K.H., Choi, H.J., and Lee, D.S. (2005). Anti-diabetic activity of beta-glucans and their enzymatically hydrolyzed oligosaccharides from Agaricus blazei. *Biotechnol. Lett.* 27 (7): 483–487.

Kim, J.W., Kim, B.C., Lee, J.H. et al. (2013). Protein content and composition of waxy rice grains. *Pak. J. Bot.* 45 (1): 151–156.

Kimball, S.R. and Jefferson, L.S. (2006). Signaling pathways and molecular mechanisms through which branched-chain amino acids mediate translational control of protein synthesis. *J. Nutr. 136* (1 Suppl): 227S–231S. https://doi.org/10.1093/jn/136.1.227S.

Kirk, S.J., Hurson, M., Regan, M.C. et al. (1993). Arginine stimulates wound healing and immune function in elderly human beings. *Surgery* 114 (2): 155–159.

Klahr, S. (1999). Can l-arginine manipulation reduce renal disease? *Semin. Nephrol.* 19 (3): 304–309.

Ko, K.Y. and Ahn, D.U. (2008). An economic and simple purification procedure for the large scale production of ovotransferrin from egg white. *Poult. Sci.* 87: 1441–1450.

Ko, S.C., Kang, N., Kim, E.A. et al. (2012). A novel angiotensin I-converting enzyme (ACE) inhibitory peptide from a marine Chlorella ellipsoidea and its antihypertensive effect in spontaneously hypertensive rats. *Process Biochem.* 47 (12): 2005–2011.

Kong, H. and Mooney, D. (2005). Polysaccharide-based hydrogels in tissue engineering. In: *Polysaccharides Structural Diversity and Functional Versatility* (ed. S. Dumitriu), 817–837. BocaRaton, FL: CRC Press.

Kovacs-Nolan, J.K.N., Zhang, J.W., Hayakawa, S., and Mine (2000). Immunoch emical and structural analysis of pepsin-digested egg white ovomucoid. *J. Agric. Food Chem.* 48: 6261–6266.

Kovacs-Nolan, J.K.N., Phillips, M., and Mine, Y. (2005). Advances in the value of eggs and egg components for human health. *J.Agric. Food Chem* 53: 8421–8431.

Kratz, F. (2008). Albumin as a drug carrier: design of prodrugs, drug conjugates and nanoparticles. *J. Control. Release* 132: 171–183.

Krishnan, H.B., Kim, W.S., Jang, S.C., and Kerley, M.S. (2009). All three subunits of soybean β-conglycinin are potential food allergens. *J. Agric. Food Chem.* 57 (3): 938–943.

Kuhara, T., Iigo, M., and Itoh, T. (2000). Orally administered lactoferrin exerts an antimetastatic effect and enhances production of IL-18 in the intestinal epithelium. *Nutr. Cancer* 38: 192–199.

Kumar, S., Sugihara, F., Suzuki, K. et al. (2015). A double-blind, placebo-controlled, randomised, clinical study on the effectiveness of collagen peptide on osteoarthritis. *J. Sci. Food Agric.* 95 (4): 702–707. https://doi.org/10.1002/jsfa.6752.

Labeit, S. and Kolmerer, B. (1995). Titins:giant proteins incharge of muscle ultrastructure and elasticity. *Science* 270: 293–296.

Lafarga, T. and Hayes, M. (2014). Bioactive peptides from meat muscle and by-products: eneration, functionality and application as functional ingredients. *Meat Sci.* 98 (2): 227–239.

Lahov, E. and Regelson, W. (1996). Antibacterial and immunostimulating casein-derived substances from milk: casecidin, isracidin peptides. *Food Chem. Toxicol.* 34: 131–145.

Lahtinen, S.J., Knoblock, K., Drakoularakou, A. et al. (2010). Effect of molecule branching and glycosidic linkage on the degradation of polydextrose by gut microbiota. *Biosci. Biotechnol. Biochem.* 74 (10): 2016–2021.

Lasztity, R. (1999). *The Chemistry of Cereal Proteins*. Akademiai Kiado.

Latif, S., Pfannstiel, J., Makkar, H.P., Becker, K. (2013). Amino acid composition, antinutrients and allergens in the peanut protein fraction obtained by an aqueous enzymatic process. *Food Chem.*, 136(1), 213–217. doi:https://doi.org/10.1016/j.foodchem.2012.07.120)

Laursen, I., Briand, P., and Lykkesfeldt, A.E. (1990). Serum albumin as a modulator on growth of the human breast cancer cell line MCF-7. *Anticancer Res.* 10: 343–351.

Lawrie, R.A. (2006). Chemical and biochemical constitution of muscle. In: Lawrie, R.A., Ledward, D. (Eds.), Lawrie's Meat Science, seventh ed. Woodhead Publishing, Cambridge UK, pp. 75–127.

LeDuy, A., Choplin, L., Zajic, J.E., and Luong, J.H. (2002). Pullulan: properties, synthesis, and applications. In: *Encyclopedia of Polymer Science and Technology* (ed. K. Matyjaszewski), 1–14. New York: Wiley.

Lee, K.Y. and Mooney, D.J. (2012). Alginate: properties and biomedical applications. *Prog. Polym. Sci.* 37 (1): 106–126.

Lefranc-Millot, C., Guérin-Deremaux, L., Wils, D. et al. (2012). Impact of a resistant dextrin on intestinal ecology: how altering the digestive ecosystem with NUTRIOSE®, a soluble fibre with prebiotic properties, may be beneficial for health. *J. Int. Med. Res.* 40 (1): 211–224. https://doi.org/10.1177/147323001204000122.

Lehman, W. and Craig, R. (2008). Tropomyosin and the steric mechanism of muscleregulation. In: *Tropomyosin* (ed. P. Gunning), 95–109. New York: Springer.

Lesile, M., Stephen, M., and Robert, S. (2003). Cotton and wool outlook. Econ Res Service USDA. (USDA publication; no. CWS-0303), 1–5.

Lina, B.A., Jonker, D., and Kozianowski, G. (2002). Isomaltulose (Palatinose): a review of biological and toxicological studies. *Food Chem. Toxicol.* 40 (10): 1375–1381. https://doi.org/10.1016/s0278-6915(02)00105-9.

Lisiewska, Z., Kmiecik, W., Gębczyński, P., and Sobczyńska, L. (2011). Amino acid profile of raw and as-eaten products of spinach (Spinacia oleracea L). *Food Chem.* 126 (2): 460–465.

Liu, H.T., He, J.L., Li, W.M., Yang, Z., Wang, Y.X., Bai, X.F., Yu, C., Du, Y.G. (2010). Chitosan oligosaccharides protect human umbilical vein endothelial cells from hydrogen peroxide induced apoptosis. *Carbohydr. Polym.*, 80, 1062–71. doi:https://doi.org/10.1016/j.carbpol.2010.01.025.

Liu, J., Zhang, B., Song, S., (2014). Bovine collagen peptides compounds promote the proliferation and differentiation of MC3T3-E1 pre-osteoblasts. *PLoS One*, 9(6),99920. doi:https://doi.org/10.1371/journal.pone.0099920

Liu, J., Zhan, X., Wan, J. et al. (2015). Review for carrageenan-based pharmaceutical biomaterials: favourable physical features versus adverse biological effects. *Carbohydr. Polym.* 121: 27–36.

Yang Liu., Guowan Su., Feibai Zhou., Jianan Zhang., Lin Zheng., and Mouming Zhao. (2018). Protective effect of Bovine Elastin Peptides against Photoaging in mice and identification of novel Antiphotoaging Peptides. *J. Agric. Food Chem.*, 66(41), 10760–10768. DOI: https://doi.org/10.1021/acs.jafc.8b04676.

Livney, Y.D. (2010). Milk proteins as vehicles for bioactives. *Curr. Opin. Colloid Interface Sci.* 15: 73–83.

Lule, V.K., Garg, S., Pophaly, S.D., and Tomar, S.K. (2015). Potential health benefits of lunasin: a multifaceted soy-derived bioactive peptide. *J. Food Sci.* 80 (3): R485–R494.

Ma, J., Stevens, J.E., Cukier, K. et al. (2009). Effects of a protein preload on gastric emptying, glycemia, and gut hormones after a carbohydrate meal in diet-controlled type 2 diabetes. *Diabetes Care* 32 (9): 1600–1602. https://doi.org/10.2337/dc09-0723.

Macfarlane, S., Macfarlane, G.T., and Cummings, J.H. (2006). Review article: prebiotics in the gastrointestinal tract. *Aliment. Pharmacol. Ther.* 24 (5): 701–714. https://doi.org/10.1111/j.1365-2036.2006.03042.

Madhukumar, M.S. and Muralikrishna, G. (2010). Structural characterization and determination of prebiotic activity of purified xylooligosaccharides obtained from Bengal gram husk (*Cicer arietinum* L.) and wheat bran (*Triticum aestivum*). *Food Chem.* 118: 215–222.

Madureira, A.R., Pereira, C.I., Gomes, A.M.P. et al. (2007). Bovine whey proteins-overview on their main biological properties. *Food Res. Int.* 40: 1197–1211.

Mäkeläinen, H.S., Forssten, s., Saarinen, M. et al. (2010). Xylo-oligosaccharides enhance the growth of bifidobacteria and *Bifidobacterium lactis* in a simulated colon model. *Benefic. Microbes* 1 (1): 81–91.

Manso, M.A., Miguel, M., Even, J. et al. (2008). Effect of the long-term intake of egg white hydrolysates on the oxidative status and blood lipid profile of pontaneously hypertensive rats. *Food Chem.* 109: 361–367.

Martínez-Cuesta, S., Rahman, S.A., Furnham, N., and Thornton, J.M. (2015). The classification and evolution of enzyme function. *Biophys. J. 109* (6): 1082–1086. https://doi.org/10.1016/j.bpj.2015.04.020.

Martínez-Montero, C., Rodríguez Dodero, M.C., Guillén Sánchez, D.A., and Barroso, C.G. (2004). Analysis of low molecular weith carobohydrates in food and beverages: a review. *Chromatographia* 59: 15–30.

Mathews, R.S. (2011). Current and potential health claims for oat products. In: *Oats: Chemistry and Technology* (ed. H.H. Webster and P.J. Wood), 275–300. St. Paul, MN, USA: AAAC International Press.

Matsumoto, S., Noguichi, H., Shimoda, M. et al. (2010). Seven consecutive successful clinical islet isolations with pancreatic ductal injection. *Cell Transplant. 19* (3): 291–297. https://doi.org/10.3727/096368909X481773.

Matsuo, T. (2004). Trehalose versus hyaluronan or cellulose in eyedrops for the treatment of dry eye. *Jpn. J. Ophthalmol. 48* (4): 321–327. https://doi.org/10.1007/s10384-004-0085-8.

Matsuo, T., Tsuchida, Y., and Morimoto, N. (2002). Trehalose eye drops in the treatment of dry eye syndrome. *Ophthalmology 109* (11): 2024–2029. https://doi.org/10.1016/s0161-6420(02)01219-8.

Maxwell, A.J., Anderson, B.E., and Cooke, J.P. (2000). Nutritional therapy for peripheral arterial disease: a double-blind, placebo-controlled, randomized trial of HeartBarReg. *Vasc. Med.* 5 (1): 11–19.

Mazumder, K., York, W.S. (2010). Structural analysis of arbinoxylan isolated from ball-milled switchgrass biomass. *Carbohydr. Res.*, 345, 2183–2193. doi: https://doi.org/10.1016/j.carres.2010.07.034.

McBurney, M.I. and Thompson, L.U. (1989). in vitro ferment abilities of purified fiber supplements. *Food Sci.* 54: 347–335.

McLachlan, C. (2001). Beta-casein A1, ischaemic heart disease mortality, and other illnesses. *Med. Hypotheses* 56: 262–272.

Middlebos, I.S. and Fahey, G.C. Jr. (2008). Soybean carbohydrates. In: *Soybeans: Chemistry, Production, Processing, and Utilization*, Monograph Series on Oilseeds (ed. L.A. Johnson, P.J. White and R. Galloway). Urbana, IL: AOCS Press.

Miguel, M. and Aleixandre, A. (2006). Antihypertensive peptides derived from egg proteins. *J. Nutr.* 136: 1457–1460.

Miguel, M., Alvarez, Y., López-Fandiño, R., Alonso, M. J., & Salaices, M. (2007). Vasodilator effects of peptides derived from egg white proteins. *Regulatory Peptides*, 140 (3), 131–135.

Mine, Y. (2008). *Egg Bioscience and Biotechnology*. Hoboken, NJ: Wiley.

Mitchell, H. (2006). *Sweeteners and Sugar Alternatives in Food Technology*, vol. 2, 87. Oxford, England: Blackwell Publishing Ltd.

Moon, S.H., Lee, J.H., Lee, Y.J. et al. (2013). Screening for cytotoxic activity of ovotransferrin and its enzyme hydrolysates. *Poult. Sci.* 92 (2): 424–434.

Mountzouris, K.C., Gilmour, S.G., and Rastall, R.A. (2002). Continuous production of oligodextrans via controlled hydrolysis of dextran in an enzyme membrane reactor. *J. Food Sci.* 67: 1767–1771. https://doi.org/10.1111/j.1365-2621.2002.tb08720.x.

Muir, J.G., Shepherd, S.J., Rosella, O. et al. (2007). Fructan and free fructose content of common Australian vegetables and fruit. *J. Agric. Food Chem.* 55: 6619–6662.

Muir, J.G., Rose, R., Rosella, O. et al. (2009). Measurement of short-chain carbohydrates in common Australian vegetables and fruits by high-performance liquid chromatography (HPLC). *J. Agric. Food Chem.* 57 (2): 554–565. https://doi.org/10.1021/jf802700e.

Nagata, K. and Yoshida, N. (1984). Interaction between Trypsin-like enzyme from *Streptomyces erythraeus* and chicken ovomucoid. *J.Biochem.* 96: 1041–1049.

Nakagawa, T., Watabe, S., and Hashimoto, K. (1998). Identification of three major components in fish sarcoplasmic proteins. *Nippon Suisan Gakkaishi* 54 (6): 999–1004.

Nasri, H., Baradaran, A., Shirzad, H., and Rafieian-Kopaei, M. (2014). New concepts in nutraceuticals as alternative for pharmaceuticals. *Int. J. Prev. Med.* 5 (12): 1487–1499.

Nehete, J.Y., Bhambar, R.S., Narkhede, M.R., and Gawali, S.R. (2013). Natural proteins: sources, isolation, characterization and applications. *Phcog Rev* 7: 107–116.

Nisbet, A.D., Saundry, R.H., Moir, A.J.G. et al. (1981). The complete amino-acid sequence of hen ovalbumin. *Eur. J. Biochem.* 115: 335–345.

Numata, K. and Kaplan, D.L. (2010). Silk-based delivery systems of bioactive molecules. *Adv. Drug Deliv. Rev.* 62: 1497–1508.

Obinata, T., Maruyama, K., Sugita, H. et al. (1981). Dynamic aspects of structural proteins invertebrate skeletal muscle. *MuscleNerve* 4: 456–488.

Oe, H., Doi, E., and Hirose, M. (1988). Amino-terminal and carboxylterminal half-molecules of ocotransferrin: preparation by a novel procedure and their interactions. *J. Biochem.* 103: 1066–1072.

Oguro, T., Watanabe, K., Tani, H. et al. (2000). Morphological observations on antitumour activities of 710 kDa fragment in α-subunit from pronase treated ovomucin in a double grated tumor system. *Food Sci. Technol. Res.* 6: 179–185.

Ohtsuka, Y. and Nakaya, J. (2000). Effect of oral administration of l-arginine on senile dementia. *Am. J. Med.* 108 (5): 439.

Olano-Martin, E., Rimbach, G.H., Gibson, G.R., and Rastall, R.A. (2003). Pectin and pectic-oligosaccharides induce apoptosis in in vitro human colonic adenocarcinoma cells. *Anticancer Res.* 23 (1A): 341–346.

Oliveira, F.C., Coimbra, J.S.R., Silva, L.H.M.E. et al. (2009). Ovomucoid partitioning in aqueous two-phase system. *Biochem. Eng. J.* 47: 55–60.

Omana, D.A., Wang, J., and J, W. (2010). Co-extraction of egg white proteins using ion-exchange chromatography from ovomucin-removed egg white. *J. Chromatogr. B Anal. Technol. Biomed. Life Sci.* 878: 1771–1776.

Osborne, T.B. (1924). *The Vegetable Proteins*. London: Longmans, Green and Co.

Osmałek, T., Froelich, A., and Tasarek, S. (2014). Application of gellan gum in pharmacy and medicine. *Int. J. Pharm.* 466 (1): 328–340.

Paddon-Jones, D. and Rasmussen, B.B. (2009). Dietary protein recommendations and the prevention of sarcopenia. *Curr. Opin. Clin. Nutr. Metab. Care* 12 (1): 86–90. https://doi.org/10.1097/MCO.0b013e32831cef8b.

Pal, S. and Ellis, V. (2010). The chronic effects of whey proteins on blood pressure, vascular function, and inflammatory markers in overweight individuals. *Obesity (Silver Spring, Md.)* 18 (7): 1354–1359. https://doi.org/10.1038/oby.2009.397.

Pancholy, S. K., Deshpande, A. S., & Krall, S. (1978). Amino acids, oil and protein content of some selected peanut cultivars [Nutrient analysis]. *Proceedings American Peanut Research and Education Association, Inc.* 10: 30–37.

Panesar, P., Kumari, S., and Panesar, R. (2011). Prebiotics: current status and perspectives. *Int. J. Food Sci. Technol.* 1 (1): 181–192.

Panos, I., Acosta, N., and Heras, A. (2008). New drug delivery systems based on chitosan. *Curr. Drug Discov. Technol.* 5 (4): 333–341.

Park, Y.K. and Yetley, E.A. (1993). Intakes and food sources of fructose in the United States. *Am.J. Clin. Nutr.* 58: 737S–747S.

Park, K.G., Hayes, P.D., Garlick, P.J. et al. (1991). Stimulation of lymphocyte natural cytotoxicity by l-arginine. *Lancet* 337 (8742): 645–646.

Parodi, P. (1998). A role for milk proteins in cancer prevention. *Aust. J. Dairy Technol.* 53: 37–47.

Parodi, P.A. (2007). Role for milk proteins and their peptides in cancer prevention. *Curr. Pharma. Des* 3: 813–828.

Du, B., Bian, Z., and Xu, B. (2014). Skin health promotion effects of natural beta-glucan derived from cereals and microorganisms: a review. *Phytother. Res.* 28: 159–166.

Pawar, S.N. (2011). Chemical modification of alginates in organic solvent systems. *Biomacromolecules* 12 (11): 4095–4103.

Pelzer, S., Zurek, C., Rose, T., et al. (2012). Microorganisms having enhanced sucrose mutase activity. US Patent 8790900 B2.

Pennings, B., Boirie, Y., Senden, J.M. et al. (2011). Whey protein stimulates postprandial muscle protein accretion more effectively than do casein and casein hydrolysate in older men. *Am. J. Clin. Nutr. 93* (5): 997–1005. https://doi.org/10.3945/ajcn.110.008102.

Pessi, T., Isolauri, E., Sütas, Y. et al. (2001). Suppression of T-cell activation by *Lactobacillus rhamnosus* GG-degraded bovine casein. *Int. Immunopharmacol.* 1: 211–218.

Peterson, D.M. (2011). Storage proteins. In: *Oats: Chemistry and Technology* (ed. H.H. Webster and P.J. Wood), 123–142. St. Paul, MN, USA: AAAC International Press.

Petri, D.F.S. (2015). Xanthan gum: a versatile biopolymer for biomedical and technological applications. *J. Appl. Polym. Sci.* 132 (23): 1–13.

Pienta, K.J., Naik, H., Akhtar, A. et al. (1995). Inhibition of spontaneous metastasis in a rat prostate cancer model by oral administration of modified citrus pectin. *J. Natl. Cancer Inst. 87* (5): 348–353. https://doi.org/10.1093/jnci/87.5.348.

Pihlanto, A. (2011). Whey proteins and peptides. *Nutrafoods* 10: 29–42.

Platt, D. and Raz, A. (1992). Modulation of the lung colonization of B16-F1 melanoma cells by citrus pectin. *J. Natl. Cancer Inst. 84* (6): 438–442. https://doi.org/10.1093/jnci/84.6.438.

Playne, M.J. and Crittenden, R.G. (2004). Prebiotics from lactose, sucrose, starch and plant polysaccharides. *Nutr. Sci. Technol.* 2: 99–134.

Playne, M.J. and Crittenden, R.G. (2009). Galacto-oligosaccharides and other products derived from lactose. In: *Lactose, Water, Salts and Minor Constituents*, 3e (ed. P.L.H. McSweeney and P.F. Fox), 121–201. New York: Springer.

Poesen, R., Evenepoel, P., de Loor, H., Delcour, J.A., Courtin, C.M., Kuypers, D., Augustijns, P., Verkeke, K., Meijers, B. (2016). The influence of prebiotic rabinoxylan oligosaccharides on microbiota derived uremic retention solutes in patients with chronic kidney disease: a randomized controlled trial. *PLoS One*, 11 (4), e0153893. doi: https://doi.org/10.1371/journal.pone.0153893.

Prajapati, V.D., Maheriya, P.M., Jani, G.K., and Solanki, H.K. (2014). RETRACTED: carrageenan: a natural seaweed polysaccharide and its applications. *Carbohydr. Polym.* 105: 97–112.

Qin, Z. (2015). Soluble elastin peptides in cardiovascular homeostasis: foe or ally. *Peptides* 67: 64–73. https://doi.org/. doi: 10.1016/j.peptides.2015.03.006.

Rapoport, S.I. (2000). Osmotic opening of the blood-brain barrier: principles, mechanism, and therapeutic applications. *Cell. Mol. Neurobiol. 20* (2): 217–230. https://doi.org/10.1023/a:1007049806660.

Rathore, A.S. and Gupta, R.D. (2015). Chitinases from bacteria to human: properties, applications, and future perspectives. *Enzyme Res* 2015: https://doi.org/10.1155/2015/791907.2019.

Reddy, B.S., Simi, B., and Engle, A. (1994). Biochemical epidemiology of colon cancer: effect of types of dietary fiber on colonic diacylglycerols in women. *Gastroenterology* 106: 883–889.

Rekha, M. and Sharma, C.P. (2007). Pullulan as a promising biomaterial for biomedical applications: a perspective. *Trends Biomater. Artif. Organs* 20: 116–121.

Rinaudo, M. (2014). Biomaterials based on a natural polysaccharide: alginate. *Rev. Esp. en Cienc. Químico-Biológicas* 17 (1): 92–96.

Robert, H.S. (2016). *The Latest on Glucosamine/Chondroitin Supplement.* Harvard University Medical School: Harvard Health Publishing.

Ruiz-Matute, A.I., Montilla, A., del Castillo, M.D. et al. (2007). AGC method for simultaneous analysis of bornesitol, other polyalcohols and sugars in coffee and its substitutes. *J. Sep. Sci.* 30: 557–562.

Rutherfurd, S.M., Fanning, A.C., Miller, B.J., and Moughan, P.J. (2015). Protein digestibility-corrected amino acid scores and digestible indispensable amino acid scores differentially describe protein quality in growing male rats. *J. Nutr.* 145: 372–379.

Rycroft, C.E., Jones, M.R., Gibson, G.R., Rastall, R.A. (2001). A comparative *in vitro* evaluation of the fermentation properties of prebiotic oligosaccharides. *J. Appl. Microbiol.* 91, 878–887. doi: https://doi.org/10.1046/j.1365-2672.2001.01446.x.

Sajilata, M. G., Singhal, Rekha S., Kulkarni, Pushpa R. (2006). Resistant starch – a review. *Compr. Rev. Food Sci. Food Saf.*, 5 (1), 1–17. doi:https://doi.org/10.1111/j.1541-4337.2006.tb00076.x.

Sako, T., Matsumoto, K., and Tanaka, R. (1999). Recent progress on research and applications of non-digestible galacto-oligosaccharides. *Int. Dairy J.* 9: 69–80.

Sangeetha, P.T., Ramesh, M.N., and Prapulla, S.G. (2005). Recent trends in the microbial production, analysis and application of fructooligosaccharides. *Trends Food Sci. Technol.* 16: 442–457.

Sarmadi, B.H. and Ismail, A. (2010). Antioxidative peptides from food proteins:a review. *Peptides* 31 (10): 1949–1956.

Sayago-Ayerdi, S.G., Torvar, J., Blancas-Benitez, F.J., and Bello-Perez, L.A. (2011). Resistant starch in common starchy foods as an alternative to increase dietary fibre intake. *J. Food Nutr. Res.* 50 (1): 1–12.

Shariatinia, Z. (2019). Pharmaceutical applications of chitosan. *Adv. Colloid Interf. Sci.* 263: 131–194.

Shukla, S., Shukla, A., Mehboob, S., and Guha, S. (2011). Meta-analysis: the effects of gut flora modulation using prebiotics, probiotics and synbiotics on minimal hepatic encephalopathy. *Aliment. Pharmacol. Ther.* 33 (6): 662–671.

Siddiqui, I.R. and Furgala, B. (1967). Isolation and characterization of oligosaccharides from honey. Part I disaccharides. *J. Apic. Res.* 6 (3): 139–145.

Silva TH, Moreira-Silva, J., Marques. A.L., Domingues. A., Bayon. Y., Reis. R.L. (2014). Marine origin collagens and its potential applications *Mar. Drugs*, 12(12),5881–901. doi: https://doi.org/10.3390/md12125881.

Singh, B.P., Vij, S., and Hati, S. (2014). Functional significance of bioactive peptides derived from soybean. *Peptides* 54: 171–179.

Slavin, J. (2013). Fiber and prebiotics: mechanisms and health benefits. *Nutrients* 5: 1417–1435.

Slizewska, K. (2013). The citric acid-modified, enzyme-resistant dextrin from potato starch as a potential prebiotic. *Acta Biochim. Pol.* 60 (4): 671–675.

Song, H., Zhang, S., and Li, B. (2018). Effect of collagen hydrolysates from silver carp skin (*Hypophthalmichthys molitrix*) on osteoporosis in chronologically aged mice: increasing bone remodeling. *Nutrients* 10.

Spiller, G.A., Chernoff, M.C., Hill, R.A. et al. (1980). Effect of purified cellulose, pectin, and a low-residue diet on fecal volatile fatty acids, transit time, and fecal weight in humans. *Am. J. Clin. Nutr.* 33 (4): 754–759. https://doi.org/10.1093/ajcn/33.4.754.

Sprange, K.U. (1975). The Bombyx mori silk proteins: characterization of large polypeptides. *Biochemistry* 14 (5): 925–931.

Stadelman, W.J. and Cotterill, O.J. (2001). *Egg Science and Technology*, 4e. Westport, CT: Avi Publishing Company.

Strasburg, G., Xiong, Y.L., and Chiang, W. (2008). Physiology and chemistry of edible muscle tissues. In: *Fennema's Food Chemistry*, 4e (ed. S. Damodaran, K.L. Parkin and O.R. Fennema), 923–973. Boca Raton FL: CRC Press.

Sun, J., Zhao, R., Zeng, J. et al. (2010). Characterization of dextrins with different dextrose equivalents. *Molecules* 15: 5162–5173.

Swartz, D., Greaser, M., and Cantino, M. (2009). Muscle structure and function. In: *Applied Muscle Biology and Meat Science* (ed. M. Du and R.J. McCormick), 1–45. Boca Raton FL: CRC Press.

Takazoe, I. (1985). New trends on sweeteners in Japan. *Int. Dent. J. 35* (1): 58–65.

Tanimura, J. (1967). Studies on arginine in human semen. II. The effects of medication with l-arginine-HCL on male infertility. *Bull. Osaka Med. Sch.* 13 (2): 84–89.

Tapsas, D., Fälth-Magnusson, K., Högberg, L., Hammersjö, J.-Å., Hollén, E. (2014). Swedish children with celiac disease comply well with a gluten-free diet, and most include oats without reporting any adverse effects: a long-term follow-up study. *Nutr. Res.*34, 436–441. doi: https://doi.org/10.1016/j.nutres.2014.04.006.

Tecson, E.M.S., Esmama, B.V., Lontok, L.P., and Juliano, B.O. (1971). Studies on the extraction and composition of rice endosperm, glutelin, and prolamin. *Cereal Chem.* 48 (2): 168–181.

Tester, R.F., Karkalas, J., and Qi, X. (2004). Starch – composition, fine structure and architecture. *J. Cereal Sci.* 39: 151–165.

The American Society of Health-System Pharmacists. (2015). Archived from the original on 2017-09-04 Retrieved 11 August 2015.

Tiihonen, K.K., Roÿotiö, H., Putaala, H., and Ouwehand, A.C. (2011). Polydextrose functional fibre improving digestive health, satiety and beyond. *Nutrafoods* 10: 23–28.

Tiwari, U. and Cummings, E. (2009). Review. Factors influencing β-glucan levels and molecular weight in cereal-based products. *Cereal Chem.* 86 (3): 290–301.

Tömösközi, S., Lásztity, R., Haraszi, R., and Baticz, O. (2010). Isolation and study of the functional properties of pea proteins. *Nahrung* 45 (6): 399–401.

Tonstad, S., Smerud, K., and Høie, L. (2002). A comparison of the effects of 2 doses of soy protein or casein on serum lipids, serum lipoproteins, and plasma total homocysteine in hypercholesterolemic subjects. *Am. J. Clin. Nutr.* 76: 78–84.

Tsuji, Y., Yamada, K., Hosoya, N., and Moriuchi, S. (1986). Digestion and absorption of sugars and sugar substitutes in rat small intestine. *J. Nutr. Sci. Vitaminol.* 32 (1): 93–100.

Tuohy, K.M., Ziemer, C.J., Klinder, A. et al. (2002). A human volunteer study to determine the prebiotic effects of lactulose powder on human colonic microbiota. *Microb. Ecol. Health Dis.* 14: 165–173.

U.S. Agricultural Research Service Food Data Central

Vacca-Smith, A., Van Wuyckhuyse, B., Tabak, L., and Bowen, W. (1994). The effect of milk and casein proteins on the adherence of Streptococcus mutans to saliva-coated hydroxyapatite. *Arch. Oral Biol.* 39: 1063–1069.

Van Creaeyveld, V., Swennen, K., van de Wiele, T., Marzorati, M., Verstraete, W., Delaedt, Y., Onagbesan, O., Decuypere, E., Buyse, J., De Ketelaere, B., Borekaert, W.F., Delcour, J.A., Courtin, C.M. (2008). Structurally different wheat-derived arabinoxylanoligosaccharides have different prebiotic and fermentation properties in rats. *J. Nutr.*, 138 (12), 2348–2355. doi: https://doi.org/10.3945/jn.108.094367.

Van Den Heuvel, E.G.H.M., Schoterman, M.H.C., and Muijs, T. (2000). Transgalactooligosaccharides stimulate calcium absorption in postmenopausal women. *J. Nutr.* 130 (12): 2938–2942.

Varshosaz, J. (2012). Dextran conjugates in drug delivery. *Expert Opin. Drug Deliv.* 9 (5): 509–523.

Varzakas, T., Labropoulos, A., and Anestis, S. (2012). *Sweeteners: Nutritional Aspects, Applications, and Production Technology*, 59–60. CRC Press.

Vincken, J.P., Schols, H.A., Oomen, R.J. et al. (2003). If homogalacturonan were a side chain of rhamnogalacturonan I. Implications for cell wall architecture. *Plant Physiol.* 132 (4): 1781–1789.

Vogel, M. (1991). Alternative utilisation of sugar beet pulp. *Zuckerindustrie* 116: 266–270.

Vollmer, D.L., West, V.A., and Lephart, E.D. (2018). Enhancing skin health: by oral administration of natural compounds and minerals with implications to the dermal microbiome. *Int. J. Mol. Sci.* 19 (10): 3059. https://doi.org/10.3390/ijms19103059.

Waisbren, S.E., Potter, N.L., and Gordon, C.M. (2012). The adult galactosemic phenotype. *J. Inherit. Metab. Dis.* 35: 279–286.

Wakai, A., McCabe, A., Roberts, I., and Schierhout, G. (2013). Mannitol for acute traumatic brain injury. *Cochrane Database Syst. Rev.* 8 (8): CD001049.

Waldron, K.W., Parker, M.L., and Smith, A.C. (2003). Plant cell walls and food quality. *Compr. Rev. Food Sci. Food Saf.* 2: 101–119.

Wan, Y., Lu, J., and Cui, Z. (2006). Separation of lysozyme from chicken egg white using ultrafiltration. *Sep. Purif. Technol.* 48: 133–142.

Watanabe, G., Tomiyama, H., and Doba, N. (2000). Effects of oral administration of l-arginine on renal function in patients with heart failure. *J. Hypertens.* 18 (2): 229–234.

Watford, M. (1991). The urea cycle: a two-compartment system. *Essays Biochem.* 26: 49–58.

White, P.J. (2011). Oat starch: physicochemical properties and function. In: *Oats: Chemistry and Technology* (ed. H.H. Webster and P.J. Wood), 109–122. St. Paul, MN, USA: AAAC International Press.

Wichienchot, S., Prasertsan, P., Hongpattarakere, T., and Rastall, R.A. (2009). Manufacture of glucooligosaccharide prebiotic by Gluconobacter oxydans NCIMB 4943. *Songklanakarin J. Sci. Technol.* 31 (6): 597–603.

Wijesekara, I. and Kim, S.K. (2010). Angiotensin-I-converting enzyme (ACE) inhibitors from marine resources: prospects in the pharmaceutical industry. *Mar. Drugs* 8 (4): 1080–1093.

Wijnands, M.V.W., Schoterman, H.C., Bruijntjes, J.P., Hollanders, V.M.H., Woutersen, R.A. (2001). Effect of dietary galacto-oligosaccharides (GOS) on azoxymethane-induced aberrant crypt foci and colorectal cancer in Fischer 344 rats. *Carcinogenesis*, 22 (1), 127–132. doi: https://doi.org/10.1093/carcin/22.1.127.

Willats, W.G.T., Knox, J.P., and Mikkelsen, J.D. (2006). Pectin: new insights into an old polymer are starting to gel. *Trends Food Sci. Technol.* 17: 97–104.

Williams, J. (1968). A comparison of glycopeptides from the ovotransferrin and serum transferrin of the hen. *Biochem. J.* 108 (5): 7–67.

Wu, J. and Acero-Lopez, A. (2012). Ovotransferrin: structure, bioactivities and preparation. *Food Res. Int.* 46: 480–487.

Xia, W., Liu, P., Zhang, J., and Chen, J. (2011). Biological activities of chitosan and chitooligosaccharides. *Food Hydrocoll.* 25 (2): 170–179.

Xin-Zhong, H., Xia-lu, S., Xiao-ping, L. et al. (2015). Effect of dietary oat β-glucan on high-fat diet induced obesity in HFA mice. *Bioact. Carbohydr. Diet. Fibre* 5 (1): 79–85.

Xiong, Y. (1997). Structure-function relationships of muscle proteins. In: *Food Proteins and Their Applications* (ed. S. Damodaran and A. Paraf), 341–392. New York: Marcel Dekker.

Yamamoto, T., Unno, T., Watanabe, Y. et al. (2004). Purification and characterization of Acremonium implicatum a-glucosidase having regioselectivity for α-(1,3)- glucosidic linkage. *Biochim. Biophys. Acta* 1700: 189–198.

Yi, Y., Neufeld, R., and Poncelet, D. (2005). Immobilization of cells in polysaccharide gels. In: *Polysaccharides: Structural Diversity and Functional Versatility*, vol. 86 (ed. S. Dumitriu), 7–91. New York: Marcel Dekker.

Yi, J., Horky, L.L., Friedlich, A.L. et al. (2009). L-arginine and Alzheimer's disease. *Int. J. Clin. Exp. Pathol. 2* (3): 211–238.

Yoo, Y.C., Watanabe, S., and Watanabe, R. (1998). Bovine lactoferrin and lactoferricin inhibit tumor metastasis in mice. *Adv. Exp. Med. Biol.* 443: 285–291.

Yu, Z., Liu, B., Zhao, W., Yin, Y., Liu, J., & Chen, F. (2012). Primary and secondary structure of novel ACE-inhibitory peptides from egg white protein. Food Chemistry, 133(2), 315-322.

Yun, J., Suh, J.H., and Song, S. (1994). Kinetic study and mathematical model for the production of isomalto-oligosaccharides from maltose by transglucosylation of Aureobasidium pullulans. *J. Korean Inst. Chem. Eng.* 32 (6): 875–880.

Zhou, L.M., Xu, J.Y., Rao, C.P. et al. (2015). Effect of whey supplementation on circulating C-reactive protein: a meta-analysis of randomized controlled trials. *Nutrients 7* (2): 1131–1143. https://doi.org/10.3390/nu7021131.

Zhu, F., Du, B., and Xu, B. (2016). Review. A critical review on production and industrial applications of betaglucans. *Food Hydrocoll.* 52: 275–288.

9

Genetically Modified Products and Non-GMO Products in Nutraceuticals

D. Prabavathy, S. Sudha, and L. Inbathamizh

Department of Biotechnology, School of Bio and Chemical Engineering, Sathyabama Institute of Science and Technology, Chennai, Tamil Nadu, India

9.1 Introduction

There is a great need to intensify the food production to overcome the challenges of food security globally. As the world population increases steadily, the agricultural production must also keep pace with it. If the current global processes continue and population growth tendencies remain unchanged, another 2.4 billion people will live in developing countries by 2050. A substantial increase in productivity, structural changes in the livestock sector, and increased animal products are required to meet the demand. According to forecasts, the average daily intake per capita is projected to exceed 3000 kcal globally by 2050 to reach 3500 kcal in developed countries (Frona et al. 2019).

On the other hand, globally, at least one in three children under five years are not receiving adequate nutrition for optimum growth and development. At least 340 million children under five years – around one in two children – suffer from "hidden" hunger due to micronutrient deficiencies (UNICEF 2019). The 2019 Joint Malnutrition Estimates report indicates that globally 49.5 million children under five years suffer from wasting, with 16.6 million of them severely wasted, and almost 149 million are stunted (UNICEF, WHO, WB, 2019).

These reports warrant that the eradication of hunger and malnutrition should be a priority of policy-making. FAO predicted that the finite amount of arable land available for food production per person will decrease from the current 0.242 to 0.18 ha by 2050 (Alexandratos and Bruinsma 2012). The scenario is further compounded by several complicating factors such as:

1) the increased demand for biofuel and feedstock production;
2) accelerated urbanization;
3) land desertification, salinization, and degradation;
4) altered land use from staple foods to pasture, driven by socioeconomic considerations;
5) climate change;
6) water resource limitation.

These factors emphasize a need in overproduction and a desired nutritional trait in the crops such that supply meets demand. Conventional breeding relies on sexual crossing of one parental line with another parental line to obtain desired traits in crop. However, the process usually takes several years before actual expression of the desired trait that can be assessed and further expanded to commercial use. The emergent biological technologies and the development of genetically modified (GM) foods promise to reduce dramatically the production timelines to new strains and to provide us with optional strategies to achieve sustainable global food security.

According to the regulation 1829/2003 of the European Parliament, the term "genetically modified food" denotes food which itself is a "food containing or composed of a GMO, or food produced using GMO." The pioneer plants subjected to the process of transgenesis involved tobacco and petunia, but the breakthrough was the introduction of a modified FlavrSavr tomato plant to the market in 1994. The range of genetically modified food includes all plants and much narrower range of animals and microbes.

Among numerous modifications induced in plants, transformations aimed at altered chemical composition of food products for nutrient enrichment and/or therapeutic value. Such foods are denoted as "nutraceuticals." Nutraceuticals include isolated nutrients, herbal products, dietary supplements, genetically engineered "designer" foods, and processed products. This chapter highlights the GM products and non-GMO products in nutraceuticals.

9.2 Nutraceuticals – Definition and Types

Till date, a certain and unambiguous definition of the term nutraceutical is not available. The term "nutraceutical" was invented in 1989 by Stephen L. Defelice, who established The Foundation for Innovation in Medicine in 1976. Health Canada working definition states, "A nutraceutical is a product isolated or purified from foods that is generally sold in medicinal forms not usually associated with food and demonstrated to have a physiological benefit or provide protection against chronic disease" (Health Canada 1998).

The US Nutraceutical Research and Education Act presented to the House of Representatives in the first session of the 106th Congress of 1999–2000 defined nutraceuticals as "a dietary supplement, food or medical food . . . that (i) has a benefit which prevents or reduces the risk of a disease or health condition, including the management of a disease or health condition or the improvement of health; and (ii) is safe for human consumption in the quantity, and with the frequency required to realize such properties."

The European Nutraceutical Association defines nutraceuticals as "nutritional products which have effects that are relevant to health . . . which are not synthetic substances or chemical compounds formulated for specific indications. . . contain[ing] nutrients (partly in concentrated form)" (Aronson 2017).

A broad classification of nutraceutical groups them in to:

1) potential nutraceutical
2) established nutraceutical

A potential nutraceutical could become an established one only after efficient clinical data of its health and medical benefits are obtained (DeFelice 1995). Nutraceuticals from the natural sources can be classified as (Das et al. 2012)

1) dietary fiber
2) probiotics
3) prebiotics
4) polyunsaturated fatty acids

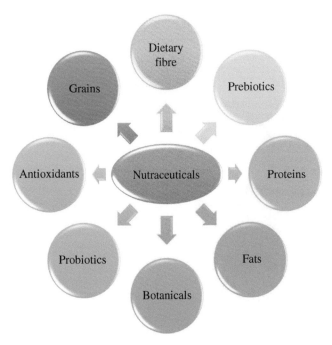

Figure 9.1 Overview of functional ingredients of nutraceuticals.

5) antioxidant, vitamins
6) polyphenols
7) spices

The functional ingredients in commercial nutraceuticals include a range of food products (see Figure 9.1).

9.3 Genetically Modified Products in Nutraceuticals

A major application and focus of biotechnology in the field of agriculture has been improvement of crop yield and pest resistance. Food crops or the improvement of food quality and functional foods garnered much less attention due to the myths and conceptions associated with GM foods. Though there has been a widespread public reluctance in the acceptability and adoption of biotechnology products, genetic modification techniques are increasingly being optimized for the production and development of healthy foods, and improvement in the levels and activity of biologically active components in food plants (phytochemicals). This change in public perception in developing countries has been made possible by the development of high-vitamin A rice.

The techniques applied in genetic modification include mutation breeding, improved conventional breeding, transgenic modifications, DNA insertion, gene transfer, and somatic hybridization (Bouis et al. 2003; Mazur 2001; Yan and Kerr 2002). The outcome of genetic modification for nutraceutical production is represented in Figure 9.2.

Modifications that have been targeted and developed by various biotechnology companies include improvement in the oil content and composition of oilseeds such as legumes (Mazur 2001;

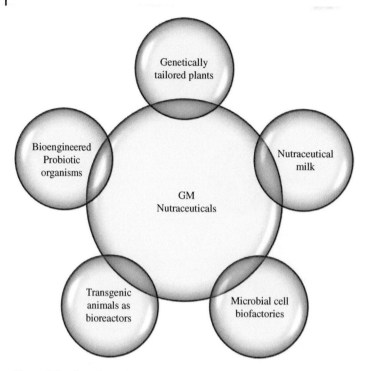

Figure 9.2 Overview of genetically modified nutraceuticals.

Uzogara 2000). Improvement in soybean oil quality includes stabilization of the unsaturated fatty acids by increasing the levels of the antioxidant, vitamin E (Yan and Kerr 2002). These technological developments indicate a relevant and important role for genetic modification in improving food quality targeted at nutritionally deprived population. GM foods are classified based on their application and legal policies as (Mishra and Singh 2013):

1) Food is genetically modified (potato, tomato, soya, maize, sunflowers, rice, pumpkins, melons, rape, etc.);
2) Food comprises of components of genetically tailored plants (starch, sugar oil, vitamins proteins, amino acids, antioxidants, minerals, etc.);
3) Food comprises of genetically adapted organisms.

The primary and secondary metabolites naturally found in plants, animals, bacteria, fungi, and microalgae constitute the bioactive components in functional food and nutraceutical products. Primary metabolites, which include amino acids, nucleic acids, and fatty acids (FAs), are required for normal healthy growth and development, while secondary metabolites, such as carotenoids, terpenoids, and alkaloids, are synthesized in specialized cell types under specific conditions. Some generally regarded as safe microorganisms (GRAS) in dairy and nondairy products exert probiotic effect directly or indirectly and enrich the food by liberating peptides and vitamins by fermentation. These natural food sources could act as substitutes for synthetic pharmaceutical products for clinical intervention of diseases, provided the health benefits are proven (Aryee and Boye 2015).

The following sections discuss the role GM products in the major functional ingredients of nutraceuticals which were listed in the earlier section.

9.3.1 Antioxidants and Vitamins

Antioxidants occur in different forms, phenolic compounds such as flavonoids and tocopherols being the most common. Antioxidants are defending compounds neutralizing the scavenging activity of free radicals and play an essential role in maintaining normal metabolism status. Vitamins are organic compounds required by human as micronutrients in trace amounts. They are found in most fruits and vegetables such as cabbage, carrots, broccoli, aubergine, berries, and potatoes and are plentiful in coffee, tea, and red wine. Vitamin deficiency causes distinguishable clinical symptoms (Srivastava 2018; Zhao 2007). Therefore, most nutraceutical or nutritional therapy products contain some vitamins, common vitamins such as vitamin A, vitamin B, vitamin C, vitamin D, and vitamin E. Biofortification, a type of micronutrient intervention, aims to increase micronutrients in seeds, tubers, and leafy vegetables of food crops and has the potential to reach the group that is often at the highest risk of micronutrient deficiencies (Hotz and McClafferty 2007). A comprehensive list on the genetic modification on the crops and their nutritional benefits are listed in Table 9.1.

These vitamin-overproducing crops not only increase nutritional value of foods but also clinically supplement vitamins in micronutrient-deficient people.

9.3.2 Prebiotics and Probiotics

The modern definition of the probiotic was given by Hanenaar and Huisint "as a viable mono or mixed culture of bacteria which, when applied to animal or man, affects the host beneficially by improving the properties of the indigenous flora" (George Kerry et al. 2018) while a *prebiotic* has been defined as a nondigestible food ingredient that beneficially affects the host by selectively stimulating the growth or activity of one or a limited number of bacteria in the colon and thus improving host health (Gibson 2004). Probiotics and prebiotics as nutraceuticals improve the intestinal microflora and inhibit the growth of pathogenic strains such as *Escherichia coli* and *Salmonella*, allergic disorders, diarrhea, and inflammatory bowel disease. Prebiotics and probiotics in foods and beverages and as supplements may enhance health independently or in combination be referred to as *synbiotics* (Champagne et al. 2005; Di Criscio et al. 2010).

Examples of some of probiotics are:

1) Lactobacilli: *L. aciacidophilus, L. casei, L. delbrueckii* subsp. *bulgaricus, L. brevis,* and *L. cellobiosus*
2) Gram-positive Cocci: *Lactococcus alctis, Streptococcus salivaritus* subsp. *thermophilus,* and *Enterococcus faecium*
3) Bifidobacteria: *B. bifidun, B. adolescentis, B. infantis, B. longum,* and *B. thermophilum*

Prebiotics are short-chain polysaccharides that have unique chemical structure and are not digested by host. They alter the composition or metabolism of microorganisms present in the gut of the host and provide beneficial effects (Macfarlane et al. 2006). The limited digestibility in the small intestine and fermentation by intestinal bacteria of these nondigestible oligosaccharides in the colon may slow energy release in individuals predisposed to diabetes, increase satiety, and reduce hunger. They may also play an important role in colonic health and other GI illnesses by stimulating the beneficial activity and proliferation of specific members of the intestinal microflora, preventing colonization by potential pathogens, producing beneficial short-chain FAs (such as acetic acid, propionic acid, and butyric acid, which are used by the host organism as an energy source), and stimulating calcium absorption from food. Known examples of prebiotics include nondigestible oligosaccharides such as inulin (fruits and vegetables), fructo-oligosaccharides

Table 9.1 Genetic modification on the crops and their nutritional benefits.

Transgenic plant	Genetic modification/metabolic engineering	Nutraceutical property	References
Vitamin A			
Tomato	Overexpression of DXP synthase, a carotenoid precursor	Enhances the total carotenoid content	Enfissi et al. (2005)
Cassava	Roots expressing the bacterial *CrtB* gene accumulated up to 21 lg/g of carotenoids	34-Fold increase with respect to the wild type	Welsch et al. (2010)
Golden potato	Expression of three Erwinia genes encoding phytoene synthase (*CrtB*), phytoene desaturase (*CrtI*), and lycopene beta-cyclase (*CrtY*), leading to the diversion of carotenoid synthesis from the α- to the β-branch	Resulting in the accumulation of 47 lg/g DW of β-carotene	Diretto et al. (2007)
Potato	Expression of the cauliflower or gene in tubers	Transgenic potatoes with orange tuber flesh containing 10 times the normal amount of β-carotene	Lopez et al. (2008) and
Wheat	Introduction of the maize *PSY1* and bacterial carotene desaturases (*CrtI*) genes	High levels of carotenoids (10.8 folds)	Cong et al. (2009)
Wheat (Bobwhite)	Introduction of the bacterial phytoene synthase gene (*CrtB*) instead of the maize PSY1	Eightfold increase in total carotenoid content	Wang et al. (2014)
White maize	Introduction of bacterial *CrtB* and *CrtI* genes	Carotenoid production from undetectable levels	Aluru et al. (2008)
Golden rice	Introduction of *Pantoea ananatis* phytoene desaturase (CrtI) and a *Narcissus pseudonarcissus* phytoene synthase (PSY) into rice	Accumulation of 1.6 mg total carotenoids per gram of dry seeds	Ye et al. (2000)
Golden rice 2	Maize (Zea mays) *PSY1* gene is utilized	A maximum of 37 mg/g total carotenoids with β-carotene preferentially accumulated in the endosperm	Paine et al. (2005)
Vitamin C			
Lettuce	Overexpression of L-gulono c-lactone oxidase (GLOase)	7-Fold improvement	Jain and Nessler (2000)
Multivitamin maize	Expression of rice *dhar* gene	6 Times accumulation of ascorbate levels	Naqvi et al. (2009)
Vitamin B9			
Tomato	Crossing two transgenic tomato lines: one expressing GCH1 which enhanced the cytosolic (pterin) branch and the other ADCS1 which enhanced the PABA branch	2-Fold increase in levels of folate	Dı́az de la Garza et al. (2007)
Rice	Same strategy in rice endosperm	100-1Fold increase in levels of folate	Storozhenko et al. (2007)
Lettuce	Expression of Arabidopsis γ-tocopherol methyltransferase	Increase in the α/γ tocopherol ratio	Cho et al. (2005)

Table 9.1 (Continued)

Transgenic plant	Genetic modification/metabolic engineering	Nutraceutical property	References
Soybean	Expression of *Perilla frutescens* γ-TMT.	10.4-Fold increase in α-tocopherol levels and a 14.9-fold increase in β-tocopherol levels in soybean seeds	Tavya et al. (2007)
Maize	Constitutive expression of two *Arabidopsis* cDNA clones encoding *p*-hydroxyphenylpyruvate dioxygenase (HPPD) and 2-methyl-6-phytylplastoquinol methyltransferase (MPBQ MT)	Increase in tocopherol content by 3-fold	Naqvi et al. (2011)
Vitamin B6			
Cassava	Simultaneous overexpression of *Arabidopsis* *PDX1.1* and *PDX2* genes	Achieved a 9.0-fold increase in the leaves to 54.74 mg/g by CaMV35S promoter and a 15.4-fold increase in the roots to 16.21 mg/g by root-enhanced Patatin promoter, respectively	Li et al. (2015)
Vitamin E			
Corn	Overexpression of the barley HGGT	Increase in as much as 6-fold increase in tocotrienol and tocopherol content	Cahoon et al. (2003)

(FOS), galacto-oligosaccharides (GOS), lactulose, and resistant starch (Al-Sheraji et al. 2013; Bosscher et al. 2006).

Novel bioengineered probiotics can be produced through genetic modifications which enhance the efficacy of conventional probiotics. Studies focus on the conversion of a non-probiotic strain to a probiotic strain and improving the probiotic properties of established strains (Chua et al. 2017; Steidler 2003). These genetically engineered strains can be designed for additional applications such as a vaccine or drug delivery, mimicking surface receptors, targeting specific toxins or pathogens, and enhancement of host immune responses (Amalaradjou and Bhunia 2013). The designer probiotics could be used as therapeutic agents for the treatment of various noncommunicable diseases as well as infectious diseases through the production of antimicrobial peptides. The choice of probiotic strain for genetic modifications includes analysis of the following essential criteria (Mazhar et al. 2020):

- genotype and phenotype
- protein or carbohydrate utilization patterns
- bile or acid tolerance
- growth as well as survival
- antibiotic resistance patterns
- intestinal epithelial adhesion characteristics
- production of antimicrobials
- ability to impede known pathogens and immunogenicity

A brief summary of studies on genetic modification of probiotics is listed in Table 9.2.

Table 9.2 Genetic modification of probiotics and their applications.

Applications of GM probiotics			
Production of antimicrobial peptides			
Probiotic strain	**Genetic modification**	**Outcome**	**References**
L. lactis	Antimicrobials A3APO and alyteserin production	Successful inhibition of *E. coli* and *Salmonella*	Volzing et al. (2013)
Lactobacillus sake	Expression of hybrid bacteriocins Pediocin PA-1, Sakacin P, Curvacin A, Enterocin A, Leucocin A	Hybrid bacteriocin was active and potent with varied targeting specificity	Dash et al. (2015)
Lactobacillus salivarius	Production of Bactofencin A	Shares similarity with eukaryotic cationic AMPs, inhibitory against medically significant pathogens (*Staphylococcus aureus* and *Listeria monocytogenes*)	Forsythe et al. (2012)
Stress tolerance			
L. paracasei	Overexpression of heat shock protein chaperones (GroES and GroEL)	Increases solvent resistance as well as improved thermotolerance in probiotic strains	Mathipa and Thantsha (2017)
L. salivarius	*Listerial betaine* uptake system (BetL)	Increases the resistance of the probiotic to several stresses	Sheehan (2006)
Anticancer therapeutics			
Salmonella typhimurium A1-R	Engineered tumor-targeting variant	Metastatic cancer treatment	Hiroshima et al. (2015)
L. lactis strain sAGX0085	htff1 cassette in genome, producing hTFF1 – administration through a mouth rinse formulation in hamster model	Significantly reduces the severity and the course of radiation-induced OM	Caluwaerts et al. (2010)
Psychobiotics – probiotics for cognitive health			
Lactobacillus rhamnosus JB-1	Murine model	Immunoregulatory effects studies	Al-Nedawi et al. (2015)
Enhancement of anti-inflammatory response			
L. lactis	Expression of anti-TNF-α nanobodies	Reduces the colonic inflammation in mice with dextran sulfate sodium (DSS)-induced chronic colitis.	Vandenbroucke et al. (2010)
L. lactis	Mutant strain inactivated in its major housekeeping protease, HtrA, enhanced elafin expression	Reduces intestinal inflammation in DSS-treated mice	Bermúdez-Humarán et al. (2015)
Enhancement of colonization exclusion			
Lactococcus lactis CH	Cloning of the gene coding for the flagellin of *B. cereus* CH was performed in the lactococcal vector pNZ8110 under the control of a nisin-inducible promoter.	Inhibits competitively the adhesion of the pathogens *Escherichia coli* LMG2092 and *Salmonella enterica* ssp. *enterica* LMG15860	Sánchez et al. (2011)

Table 9.2   (Continued)

Applications of GM probiotics

Production of antimicrobial peptides

Probiotic strain	Genetic modification	Outcome	References
Immunomodulation and cytoprotection			
Lactobacillus paracasei	Expression of VHH against rotavirus	Shortened disease duration, severity, and viral load in a mouse model of rotavirus-induced diarrhea	Pant (2006)
L. lactis	Produce the rotavirus spike-protein subunit VP8* in cytoplasmic, secreted and cell wall-anchored forms	Block rotavirus infection by 50 and 100%	Marelli et al. (2011)
Lactobacillus plantarum	Expression of a long (D1–D5 [D1–D5]) and a short (D4–D5) version of the extracellular domain of invasin from the human pathogen *Yersinia pseudotuberculosis*	Surface display of invasin and were potent activators of NF-κB when interacting with monocytes in cell culture	Fredriksen et al. (2012)
Management of metabolic diseases			
Lactobacillus gasseri ATCC 33323 (L.)	Engineered to secrete GLP-1(1-37) using the SlpA promoter	Ameliorates hyperglycemia in a rat model of diabetes by reprogramming intestinal cells into glucose-responsive insulin-secreting cells.	Duan (2015)

The novel oral recombinant probiotics possess advantages such as low-cost batch preparation, increased shelf life and stability, ease of administration, low delivery costs, and facilitated technology transfer (Taylor and Lamont 2005). Yet, the possibility of reversion to virulence remains a concern. Several strategies for biological containment have been taken.

FOS, GOS, and trans-galacto-oligosaccharides (TOS) are the most common prebiotics. Fermentation of prebiotics by gut microbiota produces short-chain fatty acids (SCFAs), including lactic acid, butyric acid, and propionic acid. The effects of prebiotics on human health are mediated through their degradation products by microorganisms (Davani-Davari et al. 2019), inulin, and inulin-type fructans, also known as soluble dietary fibers, and could be produced by probiotic *Lactobacillus gasseri* strains. Anwar et al. (2010) reported an evaluation of fructan synthesis in three *L. gasseri* strains. *L. gasseri* strains DSM 20604 and 20077 synthesize inulin (and oligosaccharides) and levan products, respectively. *L. gasseri* DSM 20604 is the second *Lactobacillus* strain shown to produce inulin polymer and FOS in situ. The probiotic bacterium *L. gasseri* DSM 20243 did not produce any fructans, although a fructansucrase-encoding gene in its genome sequence was identified. Further studies showed that this *L. gasseri DSM 20243* gene was prematurely terminated by a stop codon. Exchanging the stop codon for a glutamine codon resulted in a recombinant enzyme-producing inulin and FOS. The three recombinant fructansucrase enzymes characterized from three different *L. gasseri* strains have very similar primary protein structures and yet synthesize different fructan products. An interesting feature of the *L. gasseri* strains is that they were unable to ferment raffinose, whereas their respective recombinant enzymes converted raffinose into fructan and FOS.

In the studies by Yu and O'Sullivan (2014), the *lacS* gene from the hyperthermophile *Sulfolobus solfataricus* was expressed in *Lactococcus lactis*. A synthetic gene (*lacSt*) with optimized codon usage for *L. lactis* was designed and synthesized. This hyperthermostable β-galactosidase enzyme was successfully overexpressed in *L. lactis* LM0230 using a nisin-controlled gene expression system. The total GOS yield increased with the initial lactose concentration, whereas the highest lactose conversion rate (72%) was achieved from a low lactose solution (5%). 2′-Fuco-syllactose (2′-FL) is one of the most abundant oligosaccharides in human milk and has been approved as nutritional additive in term infant and toddler formulas. By increasing the availability of GDP-L-fucose and overexpression of fucosyltransferase, 2′-FL could be largely produced from lactose and glycerol in *E. coli* (Baumgärtner et al. 2013).

Levansucrases (EC 2.4.1.10, LS) are of high interest for the synthesis of novel prebiotic FOS, but the availability is limited. Genome mining was used to explore their biodiversity using 26 characterized LSs as a reference set for a sequence-driven approach leading to a collection of 32 enzymes representative of the biodiversity for which the gene was cloned and overexpressed in *E. coli*. These enzymes underwent an initial screening process based on total activity, transfructosylation activity, and levan-forming ability which narrowed the candidates to 10 potential enzymes. These LS enzymes were found to have high levan production (33 ± 1 g levan per mg protein) and are able to produce very large polymers (Hill et al. 2019). Food scientists are continuously looking for novel enzymes from plant and microbial species to produce a variety of prebiotics for commercial applications.

9.3.3 Polyunsaturated Fatty Acids (PUFA)

PUFAs also known as "essential fatty acids" are vital to the body's function and are nutritionally supplemented (Escott-Stump and Mahan 2000). They also have crucial biological activities such as prevention of arteriosclerosis and hyperlipidemia (La Guardia et al. 2005; Swanson et al. 2012). PUFAs have two subdivisions: omega-3-(n-3) fatty acids and omega-6-(n-6) fatty acids. The major omega-3-fatty acids are:

- α-linolenic acid (ALA)
- eicosapentanoic acid (EPA)
- docosahexanoic acid (DHA)

ALA is the precursor of EPA and DHA. Omega-6-PUFAs mainly consist of

- linoleic acid (LA)
- γ-linolenic acid (GLA)
- arachidonic acid (ARA)

Fish and fish oils have been the sole PUFA sources. Alternative sources are explored due to the unstable marine sources and increasing demand. Biotechnological interventions through fermentative processes have been developed using microorganisms such as microalgae, fungi, and engineered yeasts for the production of DHA, ARA, and EPA, respectively (Hayashi et al. 2016).

Earlier studies on gene modifications in soybean and canola led to the modified expression of PUFAs (Fatima et al. 2013). In plants, o-6 desaturase-catalyzed pathway in the microsomes is a major source of polyunsaturated lipids. Introduction of the fungal (Mortierella) D6-desaturase gene in canola produced o-3 fatty acids (Ursin 2003). o-6 and GLA content was engineered in safflower oil to amounts as high as 40%, which is four times higher than the levels found in evening primrose (*Oenothera biennis*) and borage (*Borago officinalis*) (Biosciences 2008). Transformation of safflower by introducing *Saprolegnia diclina* D6-desaturase produced GLA to levels higher than 70% (v/v) (Nykiforuk et al. 2012). Domínguez et al. (2010) have overexpressed the ω-3 fatty acid desaturases *FAD3* and *FAD7* that catalyze the conversion of linoleic acid (18 : 2) to LA (18 : 3), the precursor of hexenals and its derived alcohols. Transgenic OE-FAD tomato plants exhibit altered fatty acid composition, with an increase in the 18 : 3/18 : 2 ratio in fruits.

Microorganisms are known natural producers of microbial oils similar to those obtained from plants and animals and a possible source of nutritionally important omega-3 PUFAs. In addition, microbial oils usually contain a significant level of natural antioxidants, such as carotenoids and tocopherols, which play an important role in protecting omega-3 PUFAs from oxidation and therefore improve their storage stability. The first commercial product obtained from microbial oil was a GLA (C18 : 3 *n*-6)-rich oil produced using the filamentous fungus *Mucor circinelloides* (Patel et al. 2019).

Oleaginous microalgae constitute microscopic bio-factories that are capable of producing elevated amounts of oil which can be used as feedstock for omega-3 PUFAs. A number of algal species, such as *Nitzschia, Navicula, Nannochloropsis, Phaeodactylum,* and *Porphyridium,* have been identified as producers of omega-3 PUFAs (Adarme-Vega et al. 2012; Moomaw et al. 2017; Ward and Singh 2005).

9.3.4 Phytochemicals

Phytochemicals are non-nutritive plant chemicals that have either defensive or disease protective properties. They are nonessential nutrients and mainly produced by plants to provide them protection. Phytochemicals with nutraceutical properties present in food are of enormous significance due to their beneficial effects on human health since they offer protection against numerous diseases or disorders such as cancers, coronary heart disease, diabetes, high blood pressure, inflammation, microbial, viral and parasitic infections, psychotic diseases, spasmodic conditions, ulcers, and osteoporosis and associated disorders (Prakash et al. 2012).

Phytosterols and phytostanols are cholesterol-like molecules found in all plant foods, but the highest concentrations occur in unrefined plant oils, including vegetable, nut, and olive oils. Nuts, seeds, whole grains, and legumes are also good dietary sources of phytosterols. As phytostanols are more stable than phytosterols during food processing, genetic engineering has been applied for the development of rapeseed and soybean oils with modified ratios of phytosterols to phytostanols. Plants were transformed with a gene from yeast encoding the enzyme 3-hydroxysteroid oxidase, which converts phytosterols to phytostanols (Venkatramesh et al. 2003). A species of *Arabidopsis thaliana* has been reported as sterol methyltransferase 2 mutants and found to be involved in sterol biosynthesis leading to plant innate immunity against bacterial pathogens. Arabidopsis cytochrome P450 CYP710A1 has the capability to encode C22-sterol desaturase which can convert β-sitosterol to stigmasterol due to induced inoculation with non-host pathogens. An Arabidopsis Atcyp710A1 with null mutant was developed with both nonhost and basal resistance. Overexpression of AtCYP710A1 enhanced the resistance to host pathogens via involvement of sterols in plant innate immunity against bacterial infections and also has regulated nutrient efflux into the apoplast (Wang et al. 2012; Zauber et al. 2014).

Polyphenols are also potent antioxidants and numerous studies have shown the accumulation of specific phenolics in crop plants. Most studies have used key genes to transform vegetables and fruits. Constitutive overexpression of petunia chalcone isomerase *chi-a* gene, involved in flavonol biosynthesis, resulted in a 78-fold increase in flavonol content of tomato peel. Chlorogenic acid and other flavonoids were also increased several-fold via constitutive expression of hydroxycinnamoyl transferase *HQT* gene (Schijlen et al. 2006). Plants are poor in flavones. However, genetic engineering has been able to produce novel polyphenolics/flavonoids in high concentrations in transgenic tomato fruit transformed with various, heterologous genes of flavonoid biosynthesis pathway (Shih et al. 2008). Similarly, introduction of grape stilbene synthase (*StSY*) gene in tomato generated resveratrol, which is not naturally present in tomato (Nicoletti et al. 2007).

Genetically engineered (GE) nutraceuticals include foods associated with increased health benefits and/or disease prevention (second-generation GM food products) – but also foods, plants, and animal products – that could be used to create vaccines and drugs that could treat or cure diseases (third-generation GM products). GE nutraceuticals are designed for the purpose of creating inexpensive alternative pharmaceuticals, fighting disease in developing countries, and improving consumer health through common foods such as fruits and vegetables (Britwum et al. 2018).

The biomedicines produced in plants are as follows:

- **Antigens for the production of edible vaccines**: vaccines derived from plants have so far induced immunity against rabies virus, hepatitis B, rotavirus, HIV, and other pathogens.
- **Monoclonal antibodies**: transgenic plants as bioreactors.
- **Pharmaceutical proteins**: some samples of biomedicines recently expressed in plants include *erythropoietin, interferon*, hirudin, aprotinin, Leu-enkephalin, and somatotropin of human growth hormone (Alireza and Nader 2015).

The first plant-made pharmaceutically relevant protein was the human growth hormone, expressed in transgenic tobacco in 1986. Milestone for plant-based recombinant protein production for human health use was the approval in 2012 by the US Food and Drug Administration of plant-made taliglucerase alfa, a therapeutic enzyme for the treatment of Gaucher's disease (GD), synthesized in carrot suspension cultures by Protalix BioTherapeutics. GD is a lysosomal storage disorder caused by a hereditary deficiency of the enzyme glucocerebrosidase, which is involved in glycolipid metabolism. GD creates a disabling condition curable only with permanent enzyme replacement therapy (ERT). The results demonstrated that the oral administration of proteins encapsulated in plant cells is feasible and may be a valuable alternative to intravenous administration of ERT (Massa et al. 2018).

Studies have indicated that an immune response can be mounted in individuals fed with plant material expressing a disease antigen. The first trials with plant-based vaccines were conducted with the nontoxic B subunit of heat-labile enterotoxin (LT-B) of enterotoxigenic *E. coli* contained either in raw potato or maize administered orally to healthy volunteers for safety and immunogenicity testing. No adverse effects of vaccination were noticed (Tacket 2007). Fragments encoding a chimeric protein of G protein and N protein of the rabies virus fused with that of alfalfa mosaic virus coat protein were introduced into a TMV-derived plant expression vector. The vaccine transiently expressed in spinach was orally administered (three doses of spinach; 20 g corresponding to 84 µg of chimeric rabies peptide each) in a clinical trial revealing the induction of elevated rabies-specific IgG in a group of individuals previously vaccinated with a commercial injection-type vaccine and in volunteers with no history of rabies vaccination (Yusibov et al. 2002).

Further the evolution of molecular techniques has led to the development of systems such as the gateway-mediated cloning (Dafny-Yelin and Tzfira 2007), golden gate (Binder et al. 2014), and golden braid (Sarrion-Perdigones et al. 2011) which facilitates the assembly of multi-modular constructs for the expression of multiple proteins or enzymes in plants.

9.3.5 Bioengingeered Animals and Microbes

The production of transgenic animals, which potentially can have a deep impact on the livestock and pharmaceutical chains, has proceeded much slower than genetic modification of crops. Milk is the most mature and proven transgenic system for the production of recombinant pharmaceutical proteins. The first commercial biopharmaceutical recombinant protein produced in transgenic animals – ATryn, a recombinant human antithrombin and approved for human use for the treatment of patients with hereditary antithrombin deficiency was developed by GTC Biotherapeutics – was produced in goat mammary gland. The approval by EMA in 2006 and by FDA in 2009 validated and confirmed the transgenic animal manufacturing platform (Bertolini et al. 2016).

The microbial metabolites from engineered microorganisms are of immense importance as therapeutics or nutraceuticals. Microbial metabolites combined with modern natural product research methodology has opened the way for a new era of nutraceuticals and therapeutics. A large array of nutraceutical products (carotenoids, PUFA, and flavonoids) is being explored through the use of metabolic engineering. This approach bypasses the traditional challenges of direct extraction from animals and plants and provides an environmental friendly and sustainable platform for industrial production. Microbes can be engineered to produce metabolites, known as postbiotics that have health, nutrition, and industrial applications. The postbiotics confer beneficial health effects such as inhibition of gut and genitourinary microbial infections and immunomodulation, and prevent the inflammatory gut diseases and cancer. It is desirable to discover the gastrointestinal microbiota for using them as hosts for expressing recombinant proteins intended for commercial applications (Singh et al. 2019; Yuan and Alper 2019).

9.4 Benefits and Risks Associated with Genetically Modified Food Products

The increasing number of transgenic food products on the food market provides a concentrated source of nutraceutics, or substances carrying high therapeutic and pro-health value, representing a desirable element of a differentiated diet. "Pharming" involves the use of plants and animals as bioreactors of therapeutic compounds. Yet these nutraceutics are associated with their inherent risks and negative effects on the human population (Kramkowska et al. 2013). Three major health risks potentially associated with GM foods are:

- toxicity
- allergenicity
- genetic hazards

Examples of induced food allergy include Star Link Maize and soybean enriched in methionine. Milk from genetically modified cows increased IGF 1 concentration in serum, which positively correlated with breast, lung, and colon cancer. Maize MON810 had a harmful influence on the cells of pancreas, intestines, liver, and kidney of rodents. Genetically modified potatoes with lectin content abnormalities in development and immunity in rodents (Zhang et al. 2016).

Genetically modified plants or animals can reproduce, spread, and propagate in an uncontrolled and irreversible biosphere, with unpredictable effects on the surrounding biological environment. Thus, it becomes essential to make a distinction between application of genetic engineering that takes place in a closed and isolated environment and applications that are released into the environment, without the possibility of containment (Arcieri 2016). Hence, development of nutraceuticals depends on its quality, safety, long-term adverse effects, and toxicity as well as supplementation studies and clinical trials in humans.

9.5 Public Perception of GM Food

Public attitudes toward GM food from country to country in different regions of the world continue to vary (Cui and Shoemaker 2018). The review by Van Eenennaam and Young (2018) noted that the negative view of GM food in Europe was exacerbated by the bovine spongiform encephalopathy (BSE) crisis first in the late 1980s and again in the 1990s. In contrast, the United States, Canada, and some Latin American countries have widely adopted GM crops. Though the progress is slow, there seems to be a new receptiveness for GM food among some of the African countries. In Asian countries, it has been noted that China's initial lead position in GM food has slowed over time due to global resistance to GM food. Finally, Van Eenennaam and Young compared China with other Asia countries (India and The Philippines) where bans on GM foods or vandalism on GM crops have occurred. Britwum et al. (2018) studies showed a strong preference for GE nutraceuticals that offer disease prevention or treatment benefits compared to those that offer only general health benefits, an outcome consistent even among participants opposing genetic modification.

9.6 Non-GM Products in Nutraceuticals

A wide range of food products belong to this category and have been used traditionally, such as the herbs and spices. Novel nutraceuticals have been obtained from the fruit and vegetable residues. Nanotechnology methods aim at the improvement of nutraceutical quality by increasing their stability and efficiency. Production of any such nutraceutical without the involvement of GMOs can be assigned to non-GM nutraceuticals.

9.6.1 Botanicals and Spices

Botanicals were often used as a synonym for herbs or herbal products with medicinal potency. Botanicals are nutraceuticals made from plant parts. Herbals are the products that consist of a whole, fresh plant or its part, such as dried leaf, fruit, roots, or concentrated extract (Gulati et al. 2019). Spices are a group of esoteric food adjuncts that have been in use for thousands of years to enhance the sensory quality of foods; the quantity and variety consumed in tropical countries is particularly extensive. These spice ingredients impart characteristic flavor, aroma, or piquancy and color to foods. Spices exert one or more of the following activities: antioxidant, anti-inflammatory, anticancer, antidiabetic, digestive stimulant, protection of RBC integrity, cholesterol lowering, and antilithogenic (Srinivasan 2011). Spices and botanicals have been used from time immemorable. Several recent studies have reiterated the use of these substance as nutraceuticals. Spices and herbs are in most cases harmless when used as food but may exhibit toxicity when used as medicine, because of their relative higher dose administered or rather due to the possibilities of their interactions with other pharmaceutical medications (Ernst 2003).

9.6.2 Fruit Residues as Source of Nutraceuticals

Fruit and vegetable wastes (FVW) are produced in large quantities in markets and their recovery could be used for the production of nutraceuticals and functional foods. Phenolic constituents used as nutraceuticals could be obtained from different fruit residues such as apple peel and pomace, grapes seed and skin, citrus, banana peel, and mango kernel (Varzakas et al. 2016). It is possible to obtain a valuable oil with the greatest amount of linoleic acid (70%) from grape seeds, which exerts an anticholesterolic action and contains antioxidants and vitamins (Barbieri et al. 2013). Nutritional and nutraceutical components were studied from the juices and its ready-to-serve (RTS) beverage made of residues of banana rhizome and banana pseudostem. BR juice showed higher total phenolic content (TPC) and total flavonoid content (TFC) of 341.44 mg GAE and 87.60 mg CE/200 ml, respectively, when compared to BPS juice. Moreover, it exhibited high antioxidant activity in all the assays tested. Hence, BPS and BR juices can be effectively used to produce new-generation functional beverages (Saravanan and Aradhya 2011). Akhtar et al. (2015) focused on the nutritional, functional, and anti-infective properties of pomegranate (*Punica granatum* L.) peel (PoP) and peel extract (PoPx) and on their applications as food additives, functional food ingredients, or biologically active components in nutraceutical preparations.

9.6.3 Nanocarrier-Based Nutraceuticals

Studies indicate a strong correlation between nutraceuticals and cancer prevention. For example, a study was conducted to investigate the relationship between pancreatic cancer risk and dietary carotenoids. The study revealed that consumption of lycopene decreases the pancreatic cancer risk among men by 31% and indicated that tomato-based products with high levels of lycopene could reduce pancreatic cancer risk (Nkondjock et al. 2005). Nutraceuticals prevent cancer through several mechanisms such as inhibiting cell proliferation and differentiation, inhibiting efflux transporters such as multidrug resistance protein (MRP), or by reducing the toxicity of chemotherapeutic drugs (Saneja et al. 2014). The use of nutraceuticals in cancer prevention is limited due to poor aqueous solubility and poor permeability which ultimately leads to poor bioavailability in humans. Additional factors which may also contribute for poor bioavailability of nutraceuticals are restricted release from the food matrix, formation of insoluble complexes with other components in the gastrointestinal tract, and/or bio-transformations in the GIT. These challenges are overcome by use of nanocarriers for drug delivery. Nanocarriers have the ability to modulate pharmacodynamic as well as pharmacokinetic profiles of nutraceuticals (Díaz and Vivas-Mejia 2013). Further, coadministration of nutraceuticals with chemotherapeutic agents also alleviates the toxicity of administered agents such as coadministration of co-enzyme Q10 prevents anthracycline-induced cardiotoxicity (Conklin 2005). Various kinds of nanocarriers such as polymeric nanoparticles, micelles, liposomes, etc. have been used to enhance the bioavailability and efficacy of nutraceuticals in recent years. These nanocarriers can be broadly classified into three categories based on the excipients from which they are made: (i) polymeric nanocarriers, (ii) lipid-based nanocarriers, and (iii) inorganic nanocarriers. Several studies are underway to evaluate the efficiency of nanocarrier-based nutraceuticals for cancer therapy (Arora and Jaglan 2016). The nanocarriers evaluated for nutraceutical are listed in Table 9.3.

9.7 Challenges with Nutraceuticals

Nutraceutical industry is associated with great concern and challenges ahead. A great surge has been observed in the global nutraceutical market. The major factor attributing to this surge is the absence of strict regulations to control the nutraceutical industry. The nutritional and therapeutic

Table 9.3 Examples of nanocarriers used as excipients for nutraceuticals.

Polymeric nanoparticle	
Nutraceutical	**Excipient**
Betulinic acid	PLLA poly(L-lactic acid)
Curcumin	PLGA poly(lactic-*co*-glycolic acid)
Naringenin	Chitosan
Resveratrol	Gelatin
Thymoquinone PVP, PEG	PVP – polyvinylpyrrolidone, PEG – polyethyleneglycol
Lipid-based nanocarriers	
Thymoquinone	Hydrogenated palm oil, olive oil, Polysorbate 80
Plumbagin	Phospholipid, Tween 80
Curcumin	TPGS, Brij78, GMS, Lecithin
Inorganic nanocarriers	
Apigenin	AuNPs
Plumbagin	Ag_2O
Sulforaphane	Fe_3O_4, Au

claims of the nutraceuticals are not proven as in the case of pharmaceuticals. The patients are also concerned about the use of pharmaceutical products because of their high price and several side effects. Approximately 80% of global population preferred using dietary supplements and nutraceuticals (Ekor 2014; Nounou et al. 2018), while, the in-vivo and in-vitro studies that prove the nutraceutical products claims have been neglected (Santini et al. 2018).

9.8 Conclusion

Nutraceuticals are present in most of the food ingredients with varying concentrations. Further advances in the genetic engineering has made the fortification and addition of therapeutic values to plant, animal, and microbe-based foods. The claims of the beneficial effects of the nutraceuticals available in the commercial market are not proven. The consumer should be educated with the recommended dosage and informed about the GM or non-GM status so as to make a choice. Great attention is essential in nutraceutical research to convert majority of potential nutraceuticals to established ones, thereby, truly delivering their enormous benefits. Production of personalized nutraceuticals is not far with the current gene technology available.

References

Adarme-Vega, T.C., Lim, D.K., Timmins, M. et al. (2012). Microalgal biofactories: a promising approach towards sustainable omega-3 fatty acid production. *Microbial Cell Factories* 11 (1): 96.

Akhtar, S., Ismail, T., Fraternale, D., and Sestili, P. (2015). Pomegranate peel and peel extracts: chemistry and food features. *Food Chemistry* 174: 417–425.

Alexandratos, N. and Bruinsma, J. (2012). *World Agriculture Towards 2030/2050 the 2012 Revision*. Rome: FAO.

Alireza, T. and Nader, R.E. (2015). Molecular farming in plants. In: *Plants for Future* (ed. H.L. Shemy), 25–41. London, UK: Intech Open.

Al-Nedawi, K., Mian, M.F., Hossain, N. et al. (2015). Gut commensal microvesicles reproduce parent bacterial signals to host immune and enteric nervous systems. *The FASEB Journal* 29 (2): 684–695.

Al-Sheraji, S.H., Ismail, A., Manap, M.Y. et al. (2013). Prebiotics as functional foods: a review. *Journal of Functional Foods* 5 (4): 1542–1553.

Aluru, M., Xu, Y., Guo, R. et al. (2008). Generation of transgenic maize with enhanced provitamin A content. *Journal of Experimental Botany* 59 (13): 3551–3562.

Amalaradjou, M.A.R. and Bhunia, A.K. (2013). Bioengineered probiotics, a strategic approach to control enteric infections. *Bioengineered* 4 (6): 379–387.

Anwar, M.A., Kralj, S., Pique, A.V. et al. (2010). Inulin and levan synthesis by probiotic *Lactobacillus gasseri* strains: characterization of three novel fructansucrase enzymes and their fructan products. *Microbiology* 156 (4): 1264–1274.

Arcadia Biosciences, Inc. (2008). Arcadia biosciences and bioriginal food and science corp. Enter strategic alliance to market high GLA safflower oil. *Business Wire*.

Arcieri, M. (2016). Spread and potential risks of genetically modified organisms. *Agriculture and Agricultural Science Procedia* 8: 552–559.

Aronson, J.K. (2017). Defining 'nutraceuticals': neither nutritious nor pharmaceutical. *British Journal of Clinical Pharmacology* 83 (1): 8–19.

Arora, D. and Jaglan, S. (2016). Nanocarriers based delivery of nutraceuticals for cancer prevention and treatment: a review of recent research developments. *Trends in Food Science & Technology* 54: 114–126.

Aryee, A.N. and Boye, J.I. (2015). Current and emerging trends in the formulation and manufacture of nutraceuticals and functional food products. In: *Nutraceutical and Functional Food Processing Technology*, 1–52. Germany: Wiley.

Barbieri, L., Andreola, F., Lancellotti, I., and Taurino, R. (2013). Management of agricultural biomass wastes: preliminary study on characterization and valorisation in clay matrix bricks. *Waste Management* 33 (11): 2307–2315.

Baumgärtner, F., Seitz, L., Sprenger, G.A., and Albermann, C. (2013). Construction of *Escherichia coli* strains with chromosomally integrated expression cassettes for the synthesis of 2′-fucosyllactose. *Microbial Cell Factories* 12 (1): 40.

Bermúdez-Humarán, L.G., Motta, J.P., Aubry, C. et al. (2015). Serine protease inhibitors protect better than IL-10 and TGF-β anti-inflammatory cytokines against mouse colitis when delivered by recombinant lactococci. *Microbial Cell Factories* 14 (1): 26.

Bertolini, L.R., Meade, H., Lazzarotto, C.R. et al. (2016). The transgenic animal platform for biopharmaceutical production. *Transgenic Research* 25 (3): 329–343.

Binder, A., Lambert, J., Morbitzer, R. et al. (2014). A modular plasmid assembly kit for multigene expression, gene silencing and silencing rescue in plants. *PLoS One* 9 (2): e88218.

Bosscher, D., Van Loo, J., and Franck, A. (2006). Inulin and oligofructose as functional ingredients to improve bone mineralization. *International Dairy Journal* 16: 1092–1097.

Bouis, H.E., Chassy, B.M., and Ochanda, J.O. (2003). Genetically modified food crops and their contribution to human nutrition and food quality. *Trends in Food Science & Technology* 14 (5–8): 191–209.

Britwum, K., Yiannaka, A., and Kastanek, K. (2018). Public perceptions of genetically engineered nutraceuticals. *AgBioForum* 21 (1): 13–24.

Cahoon, E.B., Hall, S.E., Ripp, K.G. et al. (2003). Metabolic redesign of vitamin E biosynthesis in plants for tocotrienol production and increased antioxidant content. *Nature Biotechnology* 21 (9): 1082–1087.

Caluwaerts, S., Vandenbroucke, K., Steidler, L. et al. (2010). AG013, a mouth rinse formulation of *Lactococcus lactis* secreting human Trefoil Factor 1, provides a safe and efficacious therapeutic tool for treating oral mucositis. *Oral Oncology* 46 (7): 564–570.

Champagne, C.P., Gardner, N.J., and Roy, D. (2005). Challenges in the addition of probiotic cultures to foods. *Critical Reviews in Food Science and Nutrition* 45: 61–84.

Cho, E.A., Lee, C.A., Kim, Y.A. et al. (2005). Expression of c-tocopherol methyltransferase transgene improves tocopherol composition in lettuce (*Latuca sativa* L.). *Molecular Cells* 19: 16–22.

Chua, K.J., Kwok, W.C., Aggarwal, N. et al. (2017). Designer probiotics for the prevention and treatment of human diseases. *Current Opinion in Chemical Biology* 40: 8–16.

Cong, L., Wang, C., Chen, L. et al. (2009). Expression of phytoene synthase 1 and carotene desaturase crtI genes result in an increase in the total carotenoids content in transgenic elite wheat (*Triticum aestivum* L.). *Journal of Agricultural and Food Chemistry* 57 (18): 8652–8660.

Conklin, K.A. (2005). Coenzyme q10 for prevention of anthracycline-induced cardiotoxicity. *Integrative Cancer Therapies* 4: 110–130.

Cui, K. and Shoemaker, S.P. (2018). Public perception of genetically-modified (GM) food: a Nationwide Chinese Consumer Study. *NPJ Science of Food* 2 (1): 1–8.

Dafny-Yelin, M. and Tzfira, T. (2007). Delivery of multiple transgenes to plant cells. *Plant Physiology* 145 (4): 1118–1128.

Das, L., Bhaumik, E., Raychaudhuri, U., and Chakraborty, R. (2012). Role of nutraceuticals in human health. *Journal of Food Science and Technology* 49 (2): 173–183.

Dash, S., Clarke, G., Berk, M., and Jacka, F.N. (2015). The gut microbiome and diet in psychiatry: focus on depression. *Current Opinion in Psychiatry* 28 (1): 1–6.

Davani-Davari, D., Negahdaripour, M., Karimzadeh, I. et al. (2019). Prebiotics: definition, types, sources, mechanisms, and clinical applications. *Foods* 8 (3): 92.

DeFelice, S.L. (1995). The nutraceutical revolution: its impact on food industry R&D. *Trends in Food Science & Technology* 6 (2): 59–61.

Di Criscio, T., Fratianni, A., Mignogna, R. et al. (2010). Production of functional probiotic, prebiotic, and symbiotic ice creams. *Journal of Dairy Science* 93: 4555–4564.

Diaz de la Garza, R., Gregory, J.F., and Hanson, A.D. (2007). Folate biofortification of tomato fruit. *Proceedings of the National Academy of Sciences of the United States of America* 104: 4218–4222.

Díaz, M.R. and Vivas-Mejia, P.E. (2013). Nanoparticles as drug delivery systems in cancer medicine: emphasis on RNAi-containing nanoliposomes. *Pharmaceuticals* 6: 1361–1380.

Diretto, G., Al-Babili, S., Tavazza, R. et al. (2007). Metabolic engineering of potato carotenoid content through tuber-specific overexpression of a bacterial mini-pathway. *PLoS ONE* 2: e350.

Domínguez, T., Hernández, M.L., Pennycooke, J.C. et al. (2010). Increasing ω-3 desaturase expression in tomato results in altered aroma profile and enhanced resistance to cold stress. *Plant Physiology* 153 (2): 655–665.

Duan, F.F., Liu, J.H., and March, J.C. (2015). Engineered commensal bacteria reprogram intestinal cells into glucose-responsive insulin-secreting cells for the treatment of diabetes. *Diabetes* 64 (5): 1794–1803.

Ekor, M. (2014). The growing use of herbal medicines: issues relating to adverse reactions and challenges in monitoring safety. *Frontiers in Pharmacology* 4: 177.

Enfissi, E.M.A., Fraser, P.D., Lois, L.M. et al. (2005). Metabolic engineering of the mevalonate and nonmevalonate isopentenyl diphosphate-forming pathways for the production of health-promoting isoprenoids in tomato. *Plant Biotechnology Journal* 3: 17–27.

Ernst, E. (2003). Complementary medicine: where is the evidence? *The Journal of Family Practice* 52: 630–634.

Escott-Stump, E. and Mahan, L.K. (2000). *Krause's Food, Nutrition and Diet Therapy*, 10e, 553–559. Philadelphia: WB Saunders Company.

Fatima, T., Handa, A.K., and Mattoo, A.K. (2013). Functional foods: genetics, metabolome, and engineering phytonutrient levels. In: *Natural Products* (ed. K.G. Ramawat and J.M. Mérillon), 1715–1749. Berlin Heidelberg: Springer-Verlag.

Forsythe, P., Kunze, W.A., and Bienenstock, J. (2012). On communication between gut microbes and the brain. *Current Opinion in Gastroenterology* 28 (6): 557–562.

Fredriksen, L., Kleiveland, C.R., Hult, L.T.O. et al. (2012). Surface display of N-terminally anchored invasin by *Lactobacillus plantarum* activates NF-κB in monocytes. *Applied and Environmental Microbiology* 78 (16): 5864–5871.

Fróna, D., Szenderák, J., and Harangi-Rákos, M. (2019). The challenge of feeding the world. *Sustainability* 11 (20): 5816.

George Kerry, R., Patra, J. K., Gouda, S., Park, Y., Shin, H.-S., & Das, G. (2018). Benefaction of probiotics for human health: a review. *Journal of Food and Drug Analysis* 26(3):927–939. doi: https://doi.org/10.1016/j.jfda.2018.01.002

Gibson, G.R. (2004). Fiber and effects on probiotics (the prebiotic concept). *Clinical Nutrition Supplements* 1 (2): 25–31.

Gulati, O.P., Ottaway, P.B., Jennings, S. et al. (2019). Botanical nutraceuticals (food supplements and fortified and functional foods) and novel foods in the EU, with a main focus on legislative controls on safety aspects. In: *Nutraceutical and Functional Food Regulations in the United States and Around the World* (ed. D. Bagchi), 277–321. Academic Press.

Hayashi, S., Satoh, Y., Ujihara, T. et al. (2016). Enhanced production of polyunsaturated fatty acids by enzyme engineering of tandem acyl carrier proteins. *Scientific Reports* 6: 35441.

Health Canada (1998). *Nutraceuticals/Functional Foods and Health Claims on Foods (Policy Paper)*. Health Canada: Therapeutic Products Programme and the Food Directorate from the Health Protection Branch http://www.hc-sc.gc.ca/hpb-dgps/therapeut/htmleng/ffn.html.

Hill, A., Chen, L., Mariage, A. et al. (2019). Discovery of new levansucrase enzymes with interesting properties and improved catalytic activity to produce levan and fructooligosaccharides. *Catalysis Science & Technology* 9 (11): 2931–2944.

Hiroshima, Y., Zhao, M., Zhang, Y. et al. (2015). Tumor-targeting Salmonella typhimurium A1-R arrests a chemo-resistant patient soft-tissue sarcoma in nude mice. *PloS one* 10 (8): e0134324.

Hotz, C., and McClafferty, B. (2007). From harvest to health: challenges for developing biofortified staple foods and determining their impact on micronutrient status. *Food and Nutrition Bulletin* 28(2 Suppl), S271–S279. doi: https://doi.org/10.1177/15648265070282S206

Jain, A.K. and Nessler, C.L. (2000). Metabolic engineering of an alternative pathway for ascorbic acid biosynthesis in plants. *Molecular Breeding* 6: 73–78.

Kramkowska, M., Grzelak, T., and Czyzewska, K. (2013). Benefits and risks associated with genetically modified food products. *Annals of Agricultural and Environmental Medicine* 20 (3): 413–419.

La Guardia, M., Giammanco, S., Di Majo, D. et al. (2005). Omega 3 fatty acids: biological activity and effects on human health. *Panminerva Medica* 47 (4): 245.

Li, K. T., Moulin, M., Mangel, N., Albersen, M., Verhoeven-Duif, N. M., Ma, Q., et al. (2015). Increased bioavailable vitamin B6 in field-grown transgenic cassava for dietary sufficiency. *Nature Biotechnology* 33, 1029–1032. doi:https://doi.org/10.1038/nbt.3318

Lopez, A.B., Eck, J.V., Conlin, B.J. et al. (2008). Effect of the cauliflower or transgene on carotenoid accumulation and chromoplast formation in transgenic potato tubers. *Journal of Experimental Botany* 59: 213–223.

Macfarlane, S., Macfaelane, G. T., & Cummings, J. H. (2006). Review article: prebiotics in the gastrointestinal tract. *Alimentary Pharmacology and Therapeutics* 24(5): 701–714. doi:https://doi.org/10.1111/j.1365-2036.2006.03042.x

Marelli, B., Perez, A.R., Banchio, C. et al. (2011). Oral immunization with live *Lactococcus lactis* expressing rotavirus VP8* subunit induces specific immune response in mice. *Journal of Virological Methods* 175 (1): 28–37.

Massa, S., Presenti, O., and Benvenuto, E. (2018). Engineering plants for the future: farming with value-added harvest. In: *Progress in Botany*, vol. 80 (ed. F.M. Cánovas, U. Lüttge and R. Mat), 65–108. Cham: Springer.

Mathipa, M.G. and Thantsha, M.S. (2017). Probiotic engineering: towards development of robust probiotic strains with enhanced functional properties and for targeted control of enteric pathogens. *Gut Pathogens* 9 (1): 28.

Mazhar, S.F., Afzal, M., Almatroudi, A. et al. (2020). The prospects for the therapeutic implications of genetically engineered probiotics. *Journal of Food Quality* 2020: Article ID 9676452, 11 pages.

Mazur, B.J. (2001). Developing transgenic grains with improved oils, proteins and carbohydrates. In: *Novartis Foundation Symposium*, vol. 1999 (ed. D.J. Chadwick and J.A. Goode), 233–239. Chichester; New York: Wiley.

Mishra, S. and Singh, R.B. (2013). Physiological and biochemical significance of genetically modified foods: an overview. *The Open Nutraceuticals Journal* 6 (1): 18–26.

Moomaw, W., Berzin, I., and Tzachor, A. (2017). Cutting out the middle fish: marine microalgae as the next sustainable omega-3 fatty acids and protein source. *Industrial Biotechnology* 13 (5): 234–243.

Naqvi, S., Zhu, C., Farre, G. et al. (2009). Transgenic multivitamin corn through biofortification of endosperm with three vitamins representing three distinct metabolic pathways. *Proceedings of the National Academy of Sciences of United States of America* 106: 7762–7767.

Naqvi, S., Farré, G., Zhu, C. et al. (2011). Simultaneous expression of *Arabidopsis* q-hydroxyphenylpyruvate dioxygenase and MPBQ methyltransferase in transgenic corn kernels triples the tocopherol content. *Transgenic Research* 20: 177–181.

Nicoletti, I., De Rossi, A., Giovinazzo, G., and Corradini, D. (2007). Identification and quantification of stilbenes in fruits of transgenic tomato plants (*Lycopersicon esculentum* Mill.) by reversed phase HPLC with photodiode array and mass spectrometry detection. *Journal of Agricultural and Food Chemistry* 55 (9): 3304–3311.

Nkondjock, A., Ghadirian, P., Johnson, K.C. et al. (2005). Dietary intake of lycopene is associated with reduced pancreatic cancer risk. *The Journal of Nutrition* 135: 592–597.

Nounou, M.I., Ko, Y., Helal, N.A., and Boltz, J.F. (2018). Adulteration and counterfeiting of online nutraceutical formulations in the United States: time for intervention? *Journal of Dietary Supplements* 15 (5): 789–804.

Nykiforuk, C.L., Shewmaker, C., Harry, I. et al. (2012). High level accumulation of gamma linolenic acid (C18: 3Δ6. 9, 12 cis) in transgenic safflower (*Carthamus tinctorius*) seeds. *Transgenic Research* 21 (2): 367–381.

Paine, J. A., Shipton, C. A., Chaggar, S., Howells, R. M., Kennedy, M. J., Vernon, G., et al. (2005). Improving the nutritional value of Golden Rice through increased pro-vitamin A content. *Nature Biotechnology* 23, 482–487.doi: https://doi.org/10.1038/nbt1082

Pant, N., Hultberg, A., Zhao, Y. et al. (2006). Lactobacilli expressing variable domain of llama heavy-chain antibody fragments (lactobodies) confer protection against rotavirus-induced diarrhea. *The Journal of Infectious Diseases* 194 (11): 1580–1588.

Patel, A., Matsakas, L., Hrůzová, K. et al. (2019). Biosynthesis of nutraceutical fatty acids by the oleaginous marine microalgae *Phaeodactylum tricornutum* utilizing hydrolysates from organosolv-pretreated birch and spruce biomass. *Marine Drugs* 17 (2): 119.

Prakash, D., Gupta, C., and Sharma, G. (2012). Importance of phytochemicals in nutraceuticals. *Journal of Chinese Medicine Research and Development* 1 (3): 70–78.

Sánchez, B., López, P., González-Rodríguez, I. et al. (2011). A flagellin-producing *Lactococcus* strain: interactions with mucin and enteropathogens. *FEMS Microbiology Letters* 318 (2): 101–107.

Saneja, A., Khare, V., Alam, N. et al. (2014). Advances in Pglycoprotein- based approaches for delivering anticancer drugs: pharmacokinetic perspective and clinical relevance. *Expert Opinion on Drug Delivery* 11: 121–138.

Santini, A., Cammarata, S.M., Capone, G. et al. (2018). Nutraceuticals: opening the debate for a regulatory framework. *British Journal of Clinical Pharmacology* 84 (4): 659–672.

Saravanan, K. and Aradhya, S.M. (2011). Potential nutraceutical food beverage with antioxidant properties from banana plant bio-waste (pseudostem and rhizome). *Food & Function* 2 (10): 603–610.

Sarrion-Perdigones, A., Falconi, E.E., Zandalinas, S.I. et al. (2011). GoldenBraid: an iterative cloning system for standardized assembly of reusable genetic modules. *PLoS One* 6 (7): e21622.

Schijlen, E., Ric de Vos, C.H., Jonker, H. et al. (2006). Pathway engineering for healthy phytochemicals leading to the production of novel flavonoids in tomato fruit. *Plant Biotechnology Journal* 4 (4): 433–444.

Sheehan, V.M., Sleator, R.D., Fitzgerald, G.F., and Hill, C. (2006). Heterologous expression of BetL, a betaine uptake system, enhances the stress tolerance of *Lactobacillus salivarius* UCC118. *Applied and Environmental Microbiology* 72 (3): 2170–2177.

Shih, C.H., Chen, Y., Wang, M. et al. (2008). Accumulation of isoflavone genistin in transgenic tomato plants overexpressing a soybean isoflavone synthase gene. *Journal of Agricultural and Food Chemistry* 56 (14): 5655–5661.

Singh, B., Mal, G., Gautam, S.K., and Mukesh, M. (2019). Nutraceuticals from bioengineered microorganisms. In: *Advances in Animal Biotechnology*, 59–69. Cham: Springer.

Srinivasan, K. (2011). Spices for taste and flavour: Nutraceuticals for human health. In: *Spices: The elixir of life.* (ed. Amit Krishna De), 29–48. New Delhi: Originals.

Srivastava, R.K. (2018). Need of nutraceuticals/functional food products for health benefits to world-wide people. *Journal of Biotechnology and Biomedical Science* 1 (4): 1.

Steidler, L. (2003). Genetically engineered probiotics. *Best Practice & Research Clinical Gastroenterology* 17 (5): 861–876.

Storozhenko, S., De Brouwer, V., Volckaert, M. et al. (2007). Folate fortification of rice by metabolic engineering. *Nature Biotechnology* 25: 1277–1279.

Swanson, D., Block, R., and Mousa, S.A. (2012). Omega-3 fatty acids EPA and DHA: health benefits throughout life. *Advances in Nutrition* 3 (1): 1–7.

Tacket, C.O. (2007). Plant-based vaccines against diarrheal diseases. *Transactions of the American Clinical and Climatological Association* 118: 79–87.

Tavya, V., Kim, Y., Kagan, I. et al. (2007). Increased a-tocopherol content in soybean seed overexpressing the *Perilla frutescens* c tocopherol methyltransferase gene. *Plant Cell Reports* 26: 61–70.

Taylor, C.P. and Lamont, J.T. (2005). Genetically engineered probiotics: a new twist on an old remedy. *Gastroenterology* 128 (5): 1509–1512.

Ursin, V.M. (2003). Modification of plant lipids for human health: development of functional land-based omega-3 fatty acids. *The Journal of Nutrition* 133 (12): 4271–4274.

Uzogara, S.G. (2000). The impact of genetic modification of human foods in the 21st century: a review. *Biotechnology Advances* 18 (3): 179–206.

Van Eenennaam, A.L. and Young, A.E. (2018). Public perception of animal biotechnology. In: *Animal Biotechnology*, vol. 2 (ed. H. Niemann and C. Wrenzycki), 275–303. Cham: Springer.

Vandenbroucke, K., De Haard, H., Beirnaert, E. et al. (2010). Orally administered *L. lactis* secreting an anti-TNF nanobody demonstrate efficacy in chronic colitis. *Mucosal Immunology* 3 (1): 49–56.

Varzakas, T., Zakynthinos, G., and Verpoort, F. (2016). Plant food residues as a source of nutraceuticals and functional foods. *Foods* 5 (4): 88.

Venkatramesh, M., Karunanandaa, B., Sun, B. et al. (2003). Expression of a *Streptomyces* 3-hydroxysteroid oxidase gene in oilseeds for converting phytosterols to phytostanols. *Phytochemistry* 62 (1): 39–46.

Volzing, K., Borrero, J., Sadowsky, M.J., and Kaznessis, Y.N. (2013). Antimicrobial peptides targeting gram-negative pathogens, produced and delivered by lactic acid bacteria. *ACS Synthetic Biology* 2 (11): 643–650.

Wang, K., Senthil-Kumar, M., Ryu, C.M. et al. (2012). Phytosterols play a key role in plant innate immunity against bacterial pathogens by regulating nutrient efflux into the apoplast. *Plant Physiology* 158: 1789–1802.

Wang, C., Zeng, J., Li, Y. et al. (2014). Enrichment of provitamin A content in wheat (*Triticum aestivum* L.) by introduction of the bacterial carotenoid biosynthetic genes CrtB and CrtI. *Journal of Experimental Botany* 65 (9): 2545–2556.

Ward, O.P. and Singh, A. (2005). Omega-3/6 fatty acids: alternative sources of production. *Process Biochemistry* 40 (12): 3627–3652.

Welsch, R., Arango, J., Bar, C. et al. (2010). Provitamin A accumulation in cassava (*Manihot esculenta*) roots driven by a single nucleotide polymorphism in a phytoene synthase gene. *Plant Cell* 22: 3348–3356.

Yan, L. and Kerr, P.S. (2002). Genetically engineered crops: their potential use for improvement of human nutrition. *Nutrition Reviews* 60 (5): 135–141.

Ye, X., Al-Babili, S., Kloti, A. et al. (2000). Engineering the provitamin A (beta-carotene) biosynthetic pathway into (carotenoid-free) rice endosperm. *Science* 287: 303–305.

Yu, L. and O'Sullivan, D.J. (2014). Production of galactooligosaccharides using a hyperthermophilic β-galactosidase in permeabilized whole cells of *Lactococcus lactis*. *Journal of Dairy Science* 97 (2): 694–703.

Yuan, S.F. and Alper, H.S. (2019). Metabolic engineering of microbial cell factories for production of nutraceuticals. *Microbial Cell Factories* 18 (1): 46.

Yusibov, V., Hooper, D.C., Spitsin, S.V. et al. (2002). Expression in plants and immunogenicity of plant virus-based experimental rabies vaccine. *Vaccine* 20 (25–26): 3155–3164.

Zauber, H., Burgos, A., Garapati, P., and Schulze, W.X. (2014). Plasma membrane lipid–protein interactions affect signaling processes in sterol-biosynthesis mutants in Arabidopsis thaliana. *Frontiers in Plant Science* 5: 78.

Zhang, C., Wohlhueter, R., and Zhang, H. (2016). Genetically modified foods: a critical review of their promise and problems. *Food Science and Human Wellness* 5 (3): 116–123.

Zhao, J. (2007). Nutraceuticals, nutritional therapy, phytonutrients, and phytotherapy for improvement of human health: a perspective on plant biotechnology application. *Recent Patents on Biotechnology* 1 (1): 75–97.

10

Quality Assurance of Nutraceuticals and Their Approval, Registration, Marketing

L. Inbathamizh, D. Prabavathy, and S. Sudha

Department of Biotechnology, School of Bio and Chemical Engineering, Sathyabama Institute of Science and Technology, Chennai, Tamil Nadu, India

10.1 Background

The shifting scenario from treatment to prevention urges the need for novel approaches. This change has provided avenues and impetus for the emergence of nutraceuticals in healthcare. Intelligent food in these medicinal forms offers healthier choices earlier in life to combat the impact of life-style diseases and metabolic syndromes. Increasing risk of diseases and high costs associated with healthcare treatments have accelerated the growth of these products. The words of Thomas Alva Edison, said several years ago, seem to suit the situation presently and ahead. In line with his words, doctors no longer give medicines, instead instill patients' interest in understanding the cause and prevention of disease with more care toward diet and nutrition.

Today's food is mostly a product of milling and processing with compromised nutritive value (Tovey and Hobsley 2004). These losses are compensated by additional supplements to balance today's lifestyle (Burdock et al. 2006; Choi et al. 2006; Olmedilla-Alonso et al. 2006; Sieber 2007). Nutraceuticals have set a trend in maintaining the quality of life as health promoters and defenders protecting against nearing diseases. Moreover, they are associated with minimum side effects when compared with pharmaceuticals. Further, since nutrients act as pharmaceuticals in these products, additional therapy involving nutrition or intake of nutrients is not required anymore with the arrival of nutraceuticals (Ramaa et al. 2006; Bagchi 2006; Berger and Shenkin 2006).

With the establishment of connectivity between diet, health, and well-being, food and related products have turned out to be the chief vehicles toward the path of optimal health and wellness, and no longer meant only to satisfy hunger or prevent diseases (Hasler 2000). Natural products especially those derived from plants are gaining more importance as potent resources of human foods and medicines (Bland 1996). Availability, affordability, and safety have accounted for the healing potential of plant-based natural products and food-based medicines. Nutraceuticals are preferred for their good safety profile and high bioavailability, which have been reported (Augustin and Sanguansri 2015).

With its nomenclature assigned by Stephen DeFelice, a nutraceutical can refer to any food substance that has health benefits (DeFelice 1995). It is a new paradigm in food science stretching beyond the diet but before the drugs, acting as a bridge between nutrition and medicine (Biesalski 2001; El Sohaimy 2012; Santini and Novellino 2014). It is receiving international recognition and is consumed in required levels regularly as a part of a varied diet (Mandel et al. 2005). Changes in lifestyle and advent of related health complications have included functional ingredients such as probiotics, amino acids, fatty acids, vitamins, minerals, and so on, under this category. Thus, nutraceuticals can be broadly classified as Dietary Supplements and Food and Beverages. Vitamins and Minerals, Herbals, Protein Supplements, and Probiotics constitute Dietary Supplements. Fortified Probiotics and Energy Drinks are incorporated under Food and Beverages (National Institutes of Health 2020). A functional food can turn out to be a nutraceutical based on circumstances, ingredients, and claims on label (Borchers et al. 2016). A clear distinction exists in the perspectives on these products between the Western and Eastern countries. While they are viewed commercially by the Westerners, they are influenced by cultural values in the East (Kojima 1996; Bucobo 1998).

Though nutraceuticals are mostly referred to as pharma foods, a wider overlap exists between functional foods and nutraceuticals (Volpe and Sotis 2015; Finley 2016). They lack a unique identity to be distinguished from other food-derived categories such as food supplements, pre and probiotics, fortified foods, and herbal products. Though they are rapidly developing worldwide, their definition is still unclear and lies in the gray area between food and pharmaceuticals (Da Costa 2017). The definition and regulations of these products differ from country to country. They sound contradictory at times remaining far from being accepted and shared globally (Aronson 2017).

While food products can have beneficial effects without any proven pharmacological effect, the benefits and risks of pharmaceuticals are continuously assessed throughout their life span (Rautiainen et al. 2016). With the increasing use of nutraceuticals around the world, it has become indispensable to concentrate on the quality and safety of these products. There is a lack of proper balance between the increasing number of claims and the number of new products. This has generated discussions on the impact of nutraceuticals on public health. Further, it has enhanced interest and encouraged the enforcement of policies for their approval, registration, and marketing.

Many studies have revealed the potential mechanism of the therapeutic role of bioactive components in nutraceuticals. Yet, many of the health claims are not adequately substantiated by information on safety, quality, and efficacy of these products. This may result in false expectations and miss their significant benefits. On the other hand, the ingredients present may be of unknown provenance or may even be mislabeled, which can end up in serious health consequences (The United States Pharmacopeial Convention 2016). Therefore, there is a growing need for stronger systems to frame unambiguous definition and shared regulations for the remarkable outreach of quality assured and safe nutraceuticals. This chapter outlines these features bringing out the significance of quality standards with relevance to the nutraceutical industry.

10.2 Quality Assurance (QA)

10.2.1 QA: Basic Concepts

Quality is not a value to be added but an essential basic attribute to be achieved. It is the excellence that is better than a minimum standard. A standard level of quality and consistency in the product, as well as the process, should be maintained through a systematic approach that pays attention to every stage of the process involved. QA thus focuses on providing confidence regarding the fulfillment of quality requirements. The components of QA are categorized into three major levels.

Operational level deals with the day-to-day operations. Tactic level comprises training and facilities. A strategic level is associated with quality policies. Planning is the first step in all QA programs, and quality control constitutes the major part of QA. In general, QA includes all the necessary steps to ensure that the performance of trials, data generation, and documentation are in compliance with the relevant regulatory requirements. Efficient and effective quality systems can enhance the elimination of errors and rework and ensure prompt approval, registration, and marketing of products, adding benefits to the company both financially and socially (Tyler and Foster 1996). Quality assured products greatly assist in converting customer satisfaction to a profitable market.

To achieve the desired outcomes, some of the essential QA best practices can be adopted. These include determination of quality expectations, execution against expectations, and data-driven continuous improvement. Defining quality metrics based on customer requirements and critical control points, identification and assessment of risks, and establishment of mitigations are all in the quality expectation category. If results fall out of specifications, statistical process control, grading, testing, and reviews can be used as tactics. Further, collection of data and measurement of performance help in identifying cause-and-effect relationships and handling bottlenecks. In addition to day-by-day monitoring, data on aggregate performance over the long-term is also gathered to uncover inefficiencies and recurring issues. These can be further used for setting short- and long-term goals (Safetychain 2020).

10.2.2 QA: Need and Challenges

10.2.2.1 Emphasis on QA

Throughout the world, regulatory authorities are concentrating on the quality of nutraceuticals as they are consumed by human beings. With the flow of these products across the world, maintenance of quality standards as per the government policies plays a vital role and acts as the pivot for the growth of the industry. Quality and safety need to be established in preclinical and clinical settings (Knight 2004; Gardiner 2005; Morrow et al. 2005; Yen 2005; Ziker 2005). The essential "E"s for QA of nutraceuticals are depicted in figure (See Figure 10.1).

10.2.2.2 Ingredients: Quality markers

Quality starts with the ingredients that account for the safety and acceptability of the products into the market. The quality attributes of ingredients as highlighted in figure (See Figure 10.2) play a vital role in deciding the fate of the product. To assist evaluations, ingredients are listed either positive or negative based on their acceptability for use in food supplements or nutraceuticals. In the United States, the acceptable list comes under the Generally Recognized As Safe (GRAS) category (U.S. Food and Drug Administration 2019a). In the countries of the Association of Southeast Asian Nations (ASEAN), some of the substances used in traditional medicine and health supplements have been included in the restricted list (ASEAN 2010).

10.2.2.3 Risks: Regulatory Confusion, Misbranding, Adulteration, and Contamination

Nutraceuticals may be treated as hybrids and thus may be regulated as foods or drugs. The situation may vary according to place. Coenzyme Q10 (CoQ10) is included in the Japanese Pharmacopoeia and regulated as a drug, whereas it is taken as a dietary supplement in the United States (US). Similarly, *Echinacea* is treated as a food supplement in the United States, while it is a drug as per European Pharmacopoeia (The United States Pharmacopeial Convention 2016).

Country-wise variation in ingredients if not identified and substantiated by scientific data may lead to adverse effects. While the Chinese star anise is valued as a food ingredient with health

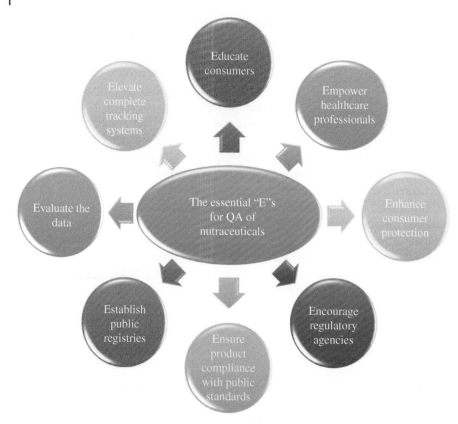

Figure 10.1   The essential "E"s for QA of Nutraceuticals.

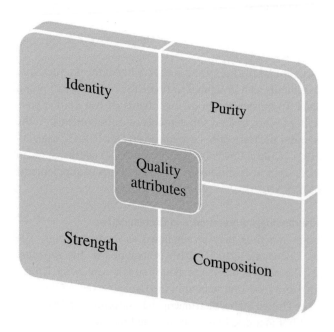

Figure 10.2   Quality attributes of nutraceutical ingredients.

benefits, Japanese star anise is toxic and can even kill the consumer (American Herbal Products Association 2014). Lack of an adequate regulatory framework seems to pose the biggest challenge for the accurate analysis of the safety aspects (Starr 2015).

Sometimes, instead of supporting health, the products have even created unexpected risks (U.S. Food and Drug Administration 2018a). Reports exist for unfavorable events due to the intake of such products for weight loss or energy, with the specific ingredients left unidentified (Geller et al. 2015). Even some of the commonly used dietary supplements such as ginseng, dehydroepian-drosterone, and feverfew were found to contain inappropriate quantities of the labeled ingredients, contaminated with the unlabeled chemicals and adulterated with the other prescription products (Heptinstall et al. 1992; Cui et al. 1994; Parasrampuria et al. 1998). One of the disastrous incidents with several deaths and over 900 reports of health issues was due to the inconsistent alkaloid composition in ephedra products. A final rule in 2004 declared these dietary supplements with ephedrine alkaloids as adulterated. Ultimately, there was a recall of all ephedra-containing dietary supplements (Gurley et al. 2000; Food and Drug Administration and HHS 2004).

DNA testing of 44 herbal products revealed that 59% of them lacked the ingredients listed on the label (Newmaster et al. 2013). Another evaluation indicated the presence of undeclared allergens (The New York Times 2015). Vitamin D products used in a research study when tested showed 52–153% of the expected dose (LeBlanc et al. 2013). Misbranding of homeopathic teething tablets with high levels of belladonna alkaloids such as atropine and scopolamine was the cause behind adverse cases of seizures and deaths. The number of alkaloids varied several folds from one lot to another and also between the tablets within the same batch (U.S. Food and Drug Administration 2016a, 2017, 2019b).

Contamination poses another major health risk. Contaminants can be of inorganic or organic origin (Filipiak-Szok et al. 2015; Gil et al. 2016). Recall of supplements with 56 times hazardous levels of lead to an exposed child has been reported in 2016 (U.S. Food and Drug Administration 2016b). Over 37 kratom herbal products were found to be contaminated with *Salmonella* in 2018 (U.S. Food and Drug Administration 2018b). Most of the tested products also contained pesticide residues beyond permitted levels (US Government Accountability Office 2010). Investigations have revealed that multiple contracted manufacturers involved in the supply of nutritional and dietary supplements, in industries such as Mericon and Major-Rugby, could not maintain quality standards (U.S. Food and Drug Administration 2020a).

10.2.3 QA Systems

10.2.3.1 Good Manufacturing Practices (GMPs)

Compendia or Policies on Quality standards guide manufacturers to follow GMPs and provide assurance of the good quality of their products. Testing and voluntary verification programs based on public standards further can help in checking the ingredients and ensuring the standard of quality of the products (The United States Pharmacopeia 2020a). Effective application of a quality management system (QMS) is essential to impart GMPs (Institute of Food Science and Technology 2012).

Manufacturers can follow the GMP guidelines that correspond to the legislation of their respective countries. A set of guidelines called "Current Good Manufacturing Practices" (cGMPs) have been enforced by the US Food and Drug Administration (FDA) under the Title 21 Code of Federal Regulations (CFR) part 111, with the amendment of the Dietary Supplement Health and Education Act (DSHEA) (U.S. Food and Drug Administration 2010, 2019c). This has triggered the progress of the natural products industry (Vitamin Retailer 2013).

GMPs enable the chances of minimizing all possible errors by controlling each step of the manufacturing process, which otherwise may turn out to be extremely difficult for checking the quality of a finished product. The routine activity followed by an organization can be in the form of a set of written instructions named as a "Standard Operating Procedure" (SOP). It is to ensure that approved procedures are followed under a QA project plan in compliance with the regulations of the company and government.

GMP measures are designed toward an effective overall approach for ensuring safety, integrity, strength, purity, and composition of the product and maintaining standards in their testing, manufacturing, storage, handling, and distribution. Thus, they help in avoiding shortfalls and rejection rates within the manufacturing processes. Consistency is followed throughout through the key elements that include place, people, process, and product. The basic elements of GMP are listed in figure (see Figure 10.3). Premises include the building and other facilities such as

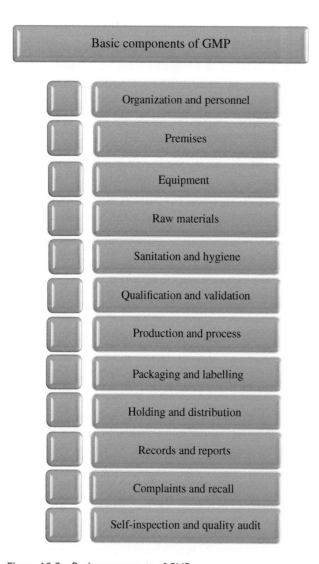

Figure 10.3 Basic components of GMP.

water, heating, ventilation, and air-conditioning systems, utilities, and pest control. Equipment ID, logbooks, preventative maintenance, qualification, calibration, and cleaning are all the programs under Equipment. Qualification, job responsibilities, training, health and hygiene, and organization chart with reporting structure, constitute the Personnel component. Besides, specifications, sampling, and stability studies are also a part of GMP (Bagchi 2006). These practices ultimately help in providing greater confidence to the manufacturers and greater security to the consumers.

10.2.3.2 International Organization for Standardization (ISO)

ISO 9000 family is a set of standards related to the fundamentals of QMS (Tsim et al. 2002). The underlying seven basic principles are customer focus, leadership, engagement of people, process approach, improvement, evidence-based decision-making, and relationship management (Beattie 1999; Tsim et al. 2002). ISO 9001 emphasizes the requirements essential to be fulfilled by a company to meet the standards (Mihail 2016; ASQ 2020). It is the most widely used quality management tool for certification. Nutraceuticals need to comply with ISO standards. ISO 9001 is a generic standard that can be applied to any organization. Systemization of work helps in improving the efficiency and effectiveness of the organization such that nothing important is left out and clarity on responsibility is sorted out. The standard is applied to the processes and not products, thus the focus is only on work and not on the result. It is indeed a substantial part of all that is required to ensure the satisfaction of customers' quality requirements. ISO certification paves way for more confidence and opportunities for international trade.

10.2.3.3 Hazard Analysis and Critical Control Points (HACCP)

HACCP offers a systemic approach to identify, evaluate, and control physical, chemical, biological, and radiological hazards that hinder food safety. Initiated in 1960, to ensure food safety for the first manned National Aeronautics and Space Administration (NASA) mission, now it has developed into a universally accepted process for food safety assurance. HACCP is also widely applied to other industries such as pharmaceuticals and further applicable for nutraceuticals. In the United States, 21 CFR part 120 and 123 regulate HACCP compliance. Food and Agriculture Organization (FAO) and the World Health Organization (WHO) have established the guidelines in the case of minor food businesses (World Health Organization and Food and Agriculture Organization of the United Nations 2006). HACCP is governed by seven principles that include the conduct of hazard analysis, determination of the critical control points, the establishment of critical limits, monitoring system, corrective action, verification procedures, and documentation. These principles are incorporated in ISO 22000 Food Safety and Management System (FSMS) 2011 that include the elements of prerequisite programs such as GMPs (ISO 2018). All these enable HACCP in contributing a major part to the overall QA in the international trade system of food and related products (World Trade Organization 1999; Lammerding and Fazil 2000; World Trade Organization 2012).

10.2.4 Reviewers of Quality: Roles and Measures

10.2.4.1 United States Pharmacopeia – National Formulary (USP – NF)

USP – NF is an official compendium of the United States. It offers a range of tools to help manufacturers and suppliers in determining the identity and quality of nutritional and natural ingredients (The United States Pharmacopeia 2019).

10.2.4.1.1 USP Standards Documentary standards and Reference standards are offered by the USP to assist the industries. The former explains specifications and tests required in the form of written monographs. The latter is applicable when highly characterized substances are used to conduct the relevant quality control tests and analytical procedures (The United States Pharmacopeia 2020b). These standards have significant control over the mixing of contaminants and adulterants. There are more than 3600 items with 800 plus monographs and about 200 reference standards in the USP catalog.

10.2.4.1.2 Third-Party Verification Services (The United States Pharmacopeia 2020a) More than 400 million dietary supplements that meet the Verification Program's criteria have been awarded the USP Verified Mark. GMP Facility Audit Program is offered to help the manufacturers to prepare for quality inspections.

10.2.4.1.3 USP Meetings and Courses USP offers different educational programs including workshops on adulteration, for practitioners, industrialists, and others in the relevant fields, through online and classroom modes (The United States Pharmacopeia 2020c).

10.2.4.1.4 Stakeholders and User Forums USP hosts forums for the exchange of ideas, learning, sharing, applying USP resources, and providing direct feedback (The United States Pharmacopeia 2020d).

10.2.4.1.5 Food Fraud Database A library of methods to detect the risk of food fraud is provided as a database (Decernis 2020).

10.2.4.1.6 E-Newsletters Periodic news and industry hot topics are shared via email (The United States Pharmacopeia 2020e).

10.2.4.2 National Sanitation Foundation (NSF)

NSF is an independent organization concerned with public health and safety. It offers standards for the registration of areas such as food, water, health, consumer products, and management systems. The NSF certification indicates the compliance of the product with quality and safety standards. It is the most frequent of all third-party verifications with the conduct of audits every 6 months to check 21 CFR 111 GMP compliance (NSF 2020).

10.2.4.3 Natural Products Association (NPA)

NPA was founded in 1936 to empower the natural products industry. It conducts audits every two years. It is the third tier indicator for quality. Certification is given as an "A" rating. More than 60 companies have received certification (Natural Products Association 2020a). But, NPA cannot evaluate the quality of individual products and hence is not meant for product labeling (Natural Products Association 2020b).

10.2.4.4 FDA

FDA's guidance is considered only as a suggestion or recommendation and not as a require-ment and thus does not establish legally enforceable responsibility (U.S. Food and Drug Administration 2012). FDA is in fact the lowest tier indicator for the quality of dietary supplements and nutrient products due to accumulating issues with the auditing systems. The audits done so far have indicated 48–70% GMP deficiency (Newsday 2013; Marcus 2016; Nutraceuticals World 2018).

10.2.4.5 Certificate of Analysis (CoA)

CoA provides valuable information about the ingredients present in a specific batch of a dietary supplement product.

10.2.4.6 Dietary Supplement Policy (DSP)

DSP can be developed in every institution supported by the American Society of Health-System Pharmacists (ASHP). According to DSP, the product should undergo the same rigorous evaluation process as pharmaceuticals (Kroll et al. 2004).

10.3 Regulations

10.3.1 Need for Globalization

The underlying regulatory policies for any consumer product should always target toward maintaining an appropriate balance between benefits, risks, and consumer access. Usually, food-like products are regulated through registration-based systems, while drug-like products need to face a premarket approval system. A major breakthrough in the assessment of the safety of foodstuffs and their derivatives was the formulation of Rome-based, Codex Alimentarius (food code) Commission by the United Nations (UN) Food and Agricultural Organization (FAO) and the World Health Organization (WHO) in 1962. Codex became the global reference point for the manufacturers, consumers, regulatory agencies, as well as the international food trade. It was a collection of internationally recognized guidelines with more than 200 standards, which characterized health claims with respect to nutrient potential, increased efficacy, and decreased toxicity (Food and Agriculture Organization 2013). International Alliance of Dietary Food Supplement Associations (IADSA) was created in 1998 for global communication of information and ideas (International Alliance of Dietary Food Supplement Associations (IADSA) 2020).

Only better characterized and research-proven nutraceuticals can evolve successfully and gain consumer confidence. Despite the existence of commissions and associations, regulations of these products in terms of registration, approval, and marketing were unclear in the whole of the twentieth century. Still, there is a lack of common shared legislation as each country follows a unique set of regulations due to different cultural settings and heterogeneous dietary habits. This seems to pose a serious challenge for nutraceutical globalization.

The term "nutraceuticals" as such does not have any regulatory definition. In general, the word is applied to a range of products including specific diets and processed foods (NutraIngredients-USA 2012). Traditional and nontraditional foods are also available in the market in the name of nutraceuticals (National Institutes of Health 2020; The United States Pharmacopeia 2020a). But in certain countries like India, traditional foods are not included in nutraceuticals (Jain et al. 2018). The majority of countries treat nutraceuticals as a category of food. An explicit set of regulations are framed for the registration and approval of these products. Such regulations are needed to screen out the pitfalls and bring new products to the market with quality and safety.

10.3.2 Approval and Registration: Global Scenario

Regulatory authorities can be approached either by registration-based or by notification-based systems. The registration-based approach involves a slow, lengthy, and intense review process and requires detailed information in the form of the registration dossier. The notification-based approach is characterized by a fast and minimal review process with concise information on the manufacturer, product, and label, and is meant for the introduction of the product to the market.

10.3.2.1 Regulations in the United States

The USFDA defines nutraceuticals as dietary supplements and is responsible for the regulations of these products. A different set of regulations that vary from that of conventional foods and drug products are adopted (U.S. Food and Drug Administration 2020b). Most of the nutraceuticals in the United States are the products of biotechnology (Bagchi 2006).

FDA's requirements for the manufacture, package, label, or hold of dietary supplements are released as GMP regulations (Wallace et al. 2013). These are applicable to all local as well as foreign companies. The US claims and labeling regulations seem to be more restrictive compared to countries like India (Kumar et al. 2016).

Food and Drug Cosmetic Act amended DSHEA in 1994. According to DSHEA and GMP regulations from 2007, it is the responsibility of the manufacturer to ensure the safety and quality of the nutraceutical before it is marketed. The manufacturer cannot claim the product's application in diagnosis, prevention, reduction, or treatment of a disease. But the guarantee for the identity, purity, strength, and composition of the ingredients should be given.

Health claims and nutrient claims on food labeling are enabled by the FDA Modernization Act (FDAMA) of 1997. This is based on an authoritative report from the Academy of Sciences and notification to FDA at least four months before entering the market (National Institutes of Health 1994). Manufacturers should ensure that the product label carries only true information and not misguiding (Hasler 2008). They neither have to register with FDA nor get approval from FDA for producing or selling these products. But after they reach the market, FDA can take action against any product if found unsafe, adulterated, or misbranded. FDA monitors postmarketing safety by analyzing product information that includes labeling, claims, package inserts, and relevant literature along with adverse event reports if any.

Three types of claims such as Health claims, Nutrient control claims, and Structure/Function claims can be used. Health claims authorized under the Nutrition Labelling and Education Act of 1990 (NLEA) explain the relationship between the ingredients and decreasing risk of disease (Federal Register 1997). They are further grouped into Significant Scientific Agreement (SSA) claims, FDMA claims, and Qualified Health claims. To describe the percentage of nutrients with respect to the daily value, nutrient control claims are used. Structure/function claims are associated with an effective contribution to the improvement of the structure or the physiological role of the body in preserving health.

21 CFR 190 deals with the registration of dietary supplements in the United States. The ingredients of dietary supplements are categorized into active and inactive ingredients. The active ingredients should meet the definition as given by DSHEA, 1994. For legal registration, they are also classified as Old Dietary Ingredients (ODI) or "Grandfathered," and New Dietary Ingredients (NDI). The products in the market before 15 October 1994 are ODI, and that after that date, or ODI with changes made, are considered as NDI.

Registration of the facility is done in form 3537. Centre for Food Supply and Applied Nutrition (CFSAN) is responsible to conduct premarket clearance for NDI products. NDI notification should be submitted 75 days before marketing (Kumar et al. 2016). The following documents have to be submitted for the premarket clearance:

1) Name and address of the applicant
2) Name of the product
3) Product description stating NDI level and labeling conditions
4) Evidence for safety
5) Signature of the manufacturer or distributor (U.S. Food and Drug Administration 2019d,e; Kessler et al. 2001)

10.3.2.2 Regulations in India

In India, there is no specific legal status to nutraceuticals. A legislation system in the name of the Food Safety and Standards Authority of India (FSSAI) has been established by the government of India under the Food and Safety and Standards Act (FSSA), 2006. The regulations are with effect from 2011. Nutraceuticals that do not claim to cure any disease can only be permitted by these regulations. FSSA does not separate functional foods, dietary supplements, and nutraceuticals. All these are defined in general as "Foods for special dietary uses" (Food Safety and Standards Authority of India 2016). Thereupon, various Central Acts on fruits, meat, oils, flour, milk, and their products have been repealed. The regulatory requirements in India are illustrated in figure (see Figure 10.4).

FSSAI is the regulatory authority that grants approval for the registration of nutraceuticals in India (Sharma et al. 2013). Further, it is instrumental in promoting awareness of food safety standards in India (Food Safety and Standards Authority of India 2020). Documents such as Application forms A, B and C, Self-attested declaration forms, Layout plan of the unit, Details of equipment, Food category details, Analysis report, Premises details, Food safety system, Materials, Partnership, Water report, Recall plan, and Non-objection certificates (NOCs) should all be enclosed for registration, approval, and licensing (Food Safety and Standards Authority of India 2012; Pasumarthy et al. 2014). The steps involved in the registration of manufacturing sites and manufacturing licensing in India are depicted in figures (See Figures 10.5 and 10.6).

Though the procedure for registration is provided by FSSAI, clarity of specific regulations for registration is lacking. Thus, launching nutraceuticals in India is still facing the challenges (Sharma et al. 2013; Mondaq 2013; Food Safety and Standards Authority of India 2013). Moreover, nutraceuticals manufactured in tablet or gelatin capsule form are brought under the category of drugs. Some of the colorants and additives added in the manufacture of certain nutraceutical products are absent in the permitted list (Mondaq 2013). These further add hurdles to the nutraceutical industry in the country.

10.3.2.3 Regulations in Other Countries

In the European Union, concentrated sources of nutrients and other substances with nutritional or physiological effect come under the category of food supplements. Food legislation is under the European Food and Safety Authority (EFSA). Directive 2002/46/EC is the major legislation for food supplements. Registration of products is not required but the marketing of those with vitamins and minerals not listed is prohibited (European Commission 2020). The term nutraceutical is not mentioned in the current European legislation. Nutraceuticals are brought under Foods for Particular Nutritional Uses (PARNUTS), within the regulatory framework of Directive 89/398/ EEC 1989. Foods for specific nutritional requirements and those for special medical reasons are

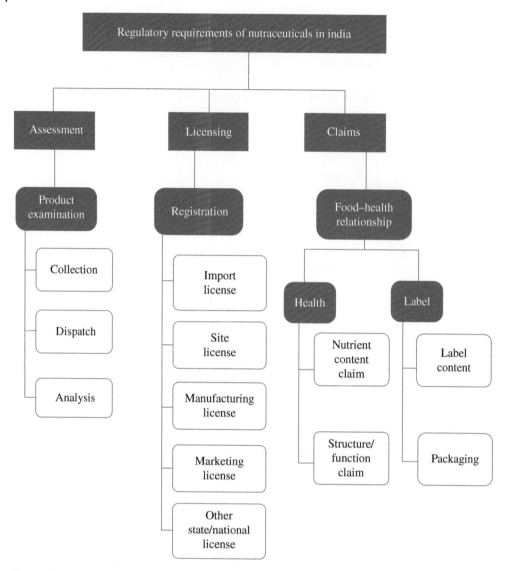

Figure 10.4 Regulatory requirements of nutraceuticals in India.

included in this category, only after the proper evaluation of their safety and efficacy through in vitro and in vivo studies (Santini et al. 2018).

Japan's regulations use two categories namely Foods for Specified Health Use (FOSHU) and Food and Nutrient Functional Claims (FNFC) (Shimizu 2003; Saito 2007). The legislation set in 1991 evolved into Health Promotion Law in 2003 (Yamada et al. 2008). FNFC claims are standardized and do not require government approval. But FOSHU claims must provide evidence to the government and are permitted only when approved by the government.

In China, "Health food" comprises food, dietary supplements, or traditional Chinese medicine (TCM). These products need to be registered with and approved by the China Food and Drug Administration (CFDA) based on the former State Food and Drug Administration (SFDA) (Yang 2008; SFDA 2020).

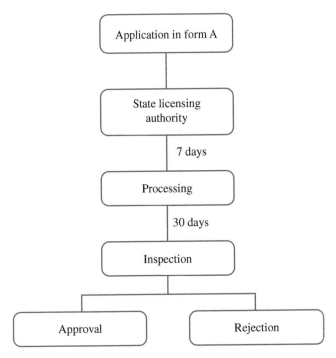

Figure 10.5   Registration of manufacturing sites in India.

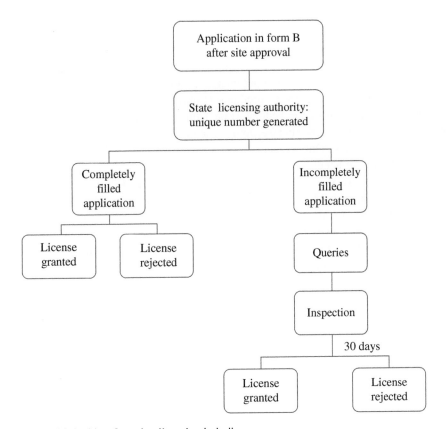

Figure 10.6   Manufacturing licensing in India.

In Australia and Canada, nutraceuticals are regulated more as drugs (L'Abbé et al. 2008). They are categorized as "Complementary medicines" in Australia (Therapeutic Goods Administration 2013) and as "Natural Health Products" in Canada (Justice Laws Website 2020). Manufacturing license and registration are required.

Russian Federal Law No 29-FZ on Quality and Safety of Food Products considers food products as a category of food supplements and uses the nomenclature "Biologically Active Food Supplements" (BAFS). The regulations are similar to that in the United States and Europe, but stricter regarding the composition of BAFS. The state registration of BAFS is run by the Rospotrebnadzor as per the requirements of Russia's sanitary legislation. Compliance of the product is assessed and the information of the registered products is stored in the State Register (Sukhanov et al. 2011).

Countries such as Argentina, Brazil, and Colombia follow a simple registration-based approach while Mexico and Chile adopt a notification-based approach addressed to the local competent authority (Mansour 2008). The situation seems to be stricter in some countries such as Brazil, China, and Taiwan where a complete animal or human clinical study is required prior to registration (Hasler 2000).

10.4 Marketing

10.4.1 Current Status

Marketing plays a key role in the success of the nutraceutical industry and lays a significant impact on consumers. Initially, the industry grew at 7% per annum but in the next few years, the growth doubled to about 14% per annum. It is estimated that around 12–15 billion dollars are being added every year. Currently, the United States has the largest nutraceutical market comprising 65% of functional food and beverages and 35% of dietary supplements (Verma and Popli 2018). Every year, about 150 million Americans are using these products (Council for Responsible Nutrition (CRN) 2019). Advertising is regulated by the Federal Trade Commission (National Institutes of Health 2013). DSHEA provides more marketing freedom to the manufacturers and more information to the customers (Bagchi 2006). Online retail stores such as Amazon and eBay flood the American market and sell the nutraceuticals with therapeutic claims (Nounou et al. 2018). The average use of these products across all age groups is found to be around 52% (Kantor et al. 2016).

Next to the United States, Japan holds second place in the nutraceutical market. China also seems to rise as the middle class of China has started focusing more on lifestyle and well-being. Countries such as the European Union with stringent regulations and approval process, lack product innovations, and are far beyond in this sector. India constitutes 1.5% of the global market. Pharmaceutical companies and the Fast Moving Consumer Goods (FMCG) suppliers are the prime players in the market. Sixty percent of the market is constituted by functional food and beverages, and 40% by dietary supplements, which include vitamin and mineral supplements, herbal supplements, protein supplements, and chyawanprash (Ganesh et al. 2015). With the availability of good quality natural products, enriched biodiversity, and traditional knowledge, India holds a firm place in the nutraceutical market.

10.4.2 Sustaining Amidst Food and Pharma Competitors

A profound competition exists between food and pharma companies for the dominance of the sector in the global market. Food companies have more expertise in reaching the mass of consumers through large-scale manufacturing and global logistics. Whereas pharma companies are stronger in their research expertise. The food industry has a deeper understanding of nutrition formulations, consumer analysis, and mass marketing than the pharma industry. Food companies with separate health sections, successful brands, and health-enhancing plans are sustaining in the market. But they struggle to cope up with the major breakthroughs due to lack of elaborate scientific resources. Though the pharma industry overcomes this difficulty with stronger research departments and wider links to the scientific community, it targets and concentrates on medical professionals and pharmacists, than on consumers.

On the other hand, nutraceutical companies try to overcome the challenges of pharma as well as food industries. Nutraceutical industry offers a new revenue source with lower Research and Development costs, health budgets, and regulatory requirements, unlike pharma companies. The industry also seems to be fast-growing with wider options for new brands, innovative products, and accepted channels for marketing, which are less likely in food companies. Nutraceuticals seem to be the prime beneficiaries of innovations such as genetic modifications, marker-assisted sections, and biofortifications (KPMG 2015).

With the increasing challenges, food and pharma companies have started taking advantage of the growing nutraceutical industry. The popular British multinational pharmaceutical company, GlaxoSmithKline, sold its nutraceutical drinks Lucozade and Ribena to Japan's Suntory in 2013 (GlaxoSmithKline (GSK) 2013). Nestle cleared out its PowerBar to cereal maker Post Holdings in the United States (Nestle 2014). Similarly, Unilever sold its SlimFast to Kainos Capital (Unilever 2014).

The convergence of industries has also occurred to improve the properties and benefits of the products. For instance, Integrity Nutraceuticals and Cornerstone Research and Development merged in April 2014 in order to combine the capsule manufacturing capability of the former with the vitamin supplement production of the latter (HIG Growth Partners 2014). There are incidences where pharma companies have also joined hands with nutraceutical companies, such as the merging of Spanish Labaratorio Reig Jofre with Natraceutical in December, 2014 (Jofre 2014).

The nutraceutical market is open. It offers an able platform for converting pharmaceuticals to be more consumer-oriented and for adding a medical image to food products. For example, Yakult, which was initially consumed as a health drink, is now medically manufactured and prescribed by physicians. Similarly, Axona was previously marketed for its medical claims and clinical dietary management in Alzheimer's disease, but now considered more as a dietary supplement (KPMG 2015). Though innovations keep arising from, either way, the nutraceutical industry should be vigilant and competent to sustain and stand firm amidst the robust food and pharma industries that have already established.

10.4.3 Success Determinants

With increasing risk and awareness of the disease, the demand for nutraceuticals is growing. Large investments are made in this area for inviting innovative products to hit the market. Only those companies which strike the bullseye in the key areas as in figure yield the blockbuster products (See Figure 10.7).

Safety and quality should be maintained throughout, using a standardized protocol. Postmarket surveillance is equally important to premarket requirements. More than 75 approved drugs were identified with safety issues during postmarketing and removed from the US market between 1962 and 2002 (Wysowski and Swartz 2005). Risks are also found in the supply chain, for example the growth of molds or toxins in sun-dried products due to carelessness and improper maintenance.

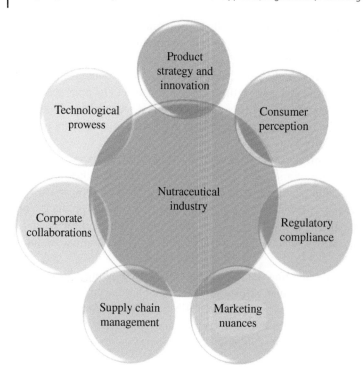

Figure 10.7 Success determinants of nutraceutical industry.

Vertical integration among companies help in achieving greater certainty of supply and developing novel products or newer applications of existing ingredients. For instance, Danone, a renowned European food company, acquired nutritional supplements manufacturer, Complan Foods in 2011 (Nutraingredients 2011), and also purchased a share of 40% in Kenya's Brookside Dairy with 140 000 milk farms in East Africa in 2014 (Bloomberg 2014).

Securing intellectual property, availability of patents, and trademark; understanding both downstream and upstream marketing, budget, advertising; and analyzing the customers' minds are all crucial in determining the success of the products. Money should be spent at the correct time. Marketing, product labeling, and regulations must harmonize with each other. The time before and during the product launch is critical for the marketing team to exhibit their best efforts (Datta 2017). A case study has revealed that user-centered design (UCD) promotes a multidisciplinary approach to the development of new and more market-oriented products (Bogue et al. 2017).

Several market trends have been identified to enhance the growth in this sector. The convergence of categories, channels, and technologies, increasing demand for sustainable and eco-friendly products, and the rise of new paradigms on health and wellness are some of the significant trends highlighted (Hilton 2017).

10.4.4 Gaps To Be Bridged

Global marketing of nutraceuticals still poses to be impractical. Confusions in distinguishing as food or drug, exaggerated health claims, and country-wise variations in regulations are all the common obstacles that block the globalization of nutraceuticals. Lack of adequate awareness, the prevalence of regulatory confusion, and poor vision of the market act as barriers preventing large companies to venture into nutraceuticals (Just Food 2008).

Government policies are not always deterrent. Sometimes, they also help in promoting the market by levying "fat taxes" on products that contain excessive quantities of fat or sugar and by funding vitamin fortification initiatives (KPMG 2015). Effective market growth ultimately is reflected by valid scientific research and international regulatory compliance.

10.5 Conclusion

The nutraceutical industry is growing at a rate outpacing the other related markets. Though several regulatory constraints on nutraceuticals are enforced around the world, there is an urge to bring together experts from a wide range of areas to derive appropriate regulations and check the efficacy of these products. The future looks promising and progressive as long as the companies take a proactive quality approach to ensure the integrity of products, protect public health, and elevate confidence. Solid clinical evidence and a more strict evaluation process need to be emphasized such that only products assured of quality and safety are approved and marketed. Increased accountability, educated consumers and effective regulations can all impact the status of the nutraceutical market significantly and further open the doors for more beneficial innovations to step in this industry.

References

American Herbal Products Association (2014). Star Anise. http://www.ahpa.org/Resources/TechnicalGuidance/ScientificAffairs/BotanicalAuthenticationProgram/Staranise.aspx (accessed 10 July 2020).

Aronson, J.K. (2017). Defining 'nutraceuticals': neither nutritious nor pharmaceutical. *British Journal of Clinical Pharmacology* 83 (1): 8–19.

ASEAN (2010). Guiding Principles for Inclusion of Active Substances into the Restricted List for Traditional Medicines and Health Supplements (TMHS). https://www.asean.org/storage/images/archive/SnC/Guiding_Principles_for_Restricted_List_of_Active_Substances.pdf (accessed 19 July 2020).

ASQ (2020). ISO 9000. https://asq.org/quality-resources/iso-9000 (accessed 16 July 2020).

Augustin, M.A. and Sanguansri, L. (2015). Challenges and solutions to incorporation of nutraceuticals in foods. *Annual Review of Food Science and Technology* 6: 463–477.

Bagchi, D. (2006). Nutraceuticals and functional foods regulations in the United States and around the world. *Toxicology (Amsterdam)* 221 (1): 439–444.

Beattie, K.R. (1999). Implementing ISO 9000: a study of its benefits among Australian organizations. *Total Quality Management* 10 (1): 95–106.

Berger, M.M. and Shenkin, A. (2006). Vitamins and trace elements: practical aspects of supplementation. *Nutrition* 22 (9): 952–955.

Biesalski, H.K. (2001). Nutraceuticals: the link between nutrition and medicine. *Oxidative Stress and Disease* 6: 1–26.

Bland, J.S. (1996). Phytonutrition, phytotherapy, and phytopharmacology. *Alternative Therapies in Health and Medicine* 2 (6): 73.

Bloomberg (2014). Danone Buys 40% of Kenya's Brookside to Expand African Footprint. https://www.bloomberg.com/news/articles/2014-07-18/danone-buys-40-of-kenya-s-brookside-to-expand-african-footprint (accessed 15 July 2020).

Bogue, J., Collins, O., and Troy, A.J. (2017). Market analysis and concept development of functional foods. In: *Developing New Functional Food and Nutraceutical Products*, 29–45. Academic Press.

Borchers, A.T., Keen, C.L., and Gershwin, M.E. (2016). The basis of structure/function claims of nutraceuticals. *Clinical Reviews in Allergy and Immunology* 51 (3): 370–382.

Bucobo, J.C. (1998). Integrative medicine. Your quick reference guide, by CM Coughlin and RM DeBusk. *Journal of Nutrition for the Elderly* 18: 67–67.

Burdock, G.A., Carabin, I.G., and Griffiths, J.C. (2006). The importance of GRAS to the functional food and nutraceutical industries. *Toxicology.* 221 (1): 17–27.

Choi, Y.M., Bae, S.H., Kang, D.H., and Suh, H.J. (2006). Hypolipidemic effect of lactobacillus ferment as a functional food supplement. *Phytotherapy Research: An International Journal Devoted to Pharmacological and Toxicological Evaluation of Natural Product Derivatives* 20 (12): 1056–1060.

Council for Responsible Nutrition (CRN) (2019). Dietary Supplements: Safe, Regulated and Beneficial. https://www.crnusa.org/resources/dietary-supplements-safe-beneficial-and-regulated (accessed 15 July 2020).

Cui, J., Garle, M., Eneroth, P., and Björkhem, I. (1994). What do commercial ginseng preparations contain? *The Lancet* 344 (8915): 134.

Da Costa, J.P. (2017). A current look at nutraceuticals – key concepts and future prospects. *Trends in Food Science and Technology* 62: 68–78.

Datta, S. (2017). Marketing challenges and strategies. In: *Developing New Functional Food and Nutraceutical Products*, 47–62. Academic Press.

Decernis (2020). Food Fraud Database. https://decernis.com/solutions/food-fraud-database/ (accessed 12 July 2020).

DeFelice, S.L. (1995). The nutraceutical revolution: its impact on food industry RandD. *Trends in Food Science and Technology.* 6 (2): 59–61.

El Sohaimy, S.A. (2012). Functional foods and nutraceuticals—modern approach to food science. *World Applied Sciences Journal* 20 (5): 691–708.

European Commission (2020). Food Supplements. https://ec.europa.eu/food/safety/labelling_nutrition/supplements_en (accessed 14 July 2020).

Federal Register (1997). Current Good Manufacturing Practice in Manufacturing, Packing, or Holding Dietary Supplements. https://www.govinfo.gov/content/pkg/FR-1997-02-06/html/97-3014.htm (accessed 14 July 2020).

Filipiak-Szok, A., Kurzawa, M., and Szłyk, E. (2015). Determination of toxic metals by ICP-MS in Asiatic and European medicinal plants and dietary supplements. *Journal of Trace Elements in Medicine and Biology* 30: 54–58.

Finley, J. (2016). The nutraceutical revolution: emerging vision or broken dream? Understanding scientific and regulatory concerns. *Clinical Research and Regulatory Affairs* 33 (1): 1–3.

Food and Agriculture Organization (2013). Codex Alimentarius Commission Procedural Manual. http://www.fao.org/3/a-i3243e.pdf (accessed 13 July 2020).

Food and Drug Administration and HHS (2004). Final rule declaring dietary supplements containing ephedrine alkaloids adulterated because they present an unreasonable risk. Final rule. *Federal Register* 69 (28): 6787.

Food Safety and Standards Authority of India (2012). Indian Food Code – Food Categorization System. https://old.fssai.gov.in/Portals/0/Pdf/INDIAN_FOOD_CODE(25-06-2012).pdf (accessed 14 July 2020).

Food Safety and Standards Authority of India (2013). Gazette Notification. https://www.fssai.gov.in/notifications.php?notification=gazette-notification (accessed 14 July 2020).

Food Safety and Standards Authority of India (2016). Regulations. https://fssai.gov.in/cms/regulations.php (accessed 14 July 2020).

Food Safety and Standards Authority of India (2020). Codex. https://fssai.gov.in/cms/codexfaq.php (accessed 14 July 2020).

Ganesh, G.N., Ramachandran, A., Suresh, K.R. et al. (2015). Nutraceuticals—a regulatory review. *International Journal of Drug Regulatory Affairs* 3 (2): 22–29.

Gardiner, P. (2005). Dietary supplement use in children: concerns of efficacy and safety. *American Family Physician* 71 (6): 1068.

Geller, A.I., Shehab, N., Weidle, N.J. et al. (2015). Emergency department visits for adverse events related to dietary supplements. *New England Journal of Medicine.* 373 (16): 1531–1540.

Gil, F., Hernández, A.F., and Martín-Domingo, M.C. (2016). Toxic contamination of nutraceuticals and food ingredients. In: *Nutraceuticals*, 825–837. Academic Press.

GlaxoSmithKline (GSK) (2013). GlaxoSmithKline Reaches Agreement to Divest Lucozade and Ribena for £1.35 Billion. https://au.gsk.com/en-au/media/press-releases/2013/glaxosmithkline-reaches-agreement-to-divest-lucozade-and-ribena-for-135-billion/ (accessed 15 July 2020).

Gurley, B.J., Gardner, S.F., and Hubbard, M.A. (2000). Content versus label claims in ephedra-containing dietary supplements. *American Journal of Health-System Pharmacy* 57 (10): 963–969.

Hasler, C.M. (2000). The changing face of functional foods. *Journal of the American College of Nutrition* 19 (sup5): 499S–506S.

Hasler, C. (2008). *Regulation of Functional Foods and Nutraceuticals: A Global Perspective ‖ (Institute of Food Technologists Series)*. Goteborgs University.

Heptinstall, S., Awang, D.V., Dawson, B.A. et al. (1992). Parthenolide content and bioactivity of feverfew (*Tanacetum parthenium* (L.) Schultz-Bip.). Estimation of commercial and authenticated feverfew products. *Journal of Pharmacy and Pharmacology.* 44 (5): 391–395.

HIG Growth Partners (2014). Integrity Nutraceuticals and Cornerstone Research and Development Merge to Form Leader in Nutraceutical Product Development and Manufacturing. https://higgrowth.com/news-release-id-734/ (accessed 15 July 2020).

Hilton, J. (2017). Growth patterns and emerging opportunities in nutraceutical and functional food categories: market overview. In: *Developing New Functional Food and Nutraceutical Products*, 1–28. Academic Press.

Institute of Food Science and Technology (2012). *Food and Drink – Good Manufacturing Practice – A Guide to Its Responsible Management*. Wiley-Blackwell.

International Alliance of Dietary Food Supplement Associations (IADSA) (2020). Resources. https://www.iadsa.org/resources/ (accessed 18 July 2020).

ISO (2018). ISO 22000:2018 Food Safety Management Systems—Requirements for Any Organization in the Food Chain. https://www.iso.org/standard/65464.html (accessed 16 July 2020).

Jain, P.N., Rathod, M.H., Jain, C.V., and Vijayendraswamy, S.M. (2018). Current regulatory requirements for registration of nutraceuticals in India and USA. *International Journal of Drug Regulatory Affairs (IJDRA)* 6 (2): 22–29.

Reig Jofre. 2014: Results Note 2015. https://www.reigjofre.com/en/noticias/item/year-2014-results-note/ (accessed 15 July 2020).

Just Food (2008). INDIA: Nutraceutical Market Sees 40% Growth. https://www.just-food.com/news/nutraceutical-market-sees-40-growth_id102784.aspx (accessed 18 July 2020).

Justice Laws Website (2020). Natural Health Products Regulations (SOR/2003-196). https://laws-lois.justice.gc.ca/eng/regulations/SOR-2003-196/ (accessed 14 July 2020).

Kantor, E.D., Rehm, C.D., Du, M. et al. (2016). Trends in dietary supplement use among US adults from 1999–2012. *JAMA* 316 (14): 1464–1474.

Kessler, R.C., Davis, R.B., Foster, D.F. et al. (2001). Long-term trends in the use of complementary and alternative medical therapies in the United States. *Annals of Internal Medicine* 135 (4): 262–268.

Knight, J. (2004). Safety concerns prompt US ban on dietary supplement. *Nature* 427 (6970): 90–90.

Kojima, K. (1996). The eastern consumer viewpoint: the experience in Japan. *Nutrition Reviews* 54 (11): S186–S188.

KPMG (2015). Nutraceuticals: The Future of Intelligent Food Report. https://home.kpmg/content/dam/kpmg/pdf/2015/05/neutraceuticals-the-future-of-intelligent-food.pdf (accessed 15 July 2020).

Kroll, D.J., Barnes, R., Bickford, C.J. et al. (2004). ASHP statement on the use of dietary supplements. *American Journal of Health-System Pharmacy* 61 (16): 1707–1711.

Kumar, P., Kumar, N., and Omer, T. (2016). A review on nutraceutical "critical supplement for building a healthy world". *World Journal of Pharmacy and Pharmaceutical Sciences* 5 (3): 579–594.

L'Abbé, M.R., Dumais, L., Chao, E., and Junkins, B. (2008). Health claims on foods in Canada. *The Journal of Nutrition* 138 (6): 1221S–1227S.

Lammerding, A.M. and Fazil, A. (2000). Hazard identification and exposure assessment for microbial food safety risk assessment. *International Journal of Food Microbiology* 58 (3): 147–157.

LeBlanc, E.S., Perrin, N., Johnson, J.D. et al. (2013). Over-the-counter and compounded vitamin D: is potency what we expect? *JAMA Internal Medicine* 173 (7): 585–586.

Mandel, S., Packer, L., Youdim, M.B., and Weinreb, O. (2005). Proceedings from the "third international conference on mechanism of action of nutraceuticals". *The Journal of Nutritional Biochemistry* 16 (9): 513–520.

Mansour, M. (2008). Codex and its competitors: the future of the global regulatory and trading regime for food and agricultural products. In: *Regulation of Functional Foods and Nutraceuticals: A Global Perspective*, vol. 28 (ed. C.M. Hasler), 377–389. Ames, IA: Blackwell Publishing.

Marcus, D.M. (2016). Dietary supplements: what's in a name? What's in the bottle? *Drug Testing and Analysis* 8 (3–4): 410–412.

Mihail, L.A. (2016). The quality management principles and their incidence within ISO 9001:2015. In: *International Congress of Automotive and Transport Engineering*, 620–628. Cham: Springer.

Mondaq (2013). Law of Nutritional and Supplemental Food Products in India – The Conflict: Food or Drug?. http://www.mondaq.com/india/food-and-drugs-law/221116/law-of-nutritional-supplemental-food-products-in-india--the-conflict-food-or-drug (accessed 14 July 2020).

Morrow, J.D., Edeki, T.I., El Mouelhi, M. et al. (2005). American Society for Clinical Pharmacology and Therapeutics position statement on dietary supplement safety and regulation. *Clinical Pharmacology and Therapeutics* 77 (3): 113–122.

National Institutes of Health (1994). Dietary Supplement Health and Education Act of 1994 Public Law, 103–417. https://ods.od.nih.gov/About/DSHEA_Wording.aspx (accessed 14 July 2020).

National Institutes of Health (2013). Office of Dietary Supplements – Health Information-frequently Asked Questions. https://ods.od.nih.gov/HealthInformation/ODS_Frequently_Asked_Questions.aspx (accessed 18 July 2020).

National Institutes of Health (2020). National Center for Complementary and Integrative Health. https://www.nccih.nih.gov/ (accessed 14 July 2020).

Natural Products Association (2020a). GMP Certified Companies. https://www.npanational.org/certifications/npa-gmp-certification-program/gmp-certified-companies/ (accessed 13 July 2020).

Natural Products Association (2020b). NPA GMP Certification Program. https://www.npanational.org/certifications/npa-gmp-certification-program/ (accessed 13 July 2020).

Nestle (2014). Nestlé Sells PowerBar. https://www.nestle.com/media/pressreleases/allpressreleases/nestle-sells-powerbar (accessed 15 July 2020).

Newmaster, S.G., Grguric, M., Shanmughanandhan, D. et al. (2013). DNA barcoding detects contamination and substitution in North American herbal products. *BMC Medicine* 11 (1): 222.

Newsday (2013). FDA Official: 70% of Supplement Companies Violate Agency Rules. https://www. newsday.com/news/health/fda-official-70-of-supplement-companies-violate-agency-rules-1.5920525 (accessed 13 July 2020).

Nounou, M.I., Ko, Y., Helal, N.A., and Boltz, J.F. (2018). Adulteration and counterfeiting of online nutraceutical formulations in the united states: time for intervention? *Journal of Dietary Supplements* 15 (5): 789–804.

NSF (2020). NSF GMP Registration Program Requirements of NSF/ANSI 173, Section 8. http://info. nsf.org/Certified/GMP/Listings.asp?program=DIETSUPP (accessed 17 July 2020).

Nutraceuticals World (2018). Data from GMP Inspections Suggests Increased Compliance. https:// www.nutraceuticalsworld.com/issues/2018-01/view_columns/data-from-gmp-inspections-suggests-increased-compliance (accessed 13 July 2020).

Nutraingredients (2011). Danone Confirms Complan Food UK Acquisition. https://www. nutraingredients.com/Article/2011/06/24/Danone-confirms-Complan-Food-UK-acquisition (accessed 15 July 2020).

NutraIngredients-USA (2012). Supplement Sales Hit $ 11.5 Billion in U.S Report Says. https://www. nutraingredients-usa.com/Article/2012/09/20/Supplement-sales-hit-11.5-billion-in-U.S.-report-says (accessed 14 July 2020).

Olmedilla-Alonso, B., Granado-Lorencio, F., Herrero-Barbudo, C., and Blanco-Navarro, I. (2006). Nutritional approach for designing meat-based functional food products with nuts. *Critical Reviews in Food Science and Nutrition* 46 (7): 537–542.

Parasrampuria, J., Schwartz, K., and Petesch, R. (1998). Quality control of dehydroepiandrosterone dietary supplement products. *JAMA* 280 (18): 1565.

Pasumarthy, N.V., Pichukala, A., Lakshmi, T. et al. (2014). Contingent analysis and evaluation of pharmaceutical product recall procedure of USA and India. *World Journal of Pharmaceutical Sciences* 2: 1728–1735.

Ramaa, C.S., Shirode, A.R., Mundada, A.S., and Kadam, V.J. (2006). Nutraceuticals—an emerging era in the treatment and prevention of cardiovascular diseases. *Current Pharmaceutical Biotechnology* 7 (1): 15–23.

Rautiainen, S., Manson, J.E., Lichtenstein, A.H., and Sesso, H.D. (2016). Dietary supplements and disease prevention—a global overview. *Nature Reviews Endocrinology* 12 (7): 407–420.

Safetychain (2020). A Guide to Quality Assurance Best Practices for the Food Industry. https://blog. safetychain.com/guide-quality-assurance-food-industry (accessed 18 July 2020).

Saito, M. (2007). Role of FOSHU (food for specified health uses) for healthier life. *Yakugaku Zasshi: Journal of the Pharmaceutical Society of Japan* 127 (3): 407–416.

Santini, A. and Novellino, E. (2014). Nutraceuticals: beyond the diet before the drugs. *Current Bioactive Compounds* 10 (1): 1–2.

Santini, A., Cammarata, S.M., Capone, G. et al. (2018). Nutraceuticals: opening the debate for a regulatory framework. *British Journal of Clinical Pharmacology* 84 (4): 659–672.

SFDA (2020). SFDA of China. http://www.sfda.com/index.html (accessed 14 July 2020).

Sharma, A., Kumar, P., Sharma, P., and Shrivastav, B. (2013). A comparative study of regulatory registration procedure of nutraceuticals in India, Canada and Australia. *International Journal of Pharmaceutical Quality Assurance* 4 (04): 61–66.

Shimizu, T. (2003). Health claims on functional foods: the Japanese regulations and an international comparison. *Nutrition Research Reviews* 16 (2): 241–252.

Sieber, C.C. (2007). Functional food in elderly persons. *Therapeutische Umschau. Revue Therapeutique.* 64 (3): 141.

Starr, R.R. (2015). Too little, too late: ineffective regulation of dietary supplements in the United States. *American Journal of Public Health* 105 (3): 478–485.

Sukhanov, B.P., Kerimova, M.G., Elizarova, E.V., and Chigireva, É.I. (2011). Sanitary and epidemiological examination of foods under carrying sanitary and epidemiological surveillance on the customer border and at in the territory of the Customers Union. *Voprosy Pitaniia* 80 (4): 25.

The New York Times (2015). Retailers are Warned Over Herbal Supplements. https://www.nytimes.com/interactive/2015/02/02/health/herbal_supplement_letters.html (accessed 12 July 2020).

The United States Pharmacopeia. USP Dietary Supplement Verification Program: Manual for Participants. 2019. https://www.usp.org/sites/default/files/usp/document/our-work/DS/dsvp-manual-participants.pdf (accessed 13 July 2020).

The United States Pharmacopeia (2020a). Verification Services. https://www.usp.org/services/verification-services (accessed 12 July 2020).

The United States Pharmacopeia (2020b). Dietary Supplement Reference Standards. https://www.usp.org/dietary-supplements/reference-standards (accessed 12 July 2020).

The United States Pharmacopeia. (2020c). Events and Training. https://www.usp.org/events-training (accessed 12 July 2020).

The United States Pharmacopeia (2020d). User Forums. https://www.usp.org/events-training/user-forums (accessed 12 July 2020).

The United States Pharmacopeia (2020e). Newsletters and Updates. https://www.usp.org/newsletter-and-information (accessed 12 July 2020).

The United States Pharmacopeial Convention (2016). USP Global Public Policy Position—Ensuring the Quality of Dietary Supplements. https://www.usp.org/sites/default/files/usp/document/about/public-policy/public-policy-dietary-supplements.pdf (accessed 10 July 2020).

Therapeutic Goods Administration (2013). An Overview of the Regulation of Complementary Medicines in Australia. https://www.tga.gov.au/overview-regulation-complementary-medicines-australia (accessed 14 July 2020).

Tovey, F.I. and Hobsley, M. (2004). Milling of wheat, maize and rice: effects on fibre and lipid content and health. *World Journal of Gastroenterology: WJG* 10 (12): 1695.

Tsim, Y.C., Yeung, V.W., and Leung, E.T. (2002). An adaptation to ISO 9001: 2000 for certified organisations. *Managerial Auditing Journal* 17 (5): 245–250.

Tyler, V.E. and Foster, F. (1996). Herbs and phytochemicals. In: *Handbook of Non-prescription Drugs* (ed. T.R. Covington, R.R. Berardi and L.L. Young). Washington, DC: American Pharmaceutical Association.

U.S. Food and Drug Administration (2010). Small Entity Compliance Guide: Current Good Manufacturing Practice in Manufacturing, Packaging, Labeling, or Holding Operations for Dietary Supplements. https://www.fda.gov/regulatory-information/search-fda-guidance-documents/small-entity-compliance-guide-current-good-manufacturing-practice-manufacturing-packaging-labeling (accessed 12 July 2020).

U.S. Food and Drug Administration (2012). Guidance for Sponsors, Investigators, and Institutional Review Boards. https://www.fda.gov/media/82634/download (accessed 18 July 2020).

U.S. Food and Drug Administration (2016a). FDA Warns Against the Use of Homeopathic Teething Tablets and Gels. https://www.fda.gov/news-events/press-announcements/fda-warns-against-use-homeopathic-teething-tablets-and-gels (accessed 12 July 2020).

U.S. Food and Drug Administration (2016b). FDA Investigates Elevated Lead Levels Linked to Ton Shen Health/Life Rising Dietary Supplements. https://www.fda.gov/food/outbreaks-foodborne-illness/fda-investigates-elevated-lead-levels-linked-ton-shen-healthlife-rising-dietary-supplements (accessed 12 July 2020).

U.S. Food and Drug Administration (2017). Laboratory Analysis of Homeopathic Teething Tablets. https://www.fda.gov/drugs/information-drug-class/laboratory-analysis-homeopathic-teething-tablets (accessed 12 July 2020).

U.S. Food and Drug Administration (2018a). Tips for Dietary Supplement Users. https://www.fda.gov/food/information-consumers-using-dietary-supplements/tips-dietary-supplement-users (accessed 10 July 2020).

U.S. Food and Drug Administration (2018b). FDA Investigated Multistate Outbreak of Salmonella Infections Linked to Products Reported to Contain Kratom. https://www.fda.gov/food/outbreaks-foodborne-illness/fda-investigated-multistate-outbreak-salmonella-infections-linked-products-reported-contain-kratom (accessed 12 July 2020).

U.S. Food and Drug Administration (2019a). Generally Recognized as Safe (GRAS). https://www.fda.gov/food/food-ingredients-packaging/generally-recognized-safe-gras (accessed 19 July 2020).

U.S. Food and Drug Administration (2019b). FDA Adverse Events Reporting System (FAERS) Public Dashboard. https://www.fda.gov/drugs/questions-and-answers-fdas-adverse-event-reporting-system-faers/fda-adverse-event-reporting-system-faers-public-dashboard (accessed 12 July 2020).

U.S. Food and Drug Administration (2019c). CFR – Code of Federal Regulations Title 21. https://www.accessdata.fda.gov/scripts/cdrh/cfdocs/cfcfr/cfrsearch.cfm?cfrpart=111 (accessed 12 July 2020).

U.S. Food and Drug Administration (2019d). Dietary Supplements. https://www.fda.gov/food/dietary-supplements (accessed 14 July 2020).

U.S. Food and Drug Administration (2019e). Questions and Answers on Dietary Supplements. https://www.fda.gov/food/information-consumers-using-dietary-supplements/questions-and-answers-dietary-supplements (accessed 14 July 2020).

U.S. Food and Drug Administration (2020a). Inspection Classification Database Search. https://www.accessdata.fda.gov/scripts/inspsearch/ (accessed 13 July 2020).

U.S. Food and Drug Administration (2020b). Guidance, Compliance, and Regulatory Information. https://www.fda.gov/drugs/guidance-compliance-regulatory-information (accessed 18 July 2020).

Unilever (2014). Unilever Sells Slim-Fast to Kainos Capital. https://www.unilever.com/news/press-releases/2014/14-07-10-Unilever-sells-Slim-Fast-to-Kainos-Capital.html (accessed 15 July 2020).

US Government Accountability Office (2010). Herbal Dietary Supplements: Examples of Deceptive Marketing and Practices and Potentially Dangerous Advice. https://www.gao.gov/products/GAO-10-662T (accessed 13 July 2020).

Verma, B. and Popli, H. (2018). Regulations of nutraceuticals in India and US. *Pharma Innovation* 7 (7): 811–816.

Vitamin Retailer (2013). Best New Products. 2013. https://vitaminretailer.com/2013-best-new-products/ (accessed 12 July 2020).

Volpe, R. and Sotis, G. (2015). Nutraceuticals: definition and epidemiological rationale for their use in clinical practice. *High Blood Pressure and Cardiovascular Prevention* 22 (3): 199–201.

Wallace, T.C., MacKay, D., Al-Mondhiry, R. et al. (2013). Dietary supplement regulation in the United States. In: *Dietary Supplement Regulation in the United States*, 1–38. Cham: Springer.

World Health Organization and Food and Agriculture Organization of the United Nations (2006). FAO/WHO guidance to governments on the application of HACCP in small and/or less-developed food businesses. *FAO Food and Nutrition Paper* 86: 1–74.

World Trade Organization (1999). Review of the Operation and Implementation of the Agreement on the Application of Sanitary and Phytosanitary Measures. https://www.wto.org/english/tratop_e/sps_e/gsps12_e.htm (accessed 17 July 2020).

World Trade Organization (2012). World Trade Report 2012. Trade and Public Policies: A Closer Look at Nontariff Measures in the 21st Century. https://www.wto.org/english/res_e/booksp_e/anrep_e/world_trade_report12_e.pdf (accessed 17 July 2020).

Wysowski, D.K. and Swartz, L. (2005). Adverse drug event surveillance and drug withdrawals in the United States, 1969–2002: the importance of reporting suspected reactions. *Archives of Internal Medicine* 165 (12): 1363–1369.

Yamada, K., Sato-Mito, N., Nagata, J., and Umegaki, K. (2008). Health claim evidence requirements in Japan. *The Journal of Nutrition* 138 (6): 1192S–1198S.

Yang, Y. (2008). Scientific substantiation of functional food health claims in China. *The Journal of Nutrition* 138 (6): 1199S–1205S.

Yen, P.K. (2005). Food and supplement safety. *Geriatric Nursing (New York, NY)* 26 (5): 279–280.

Ziker, D. (2005). What lies beneath: an examination of the underpinnings of dietary supplement safety regulation? *American Journal of Law and Medicine* 31 (2–3): 269–284.

11

Phytochemical, Pharmacological, and Health Benefits of *Glycyrrhiza glabra*

Hassan Esmaeili[1,2] and Akbar Karami[1]

[1] *Department of Horticultural Science, School of Agriculture, Shiraz University, Shiraz, Iran*
[2] *Department of Agriculture, Medicinal Plants and Drugs Research Institute, Shahid Beheshti University, Tehran, Iran*

11.1 Introduction

Licorice (*Glycyrrhiza glabra* L.) is a perennial subshrub of Fabaceae family with multiple underground stems, violet to purple flowers, composite leaves, and a pod encompasses three to five brown seeds, distributed from southern Europe to eastern Asia (Esmaeili et al. 2020). The plant cultivated in Germany, Italy, England, Belgium, France, Greece, Iraq, Turkey, Spain, Egypt, Syria, and recently in Iran. About 7500 tons of licorice roots were exported annually from Iran with a financial value of $44 million, which makes it a valuable economic medicinal plant (Esmaeili et al. 2020). *Glycyrrhiza* genus have posited important and valuable glycyrrhizin-producing species including *G. glabra* L., *Glycyrrhiza uralensis* Fisch., and *Glycyrrhiza inflata* Batal (Hayashi and Sudo 2009). By reviewing old document versions from India and China, it has been found that licorice root has been used since ancient times for treatment of the respiratory tract infections and hepatitis (Gupta et al. 2008). Decoction of licorice dried root has been consumed for many years to cure the sore throat, bronchitis, cough, as well as larynx inflammation in Iran. Glycyrrhizin was known in Japan for the treatment of liver disorders (Fujisawa 1980) and glabridin was useful for CNS and CVS complaint (Cao et al. 2007). Licorice has employed extensively in the food and confectionery, tobacco, chewing gum, beer and beverages, pharmacology and cosmetic industries. Licorice is consumed for enhancing qualitative characteristics of cigarettes by strengthening the aroma and moisture of cigarettes in tobacco industry. Several types of sweets are manufactured in different parts of the world, for example black licorice in North America, licorice allsorts in England, salty licorice candy in Dutch and Nordic countries. Licorice moderate the bitter and astringent taste of many medicines such as chloride of aluminum, hyoscyamus, senna, senega, and so on. It is also added to beer to raise its flavor. This miraculous plant has extensive pharmacological effects such as anti-ulcer, hepatoprotective, antioxidant, antimicrobial, anticancer, anti-inflammatory, memory enhancing, antidepressant effect, and hypocholesterolemic activity. This review provides a comprehensive survey emphasizing the phytochemical, pharmacological, and health benefits of *G. glabra*.

Handbook of Nutraceuticals and Natural Products: Biological, Medicinal, and Nutritional Properties and Applications,
Volume 2, First Edition. Edited by Preetha Balakrishnan and Sreerag Gopi.
© 2022 John Wiley & Sons, Inc. Published 2022 by John Wiley & Sons, Inc.

11.2 Phytochemical Compositions

The constituents of licorice root are reported to be 20% moisture, 3–16% sugars, 5–24% glycyrrhizin (as a main component), 30% starch, and 6% cinder (Duke 2002). The *G. glabra* underground extract may possess about 4–25% of the saponin. Many compositions like amino acids, volatile oil, flavonoids, inorganic salts, bitter substances, fat, sterols, asparagines, tannins, mucilage, glycosides, estrogen, protein, and resin have been separated from the roots and rhizomes of this plant (Bradley 1992; Damle 2014). The amount of constitutes in underground part of plant fluctuate with season, age, and root and rhizome diameter (Hayashi et al. 1993, 1998a). Ronbiquet in 1809 for the first time identified valuable substance glycyrrhizin from *G. glabra* roots. It is a triterpenoid saponin, which liberates two molecules of D-glucuronic acid and the aglycone 18β-glycyrrhetic acid (enoxolone) by the process of hydrolysis. The α-form of glycyrrhetinic acid has also been recognized in very small amounts in the plant (Claude et al. 2008). Beside of glycyrrhizin (glycyrrhizinic acid or glycyrrhizic), which is the most important triterpenoid in licorice root, other triterpenes such as glycyrretol, glabrolide, liquiritic acid, and isoglaborlide have been identified in the plant (Isbrucker and Burdock 2006).

So far, 70 flavonoids were identified from underground part of *G. glabra* (Nomura and Fukai 1998). Moreover, some publications have exhibited flavononids diversity in licorice leaves (Fukui et al. 1988; Hayashi et al. 2000, 2003c). The yellowish color of the licorice root indicates the presence of flavonoids such as liquirtin, isoliquertin, rhamnoliquirilin, liquiritigenin, shinflavanone, shinpterocarpin, glucoliquiritin apioside, 1-methoxyphaseolin and prenyllicoflavone A, glabridin (species-specific flavonoid), glabrene and hispaglabridins A and B (Damle 2014). Other flavonoids include: licoagrodin, licoagrochalcone A, B, C and D, licoagrocarpin, licoagrone, licochalcone C, licoagroaurone, kanzonol Y, glyinfanin B, glycyrdione A licoagroside A, ononin, calycosin 7-O-glucoside, wistin, afrormosin 7-O-(6″-malonylglucoside), vicenin-2 and isoschaftoside (Kitagawa et al. 1994; Asada et al. 1998, 1999; Li et al. 1998, 2000). Ammar et al. (2012) isolated licuraside2-(5-P-coumaryl apiosyl), liquiriteginin, liquiritin apioside, isoliquiritin, isoliquritin apioside, and neoliquiritin apioside from *G. glabra*. Also eleven phenolic constitutes named glycybridins A–K were identified by Li et al. (2017). Glabrocoumarone A and B, liqcoumarin, umbelliferone, herniarin, glycyrin, glycocoumarin, licopyranocoumarin, glabrocoumarin, and licofuranocoumarin have been discovered in *G. glabra* species (Haraguchi 2001, De Simone et al. 2001; Williamson 2003; Kinoshita et al. 2005) (See Figure 11.1).

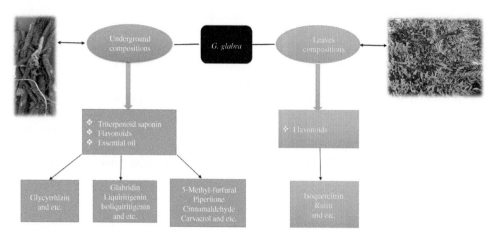

Figure 11.1 The main composition in underground and leaves of *G. glabra*.

Farag and Wessjohann (2012) collected licorice samples from Afghanistan, Egypt, and Syria and analyzed root volatile compounds, which 5-methyl-furfural, (4E)-decenal, piperitone, (E)-cinnamaldehyde, thymol, carvacrol, p-vinyl-guaiacol, eugenol, and γ-Nonalactone were the main constitutes of essential oil. In a study conducted by Ali (2013), α-pinene, β-pinene, octanol, γ-terpinene, stragole, isofenchon, β-caryophyllene, citronellyl acetate, caryophyllene oxide, and geranyl hexanolate were discovered in essential oil of licorice. It should be noted that about 10–25% of glycyrrhizin is detected in the licorice essential oil (Carmines et al. 2005) (see Figure 11.2). Although many of the plant's compounds have been reported and isolated, two group of compounds saponins and flavonoids are of particular importance to humans (See Figure 11.3). *Glycyrrhizinic acid* as a triterpenoid saponin and glabridin as a flavonoid are two valuable and biologically active compounds with extensive applications. Three saponins including licorice saponin K2/H2, licorice saponin B2 and licorice saponin G2/yunganoside K2 have been introduced as biomarkers for *G. glabra* species (Rizzato et al. 2017).

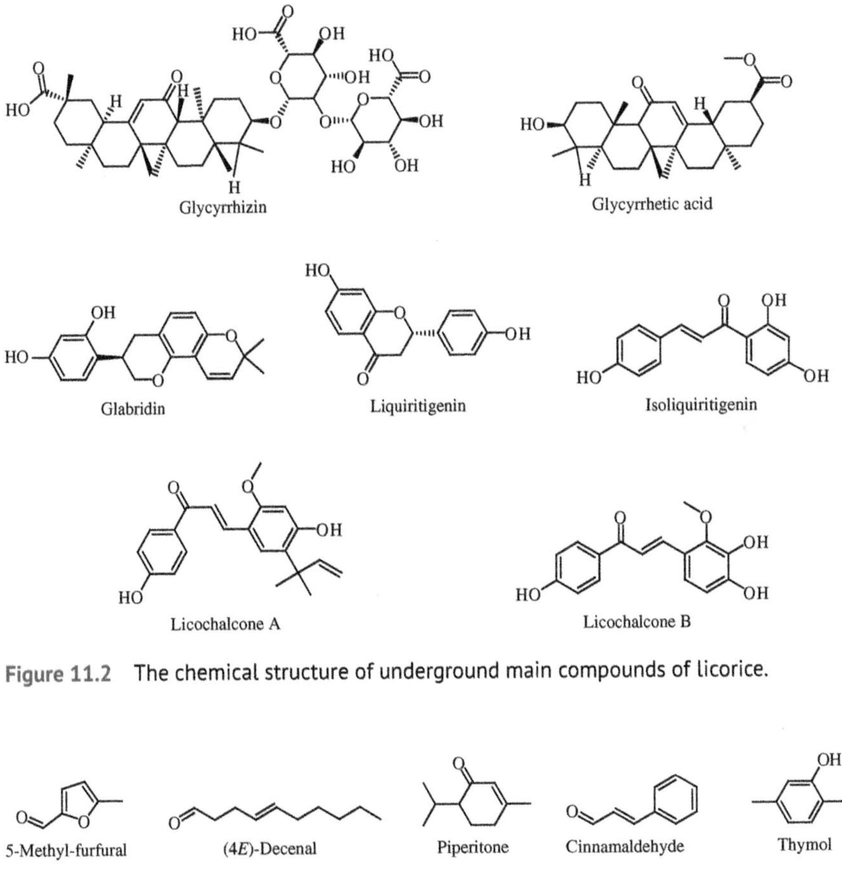

Figure 11.2 The chemical structure of underground main compounds of licorice.

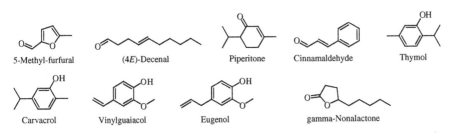

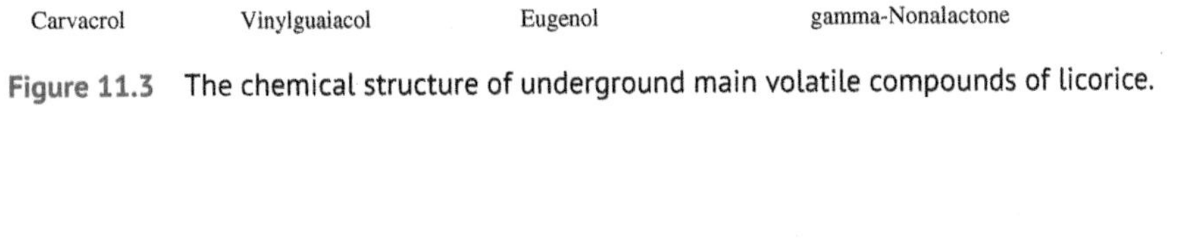

Figure 11.3 The chemical structure of underground main volatile compounds of licorice.

Some studies investigated the chemical compositions in licorice leaves and showed the existence of two categories of *G. glabra* according to main flavonol glycosides in the leaves where licorice samples divided into isoquercitrin (collected from Turkey, Italy, and Spain) and rutin (collected from Kazakhstan) groups (Hayashi et al. 1995, 1998b; Hayashi et al. 2003a, b). Hayashi et al. (2003a) also reported a mixed population based on both flavonol glycosides mentioned above for licorice plants collected from Uzbekistan. They also recognized the three flavanones, namely, pinocembrin, licoflavanone, and glabranin as major compositions common to both categories among all samples from different countries. According to this classification, our study on collected licorice populations revealed that Iranian licorice can be grouped in rutin category and ranged between 1.98 and 6.53 mg/g dry weight (Esmaeili et al. 2019). In addition, two groups of chemical compounds, namely, flavonoids and dihydrostilbenes were identified and isolated from *G. glabra* leaves (Hayashi et al. 1996; Fukai et al. 1998; Biondi et al. 2003, 2005) (see Figure 11.4).

Many factors, such as genetics, growing environment, root diameter, physicochemical properties of soil, processing procedures, and harvesting time affect the quantity and quality of the active ingredients of licorice root (Kovalenko et al. 2004; Zhang et al. 2011; Hosseini et al. 2014). It has been found that the highest amount of glycyrrhizic acid in licorice is obtained in the third year of plant growth (Muchnik 1976). It was shown in a study on some licorice populations from Iran that glycyrrhizic acid (GA) content varied between 1.38 and 3.40%. Our study on 28 different *G. glabra* populations from different wild habitat showed that GA varied between 1.34 and 7.4% The average amount of GA content in Italy (1.6–3%), Uzbekistan (4.76–6.13%), and Spain (0.7–4.4%) were less than average quantity of GA in Iranian licorice (Hayashi et al. 1998b, 2003a). The quantity of glabridin in Italy (0.07–0.27%), Spain (0.21–0.80%), Uzbekistan (0.08–0.35%), and Iran (0–1.3%)

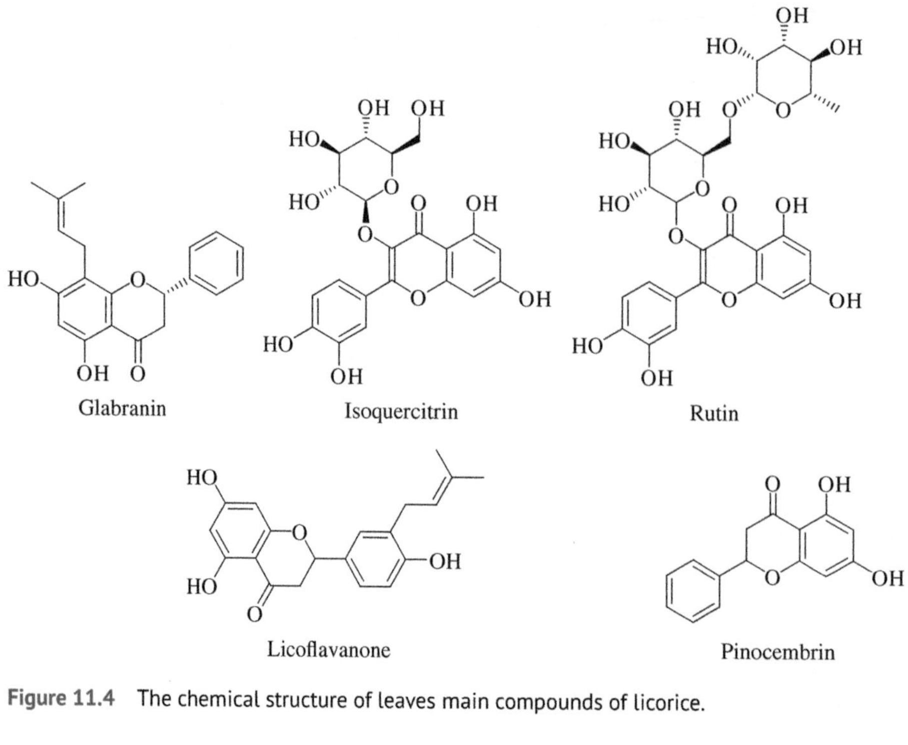

Figure 11.4 The chemical structure of leaves main compounds of licorice.

have also been reported previously (Hayashi et al. 1998b, 2003a; Esmaeili et al. 2019). The glycyrrhizin and glabridin value in the underground parts of *G. glabra* collected in Tajikestan varied from 2.56 to 9.29% and 0.09 to 0.92% of the dry weight, respectively (Hayashi et al. 2016). According to our result maximum value of glabridin in Iranian licorice (1.3%) was higher than the glabridin amount of *G. glabra* in Tajisektan (0.92% dry weight) in Spain (0.07–0.80%), Turkey (0.15–0.70%), Uzbekistan (0.03–0.35%), and Kazakhstan (0.28–0.34%) (Hayashi et al. 1995, 1998b, 2003a, b, 2016). Liquiritin and liquiritigenin with an average of less than 1 mg/g dry weight and total sugar with an average of 3.18% were estimated among studied Iranian licorice populations (Esmaeili et al. 2019).

11.3 Pharmacological and Health Benefits

Herbal have been investigated and consumed from ancient times for treatment of different diseases, and today, they have become one of the main sources of discovery for new pharmaceutical compounds. Licorice has been traditionally used to treat tuberculosis, wound diabetes, cough kidney stones, lung irritation, and diabetes (Asl and Hosseinzadeh 2008; Al-Snafi. 2018). It has also been used in China and Japan as a treatment for liver disorders (Hirayama et al. 1989; Li and Luo 2003). Although most of the health benefits of licorice are related to the underground organs, the leaves of this plant have also been traditionally used to heal wounds (Al-Snafi 2018). In traditional Iranian medicine, the plant has been applied to treat the inflammation of the stomach lining, respiratory, and gastric diseases, as well as sore throat (Esmaeili et al. 2009; Zargaran et al. 2013).

Licorice is a wondrous herb that is not only widely used in traditional medicine but also in modern medicine and industry (See Figure 11.5). Licorice root has the capability to be consumed orally to treat duodecimal, stomachic and gullet ulcers, bronchitis, inflammation, bruising, sedative, swelling, and spasm. Licorice moderate the bitter and astringent taste of many medicines such as chloride of aluminum, hyoscyamus, senna, senega, and so on (Dastagir and Rizvi 2016). Licorice bear many medicinal properties such as antioxidant, anticancer, antiviral, antibacterial, reducing fever, neurological and cardiovascular effects, antiulcer, analgesic, and anti-inflammatory, which an active ingredient or a set of active ingredients are involved in occurrence of these pharmacological properties. Recently, El-Saber Batiha et al. (2020) reported the pharmacological activity of each isolated compounds along with their category of *G. glabra* (El-Saber Batiha et al. 2020).

Some formulations are manufactured from licorice in Iran such as "D-Reglis" for inhibition of ulcer, "Mentazin" pill for treatment of gastric ulcer and to console stomach pain, "Reglis" tablets to treat duodenal bloating, "Gastrin" as anti-inflammatory and painkiller tablets for stomach swelling, "Licophar" tablet as cough medicine and phlegm removal, "Altadin" chewy pill for treatment of throat vexation, "Shirinnoush" as cough syrup and cure of duodenal ulcer (Bahmani et al. 2014). The most valuable and important ingredient in licorice is glycyrrhizin, which is 30–50 (Graebin et al. 2010) times or 33–200 (Scientific Committee on Food 2003) times sweeter than sucrose. Hepatoprotective effect of glycyrrhizic acid and 18β-glycyrrhetinic acid has already been proven (Gumpricht et al. 2005; Kao et al. 2014). Intravenous administration of glycyrrhizic acid has been shown to reduce the formation of fibrosis in the liver (Manns et al. 2012). There is also evidence that these substances are used to treat Parkinson's and ischemic diseases (Tabuchi et al. 2012; Kao et al. 2014). By boiling the root of the licorice plant in water and evaporating most of its moisture, a blackish-brown extract is obtained. It is available in both solid and paste forms. Licorice extract has many uses in medicine, pharmaceuticals, food, and cosmetic industries.

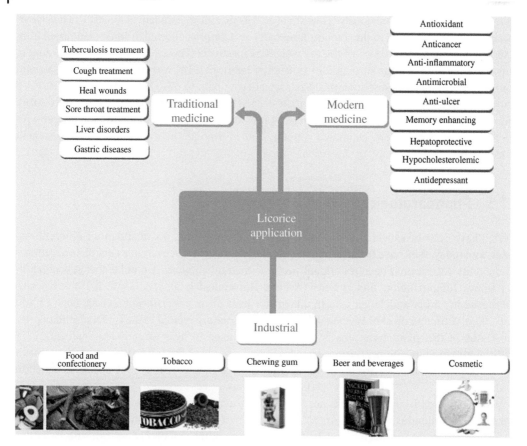

Figure 11.5 Different applications of licorice.
Sources: Antonio Gravante/123 RF; David Buffington/Photodisc/Getty Images; TravisStaton/iStock/Getty Images.

11.4 Anti-Ulcer Activity

Most likely, the most important property of licorice is its effect on the gastrointestinal tract. This plant cures inflammation and ulcers of the stomach and duodenum and has a positive effect on preventing the gastric cancer. Carbenoxolone, which is synthesized and derived from glycyrrhetic acid, is widely used to treat gastric ulcers (Isbrucker and Burdock 2006). Clinical trials using carbenoxolone disclosed significant effect on treatment of gastric and duodenal ulcers (Young et al. 1979; Ganguli and Mohamed 1980; Schwamberger and Reissigl 1980; Cook et al. 1980; Bianchi et al. 1985). As the first researcher, Revers (1956) administered licorice extract for a number of patients suffering gastric ulcers to investigate licorice effect on this disease. Positive results were achieved using 10 g/day of the licorice extract, but some of these patients showed symptoms such as headaches, dizziness, inflammation, and hypertension. However, with a dose reduction of 10–3 g/day, the symptoms of inflammation decreased. Further experiments showed that glycyrrhizin was a causative agent of these side effects (Isbrucker and Burdock 2006).

Helicobacter pylori is known to cause many gastroduodenal ailments (Dunn et al. 1997). Flavonoids, glycyrrhizic acid, and glycyrrhetinic acid extracted from liquorice have been noticed as anti-growth compounds against *H. pylori* (Chung 1998; Kim et al. 2000; Fukai et al. 2002a).

The in vitro growth of two strains of *H. pylori* (sensitive, and clarithromycin- and amoxicillin-resistant strains) was terminated by two flavonoids glabridin and glabrene isolated from licorice roots (Fukai et al. 2002a). Hydroalcohol extract from licorice root was more effective than omeprazole in terms of anti-ulcer properties (Jalilzadeh-Amin et al. 2015). It has been reported that glycyrrhetinic acid is the most active compound against *H. pylori* (Kim et al. 2000; Krausse et al. 2004). It has been reported that glycyrrhizinic acid possesses antiulcer activity via increasing the concentration of prostaglandins, which encourage mucous secretion and cell multiplication in the stomach (Maurya et al. 2009).

GutGard is a flavonoid-rich drug from licorice root donate antioxidant properties and protecting effect against gastric and gut ulcers (Mukherjee et al. 2010). In addition, this drug represented a positive performance against *H. pylori* infection, as well as relieving indigestion (Raveendra et al. 2012; Puram et al. 2013). Bennett et al. (1980) indicated that deglycyrrhizinated licorice in blend manner with cimetidine propound higher protective activity against aspirin-induced gastric ulcers in rats than low doses of either drug alone. Occasionally, clinical trials show conflicting results, for example although deglycyrrhizinated licorice did not possess a significant positive effect on British patients (Bardhan et al. 1978), Brogden et al. (1974) had reported its positive effect for the treatment of gastric ulcers. Glycyrrhetinic acid through interdiction of phosphodiesterase (PDE) activity, thereby enhancing amount of cyclic adenosine monophosphate (cAMP) of gastric mucosa of the pylorus and cardia, and repression gastric acid secretion fulfills its anti-ulcer activity role (Akbar 2020).

11.5 Hepatoprotective Activity

The hepatoprotective potential of the licorice extract may be due to its antioxidant properties, because of the fact that liver damage occurs mainly due to oxidative stress. *Glycyrrhiza glabra* has long been used to treat liver disease. *Glycyrrhiza glabra* extract was able to show hepatoprotective potential through interference in P4502E1 enzyme resulting blocking the activity of carbon tetrachloride (Jeong et al. 2002). In a study conducted by Al-Razzuqi et al. (2012), aqueous extract of *G. glabra* in a dose of 2 g/kg per day exhibited hepatic tissue restoring activity in acute liver diseases. Also *G. glabra* extract showed significant hepatoprotective activity in Swiss albino mice, which may be due to the effect of one substance or a combination of known compounds in the extract (Sharma and Agrawal 2014). About 180 chemical compounds isolated from three species *G. uralensis*, *G. glabra*, and *G. inflate* were *in vitro* assayed for their hepatoprotective potential, which some specialized compounds such as licoflavone A, xambioona, 3,4-didehydroglabridin, isoliquiritigenin, licochalcone B, licoagrochalcone A, and 2'-*O*-demethybidwillol B have remarkable protective potential against both APAP and CCl₄ induced HepG2 cells injury (Kuang et al. 2017). It has been documented that licorice compounds decreased degeneration of liver cells in chronic hepatitis B and C, and they also alleviated the hepatocellular cancer in hepatitis C virus-induced fibrosis (Fiore et al. 2008).

Previously, glycyrrhetinic acid and glycyrrhizin were investigated for hepatoprotective activity. Some publication suggested that glycyrrhetinic acid was more potent than glycyrrhizin (Hwang et al. 2006; Chen et al. 2014). Some function and process have been reported for these two compounds in their role in protection of liver such as inactivating NF-κB and inducible nitric oxide synthase, decrement free fatty acid-induced oxidative stress, reducing the Bax/Bcl-2 ratio and cleaved caspase-9, inhibiting cytochrome c and Smac release from the mitochondria to cytoplasm and prevent the mitochondrial membrane depolarization (Wu et al. 2008; Tripathi et al. 2009; Guo et al. 2013; Chen et al. 2014; Hasan et al. 2015). Hence, it can be concluded that ingredients in licorice extract protect the liver through reducing the oxidative stress, adjustment of CYP enzymes expression, helping cell to maintain its membrane structure, etc. Japan has benefitted glycyrrhizin to treat liver disease where a glycyrrhizin-containing product, Stronger Neo-Minophagen C®, extremely used for chronic hepatic diseases, and it is also consumed in Korea, China, India, and Taiwan (Lee et al. 2007; Kim et al. 2011a).

11.6 Antioxidant Activity

Reactive oxygen species (ROS) are responsible for many diseases in the human body. Minerals, polyphenols, vitamins, and some extracts of medicinal plant prevent the formation of ROS or scavenge the free radicals. The various licorice extracts obtained by using different solvents have shown great radical-scavenging activity (Wojcikowski et al. 2007; Visavadiya et al. 2009). Glycyrrhizic acid is one of the most potent hydroxyl radical scavengers (Akbar 2020). Some studies have focused on antioxidant activity of methanolic extract of licorice (Sultana et al. 2010; Chopra et al. 2013; Karahan et al. 2016; Esmaeili et al. 2019). Ethanolic extracts of licorice root exhibited a considerable scavenging activity against superoxide, nitric oxide, hydroxyl, DPPH and ABTS and showed better antioxidant activity than aqueous extract (Visavadiya et al. 2009). Quintana et al. (2019) applied supercritical CO_2 method to obtain the licorice extract, then measured its antioxidant activity resulting in higher antioxidant potential than liquid solvents. The high amount of phenolic compounds and glabridin obtained from root extract were responsible for outstanding antioxidant activity in this extraction method. Malekinejad et al. (2011) reported the antioxidant properties of licorice extract where ochratoxin A-induced damages were reduced by using the extract. Antioxidant properties of some isolated compounds of licorice root were examined, which specified that isoliquiritigenin, isoprenylchalcone derivative, hispaglabridin A, hispaglabridin B, 4′-O-methylglabridin, and glabridin possess substantial antioxidant activity. Among these compounds, glabridin displayed more potent antioxidant than other (Vaya et al. 1997).

11.7 Antimicrobial Activity

Because of the acquired resistance of microbes to antibiotics and the side effects of antibiotics, the discovery of new natural compounds and extract with proper antimicrobial properties has always been of interest to scientists. For these reasons, numerous studies have examined the antibacterial potential of plant natural compound, especially in licorice (Mitscher et al. 1980; Demizu et al. 1988; Okada et al. 1989; Haraguchi et al. 1998; Fukai et al. 2002b; Gupta et al. 2008; Bassyouni et al. 2012; Rodino et al. 2015; Najeeb and Al-Refai 2015; Wang et al. 2020). Various extracts obtained from *G. glabra* showed outstanding antibacterial activity; for instance, ethanolic extracts of *G. glabra* demonstrated remarkable inhibition potential against *Escherichia coli, Pseudomonas fluorescens Staphylococcus aureus,* and *Bacillus cereus* (Rodino et al. 2015). The disc diffusion method was applied by Sultana et al. (2010) to examine antimicrobial potential of *G. glabra* extract against 12 bacteria including *S. aureus, Bacillus megaterium, Bacillus subtilis, E. coli, Sarcina lutea, Pseudomonas aeruginosa, Salmonella typhi, Salmonella paratyphi, Shigella boydii, Salmonella dysenteriae, Vibrio parahemolyticus,* and *Vibrio mimicus* indicated highest inhibition activity against *S. aureus* and minimum effect on *P. aeruginosa*. Phytochemical and antibacterial activity of *G. glabra* ethanolic extract showed that glabridin was the active compound and hispaglabridin B was ineffective constituent against *Mycobacterium tuberculosis.* Having two free phenolic hydroxyls in glabridin structure may be important for this activity (Gupta et al. 2008). Kim et al. (2013) indicated that 18α-glycyrrhetinic acid extracted from licorice root was effective to inhibit the main periodontal pathogen *Porphyromonas gingivalis* both *in vitro* and *in vivo*. It is also reported that 18β-glycyrrhetinic acid at 0.223 µM concentration decrease the expression of genes associated with the *S. aureus* virulence resulted in *in vitro* antibacterial activity.

Flaviviruses cause many diseases in humans, including hepatic, bloodshed, encephalitic, pyretic illnesses (Crance et al. 2003). According to Crance et al. (2003), glycyrrhizin was active against flaviviruses at high non-cytotoxic concentrations. Glycyrrhizin and glycyrrhetinic acid have expressed an repressive effect on HIV-1 (Pompei et al. 1979; Ito et al. 1987) and varicella zoster viruses (Baba and Shigeta 1987) in *in vitro* condition. It has been shown that glycyrrhizin suppresses the absorption of the HIV-1 into the cell by inhibiting protein kinase C (PKC) activity (Ito et al. 1988). Cinatl et al. (2003) tested antiviral activity of pyrazofurin, ribavirin, mycophenolic acid, 6-azauridine, and glycyrrhizin against two clinical isolates of SARS-associated coronavirus, and they found that glycyrrhizin had the highest inhibitory effect on the virus. It is also specified that glycyrrhizin restrain the hepatitis C virus in a dose-dependent manner and showed synergistic efficacy with interferon (Ashfaq et al. 2011). It has been suggested that glycyrrhizin may play a role in antiviral activity by inducing interferon production (Abe et al. 1982; Utsunomiya et al. 1997). Interferon is an endogenous lymphokine, which prevent the viral replication. Clinical trials have also confirmed the role of glabridin in the treatment of hepatitis B (Zhang and Wang 2002, Sumiyama et al. 1991).

The hydroalcoholic licorice extract was efficient against all studied *Candida albicans, Candida glabrata, Candida Parapsilosis,* and *Candida tropicalis* using the disc diffusion assay resulted in inhibitory zones equal to 1.0–1.2 cm for *C. albicans* and *C. parapsilosis*, 1.0–1.3 cm for *C. tropicalis,* and 1.2 cm for *C. glabrata* after 24 hours (Martins et al. 2014).

11.8 Anticancer Activity

Inflammation and oxidative stress lead to disruption of cell signaling systems resulting in some chronic disorders such as cancer. In fact, reactive oxygen species (ROS), cyclooxygenase-2 (COX-2), and nuclear factor kappa B (NFB) influence the cell proliferation, and apoptotic pathways cause incursion, tumor angiogenesis, and metastasis (Toyokuni 2008; Luqman and Pezzuto 2010). *N*-Acetyltransferase is suggested to have toxicity and carcinogenesis potential. In a study conducted by Chung et al. (2000) indicated that glycyrrhizic acid was efficient against human colon tumor cells via inhibiting the *N*-acetyltransferase activity. Exposure to short-wavelength UVB-radiation can cause irreparable damage to the skin like cutaneous squamous cell carcinoma. It has been proved that oral consumption of glycyrrhizic acid reduce tumor numbers and shrinkage of tumor size in SKH-1 hairless mice. In fact, glycyrrhizic acid prevented the UVB-radiation-induced carcinogenesis and diminished some radiation-induced biomarkers (Cherng et al. 2011). Also anti-cancer activity of glycyrrhizinic acid against gastric cancer cell line BCG-823 (Wang et al. 2015a) and lung adenocarcinoma A549 cell lines (Huang et al. 2014b) has been reported. Several studies have focused on the anticancer properties of glycyrrhetinic acid, for instance cytotoxic and cell-death effect on non-small-cell lung cancer (Huang et al. 2014a), human myeloma cell line (U266) (Xu et al. 2011), human lung adenocarcinoma cell (Kim et al. 2011b), prostate cancer cell line LNCaP (Hawthorne and Gallagher 2008), breast cancer cell line MCF-7 (Sharma et al. 2012), and pituitary adenoma cancer cell lines MMQ and GH3 (Wang et al. 2014).

Anti-mutagenicity of licorice total extracts or its pure constitute have also been documented (Shankel and Clarke 1990; Zani et al. 1993; Mitscher et al. 1996; Kaur et al. 2012; Khan and Ahmad 2020; Akram et al. 2020).

11.9 Anti-Inflammatory Activity

Kiso et al. (1984) stated that glycyrrhizin donate anti-inflammatory activity through scavenge the reactive oxygen species (ROS), but Akamatsu et al. (1991) indicated that glycyrrhizin is not a scavenger of ROS but demonstrate an anti-inflammatory activity via prohibiting the formation of ROS generated by neutrophils. *in vitro* and *in vivo* studies have displayed that isoflurane or sevoflurane (anesthesia-induced agents) can induce some pro-inflammatory factors such as TNF-α and IL-1β that may involve with cognitive impairment in the maturity (Lu et al. 2010; Shen et al. 2013; Zhang et al. 2013).

Glycyrrhizinic acid brought down the amount of tumor necrosis factor-α (TNF-α) and interleukin 1β (IL-1β) in hippocampus of neonatal rats (Wang et al. 2015b). This decrease in levels of pro-inflammatory factors was also observed in model rats (Chang et al. 2015; Wang et al. 2016). The restraining power of a compound or extract on carrageenan-induced inflammation in rats is one of the most appropriate examination to express the anti-inflammatory of the compound. Hydro alcoholic extract of *G. glabra* root revealed a maximum of 46.86% inhibitory on carrageenan induced paw swelling which this anti-inflammatory potential was comparable to the indomethacin as standard anti-inflammatory medicine (Nirmala and Selvaraj 2011).

Lipid peroxidation of dioleoyl phosphatidylcholine (DOPC) liposomes leads to the production of compounds that are related to the inflammation. Račková et al. (2007) showed that licorice extract possesses prevention property on lipid peroxidation of artificial membranes. They also stated that anti-inflammatory effect of glycyrrhizin is most likely originated neither by its capability to reduce the formation of ROS by neutrophils nor by direct scavenging of free radicals, and this substance is not responsible for the inhibitory properties of licorice extract on neutrophil functions. Glabridin and α-glycyhrritinic acid represent anti-inflammatory potential by inhibiting glucocorticoid metabolism and tyrosinase activity of melanocytes, respectively (Maurya et al. 2009). β-Glycyrrhetinic acid and iquiritigenin are introduced as anti-inflammatory and anti-allergic potential compounds (Kroes et al. 1997; Shin et al. 2007). In addition, glyderinine is a derivative of glycyrrhizic acid, and it has been identified and introduced as an anti-inflammatory agent even better than amidopyrine and hydrocortisone (Azimov et al. 1988).

11.10 Memory Enhancing Activity

Several studies have been conducted to investigate the effect of licorice extract on mice and humans memory (Parle et al. 2004; Dhingra et al. 2004; Cui et al. 2008; Zhu et al. 2010; Chakravarthi et al. 2012; Desai et al. 2012; Chakravatjo and Avadhani 2013; Teltumbde et al. 2013). Dhingra et al. (2004) administered various doses of licorice aqueous extract to mice and observed the dose of 150 mg/kg ameliorated learning and memory enhancement of mice. They also stated that this feature of licorice extract could be due to its antioxidant and anti-inflammatory properties and simplification of cholinergic transmission in the brain of mice.

It has been made clear that glabridin has memory enhancement effect in mice through disaccorded with amnesia induced by scopolamine and diazepam (Cui et al. 2008; Desai et al. 2012).

Mental understanding and memory action of male teenagers was examined by licorice tablets. The results showed that the usage of *G. glabra* pills increased memory function among male teenager students compared to placebo (Teltumbde et al. 2013). Probably, the scavenging properties of free radicals by licorice extract reduce oxidative stress in brain cells and increase brain ability and productivity (Dhingra et al. 2004).

11.11 Hypocholesterolemic Activity

It is documented that *G. glabra* root powder and extract reveal hypocholesterolemic and antidyslipidemic activity in rat and golden hamsters, respectively (Visavadiya and Narasimhacharya 2006; Maurya et al. 2009). The administration of licorice ethanolic extract indicated a considerable reduce in cholesterol of serum in dyslipidemic golden hamster, which is most likely related to cholesterol deletion role of saponins and phytosterols in licorice root. It is expressed that phytosterols by translocation of intestinal cholesterol and saponin by precipitating of cholesterol, making it unavailable for absorption in intestine (Oakenfull and Sidhu 1990; Harwood et al. 1993; Ikeda and Sugano 1998; Howell et al. 1998).

11.12 Antidepressant Effect

The aqueous extract of *G. glabra* revealed antidepression activity, which was comparable to two antidepression synthetic compounds imipramine and fluoxetine. Dhingra and Sharma (2006) concluded that antidepressant-like activity of licorice extract in mouse models seems to be mediated via increment in dopamine and norepinephrine of brain.

11.13 Other Functions

Isoliquiritigenin demonstrated inhibitory effect on the intestine at low dose and prokinetic effect at high dose through blockade of calcium channels and activation of muscarinic receptors, respectively (Chen et al. 2009). Antitussic and expectorant activity of glycyrrhizin, liquiritin apioside, and carbenoxolone have been demonstrated (Pastorino et al. 2018).

The positive effects of glycyrrhizin and licorice extract on diabetogenic effects of streptozocin have been reported in rats (Kataya et al. 2011). Cardioprotective effects of *G. glabra* have also been identified in rats (Ojha et al. 2013). Recently, Bailly and Vergoten (2020) proved the anti-coronaviruses of glycyrrhizin and suggested that it can be the appropriate drug for testing against SARS-CoV-2 coronavirus due to its relative safety.

11.14 Conclusion

Licorice and its important compounds have been used in traditional medicine since ancient times. In recent years, extensive studies have been conducted to accurately understand the effectiveness of the plant's compounds. It has led to the production of a wide range of products from this plant, which is widely used in various industries such as food, medicine, and cosmetics. As we have pointed out in this review, licorice possess high potential for treating many abnormalities and disorders, which an active ingredient or a set of active ingredients are involved in occurrence of these properties. Since the exact mechanism of action for some licorice compounds to treat different diseases has not yet been clearly elucidated, more detailed studies are needed. The review highlighted the phytochemical, pharmacological, and health benefits of *G. glabra* to be used by other researchers for further and more comprehensive studies on the plant.

References

Abe, N., Ebina, T., and Ishida, N. (1982). Interferon induction by glycyrrhizin and glycyrrhetinic acid in mice. *Microbiology and Immunology* 26 (6): 535–539.

Akamatsu, H., Komura, J., Asada, Y., and Niwa, Y. (1991). Mechanism of anti-inflammatory action of glycyrrhizin: effect on neutrophil functions including reactive oxygen species generation. *Planta Medica* 57 (02): 119–121.

Akbar, S. (2020). *Glycyrrhiza glabra* L. (Fabaceae/Leguminosae). In: *Handbook of 200 Medicinal Plants*, 963–980. Cham: Springer.

Akram, M., Riaz, M., Wadood, A.W.C. et al. (2020). Medicinal plants with anti-mutagenic potential. *Biotechnology & Biotechnological Equipment* 34 (1): 309–318.

Ali, E.M. (2013). Phytochemical composition, antifungal, antiaflatoxigenic, antioxidant, and anticancer activities of *Glycyrrhiza glabra* L. and *Matricaria chamomilla* L. essential oils. *Journal of Medicinal Plants Research* 7 (29): 2197–2207.

Al-Razzuqi, R., Al-Jawad, F.H., Al-Hussaini, J.A., and Al-Jeboori, A. (2012). Hepatoprotective effect of *Glycyrrhiza glabra* in carbon tetrachloride-induced model of acute liver injury. *Journal of Physiology and Pharmacology Advances* 2 (7): 259–263.

Al-Snafi, A.E. (2018). *Glycyrrhiza glabra*: a phytochemical and pharmacological review. *IOSR Journal of Pharmacy* 8 (6): 1–17.

Ammar, N.M., El-Hawary, S.S.E.D., El-Anssary, A.A. et al. (2012). Phytochemical and clinical studies of the bioactive extract of *Glycyrrhiza glabra* L. Family Leguminosae. *International Journal of Phytomedicine* 4 (3): 429.

Asada, Y., Li, W., and Yoshikawa, T. (1998). Isoprenylated flavonoids from hairy root cultures of *Glycyrrhiza glabra*. *Phytochemistry* 47 (3): 389–392.

Asada, Y., Li, W., and Yoshikawa, T. (1999). The first prenylated biaurone, licoagrone from hairy root cultures of *Glycyrrhiza glabra*. *Phytochemistry* 50 (6): 1015–1019.

Ashfaq, U.A., Masoud, M.S., Nawaz, Z., and Riazuddin, S. (2011). Glycyrrhizin as antiviral agent against hepatitis C virus. *Journal of Translational Medicine* 9 (1): 112.

Asl, M.N. and Hosseinzadeh, H. (2008). Review of pharmacological effects of *Glycyrrhiza* sp. and its bioactive compounds. *Phytotherapy Research: An International Journal Devoted to Pharmacological and Toxicological Evaluation of Natural Product Derivatives* 22 (6): 709–724.

Azimov, M.M., Zakirov, U.B., and Radzhapova, S.H.D. (1988). Pharmacological study of the anti-inflammatory agent glyderinine. *Farmakologiia i toksikologiia* 51 (4): 90–93.

Baba, M. and Shigeta, S. (1987). Antiviral activity of glycyrrhizin against varicella-zoster virus in vitro. *Antiviral Research* 7 (2): 99–107.

Bahmani, M., Rafieian-Kopaei, M., Jeloudari, M. et al. (2014). A review of the health effects and uses of drugs of plant licorice (*Glycyrrhiza glabra* L.) in Iran. *Asian Pacific Journal of Tropical Disease* 4 (S2): 847–849.

Bailly, C. and Vergoten, G. (2020). Glycyrrhizin: an alternative drug for the treatment of COVID-19 infection and the associated respiratory syndrome? *Pharmacology & Therapeutics* 214: 107618.

Bardhan, K.D., Cumberland, D.C., Dixon, R.A., and Holdsworth, C.D. (1978). Clinical trial of deglycyrrhizinised liquorice in gastric ulcer. *Gut* 19 (9): 779–782.

Bassyouni, R.H., Kamel, Z., Megahid, A., and Samir, E. (2012). Antimicrobial potential of licorice: leaves versus roots. *African Journal of Microbiological Research* 6 (49): 7485–7493.

Bennett, A., Clark-Wibberley, T., Stamford, I.F., and Wright, J.E. (1980). Aspirin-induced gastric mucosal damage in rats: cimetidine and deglycyrrhizinated liquorice together give greater protection than low doses of either drug alone. *Journal of Pharmacy and Pharmacology* 32: 151.

Bianchi, G.P., Petrillo, M., Lazzaroni, M. et al. (1985). Comparison of pirenzepine and carbenoxolone in the treatment of chronic gastric ulcer. A double-blind endoscopic trial. *Hepato-Gastroenterology* 32 (6): 293–295.

Biondi, D.M., Rocco, C., and Ruberto, G. (2003). New dihydrostilbene derivatives from the leaves of *Glycyrrhiza glabra* and evaluation of their antioxidant activity. *Journal of Natural Products* 66 (4): 477–480.

Biondi, D.M., Rocco, C., and Ruberto, G. (2005). Dihydrostilbene derivatives from *Glycyrrhiza glabra* leaves. *Journal of Natural Products* 68 (7): 1099–1102.

Bradley, P.R. (1992). *British Herbal Compendium. Volume 1. A Handbook of Scientific Information on Widely Used Plant Drugs. Companion to Volume 1 of the British Herbal Pharmacopoeia*. British Herbal Medicine Association.

Brogden, R.N., Speight, T.M., and Avery, G.S. (1974). Deglycyrrhizinised liquorice: A report of its pharmacological properties and therapeutic efficacy in peptic ulcer. *Drugs* 8 (5): 330–339.

Cao, J., Chen, X., Liang, J. et al. (2007). Role of P-glycoprotein in the intestinal absorption of glabridin, an active flavonoid from the root of *Glycyrrhiza glabra*. *Drug Metabolism and Disposition* 35 (4): 539–553.

Carmines, E.L., Lemus, R., and Gaworski, C.L. (2005). Toxicologic evaluation of licorice extract as a cigarette ingredient. *Food and Chemical Toxicology* 43 (9): 1303–1322.

Chakravarthi, K.K. and Avadhani, R. (2013). Beneficial effect of aqueous root extract of Glycyrrhiza glabra on learning and memory using different behavioral models: An experimental study. *Journal of Natural Science, Biology, and Medicine* 4 (2): 420.

Chakravarthi, K.K., Avadhani, R., and Narayan, R.S. (2012). Effects of *Glycyrrhiza glabra* root extract on learning and memory in Wistar albino rats. *Drug Invention Today* 4 (7): 387–390.

Chang, C.Z., Wu, S.C., and Kwan, A.L. (2015). Glycyrrhizin attenuates proinflammatory cytokines through a peroxisome proliferator-activated receptor-γ-dependent mechanism and experimental vasospasm in a rat model. *Journal of Vascular Research* 52 (1): 12–21.

Chen, G., Zhu, L., Liu, Y. et al. (2009). Isoliquiritigenin, a flavonoid from licorice, plays a dual role in regulating gastrointestinal motility in vitro and in vivo. *Phytotherapy Research: An International Journal Devoted to Pharmacological and Toxicological Evaluation of Natural Product Derivatives* 23 (4): 498–506.

Chen, H.J., Kang, S.P., Lee, I.J., and Lin, Y.L. (2014). Glycyrrhetinic acid suppressed NF-κB activation in TNF-α-induced hepatocytes. *Journal of Agricultural and Food Chemistry* 62 (3): 618–625.

Cherng, J.M., Tsai, K.D., Yu, Y.W., and Lin, J.C. (2011). Molecular mechanisms underlying chemopreventive activities of glycyrrhizic acid against UVB-radiation-induced carcinogenesis in SKH-1 hairless mouse epidermis. *Radiation Research* 176 (2): 177–186.

Chopra, P.K.P.G., Saraf, B.D., Inam, F., and Deo, S.S. (2013). Antimicrobial and antioxidant activities of methanol extract roots of *Glycyrrhiza glabra* and HPLC analysis. *International Journal of Pharmacy and Pharmacological Sciences* 5 (2): 157–160.

Chung, J.G. (1998). Inhibitory actions of glycyrrhizic acid on arylamine *N*-acetyltransferase activity in strains of *Helicobacter pylori* from peptic ulcer patients. *Drug and Chemical Toxicology* 21 (3): 355–370.

Chung, J.G., Chang, H.L., Lin, W.C. et al. (2000). Inhibition of *N*-acetyltransferase activity and DNA-2-aminofluorene adducts by glycyrrhizic acid in human colon tumour cells. *Food and Chemical Toxicology* 38 (2–3): 163–172.

Cinatl, J., Morgenstern, B., Bauer, G. et al. (2003). Glycyrrhizin, an active component of liquorice roots, and replication of SARS-associated coronavirus. *The Lancet* 361: 2045–2046.

Claude, B., Morin, P., Lafosse, M. et al. (2008). Selective solid-phase extraction of a triterpene acid from a plant extract by molecularly imprinted polymer. *Talanta* 75 (2): 344–350.

Cook, P.J., Vincent-Brown, A., Lewis, S.I. et al. (1980). Carbenoxolone (duogastrone) and cimetidine in the treatment of duodenal ulcer—a therapeutic trial. *Scandinavian Journal of Gastroenterology Supplement* 65: 93–101.

Crance, J.M., Scaramozzino, N., Jouan, A., and Garin, D. (2003). Interferon, ribavirin, 6-azauridine and glycyrrhizin: antiviral compounds active against pathogenic flaviviruses. *Antiviral Research* 58 (1): 73–79.

Cui, Y.M., Ao, M.Z., Li, W., and Yu, L.J. (2008). Effect of glabridin from *Glycyrrhiza glabra* on learning and memory in mice. *Planta Medica* 74 (04): 377–380.

Damle, M. (2014). *Glycyrrhiza glabra* (Liquorice)—a potent medicinal herb. *International Journal of Herbal Medicine* 2 (2): 132–136.

Dastagir, G. and Rizvi, M.A. (2016). *Glycyrrhiza glabra* L. (Liquorice). *Pakistan Journal of Pharmaceutical Sciences* 29 (5): 1727–1733.

De Simone, F., Aquino, R., De Tommasi, N. et al. (2001). Anti-HIV aromatic compounds from higher plants. *Bioactive Compounds from Natural Sources* 305: 305–336.

Demizu, S., Kajiyama, K., Takahashi, K. et al. (1988). Antioxidant and antimicrobial constituents of licorice: isolation and structure elucidation of a new benzofuran derivative. *Chemical and Pharmaceutical Bulletin 36* (9): 3474–3479.

Desai, S.K., Pandey, C.H., and Mulgaonkar, S.S. (2012). Memory-strengthening activity of aqueous liquorice extract and glabridin extract in behavioral models. *International Journal of Pharmaceutical Sciences Review and Research* 16 (1): 120–124.

Dhingra, D. and Sharma, A. (2006). Antidepressant-like activity of *Glycyrrhiza glabra* L. in mouse models of immobility tests. *Progress in Neuro-Psychopharmacology and Biological Psychiatry* 30 (3): 449–454.

Dhingra, D., Parle, M., and Kulkarni, S.K. (2004). Memory enhancing activity of *Glycyrrhiza glabra* in mice. *Journal of Ethnopharmacology* 91 (2–3): 361–365.

Duke, J.A. (2002). *Handbook of Medicinal Herbs*. CRC Press.

Dunn, B.E., Cohen, H., and Blaser, M.J. (1997). *Helicobacter pylori*. *Clinical Microbiology Reviews* 10: 720–741.

El-Saber Batiha, G., Magdy Beshbishy, A., El-Mleeh, A. et al. (2020). Traditional uses, bioactive chemical constituents, and pharmacological and toxicological activities of *Glycyrrhiza glabra* L. (Fabaceae). *Biomolecules* 10 (3): 352.

Esmaeili, S., Naghibi, F., Mosaddegh, M. et al. (2009). Screening of antiplasmodial properties among some traditionally used Iranian plants. *Journal of Ethnopharmacology* 121 (3): 400–404.

Esmaeili, H., Karami, A., Hadian, J. et al. (2019). Variation in the phytochemical contents and antioxidant activity of *Glycyrrhiza glabra* populations collected in Iran. *Industrial Crops and Products* 137: 248–259.

Esmaeili, H., Karami, A., Hadian, J. et al. (2020). Genetic structure and variation in Iranian licorice (*Glycyrrhiza glabra* L.) populations based on morphological, phytochemical and simple sequence repeats markers. *Industrial Crops and Products* 145: 112140.

Farag, M.A. and Wessjohann, L.A. (2012). Volatiles profiling in medicinal licorice roots using steam distillation and solid-phase microextraction (SPME) coupled to chemometrics. *Journal of Food Science* 77 (11): 1179–1184.

Fiore, C., Eisenhut, M., Krausse, R. et al. (2008). Antiviral effects of *Glycyrrhiza* species. *Phytotherapy Research: An International Journal Devoted to Pharmacological and Toxicological Evaluation of Natural Product Derivatives* 22 (2): 141–148.

Fujisawa, K. (1980). Therapeutic approach to chronic active hepatitis with glycyrrhizin. *Asian Medical Journal* 23: 745–756.

Fukai, T., Cai, B.S., Maruno, K. et al. (1998). An isoprenylated flavanone from *Glycyrrhiza glabra* and rec-assay of licorice phenols. *Phytochemistry* 49 (7): 2005–2013.

Fukai, T., Marumo, A., Kaitou, K. et al. (2002a). Anti-*Helicobacter pylori* flavonoids from licorice extract. *Life Sciences* 71 (12): 1449–1463.

Fukai, T., Marumo, A., Kaitou, K. et al. (2002b). Antimicrobial activity of licorice flavonoids against methicillin-resistant *Staphylococcus aureus*. *Fitoterapia* 73 (6): 536–539.

Fukui, H., Goto, K., and Tabata, M. (1988). Two antimicrobial flavanones from the leaves of *Glycyrrhiza glabra*. *Chemical and Pharmaceutical Bulletin* 36 (10): 4174–4176.

Ganguli, P.C. and Mohamed, S.D. (1980). Long-term therapy with carbenoxolone in the prevention of recurrence of gastric ulcer. Natural history and evolution of important side-effects and measures to avoid them. *Scandinavian Journal of Gastroenterology Supplement* 65: 63–71.

Graebin, C.S., Verli, H., and Guimarães, J.A. (2010). Glycyrrhizin and glycyrrhetic acid: scaffolds to promising new pharmacologically active compounds. *Journal of the Brazilian Chemical Society* 21 (9): 1595–1615.

Gumpricht, E., Dahl, R., Devereaux, M.W., and Sokol, R.J. (2005). Licorice compounds glycyrrhizin and 18β-glycyrrhetinic acid are potent modulators of bile acid-induced cytotoxicity in rat hepatocytes. *Journal of Biological Chemistry* 280 (11): 10556–10563.

Guo, X.L., Liang, B., Wang, X.W. et al. (2013). Glycyrrhizic acid attenuates CCl4-induced hepatocyte apoptosis in rats via a p53-mediated pathway. *World Journal of Gastroenterology: WJG* 19 (24): 3781.

Gupta, V.K., Fatima, A., Faridi, U. et al. (2008). Antimicrobial potential of *Glycyrrhiza glabra* roots. *Journal of Ethnopharmacology* 116 (2): 377–380.

Haraguchi, H. (2001). Antioxidative plant constituents. In: *Bioactive Compounds from Natural Sources* (ed. C. Tringali), 337–378. London: Taylor & Francis.

Haraguchi, H., Tanimoto, K., Tamura, Y. et al. (1998). Mode of antibacterial action of retrochalcones from *Glycyrrhiza inflata*. *Phytochemistry* 48 (1): 125–129.

Harwood, H.J., Chandler, C.E., Pellarin, L.D. et al. (1993). Pharmacologic consequences of cholesterol absorption inhibition: alteration in cholesterol metabolism and reduction in plasma cholesterol concentration induced by the synthetic saponin *beta*-tigogenin cellobioside (CP-88818; tiqueside). *Journal of Lipid Research* 34 (3): 377–395.

Hasan, S.K., Khan, R., Ali, N. et al. (2015). 18-β glycyrrhetinic acid alleviates 2-acetylaminofluorene-induced hepatotoxicity in Wistar rats: role in hyperproliferation, inflammation and oxidative stress. *Human & Experimental Toxicology* 34 (6): 628–641.

Hawthorne, S. and Gallagher, S. (2008). Effects of glycyrrhetinic acid and liquorice extract on cell proliferation and prostate-specific antigen secretion in LNCaP prostate cancer cells. *Journal of Pharmacy and Pharmacology* 60 (5): 661–666.

Hayashi, H. and Sudo, H. (2009). Economic importance of licorice. *Plant Biotechnology* 26 (1): 101–104.

Hayashi, H., Fukui, H., and Tabata, M. (1993). Distribution pattern of saponins in different organs of *Glycyrrhiza glabra*. *Planta Medica* 59 (04): 351–353.

Hayashi, H., Honda, G., Tabata, M. et al. (1995). A survey of distribution and characteristics of *Glycyrrhiza glabra* L. in Turkey. *Natural Medicines* 49: 129–132.

Hayashi, H., Yasuma, M., Hiraoka, N. et al. (1996). Flavonoid variation in the leaves of *Glycyrrhiza glabra*. *Phytochemistry* 42 (3): 701–704.

Hayashi, H., Hiraoka, N., Ikeshiro, Y. et al. (1998a). Seasonal variation of glycyrrhizin and isoliquiritigenin glycosides in the root of *Glycyrrhiza glabra* L. *Biological and Pharmaceutical Bulletin* 21 (9): 987–989.

Hayashi, H., Shibano, M., Kusano, G. et al. (1998b). A field survey of *Glycyrrhiza glabra* L. *Sicily and Spain*. *Natural Medicines* 52: 259–264.

Hayashi, H., Hosono, N., Kondo, M. et al. (2000). Phylogenetic relationship of six *Glycyrrhiza* species based on rbcL sequences and chemical constituents. *Biological and Pharmaceutical Bulletin* 23 (5): 602–606.

Hayashi, H., Hattori, S., Inoue, K. et al. (2003a). Field survey of *Glycyrrhiza* plants in Central Asia (3). Chemical characterization of *G. glabra* collected in Uzbekistan. *Chemical and Pharmaceutical Bulletin* 51 (11): 1338–1340.

Hayashi, H., Hattori, S., Inoue, K. et al. (2003b). Field survey of *Glycyrrhiza* plants in central Asia (1). Characterization of *G. uralensis*, *G. glabra* and the putative intermediate collected in Kazakhstan. *Biological and Pharmaceutical Bulletin* 26 (6): 867–871.

Hayashi, H., Zhang, S.L., Nakaizumi, T. et al. (2003c). Field survey of *Glycyrrhiza* plants in central Asia (2). Characterization of phenolics and their variation in the leaves of *Glycyrrhiza* plants collected in Kazakhstan. *Chemical and Pharmaceutical Bulletin* 51 (10): 1147–1152.

Hayashi, H., Tamura, S., Chiba, R. et al. (2016). Field survey of glycyrrhiza plants in Central Asia (4). Characterization of *G. glabra* and *G. bucharica* collected in Tajikistan. *Biological and Pharmaceutical Bulletin* 39 (11): 1781–1786.

Hirayama, C., Okumura, M., Tanikawa, K. et al. (1989). A multicenter randomized controlled clinical trial of Shosaiko-to in chronic active hepatitis. *Gastroenterologia Japonica* 24 (6): 715–719.

Hosseini, S.M.A., Souri, M.K., Farhadi, N.A.S.R.I.N. et al. (2014). Changes in glycyrrhizin content of Iranian licorice (*Glycyrrhiza glabra* L.) affected by different root diameter and ecological conditions. *Agricultural Communication* 2: 27–33.

Howell, T.J., MacDougall, D.E., and Jones, P.J. (1998). Phytosterols partially explain differences in cholesterol metabolism caused by corn or olive oil feeding. *Journal of Lipid Research* 39 (4): 892–900.

Huang, R.Y., Chu, Y.L., Huang, Q.C. et al. (2014a). 18β-Glycyrrhetinic acid suppresses cell proliferation through inhibiting thromboxane synthase in non-small cell lung cancer. *PLoS One* 9 (4): e93690.

Huang, R.Y., Chu, Y.L., Jiang, Z.B. et al. (2014b). Glycyrrhizin suppresses lung adenocarcinoma cell growth through inhibition of thromboxane synthase. *Cellular Physiology and Biochemistry* 33 (2): 375–388.

Hwang, I.K., Lim, S.S., Choi, K.H. et al. (2006). Neuroprotective effects of roasted licorice, not raw form, on neuronal injury in gerbil hippocampus after transient forebrain ischemia 1. *Acta Pharmacologica Sinica* 27 (8): 959–965.

Ikeda, I. and Sugano, M. (1998). Inhibition of cholesterol absorption by plant sterols for mass intervention. *Current Opinion in Lipidology* 9 (6): 527–531.

Isbrucker, R.A. and Burdock, G.A. (2006). Risk and safety assessment on the consumption of Licorice root (*Glycyrrhiza* sp.), its extract and powder as a food ingredient, with emphasis on the pharmacology and toxicology of glycyrrhizin. *Regulatory Toxicology and Pharmacology* 46 (3): 167–192.

Ito, M., Nakashima, H., Baba, M. et al. (1987). Inhibitory effect of glycyrrhizin on the *in vitro* infectivity and cytopathic activity of the human immunodeficiency virus [HIV (HTLV-III/LAV)]. *Antiviral Research* 7 (3): 127–137.

Ito, M., Sato, A., Hirabayashi, K. et al. (1988). Mechanism of inhibitory effect of glycyrrhizin on replication of human immunodeficiency virus (HIV). *Antiviral Research* 10 (6): 289–298.

Jalilzadeh-Amin, G., Najarnezhad, V., Anassori, E. et al. (2015). Antiulcer properties of *Glycyrrhiza glabra* L. extract on experimental models of gastric ulcer in mice. *Iranian Journal of Pharmaceutical Research: IJPR* 14 (4): 1163.

Jeong, H.G., You, H.J., Park, S.J. et al. (2002). Hepatoprotective effects of 18β-glycyrrhetinic acid on carbon tetrachloride-induced liver injury: inhibition of cytochrome P450 2E1 expression. *Pharmacological Research* 46 (3): 221–227.

Kao, T.C., Wu, C.H., and Yen, G.C. (2014). Bioactivity and potential health benefits of licorice. *Journal of Agricultural and Food Chemistry* 62 (3): 542–553.

Karahan, F., Avsar, C., Ozyigit, I.I., and Berber, I. (2016). Antimicrobial and antioxidant activities of medicinal plant *Glycyrrhiza glabra* var. *glandulifera* from different habitats. *Biotechnology & Biotechnological Equipment* 30 (4): 797–804.

Kataya, H.H., Hamza, A.A., Ramadan, G.A., and Khasawneh, M.A. (2011). Effect of licorice extract on the complications of diabetes nephropathy in rats. *Drug and Chemical Toxicology* 34 (2): 101–108.

Kaur, P., Sharma, N., Singh, B. et al. (2012). Modulation of genotoxicity of oxidative mutagens by glycyrrhizic acid from *Glycyrrhiza glabra* L. *Pharmacognosy Research* 4 (4): 189.

Khan, M.S. and Ahmad, I. (2020). Diversity of antimutagenic phytocompounds from Indian medicinal plants. In: *Herbal Medicine in India*, 401–412. Singapore: Springer.

Kim, D.H., Hong, S.W., Kim, B.T. et al. (2000). Biotransformation of glycyrrhizin by human intestinal bacteria and its relation to biological activities. *Archives of Pharmacal Research* 23 (2): 172.

Kim, S.W., Lim, C.M., Lee, H.K., and Lee, J.K. (2011a). The use of stronger neo-minophagen C, a glycyrrhizin-containing preparation, in robust neuroprotection in the postischemic brain. *Anatomy & Cell Biology* 44 (4): 304–313.

Kim, H.Y., Kim, S.Y., Lee, J.H., and Han, Y.M. (2011b). Antitumor effect of 18β-glycyrrhetinic acid against human tumor xenografts caused by A549 cancer cell. *Yakhak Hoeji* 55 (1): 39–44.

Kim, S.R., Jeon, H.J., Park, H.J. et al. (2013). Glycyrrhetinic acid inhibits *Porphyromonas gingivalis* lipopolysaccharide-induced vascular permeability via the suppression of interleukin-8. *Inflammation Research* 62 (2): 145–154.

Kinoshita, T., Tamura, Y., and Mizutani, K. (2005). The isolation and structure elucidation of minor isoflavonoids from licorice of *Glycyrrhiza glabra* origin. *Chemical and Pharmaceutical Bulletin* 53 (7): 847–849.

Kiso, Y., Tohkin, M., Hikino, H. et al. (1984). Mechanism of antihepatotoxic activity of glycyrrhizin, I: effect on free radical generation and lipid peroxidation. *Planta Medica* 50 (04): 298–302.

Kitagawa, I., Chen, W.Z., Hori, K. et al. (1994). Chemical studies of Chinese licorice-roots. I. Elucidation of five new flavonoid constituents from the roots of *Glycyrrhiza glabra* L. collected in Xinjiang. *Chemical and pharmaceutical bulletin* 42 (5): 1056–1062.

Kovalenko, P.G., Antonjuk, V.P., and Maliuta, S.S. (2004). Secondary metabolites synthesis in transformed cells of *Glycyrrhiza glabra* L. and *Potentilla alba* L. as producents of radioprotective compounds. *Ukr. Bioorg Acta* 1 (2): 13–22.

Krausse, R., Bielenberg, J., Blaschek, W., and Ullmann, U. (2004). in vitro anti-*Helicobacter pylori* activity of *Extractum liquiritiae*, glycyrrhizin and its metabolites. *Journal of Antimicrobial Chemotherapy* 54 (1): 243–246.

Kroes, B.H., Beukelman, C.J., Van Den Berg, A.J.J. et al. (1997). Inhibition of human complement by β-glycyrrhetinic acid. *Immunology* 90 (1): 115–120.

Kuang, Y., Lin, Y., Li, K. et al. (2017). Screening of hepatoprotective compounds from licorice against carbon tetrachloride and acetaminophen induced HepG2 cells injury. *Phytomedicine* 34: 59–66.

Lee, C.H., Park, S.W., Kim, Y.S. et al. (2007). Protective mechanism of glycyrrhizin on acute liver injury induced by carbon tetrachloride in mice. *Biological and Pharmaceutical Bulletin* 30 (10): 1898–1904.

Li, S. and Luo, X. (2003). *Compendium of Materia Medica: (Bencao Gangmu)*. Beijing, China: Foreign Languages Press.

Li, W., Asada, Y., and Yoshikawa, T. (1998). Antimicrobial flavonoids from *Glycyrrhiza glabra* hairy root cultures. *Planta Medica* 64 (08): 746–747.

Li, W., Asada, Y., and Yoshikawa, T. (2000). Flavonoid constituents from *Glycyrrhiza glabra* hairy root cultures. *Phytochemistry* 55 (5): 447–456.

Li, K., Ji, S., Song, W. et al. (2017). Glycybridins A–K, bioactive phenolic compounds from *Glycyrrhiza glabra*. *Journal of Natural Products* 80 (2): 334–346.

Lu, Y., Wu, X., Dong, Y. et al. (2010). Anesthetic sevoflurane causes neurotoxicity differently in neonatal naïve and Alzheimer's disease transgenic mice. *Anesthesiology* 112 (6): 1404.

Luqman, S. and Pezzuto, J.M. (2010). NFκB: a promising target for natural products in cancer chemoprevention. *Phytotherapy Research* 24 (7): 949–963.

Malekinejad, H., Mirzakhani, N., Razi, M. et al. (2011). Protective effects of melatonin and *Glycyrrhiza glabra* extract on ochratoxin A—induced damages on testes in mature rats. *Human & Experimental Toxicology* 30 (2): 110–123.

Manns, M.P., Wedemeyer, H., Singer, A. et al. (2012). Glycyrrhizin in patients who failed previous interferon alpha-based therapies: biochemical and histological effects after 52 weeks. *Journal of Viral Hepatitis* 19 (8): 537–546.

Martins, N., Silva, S., Barros, L., Ferreira, I.C., and Henriques, M. (2014). in vitro study of the antifungal potential of Glycyrrhiza glabra L. against Candida species. *Proceedings of the 62th International Congress and Annual Meeting of the Society for Medicinal Plant and Natural Product Research-GA*, Guimaraes, Portugal (31 August 2014).

Maurya, S.K., Raj, K., and Srivastava, A.K. (2009). Antidyslipidaemic activity of *Glycyrrhiza glabra* in high fructose diet induced dsyslipidaemic Syrian golden hamsters. *Indian Journal of Clinical Biochemistry* 24 (4): 404.

Mitscher, L.A., Park, Y.H., Clark, D., and Beal, J.L. (1980). Antimicrobial agents from higher plants. Antimicrobial isoflavanoids and related substances from *Glycyrrhiza glabra* L. var. *typica*. *Journal of Natural Products* 43 (2): 259–269.

Mitscher, L.A., Telikepalli, H., McGhee, E., and Shankel, D.M. (1996). Natural antimutagenic agents. *Mutation Research/Fundamental and Molecular Mechanisms of Mutagenesis* 350 (1): 143–152.

Muchnik, Z.S. (1976). Content of glycyrrhizic acid, sugars and extractive substances from the subsoil organs of liquorice cultivated in Moldavia. *Ratit Resur* 12: 78–84.

Mukherjee, M., Bhaskaran, N., Srinath, R. et al. (2010). Anti-ulcer and antioxidant activity of GutGard. *Indian Journal of Experimental Biology* 48: 269–274.

Najeeb, V.D. and Al-Refai, A.S. (2015). Antibacterial effect and healing potential of topically applied licorice root extract on experimentally induced oral wounds in rabbits. *Saudi Journal of Oral Sciences* 2 (1): 10.

Nirmala, P. and Selvaraj, T. (2011). Anti-inflammatory and anti-bacterial activities of *Glycyrrhiza glabra* L. *Journal of Agricultural Technology* 7 (3): 815–823.

Nomura, T. and Fukai, T. (1998). Phenolic constituents of licorice (*Glycyrrhiza* species). In: *Fortschritte der Chemie organischer Naturstoffe/Progress in the Chemistry of Organic Natural Products*, 1–140. Vienna: Springer.

Oakenfull, D. and Sidhu, G.S. (1990). Could saponins be a useful treatment for hypercholesterolaemia? *European Journal of Clinical Nutrition* 44 (1): 79–88.

Ojha, S., Golechha, M., Kumari, S. et al. (2013). *Glycyrrhiza glabra* protects from myocardial ischemia–reperfusion injury by improving hemodynamic, biochemical, histopathological and ventricular function. *Experimental and Toxicologic Pathology* 65 (1–2): 219–227.

Okada, K., Tamura, Y., Yamamoto, M. et al. (1989). Identification of antimicrobial and antioxidant constituents from Licorice of Ussian and Xinjiang origin. *Chemical and Pharmaceutical Bulletin* 37 (9): 2528–2530.

Parle, M., Dhingra, D., and Kulkarni, S.K. (2004). Memory-strengthening activity of *Glycyrrhiza glabra* in exteroceptive and interoceptive behavioral models. *Journal of Medicinal Food* 7 (4): 462–466.

Pastorino, G., Cornara, L., Soares, S. et al. (2018). Liquorice (*Glycyrrhiza glabra*): a phytochemical and pharmacological review. *Phytotherapy Research* 32 (12): 2323–2339.

Pompei, R., Flore, O., Marccialis, M.A. et al. (1979). Glycyrrhizic acid inhibits virus growth and inactivates virus particles. *Nature* 281 (5733): 689–690.

Puram, S., Suh, H.C., Kim, S.U. et al. (2013). Effect of GutGard in the management of *Helicobacter pylori*: a randomized double blind placebo controlled study. *Evidence-Based Complementary and Alternative Medicine* 2013: 1–8.

Quintana, S.E., Cueva, C., Villanueva-Bermejo, D. et al. (2019). Antioxidant and antimicrobial assessment of licorice supercritical extracts. *Industrial Crops and Products* 139: 111496.

Račková, L., Jančinová, V., Petríková, M. et al. (2007). Mechanism of anti-inflammatory action of liquorice extract and glycyrrhizin. *Natural Product Research* 21 (14): 1234–1241.

Raveendra, K.R., Srinivasa, V., Sushma, K.R. et al. (2012). An extract of *Glycyrrhiza glabra* (GutGard) alleviates symptoms of functional dyspepsia: a randomized, double-blind, placebo-controlled study. *Evidence-Based Complementary and Alternative Medicine* 2012: 1–9.

Revers, F.E. (1956). Clinical and pharmacological investigations on extract of licorice. *Acta Medica Scandinavica* 154: 749–751.

Rizzato, G., Scalabrin, E., Radaelli, M. et al. (2017). A new exploration of licorice metabolome. *Food Chemistry* 221: 959–968.

Rodino, S., Butu, A., Butu, M., and Cornea, P.C. (2015). Comparative studies on antibacterial activity of licorice, elderberry and dandelion. *Digest Journal of Nanomaterials and Biostructures* 10 (3): 947–955.

Schwamberger, K. and Reissigl, H. (1980). Carbenoxolone patients with gastric ulcers. A double-blind trial. *Scandinavian Journal of Gastroenterology. Supplement* 65: 59–62.

Scientific Committee on Food (2003). *Opinion of the Scientific Committee on Food on Glycyrrhizinic Acid and its Ammonium Salt*.

Shankel, D.M. and Clarke, C.H. (1990). Specificity of antimutagens against chemical mutagens in microbial systems. In: *Antimutagenesis and Anticarcinogenesis Mechanisms II*, 457–460. Boston, MA: Springer.

Sharma, V. and Agrawal, R.C. (2014). *in vivo* antioxidant and hepatoprotective potential of *Glycyrrhiza glabra* extract on carbon tetra chloride (CCl4) induced oxidative-stress mediated hepatotoxicity. *International Journal of Research in Medical Sciences* 2 (1): 314–320.

Sharma, G., Kar, S., Palit, S., and Das, P.K. (2012). 18β-glycyrrhetinic acid induces apoptosis through modulation of Akt/FOXO3a/Bim pathway in human breast cancer MCF-7 cells. *Journal of Cellular Physiology* 227 (5): 1923–1931.

Shen, X., Dong, Y., Xu, Z. et al. (2013). Selective anesthesia-induced neuroinflammation in developing mouse brain and cognitive impairment. *Anesthesiology: The Journal of the American Society of Anesthesiologists* 118 (3): 502–515.

Shin, Y.W., Bae, E.A., Lee, B. et al. (2007). *in vitro* and *in vivo* antiallergic effects of *Glycyrrhiza glabra* and its components. *Planta Medica* 73 (03): 257–261.

Sultana, S., Haque, A., Hamid, K. et al. (2010). Antimicrobial, cytotoxic and antioxidant activity of methanolic extract of *Glycyrrhiza glabra*. *Agriculture and Biology Journal of North America* 1 (5): 957–960.

Sumiyama, K., Kobayashi, M., Miyashiro, E., and Koike, M. (1991). Combination therapy with transfer factor and high dose stronger neo-minophagen C in chronic hepatitis B in children (HBe Ag positive). *Acta Paediatrica Japonica: Overseas Edition* 33 (3): 327–334.

Tabuchi, M., Imamura, S., Kawakami, Z. et al. (2012). The blood–brain barrier permeability of 18β-glycyrrhetinic acid, a major metabolite of glycyrrhizin in *Glycyrrhiza* root, a constituent of the traditional Japanese medicine yokukansan. *Cellular and Molecular Neurobiology* 32 (7): 1139–1146.

Teltumbde, A.K., Wahurwagh, A.K., Lonare, M.K., and Nesari, T.M. (2013). Effect of Yashtimadhu (*Glycyrrhiza glabra*) on intelligence and memory function in male adolescents. *Scholars Journal of Applied Medical Sciences* 1 (2): 90–95.

Toyokuni, S. (2008). Molecular mechanisms of oxidative stress-induced carcinogenesis: from epidemiology to oxygenomics. *IUBMB Life* 60 (7): 441–447.

Tripathi, M., Singh, B.K., and Kakkar, P. (2009). Glycyrrhizic acid modulates t-BHP induced apoptosis in primary rat hepatocytes. *Food and Chemical Toxicology* 47 (2): 339–347.

Utsunomiya, T., Kobayashi, M., Pollard, R.B., and Suzuki, F. (1997). Glycyrrhizin, an active component of licorice roots, reduces morbidity and mortality of mice infected with lethal doses of influenza virus. *Antimicrobial Agents and Chemotherapy* 41 (3): 551–556.

Vaya, J., Belinky, P.A., and Aviram, M. (1997). Antioxidant constituents from licorice roots: isolation, structure elucidation and antioxidative capacity toward LDL oxidation. *Free Radical Biology and Medicine* 23 (2): 302–313.

Visavadiya, N.P. and Narasimhacharya, A.V. (2006). Hypocholesterolaemic and antioxidant effects of *Glycyrrhiza glabra* (Linn) in rats. *Molecular Nutrition & Food Research* 50 (11): 1080–1086.

Visavadiya, N.P., Soni, B., and Dalwadi, N. (2009). Evaluation of antioxidant and anti-atherogenic properties of *Glycyrrhiza glabra* root using *in vitro* models. *International Journal of Food Sciences and Nutrition* 60: 135–149.

Wang, D., Wong, H.K., Feng, Y.B., and Zhang, Z.J. (2014). 18beta-glycyrrhetinic acid induces apoptosis in pituitary adenoma cells via ROS/MAPKs-mediated pathway. *Journal of Neuro-Oncology* 116 (2): 221–230.

Wang, H., Zhu, Z.F., and Gao, Y. (2015a). Effect of glycyrrhizin on gastric cancer BGC-823 cell proliferation. *Shi Jie Hua Ren Xiao Hua Za Zhi* 23: 2868–2873.

Wang, H.L., Li, Y.X., Niu, Y.T. et al. (2015b). Observing anti-inflammatory and anti-nociceptive activities of glycyrrhizin through regulating COX-2 and pro-inflammatory cytokines expressions in mice. *Inflammation* 38 (6): 2269–2278.

Wang, W., Chen, X., Zhang, J. et al. (2016). Glycyrrhizin attenuates isoflurane-induced cognitive deficits in neonatal rats via its anti-inflammatory activity. *Neuroscience* 316: 328–336.

Wang, Z.F., Liu, J., Yang, Y.A., and Zhu, H.L. (2020). A review: the anti-inflammatory, anticancer, antibacterial properties of four kinds of licorice flavonoids isolated from licorice. *Current Medicinal Chemistry* 27 (12): 1997–2011.

Williamson, E.M. (2003). *Potter's Cyclopedia of Herbal Medicine*, 269–271. Saffron Walden: *CW Daniel*.

Wojcikowski, K., Stevenson, L., Leach, D. et al. (2007). Antioxidant capacity of 55 medicinal herbs traditionally used to treat the urinary system: a comparison using a sequential three-solvent extraction process. *The Journal of Alternative and Complementary Medicine* 13 (1): 103–110.

Wu, X., Zhang, L., Gurley, E. et al. (2008). Prevention of free fatty acid–induced hepatic lipotoxicity by 18β-glycyrrhetinic acid through lysosomal and mitochondrial pathways. *Hepatology* 47 (6): 1905–1915.

Xu, S.M., Zhou, L., Liu, Z.G. et al. (2011). Glycyrrhetinic acid induces apoptosis and alters survivin gene expression in human myeloma cell line U266. *Zhongguo shi yan xue ye xue za zhi* 19 (3): 652–655.

Young, G.P., St John, D.J., and Coventry, D.A. (1979). Treatment of duodenal ulcer with carbenoxolone sodium: a double-masked endoscopic trial. *Medical Journal of Australia* 1 (1): 2–5.

Zani, F., Cuzzoni, M.T., Daglia, M. et al. (1993). Inhibition of mutagenicity in *Salmonella typhimurium* by *Glycyrrhiza glabra* extract, glycyrrhizinic acid and 18α- and 18β-glycyrrhetinic acids. *Planta Medica* 59 (6): 502–507.

Zargaran, A., Zarshenas, M.M., Mehdizadeh, A., and Mohagheghzadeh, A. (2013). Management of tremor in medieval Persia. *Journal of the History of the Neurosciences* 22 (1): 53–61.

Zhang, L. and Wang, B. (2002). Randomized clinical trial with two doses (100 and 40 ml) of Stronger Neo-Minophagen C in Chinese patients with chronic hepatitis B. *Hepatology Research* 24 (3): 220–227.

Zhang, J.Z., Gao, W.Y., Gao, Y. et al. (2011). Analysis of influences of spaceflight on chemical constituents in licorice by HPLC-ESI-MS/MS. *Acta Physiologiae Plantarum* 33 (6): 2511–2520.

Zhang, L., Zhang, J., Yang, L. et al. (2013). Isoflurane and sevoflurane increase interleukin-6 levels through the nuclear factor-kappa B pathway in neuroglioma cells. *British Journal of Anaesthesia* 110 (suppl 1): 82–91.

Zhu, Z., Li, C., Wang, X. et al. (2010). 2,2′,4′-Trihydroxychalcone from *Glycyrrhiza glabra* as a new specific BACE1 inhibitor efficiently ameliorates memory impairment in mice. *Journal of Neurochemistry* 114 (2): 374–385.

12

Therapeutic Applications of Bovine Colostrum Supplements, Omega-3 PUFAs, and Flavonoids in the Prevention of Noncommunicable Diseases

Siddhi Bagwe-Parab[1], Pratik Yadav[1], Harpal S. Buttar[2], Harvinder Popli[3], and Ginpreet Kaur[1]

[1] *Department of Pharmacology, Shobhaben Pratapbhai Patel School of Pharmacy & Technology Management, SVKM's NMIMS, Mumbai, Maharashtra, India*
[2] *Department of Pathology and Laboratory Medicine, Faculty of Medicine, University of Ottawa, Ottawa, ON, Canada*
[3] *Department of Pharmacy, Delhi Pharmaceutical Sciences and Research University, New Delhi, Delhi, India*

12.1 Introduction

Bovine colostrum (BC), which is also called bisnings, beestings, or primary milk, is the first mammary secretion in all mammalian species, including humans, and is provided to their newborns during the first 24–72 hours post-parturition. Most of the mammalian species produce colostrum few days prior to giving birth. Human colostrum or BC is a concentrated, sticky, yellowish liquid, which is comprised of numerous antibodies, growth factors, antimicrobials, anti-inflammatory lactoferrin, vitamins, minerals, and essential fatty acids at a very high concentration compared to the ordinary milk. In newborns, colostrum contributes to physical growth, immune function, and development of gastrointestinal tract. In adults, colostrum promotes healing of gut inflammation and protects against gut pathogens (bacteria, viruses, fungi, yeast, mold etc.), and leaky gut syndrome. Colostrum is well acknowledged for providing many vital health benefits to the newborn. Research has shown that the cow or buffalo colostrum is 100-fold to 1000-fold more potent as opposed to the human colostrum. Therefore, the human infants can thrive on cow or buffalo colostrum supplements to gain health benefits whose mothers are unable breastfeed after delivery. BC is an emerging nutraceutical and innovative therapeutic products that are being developed for children and adults (Bagwe et al. 2015; Buttar et al. 2017).

BC comprises of the nutrients which are needed for growth and development of the new-born calf. BC is a rich source of lipids, proteins, amino acids, minerals, and vitamins. Additionally, it is also rich in immunoglobulins, growth factor, hormones, nucleotides, peptides, enzymes, cytokines, polyamines, and other bioactive peptides. The lipids present in the BC are emulsified in the form of globules, which are coated with the lipid membranes. The proteins that are present in BC are in a colloidal dispersion form, which are called as micelles. Most of the minerals and also lactose are in the solution form. The composition of BC varies with various factors such as, age, breed, stage of lactation, nutrition, and health status of the mother. Some proteins present in the BC are involved in the development of early immunological, as well as non-immunological, response. BC contains many diverse fatty acids. It also includes some of the omega-3 fatty acids (Buttar et al. 2017).

Handbook of Nutraceuticals and Natural Products: Biological, Medicinal, and Nutritional Properties and Applications,
Volume 2, First Edition. Edited by Preetha Balakrishnan and Sreerag Gopi.
© 2022 John Wiley & Sons, Inc. Published 2022 by John Wiley & Sons, Inc.

It has also been reported that BC is 100-fold to 1000-fold more potent than human colostrum. This means that even human infants can rely on cow or buffalo colostrum to gain health benefits whose mothers are unable to breastfeed their babies. The immunoglobulins present in BC show antimicrobial activity by forming a chelated complex with bacterial and viral antigens. BC also has high anti-inflammatory activity and antioxidant properties. The oxidative stress and microbial infections lead to inflammation response and generation of free radicals such as reactive oxygen species (ROS) and reactive nitrogen intermediates (RNI), which in the absence of antioxidants can cause DNA damage. High levels of antioxidants and growth factors present in colostrum have proven beneficial in wound healing and to reduce oxidative stress in athletes due to heavy exercise. The focus of the present mini-review is to highlight the antimicrobial, anti-inflammatory, and wound healing activities of BC, as well as the gastrointestinal inflammation caused by Celiac and Crohn's disease. In standardized in vitro tests, BC at 100 µg/ml showed strong antimicrobial activity against both Gram −ve and +ve strains of bacteria (*Escherichia coli, Staphylococcus aureus, Pseudomonas vulgaris, Enterobacter aerogenes, and Salmonella typhi*). In addition, the carrageenan-induced rat paw edema was moderately reduced in BC-treated animals. It was found that the combination of BC with diclofenac produces greater anti-inflammatory effects than that of BC alone, which suggests that combination treatment may reduce or minimize the side effects of this anti-inflammatory synthetic drug. Our findings suggest that BC could be used as an alternative remedy for treating the microbial infections and inflammation-related disorders (Yadav et al. 2016). K-casein present in BC has a potent antiviral property. It is a glycosylated protein which is responsible for antiviral activity by binding directly to the viral antigens through the glycosylated residue (Inagaki et al. 2014).

An excellent review and meta-analysis by Glowka et al. (2020) has shown that BC supplementation improves immunological function and reduces the risk of upper respiratory tract infections among athletes who undergo intensive and prolonged physical training. However, further well-designed, randomized, placebo-controlled, multicenter clinical trials are needed to determine the long-term safety, effectiveness, and optimal doses of BC supplements in athletes and physically active people (Główka et al. 2020).

Omega-3 fatty acids (W-3 FAs), which are also called as ω-3 polyunsaturated fatty acids (ω-3 PUFA), and their subtypes are comprised of carboxylic acid (−COOH) at one end and methyl (−CH3) group at the terminal end (Figure 12.1). The carboxylic acid (−COOH) at the beginning of the fatty acid chain is called "alpha" and the methyl (−CH3) group at the terminal end is called "omega." The name omega (ω⁻) fatty acids is derived from the location of the first double bond, which is considered from the omega (ω⁻) end. Therefore, the first double bond in the ω-3 fatty acids is in the middle of the third and fourth carbon atoms at the methyl (−CH3) end. However, the standard chemical nomenclature system according to the International Union of Pure and Applied Chemistry (IUPAC) starts from the carboxyl end (Cherian 2008). In mammals, including humans, the ω-3 fatty acids cannot be synthesized endogenously. Therefore, dietary consumption of ω-3 fatty acids is essential for the physiological functioning of human body. Humans acquire the shorter-chain ω-3 fatty acid containing 18 carbons and 3 double bonds through diet. The same shorter-chain ω-3 fatty acids can be used to synthesize the more vital long-chain ω-3 fatty acids made up of 20 carbons and 5 double bonds. The shorter-chain ω-3 fatty acids are generally called α-linolenic acid (ALA), whereas the longer-chain ω-3 fatty acids are called as eicosapentaenoic acid (EPA). The EPA can be metabolically converted to form docosahexaenoic acid (DHA), which is made up of 22 carbons and 6 double bonds. DHA is the structural part of the cell membrane phospholipids and is also involved in neuronal cell growth and differentiation, as well as in neuronal signaling mechanisms in the central nervous system (CNS). During the ageing process, the ability of humans to synthesize longer-chain

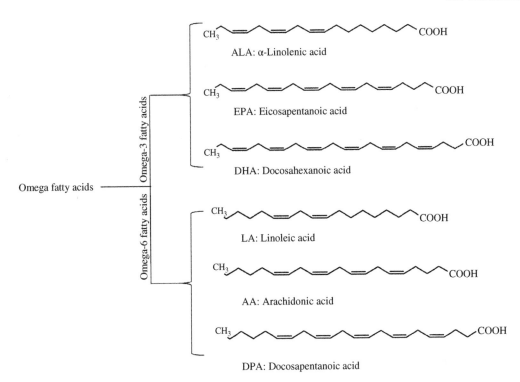

Figure 12.1 Classification of Omega fatty acids.

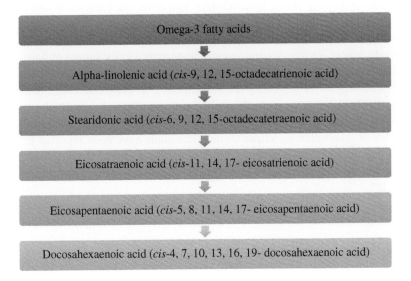

Figure 12.2 Metabolic cascade of ω-3 fatty acids (Haug et al. 2007).

ω-3 fatty acids from shorter-chain ω-3 fatty acid precursors is reduced, and therefore the health benefits from the endogenous synthesis of long-chain fatty acids is markedly decreased in elderly humans (Simopoulos 1991). Figure 12.2 shows the metabolic cascade of ω-3 fatty acids.

A number of animal studies have revealed that the chronic supplementation of *n*-3 PUFAs produce beneficial effects in neuromuscular activities. It is estimated that the alteration in the composition and fluidity of the cell membrane might be responsible for the accelerated conductance of action potentials through the neurons, thus, increasing the rate of motor unit firing on the sarcolemma (Patten et al. 2002). Similar electrical conduction pathway is predicted to occur in the skeletal muscles. Lewis et al. (2015) have reported the enhancement of muscular strength through neuromuscular recruitment during exhaustive-exercise trainings. They have suggested that such activity may be due to the increased levels of DHA, which is an essential constituent of cell membrane phospholipids of the neurons and is essential for neuronal cascades. As mentioned earlier, BC is also rich in the omega fatty acids. In future, well-designed studies should be conducted in athletes with BC supplementation to investigate the role of omega fatty acids in the neuromuscular performance.

The secondary metabolites of plants are known as flavonoids and over 10 000 different chemical structures of flavonoids have been identified till date. Flavonoids are widely distributed plant pigments that protect against the damage caused by UV radiation. Due to their strong antioxidant and anti-inflammation properties, the flavonoids capture the excessive amount of free radicals generated by oxidative stress and prevent inflammation-induced ailments. Dietary intake of flavonoids is very important for the normal physiological function of the body. There is overwhelming evidence that diets rich in flavonoids play an important role in the prevention of noncommunicable diseases (NCDs). Flavonoids also help in the prevention of metabolic abnormalities such as insulin resistance, glucose intolerance, and oxidative stress through their antioxidant and anti-inflammatory actions.

Polyphenol consists of many chemical classes, one of which is flavonoids, and it has further six subclasses: anthocyanins, flavanols, flavanones, flavones, flavonols, and isoflavones. Anthocyanins are mostly present in flowers, grains, fruits (e.g. chokeberry, elderberry juice concentrate, bilberries), vegetables (e.g. dock, kale, fennel). Flavanols are present in cocoa, chocolate, tea, and fruits. Flavones are found abundantly in parsley and oregano. Flavonols are commonly found in plants, capers, parsley, elderberry juice. Isoflavones occur in soy food (soy flour, soybeans mature seeds, natto). The most common and important dietary source of flavonoids are fruits, vegetable, seeds, tea, and cereals. The other abundant sources of the flavonoids are berries, dock, chocolate, cowpeas, parsley, oregano, and capers. Flavonoids have also been isolated from the plant parts like flowers, stems, fruits, seeds, nuts, etc. They are obtained generally from the vascular type of plants in the form of phenyl benzopyrones (phenylchromones). The most prominent source of flavonoids are citrus fruits. Flavonoids have been reported for their antioxidant, anti-inflammatory, antidiabetic, anti-obesity effects. Also, recent studies suggest the role of flavonoids in amelioration of the cardiovascular and neurodegenerative disorders (Buttar et al. 2017).

12.2 Lipid Components of Colostrum

The total amount of fatty lipids in BC is about 33 g/l. Triglycerides consist of around 95% of the lipid fraction, which are basically composed of the long chain fatty acids of different lengths. Each triacylglycerol molecule has a combination of fatty acids, which gives the liquidity to the molecule at the body temperature. Other lipids present in the BC are cholesterol (<0.5% of the lipid fraction), diacylglycerol (2% per lipid fraction), free fatty acids (<0.5% of the lipid fraction), phospholipids (1% per lipid fraction) (Haug et al. 2007). EPA and DHA are also present in BC. Different types of omega-3 polyunsaturated fatty acids (PUFAs) and their metabolic cascade are summarized in Table 12.1 and Figure 12.1.

Table 12.1 Types of omega-3-fatty acids, their source, and therapeutic uses (Simopoulos 1991).

Omega-3 fatty acids			
Types of omega-3-fatty acids	Alpha-linolenic acid	Eicosapentaenoic acid	Docosahexaenoic acid
Source	Flaxseed oil, pumpkin seeds, and walnuts	Fish oil, BC	Fish oil, BC
Therapeutic uses	Anti-inflammatory	Anti-inflammatory	Improves brain and neuronal function

Table 12.2 BC and whole milk fatty acids and percent daily requirements in humans.

BC component	**Concentration per liter of whole milk**	**Health benefits**	**References**
Fat	6.7%	Energy rich source	Bagwe et al. (2015), Yadav et al. (2016), and Buttar et al. (2017)
Saturated fatty acids	19.0 g/l	Increase HDL, decrease LDL, and total cholesterol. Inhibit bacteria, viruses	Haug et al. (2007)
Oleic acid	8.0 g/l	Induces hypotension, regulates membrane lipid structure	Terés et al. (2008)
Lauric acid	0.8 g/l	Inhibits antral and duodenal pressure waves, stimulates the pyloric motility, releases cholecystokinin, exhibits antiviral and antibacterial activity	Feltrin et al. (2007)
Myristic acid	3.0 g/l	Increases LDL and HDL	Haug et al. (2007)
Palmitic acid	8 g/l	Increases LDL and HDL	
Linoleic acid	1.2 g/l	Source of omega-6 fatty acid	
Alpha linolenic acid	0.75 g/l	Source of omega-3 fatty acid	

Source: Nagy and Tiuca (2017).

12.2.1 Role of Omega-3 PUFA in Brain Development and Function

Among its multiple dimensions, the human brain possesses intellectual and learning abilities, information processing proficiencies, cognitive and emotion functions, as well as neuroendocrine features, just to name a few. The focus of this review is on the immense role of dietary factors in the development and maintenance of diverse brain functions and synaptic plasticity of brain health and mental functions. To a large extent, the human is anatomically quite similar to other mammals (rodents, rabbits, primates), but differs in its higher functional optimal performance. The factors where the human brain functions extensively are physical training, food deficiency/abstinence, and social/scholarly/intellectual engagement. Implementation of automation technologies have eliminated the process of vigorous exercise and fasting. Therefore, it leaves only intellectual challenges to boost the brain and neuronal function. Additionally, sedentary lifestyles encourage metabolic disorders like obesity and diabetes. Also, the risk of cardiovascular disease (CVD) and cognitive impairment increases, which leads to the development of many chronic neurological disorders, including Alzheimer's disease (Mattson 2015).

Docosahaxenoic acid (DHA) is an important structural constituent of cell membrane phospholipids. It is involved in neuronal cell growth and differentiation, as well as in neuronal signaling mechanisms in the CNS. The endogenous synthesis of DHA occurs by the desaturation of ALA and AA. Maternal deficiency of ALA and AA causes fetal brain impairment and postnatal learning deficits and psychiatric problems during childhood and adult life. Lower endogenous synthesis and accumulation of DHA in the CNS is most likely to contribute in cognitive dysfunction and memory decline in elderly humans. Thus, the intake of dietary precursors of DHA, such as ALA and AA, exerts an important influence on brain development and function throughout the life span (Lauritzen et al. 2016).

12.3   Unsaturated Fatty Acids Present in BC

As shown in Table 12.2, oleic acid (OA) is present in highest concentration in BC. Therefore, the OA supplementation in humans is mainly through milk and milk products. OA lowers total cholesterol, low-density lipoprotein (LDL)-cholesterol, and triglycerides in plasma (Kris-Etherton et al. 1999). The replacement of saturated fatty acids with unsaturated fatty acids like OA reduces the risk of coronary artery disease, hyperlipidemia, etc. Several studies have also reported the chemoprotective effect of OA. The cell membranes mainly consist of the fatty acids. Lipid portion of BC is rich in OA, as well as other PUFAs. The other major PUFAs present in the BC or whole milk are linoleic acid and alpha-linoleic acid. They are further involved in the synthesis of arachidonic acid (AA) and EPA. These acids are converted to eicosanoids, which are metabolically active compounds with wide variety of cellular functions. Eicosanoids are derivatives of linoleic acid, via AA pathway, and alleviate blood platelet aggregation and risk of stroke. The eicosanoids produced from the long W-3 FAs also decrease the risk of coronary heart disease (De Lorgeril et al. 1994). EPA possesses the ability to halt the conversion of the omega-6 fatty acids to eicosanoids, which are harmful, thereby reducing myocardial risk and inhibiting tumorigenesis. PUFAs significantly affect the signal transduction mechanism and alter the gene expression. Therefore, it can be understood that the PUFAs are responsible for altering the several metabolic functions (Keenan and Patton 1995; Ontsouka et al. 2003).

12.4   Therapeutic Role of BC in Wound, Burn and Diabetic Foot Ulcer Healing

Management of wounds and burns is significant as it reduces the risk of infection and accelerate the healing process. Unattended and improper management can lead to septic shock and fatality. The reasons for these fatalities can possibly be, severe infections, traumatic shock, organ failure and nerve damage (Williams et al. 2009). Inappropriate use of drugs and nonsurgical approaches can lead to tissue gangrene, peripheral vascular disease, peripheral neuropathy, and sepsis (Enoch et al. 2006) Therefore, usage of effective, safe, and nonirritant components for the treatment of wounds and burn injuries is essential.

Colostrum is the secretion obtained post-parturition for a period of 24–48 hours from the mammary glands of female mammals (Tokuyama et al. 1990; Stelwagen et al. 2009). It acts as a laxative to deliver early stools and aids in the passage of bilirubin, which prevents constipation and jaundice in newborn, respectively (Cohen 2006; de Almeida and Draque 2007). Research on BC has revealed that it is 100–1000 times more potent than the human colostrum; therefore, it can be consumed as a supplement by the human beings for its health benefits (Sarker et al. 1998; Elfstrand et al. 2002). BC has proven to be very effective and safe in the treatment of wound and other internal, as well as external, injuries. It has been acclaimed for its antimicrobial, anti-inflammatory, wound healing, and various other properties. Historically, its applications pertaining to skin injuries, skin diseases, eye irrigation etc. are cited in the traditional medicinal books in Ayurveda. BC topical creams are used for its wound healing and antiageing properties, likewise its powder is orally administered for healing of internal wounds and abscesses. Biological dressings containing colostrum powder are used for the healing of deep wounds, which extend beyond deep fascia to the muscles and other organs. These dressings have shown to promote wound healing with more patient compliance in terms of less number of dressing requirement and less pain (Kshirsagar et al. 2015). The immunomodulatory function of colostrum has given it antibacterial, antiviral, and antifungal property. Molecular compounds like κ-casein and Bovine k-caseino glycomacropeptide (GMP) are under research for its antibacterial and antiviral properties. GMP also plays a major role in binding to *E. coli* enterotoxins and cholera toxin, which is demonstrated on the Normal Chinese hamster ovary (CHO)-K1 cells, where the normal spherical-shaped cells transformed to spindle-shaped post cholera infection. The spherical shape of the (CHO)-K1 cells were regained after treatment with GMP (Kawasaki et al. 1992). GMP also plays an important role in the prevention of dental caries by adhering to cariogenic bacteria like *Streptococcus mutans, S. sanguis,* and *S. sobrinus* present in the oral cavity (Neeser et al. 1994). Lactoferrin present in BC also exhibits antibacterial and growth promoting properties. It has bifidobacterial growth promoting factors, which is said to prevent pathogenic bacterial growth and defends human body from gastrointestinal diseases (Gyorgy et al. 1954; Petschow and Talbott 1991). Recent studies have been performed, which shows its anti-bacterial effect on Gram-positive bacteria, as well as Gram-negative bacteria. Many studies have proven lactoferrin as an antiviral, antifungal, antiparasitic, and anticancer compound (Giansanti et al. 2016).

Wound healing is a complex and dynamic process of replacing devitalized and misplaced cellular structures and tissue layers. Until now plethora of drug therapies have been studied and prescribed for wound healing, but the acceleration of healing is the important parameter, which decides the efficacy of the drug. BC is one of the most promised drug therapies for wound healing. Drugs therapies antecedent to BC lack in accelerative healing and chronic safety, which BC retains. Many preclinical studies have demonstrated the effect of BC on wound healing. Recent study on Swiss albino mice have validated the effect of BC on wound healing and repairment. The study contributed promising results stating that BC was effective in increasing tensile strength and collagen content of wound. It also accelerated the epithelialization, as well as improved the histopathological scoring. Another study reported predominance of fibroblasts, angiogenesis at the wound site, and systematic collagen fiber arrangement (Patil et al. 2015). A study on wound healing performed on 80 adult female Sprague Dawley rats suggests that BC along with honey show a better result in repairment of wound. It had demonstrated to promote wound contraction and epithelialization in rats (Tanideh et al. 2016).

BC truncated the increase in the gut permeability due to heavy exercise in athletes. In a double-blind cross over study, around 80% of the rise in permeability was reduced due to oral administration of BC 20 g/day (Marchbank et al. 2011). Oral lactoferrin supplementation decreased late onset sepsis and necrotizing enterocolitis in preterm infants. Four clinical trials conducted on 1103 preterm babies presented that oral supplementation of lactoferrin prevented sepsis, which further inhibited the development of long-term brain and lung injuries. Lactoferrin has also shown to enhance the immunity of these preterm infants, which aided in post-injury survival (Pammi and

Abrams 2015). A recent clinical trial by Kshirsagar et al. concluded that colostrum-infused dressings were more effective in wound healing than the conventional wound dressings. Seven-six percent of the patients with colostrum-infused dressings showed early recovery than the conventional wound dressings, where only 48% of the patient displayed early recovery (Kshirsagar et al. 2015). A double-blind, placebo-controlled crossover study deciphered that BC when administered in combination with zinc carnosine showed increase in the epithelial resistance and truncated the gut permeability (Davison et al. 2016).

12.5   Role of BC-Derived Omega-3 PUFA for the Prevention of Cognitive Decline and Neurodegenerative Disorders

Drug therapies that can reduce the threat of cognitive impairment in the diseases like Alzheimer, is the need of the day. Multidomain intervention is required in such conditions as the factors responsible for the diseased conditions are more. In the recent Lifestyle Interventions and Independence for Elderly (LIFE) trial, the authors have reported that beneficial activity of physical exercise did not improve the major mobility disability, which can further treat frailty (Trombetti et al. 2018). Thus, it is very important to modify the cognitive function of the elderly, which can in turn improve the frailty status (Fairhall et al. 2011). The supplementation of omega-3 PUFAs have been reported to have improved the cognitive status in the elderly (Andrieu et al. 2017; Tabue-Teguo et al. 2018). A recent study conducted on children aged 3–17 years diagnosed with attention deficit hyperactivity disorder (ADHD) and autistic spectrum disorder (ASD) suggested the lack of EPA, DHA, and AA. This study correlates the use of omega-3 PUFAs with increase in cognition (Parletta et al. 2016). W-3 FA deficiencies have been reported in patients with mental disorders such as ADHD, schizophrenia (SCZ), depression, and ASD. DHA has also been reported to exert various neuronal functions like neurogenesis, neurotransmission, and oxidative stress protection. Therefore, trials should be conducted in such patients with cognitive impairment.

12.6   Role of Omega-3 PUFA in the Prevention of CVDs

The amount of high-density lipoprotein (HDL) cholesterol rise with the intake of the omega-3 PUFA, which also improves vascular function in turn modulates the blood pressure and heart rate (Innes and Calder 2018). Triglyceride level in plasma can be reduced up to 45% with no omega-3 PUFA in the diet and the effect can be noticed in those with the highest baseline levels (Karalis 2017; Thota et al. 2018). Omega-3 PUFA causes a little rise in the high-density lipoprotein C (HDL-C) level in the body and also leads to small rise in LDL-C level in the body, which is increased in large but less amount of atherogenic particle. Omega-3 PUFA also provides cardioprotective effect by decreasing inflammation, blood pressure (BP), and have positive effect on platelet aggregation and endothelial function. Recent meta-analysis of randomized control trial (RCT) study carried out reported a considerable decrease in the cardiovascular risk in high risk of population and with increase in LDL cholesterol level in the body (Alexander et al. 2017). The recent study of VITAL trial proved that consumption of the 840 mg of the omega-3 PUFA in the age group of $\geq$50 years decreasing the risk of heart attack by 28% and reducing the risk of fatal heart attack by 50. The decrease in the plasma triglycerides without rise in the LDL cholesterol is the effect of the omega-3

PUFA from epidemiological and clinical studies. A decrease in the lipogenesis also decreases the availability of fatty acid for TG production. Significant decrease in TG level is seen in the one who consumed 3–4 g of omega-3 PUFA.

12.7 Antihypertensive Effects of Omega-3 PUFA

Studies have concluded that the consumption of supplement of omega 3-PUFA decreases systolic and diastolic blood pressure (Colussi et al. 2017). The blood pressure is reduced by the mechanism of augmentation of vagal tone, which leads to change in cardiac electrophysiology, improved autonomic function, and improved diastolic filling of cardiac ventricles. The vagal tone effect is very important because results of studies have proposed that consuming fish three times a week lead to decrease in the risk in heart rate by 3 bpm (Mozaffarian et al. 2006). Another possible mechanism of lowering blood pressure could relate to the antagonism of the vasoconstrictive effects of AA obtained prostaglandins and thromboxane (Engler 2017). Prostaglandin such as lipoxins and resolvin gained from EPA/DHA antagonize the vasoconstricting prostaglandins and enhance vascular tone. Omega-3 PUFA appears to decrease the activity of angiotensin-converting enzyme and lead to suppressing production of angiotension-2. Omega-3 PUFA also betters the vasodilatory effects of endothelial nitric oxide (Samuel et al. 2011).

12.8 Anti-inflammatory Effects of Omega-3 PUFA

Eicosanoids and AA derivative are the enzyme, which promote inflammation and which are derived from omega-6 PUFA (Rees et al. 2006). Omega-3 PUFA when consumed reduces the production of eicosanoids, which in turn reduce inflammation, and this effect is observed only when good amount of the EPA/DHA are consumed in the body approximately 2 g/day (Rees et al. 2006). Prostaglandins, which are obtain from EPA and DHA, are called resolvins, which possess potent anti-inflammatory action and has effect on neutrophils, macrophage, and dendritic cell. This anti-inflammatory effect does not have benefit toward more significant inflammation such as IBD and arthritis (Serhan et al. 2000).

12.9 Antiatherogenic Effects of Omega-3 PUFA

The indirect effects of omega-3 PUFA on atherogenesis arbitrate by the advancement of a pro-inflammatory milieu with antagonism of the anti-inflammatory omega-6 PUFA-derived prostaglandins, refinement in vascular tone by expanding nitrous oxide-arbitrate vasodilation, and direct effect of lipid and fish oil on the processes that underlie atherogenesis (Bäck 2017; Calder 2017).

12.10 Role of Flavonoids in CVD Prevention

For almost 12 years, Pozzo and his coworkers performed studies on 1658 individual that were under investigation and shown that higher amount of dietary consumption of the flavonoids resulted in the decrease in the CVD and reduces the risk up to 40–50% of nonfatal CV events

(Koch 2019). Results from numerous studies and randomized control trials (RCT) are indecisive, and the latest meta-analysis carried out by Sarrias and coworkers resulted that the flavonoids have significant effect in blood lipids. Flavanols obtained from apple, tea, and cocoa were proved to have lower the total LDL cholesterol level and significantly increase HDL level (González-Sarrías et al. 2017). Several clinical trials studies done in previous 10 years have committed that catechins possess strong antihypertensive activity and the process involved is controlling of the NADPH production and hampering of RNA expression and MMP-9 in blood patient with hypertension (Bogdanski et al. 2012; Chen et al. 2016). Fifty-six obese and hypertensive patients were under investigation by the studies done by Bogdanski and its coworker, which revealed that the green tea polyphenol are very productive in reducing the systolic and diastolic blood pressure. Catechin, which is another flavonoid, also plays a useful role in safeguarding of hypertension through the increased release of nitric oxide, which is internal relaxing factor, responsible among others, for decreasing blood pressure (Bogdanski et al. 2012).

12.11 Anti-Obesity Effects of Flavonoids

According to Huang et al, about 24 distinct trials were performed until 2013 on obese (overweight) participants, and the results have proved that tea polyphenol have properties to reduce weight (Huang et al. 2014). Studies performed on animals and in vitro have also proven to have beneficial effect of flavonoids obtained from green tea helps in weight reduction by decrease in food consumption, decline of lipid emulsification and absorption, adipogenesis, lipid synthesis suppression, and increase in energy spending via thermogenesis. Increase in fat oxidation and fecal lipid elimination were also confirmed. Commonly consumed food in daily life can also help in reduction in body weight (Nagao et al. 2007).

12.12 Antidiabetic Effects of Flavonoids

Diabetes mellitus is a chronic disease that has become major public health problem worldwide. Nearly 9% of the adult population, which is equivalent to 415 million people, are suffering from diabetes globally, and its treatment is a major medical challenge to date (Jaacks et al. 2016). Many different phenolic compounds have shown antidiabetic effects. For instance, apigenin flavone present in red pepper and lemon has depicted beneficial effects in controlling glucose and lipid metabolism through AMP (5′- adenosine monophosphate)-mediated action. It was observed that AMP activation induced by apigenin is almost 200-folds greater than AMPK (5′- adenosine monophosphate activated protein kinase) when compared to antidiabetic drug metformin. A 4mg/kg/day dose of apigenin administered for seven days showed strong antihyperglycemic effects in mice with streptozocin-induced diabetes (Rauter et al. 2010; Kawser Hossain et al. 2016). When HIT-T15 pancreatic β-cells were exposed to oxidative stress caused by 2-deoxy D-ribose, apigenin showed protective action against β-cells damage. Suh et al. (2012) reported that flavonoids produced significant reduction in intracellular ROS level and increased cell survival and decreased cell apoptosis. It appears that polyphenolic flavonoids like quercetin, myricetin, apigenin, chrysin, and luteolin have wide range of promising therapeutic abilities for the amelioration of diabetes and other NCDs.

12.13 Conclusions

Bovine and human colostrum have multiple beneficial effects in infants and adults. BC lactoferrin has anticancer effects, proline-rich polypeptides and W-3 FAs are neuroprotective and cardioprotective potential, and immunoglobulins boost immunity in children and adults. BC supplements prevent diarrhea in children, cure leaky gut syndrome, and inflammatory bowel disease in adults. A recent clinical trial in infants who were fed BC for three months showed prophylactic effects in the treatment of respiratory infections and diarrhea (Chen et al. 2020). W-3 FAs derived from BC are gaining popularity for the treatment of various chronic disorders. Many preclinical and clinical studies have reported improvement in the cognitive functions with the intake of W-3FAs. Some clinical trials have also shown improvement in the quality of life (QOL) of patients, as well as reduction in mortality (Fairhall et al. 2011).

We have also discussed potential health benefits of flavonoids, as well as treatment of cardiovascular disorders, obesity, and diabetes. No side-effects have been reported following the consumption of flavonoids. However, well-designed, randomized, placebo-controlled, multicenter clinical trials are needed to determine the long-term safety, efficacy, and optimal dose of flavonoids. Studies are also needed to understand the mechanism of action of flavonoids. From our perspective, it seems that BC, W-3 FAs, and flavonoids have a promising potential for developing nutraceuticals for curing NCDs in humans at a cost-effective manner.

Conflict of Interest

The authors declare no conflict of interest.

References

Alexander, D.D., Miller, P.E., Van Elswyk, M.E. et al. (2017). A meta-analysis of randomized controlled trials and prospective cohort studies of eicosapentaenoic and docosahexaenoic long-chain omega-3 fatty acids and coronary heart disease risk. *Mayo Clin. Proc.* 92 (1): 15–29. Elsevier.

Andrieu, S., Guyonnet, S., Coley, N. et al. (2017). Effect of long-term omega 3 polyunsaturated fatty acid supplementation with or without multidomain intervention on cognitive function in elderly adults with memory complaints (MAPT): a randomised, placebo-controlled trial. *Lancet Neurol.* 16 (5): 377–389.

Bäck, M. (2017). Omega-3 fatty acids in atherosclerosis and coronary artery disease. *Future Sci. OA.* 3 (4): FSO236.

Bagwe, S., Tharappel, L.J., Kaur, G., and Buttar, H.S. (2015). Bovine colostrum: an emerging nutraceutical. *J. Complement. Integrat. Med.* 12 (3): 175–185.

Bogdanski, P., Suliburska, J., Szulinska, M. et al. (2012). Green tea extract reduces blood pressure, inflammatory biomarkers, and oxidative stress and improves parameters associated with insulin resistance in obese, hypertensive patients. *Nutr. Res.* 32 (6): 421–427.

Buttar, H.S., Bagwe, S.M., Bhullar, S.K., and Kaur, G. (2017). Health benefits of bovine colostrum in children and adults. In: *Dairy in Human Health and Disease Across the Lifespan* (ed. R.R. Watson, R.J. Collier and V.R. Preedy), 3–20. Academic Press.

Calder, P.C. (2017). Omega-3: the good oil. *Nutr. Bull.* 42 (2): 132–140.

Chen K., Chen H., Luo J. et al. (2020). The prophylactic effect of bovine colostrum on respiratory infection and diarrhea in formula-fed infants: a randomized trial. Research Square. https://doi.org/10.21203/rs.2.20117/v1

Chen, X.Q., Hu, T., Han, Y. et al. (2016). Preventive effects of catechins on cardiovascular disease. *Molecules* 21 (12): 1759.

Cherian, G. (2008). Omega-3 fatty acids. In: *Wild-Type Food in Health Promotion and Disease Prevention* (ed. F. De Meester and R.R. Watson), 169–177. Humana Press https://doi.org/10.1007/978-1-59745-330-1_13.

Cohen, S.M. (2006). Jaundice in the full-term newborn. *Pediatr. Nurs.* 32: 202–208.

Colussi, G., Catena, C., Novello, M. et al. (2017). Impact of omega-3 polyunsaturated fatty acids on vascular function and blood pressure: relevance for cardiovascular outcomes. *Nutr. Metab. Cardiovasc. Dis.* 27 (3): 191–200.

Davison, G., Marchbank, T., March, D.S. et al. (2016). Zinc carnosine works with bovine colostrum in truncating heavy exercise-induced increase in gut permeability in healthy volunteers. *Am. J. Clin. Nutr.* 104 (2): 526–536.

De Almeida, M.F. and Draque, C.M. (2007). Neonatal jaundice and breastfeeding. *NeoReviews* 8: e282–e288.

De Lorgeril, M., Renaud, S., Salen, P. et al. (1994). Mediterranean alpha-linolenic acid-rich diet in secondary prevention of coronary heart disease. *Lancet* 343 (8911): 1454–1459.

Elfstrand, L., Lindmark-Månsson, H., Paulsson, M. et al. (2002). Immunoglobulins, growth factors and growth hormone in bovine colostrum and the effects of processing. *Int. Dairy J.* 12 (11): 879–887.

Engler, M.M. (2017). Role of dietary omega-3 fatty acids in hypertension. *Ann. Nurs. Pract.* 4 (1): 1077.

Enoch, S., Grey, J.E., and Harding, K.G. (2006). Non-surgical and drug treatments. *Br. Med. J.* 332 (7546): 900.

Fairhall, N., Langron, C., Sherrington, C. et al. (2011). Treating frailty – a practical guide. *BMC Mmed.* 9 (1): 83.

Feltrin, K.L., Little, T.J., Meyer, J.H. et al. (2007). Effects of lauric acid on upper gut motility, plasma cholecystokinin and peptide YY, and energy intake are load, but not concentration, dependent in humans. *J. Physiol.* 581 (2): 767–777.

Giansanti, F., Panella, G., Leboffe, L., and Antonini, G. (2016). Lactoferrin from milk: nutraceutical and pharmacological properties. *Pharmaceuticals.* 9 (4): 61.

Główka, N., Durkalec-Michalski, K., and Woźniewicz, M. (2020). Immunological outcomes of bovine colostrum supplementation in trained and physically active people: a systematic review and meta-analysis. *Nutrients* 12:1023. doi:https://doi.org/10.3390/nu12041023.

González-Sarrías, A., Combet, E., Pinto, P. et al. (2017). A systematic review and meta-analysis of the effects of flavanol-containing tea, cocoa and apple products on body composition and blood lipids: exploring the factors responsible for variability in their efficacy. *Nutrients* 9 (7): 746.

György, P., Norris, R.F., and Rose, C.S. (1954). Bifidus factor. I. A variant of *Lactobacillus bifidus* requiring a special growth factor. *Arch. Biochem. Biophys.* 48 (1): 193–201.

Haug, A., Høstmark, A.T., and Harstad, O.M. (2007). Bovine milk in human nutrition – a review. *Lipids Health Dis.* 6 (1): 25.

Huang, J., Wang, Y., Xie, Z. et al. (2014). The anti-obesity effects of green tea in human intervention and basic molecular studies. *Eur. J. Clin. Nutr.* 68 (10): 1075–1087.

Inagaki, M., Muranishi, H., Yamada, K. et al. (2014). Bovine κ-casein inhibits human rotavirus (HRV) infection via direct binding of glycans to HRV. *J. Dairy Sci.* 97 (5): 2653–2661.

Innes, J.K. and Calder, P.C. (2018). The differential effects of eicosapentaenoic acid and docosahexaenoic acid on cardiometabolic risk factors: a systematic review. *Int. J. Mol. Sci.* 19 (2): 532.

Jaacks, L.M., Siegel, K.R., Gujral, U.P., and Narayan, K.V. (2016). Type 2 diabetes: a 21st century epidemic. *Best Pract. Res. Clin. Endocrinol. Metab.* 30 (3): 331–343.

Karalis, D.G. (2017). A review of clinical practice guidelines for the management of hypertriglyceridemia: a focus on high dose omega-3 fatty acids. *Adv. Ther.* 34 (2): 300–323.

Kawasaki, Y., Isoda, H., Tanimoto, M. et al. (1992). Inhibition by lactoferrin and κ-casein glycomacropeptide of binding of cholera toxin to its receptor. *Biosci. Biotechnol. Biochem.* 56 (2): 195–198.

Kawser Hossain, M., Abdal Dayem, A., Han, J. et al. (2016). Molecular mechanisms of the anti-obesity and anti-diabetic properties of flavonoids. *Int. J. Mol. Sci.* 17 (4): 569.

Keenan, T.W. and Patton, S. (1995). The structure of milk: implications for sampling and storage: A. The milk lipid globule membrane. In: *Food Science and Technology, Handbook of Milk Composition* (ed. R.G. Jensen), 5–50. Academic Press.

Koch, W. (2019). Dietary polyphenols—important non-nutrients in the prevention of chronic noncommunicable diseases. A systematic review. *Nutrients* 11 (5): 1039.

Kris-Etherton, P.M., Pearson, T.A., Wan, Y. et al. (1999). High-monounsaturated fatty acid diets lower both plasma cholesterol and triacylglycerol concentrations. *Am. J. Clin. Nutr.* 70 (6): 1009–1015.

Kshirsagar, A.Y., Vekariya, M.A., Gupta, V. et al. (2015). A comparative study of colostrum dressing versus conventional dressing in deep wounds. *J. Clin. Diagn. Res.* 9 (4): PC01.

Lauritzen, L., Brambilla, P., Mazzocchi, A., Harsløf, L. B. S., Ciappolino, V., and Agostoni, C. (2016). DHA effects in brain development and function. *Nutrients* 8.6 doi:https://doi.org/10.3390/nu8010006.

Lewis, E.J.H., Radonic, P.W., Wolever, T.M.S., and Wells, G.D. (2015). 21-days mammalian omega-3 fatty acid supplementation improves aspects of neuromuscular function and performance in male athletes compared to olive oil placebo. *J. Int. Soc. Sports Nutr.* 12: 28.

Marchbank, T., Davison, G., Oakes, J.R. et al. (2011). The nutriceutical bovine colostrum truncates the increase in gut permeability caused by heavy exercise in athletes. *Am. J. Physiol. Gastrointest. Liver Physiol.* 300 (3): G477–G484.

Mattson, M.P. (2015). Lifelong brain health is a lifelong challenge: from evolutionary principles to empirical evidence. *Ageing Res. Rev.* 20: 37–45.

Mozaffarian, D., Gottdiener, J.S., and Siscovick, D.S. (2006). Intake of tuna or other broiled or baked fish versus fried fish and cardiac structure, function, and hemodynamics. *Am. J. Cardiol.* 97 (2): 216–222.

Nagao, T., Hase, T., and Tokimitsu, I. (2007). A green tea extract high in catechins reduces body fat and cardiovascular risks in humans. *Obesity* 15 (6): 1473–1483.

Nagy, K. and Tiuca, I.D. (2017). Importance of fatty acids in physiopathology of human body. In: *Fatty Acids*. IntechOpen.

Neeser, J.R., Golliard, M., Woltz, A. et al. (1994). in vitro modulation of oral bacterial adhesion to saliva-coated hydroxyapatite beads by milk casein derivatives. *Oral Microbiol. Immunol.* 9 (4): 193–201.

Ontsouka, C.E., Bruckmaier, R.M., and Blum, J.W. (2003). Fractionized milk composition during removal of colostrum and mature milk. *J. Dairy Sci.* 86 (6): 2005–2011.

Pammi, M. and Abrams, S.A. (2015). Oral lactoferrin for the prevention of sepsis and necrotizing enterocolitis in preterm infants. The Cochrane Library. *Cochr. Datab. System. Rev.* 2015 (2): CD007137.

Parletta, N., Niyonsenga, T., and Duff, J. (2016). Omega-3 and omega-6 polyunsaturated fatty acid levels and correlations with symptoms in children with attention deficit hyperactivity disorder, autistic spectrum disorder and typically developing controls. *PLoS ONE* 11 (5): e0156432.

Patil, S.U., Deshpande, P.K., Ghongane, B.B., and Rane, S.R. (2015). Assessment of healing potential of colostrum against incisional wound model in mice. *Int. J. Health Sci. Res.* 5 (12): 197–203.

Patten, G.S., Abeywardena, M.Y., McMurchie, E.J., and Jahangiri, A. (2002). Dietary fish oil increases acetylcholine- and eicosanoid-induced contractility of isolated rat ileum. *J. Nutr.* 132: 2506–2513.

Petschow, B.W. and Talbott, R.D. (1991). Response of bifidobacterium species to growth promoters in human and cow milk. *Pediatr. Res.* 29 (2): 208–213.

Rauter, A.P., Martins, A., Borges, C. et al. (2010). Antihyperglycaemic and protective effects of flavonoids on streptozotocin–induced diabetic rats. *Phytother. Res.* 24 (S2): S133–S138.

Rees, D., Miles, E.A., Banerjee, T. et al. (2006). Dose-related effects of eicosapentaenoic acid on innate immune function in healthy humans: a comparison of young and older men. *Am. J. Clin. Nutr.* 83 (2): 331–342.

Samuel, S., Peskin, B., Arondekar, B. et al. (2011). Estimating health and economic benefits from using prescription omega-3 fatty acids in patients with severe hypertriglyceridemia. *Am. J. Cardiol.* 108 (5): 691–697.

Sarker, S.A., Casswall, T.H., Mahalanabis, D. et al. (1998). Successful treatment of rotavirus diarrhea in children with immunoglobulin from immunized bovine colostrums. *Pediatr. Infect. Dis. J.* 7: 1149–1154.

Serhan, C.N., Clish, C.B., Brannon, J. et al. (2000). Novel functional sets of lipid-derived mediators with antiinflammatory actions generated from omega-3 fatty acids via cyclooxygenase 2–nonsteroidal antiinflammatory drugs and transcellular processing. *J. Exp. Med.* 192 (8): 1197–1204.

Simopoulos, A.P. (1991). Omega-3 fatty acids in health and disease and in growth and development. *Am. J. Clin. Nutr.* 54 (3): 438–463.

Stelwagen, K., Carpenter, E., Haigh, B. et al. (2009). Immune components of bovine colostrum and milk. *J. Anim. Sci.* 8: 3–9.

Suh, K.S., Oh, S., Woo, J.T. et al. (2012). Apigenin attenuates 2-deoxy-D-ribose-induced oxidative cell damage in HIT-T15 pancreatic β-cells. *Biol. Pharm. Bull.* 35 (1): 121–126.

Tabue-Teguo, M., de Souza, P.B., Christelle, C.C. et al. (2018). Effect of multidomain intervention, omega-3 polyunsaturated fatty acids supplementation or their combinaison on cognitive function in non-demented older adults according to frail status: results from the MAPT study. *J. Nutr. Health Aging* 1: 1–5.

Tanideh, N., Abdordideh, E., Yousefabad, S.L.A. et al. (2016). Evaluation of the healing effect of honey and colostrum in treatment of cutaneous wound in rat. *Comp. Clin. Pathol.* 26: 1–7.

Terés, S., Barceló-Coblijn, G., Benet, M. et al. (2008). Oleic acid content is responsible for the reduction in blood pressure induced by olive oil. *Proc. Natl. Acad. Sci.* 105 (37): 13811–13816.

Thota, R.N., Ferguson, J.J., Abbott, K.A. et al. (2018). Science behind the cardio-metabolic benefits of omega-3 polyunsaturated fatty acids: biochemical effects vs. clinical outcomes. *Food Funct.* 9 (7): 3576–3596.

Tokuyama, H., Tokuyama, Y., and Migita, S. (1990). Isolation of two new proteins from bovine colostrum which stimulate epidermal growth factor-dependent colony formation of NRK-49f cells. *Growth Fact.* 3: 105–114.

Trombetti, A., Hars, M., Hsu, F.C. et al. (2018). Effect of physical activity on frailty: secondary analysis of a randomized controlled trial. *Ann. Intern. Med.* 168 (5): 309–316.

Williams, F.N., Herndon, D.N., Hawkins, H.K. et al. (2009). The leading causes of death after burn injury in a single pediatric burn center. *Crit. Care* 13 (6): 1.

Yadav, R., Angolkar, T., Kaur, G., and Buttar, H.S. (2016). Antibacterial and antiinflammatory properties of bovine colostrum. *Recent Patents Inflamm. Allergy Drug Discov.* 10 (1): 49–53.

13

Pathophysiology of Diabetes-Induced Complications: Promising Therapeutic Role of Dietary Flavonoids and Flavonoid Supplements in the Management of Diabetic Complications

Ritu Dahiya[1], Harpal S. Buttar[2], and Suresh K. Gupta[1]

[1] *Department of Pharmacology, Delhi Pharmaceutical Science and Research University, New Delhi, Delhi, India*
[2] *Department of Pathology and Laboratory Medicine, Faculty of Medicine, University of Ottawa, Ottawa, ON, Canada*

13.1 Introduction

The term flavonoid is derived from the Latin word "flavus" meaning yellow. A large number of flavonoids have been isolated from fruits, vegetables, flowers, plant stems, herbs, spices, nuts, seeds, green tea, and red wine. Flavonoids are hydroxylated polyphenolic compounds, which possess strong ability for scavenging free radicals. They have received great attention from clinical and basic researchers for their wide range of biological effects, including antioxidant, anti-inflammation, antiaging, anti-atherosclerosis, anticancer, antidiabetic, anti-obesity, immune modulation, and neuroprotective actions. It has been suggested that due to their hypoglycemic effects in diabetes mellitus, the flavonoids have promising therapeutic applications for the prevention and management of diabetes mellitus. Chemically, flavonoids consist of three-ring nuclei (A, B, C), shown in Figure 13.1. The molecular weight of these polyphenolic compounds ranges from 270 to 320 Da (Bagwe-Parab et al. 2019).

Flavonoids are also known for their other pharmacological activities such as antiviral, antibacterial, antiallergic, and so on (Cook and Samman 1996; Testa et al. 2016; Hayat et al. 2017). They have shown antihypertensive activity and neurodegenerative actions (Chebil et al. 2006; Tsuchiya 2010). Flavonoids can inhibit lipoxygenase and cyclooxygenase, platelet aggregation, lipid peroxidation, and capillary permeability (Chebil et al. 2006; Kulkarni and Garud 2015).

13.2 Risk Factors of Diabetes Mellitus

Type 1 diabetes (TID) occur when the insulin-secreting beta cells of the pancreas get damaged or become hypoactive. TID is most common among people <30 years old, and around 10% of people suffer with TID. Since in type 1 diabetes the pancreas makes little or negligible amount of insulin, the glucose entry into the body cells is reduced and energy production is decreased. Patients with type 1 diabetes must use insulin injections to control their blood glucose levels.

In type 2 diabetes (T2D) or adult-onset diabetes, the pancreas produces enough insulin, but the patients become insulin resistant. Ninety percent people suffer from T2D. This type of diabetes

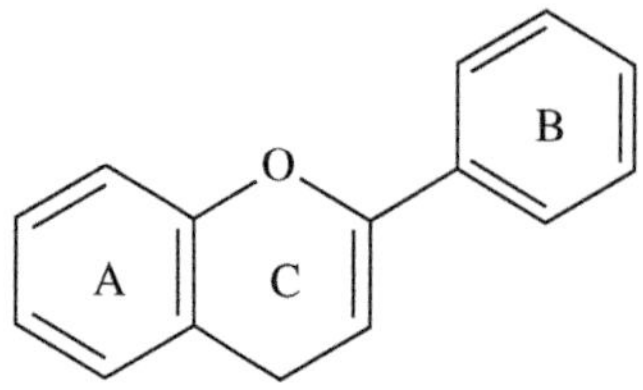

Figure 13.1 Basic ring structure of flavonoids.

mostly occurs in people >40 years old, but can also occur during childhood if risk factors are present. Several studies have shown that T2D can be controlled with a mixture of diet, weight management, and physical exercise.

Other types of diabetes might result from pregnancy (gestational diabetes), surgery, use of certain medications, various illnesses, and autoimmune disorders.

The risk factors for **type 1 diabetes** are still being explored. However, having a family member with type 1 diabetes slightly increases the risk of evolving the disease. Environmental factors and exposure to some viral infections have also been linked to the risk of developing type 1 diabetes.

Several risk factors have been associated with **type 2 diabetes** and include:

- Family history of diabetes
- Overweight
- Unhealthy diet
- Physical inactivity
- Increasing age
- High blood pressure
- Ethnicity
- Impaired glucose tolerance (IGT)*
- History of gestational diabetes
- Poor nutrition during pregnancy

Risk factors for diabetes based on the type of diabetes.

13.2.1 Risk Factors for Type 1 Diabetes

Although the exact cause of type 1 diabetes is unknown, factors that may indicate an increased risk include:

- **Family history.** The risk increases if a parent or sibling has type 1 diabetes.
- **Environmental factors.** Situations such as exposure to viral infection are likely to play some role in type 1 diabetes.
- **The presence of damaging immune system cells (autoantibodies).** Sometimes family members of people with type 1 diabetes are tested for the presence of diabetes autoantibodies. If anyone has such autoantibodies, he/she might have an increased risk of developing type 1 diabetes. But not with everyone who has such autoantibodies develops diabetes.
- **Geography.** Certain countries, such as Finland and Sweden, have higher rates of type 1 diabetes.

13.2.2 Risk Factors of Prediabetes and Type 2 Diabetes

Researchers do not fully understand why some people develop prediabetes and type 2 diabetes and others do not. It is clear that certain factors increase the risk, including:

- **Weight.** The fattier tissue, the more resistant your cells become to insulin.
- **Inactivity.** The less active you are, the greater is the risk. Physical activity helps one to control the weight, utilizes glucose as energy, and makes the cells more sensitive to insulin.
- **Family history.** The risk increases if a parent or sibling has type 2 diabetes.
- **Race.** Although it is unclear why, people of certain races – including black people, Hispanics, American Indians, and Asian-Americans – are at higher risk.
- **Age.** The risk increases as one gets older. This may be due to less physical activity, loose muscle mass, and gaining weight. But nowadays, type 2 diabetes is also increasing among children, adolescents, and younger adults.
- **Gestational diabetes.** If a person develops gestational diabetes in pregnancy, the risk of developing prediabetes and type 2 diabetes later increases. If a baby is born weighing more than 9 pounds (4 kg), the mother is also at risk of type 2 diabetes.
- **Polycystic ovary syndrome.** For women, having polycystic ovary syndrome – a common condition characterized by irregular menstrual periods, excess hair growth, and obesity – increases the risk of diabetes.
- **High blood pressure.** Having blood pressure over 140/90 millimeters of mercury (mmHg) is linked to an increased risk of type 2 diabetes.
- **Abnormal cholesterol and triglyceride levels.** If a person has low levels of high-density lipoprotein (HDL), or "good" cholesterol, the risk of type 2 diabetes is increased. Triglycerides are another type of fat carried in the blood. People with high levels of triglycerides have an increased risk of type 2 diabetes. The doctor will let you know what is the cholesterol and triglyceride levels in your body.

13.2.3 Risk Factors of Gestational Diabetes

Any pregnant woman can develop gestational diabetes, but some women are at a higher risk than others. Risk factors for gestational diabetes include:

- **Age.** Women older than age 25 are at an increased risk.
- **Family or personal history.** The risk increases if the person has prediabetes – a precursor to type 2 diabetes or if a close family member, such as a parent or sibling, has type 2 diabetes. Anyone can be at greater risk if she had gestational diabetes during a previous pregnancy, if delivered a baby with higher weight or if had an unexplained stillbirth.
- **Weight.** Being overweight before pregnancy increases your risk.
- **Race.** For reasons that are not clear, women who are black, Hispanic, American Indian, or Asian are more likely to develop gestational diabetes.

13.3 Economic Cost for Treating Diabetes and Diabetic Complications

Diabetes creates economic stress on people, families, and the health system in contrast to incidence and death. The total cost of healthcare diabetes has been measured at as much as US$825 billion. A study conducted in sub-Saharan Africa reported that the burden of diabetes in the country is equal to 1.2% (or US$19.5 billion) of total gross domestic product (or US$19.5 billion) and might increase by 2030 to around US$35–59 billion. Diabetes care costs are incurred mainly by families by out-of-pocket payments, which might create significant financial distress, especially in low-/middle-income countries. From previous studies in which information from both questionnaire surveys and provider/system analysis, outpatient costs as per-visits and medication costs were US$19 and US$460, respectively (median US$13 and 494); and inpatient costs on average (median US$464) were US$530 (Moucheraud et al. 2019).

The United States and China are among the largest healthcare expenditures on diabetes among all countries around the world. Contrary to each other, the United States had nearly threefold greater expenses on diabetes health care than China did in 2019. Given the fact that these two nations have the greatest expenses with diabetics, but these are not the nations with both the largest expenditure per patient. As of 2019, Switzerland has maximum healthcare prices per diabetic patient.

In 2017, overall global healthcare expenses linked to diabetes were assessed at US$727 billion for people between the ages 20 and 79 years. If the age range is extended to 18–99 years, the figure increases to US$850 billion. By 2045, worldwide expenses on healthcare are predicted to grow by 7% to US$776 billion (20–79 years) and US$958 billion (18–99 years). With an ID (International Dollar) of 445 billion, the North American and Caribbean region had the largest expenses on diabetes in health care (18–99 years), accounting for 52% of the overall amount spent on diabetes worldwide in the year 2017. Additionally, the Europe region (ID 224 billion) and the Western Pacific region (ID 199 billion) accounted for a substantial proportion of overall global investment. The remaining four countries accounted for just 14% of the overall regional diabetes healthcare expenses. Around 6 and 16% of overall healthcare expenditures have been dedicated to diabetes, with the least coming from Africa region with the highest coming from the Middle East and North African countries. The highest investment was in the age group for males 60–69 years (US$127 billion), along with a 7% higher share than for women. Females accounted for higher expenses than men in the 70–79 and 50–59 year sections. This is projected that healthcare expenses for the population under the age of 50 will stay constant until 2045 and will rise by 37% for the community over 70 years due to aging. Mean expenditure on health insurance per citizen was highest in the North American and Caribbean region (ID 8929) and lowest in the South East Asia region (ID 406) (Cho et al. 2018).

13.3.1 Diabetes Treatment Costs in the United States

The overall projected cost of $327 billion in 2017 for diagnosed diabetes covers $237 billion in direct care expenses and $90 billion in lost production.

The key elements of health expenses are as follows:

- In-patient health treatment (30% of gross medical expenses)
- Medicines used to treat diabetes problems (30%)
- The availability of antidiabetic agents (15%)
- Visits to the doctor clinic (13%).

People with confirmed diabetes pay an estimated annual care cost of $16752 of which about $9601 is attributed to diabetes. On average, people with confirmed diabetes had about 2.3 times greater treatment expenses than what cost would be in the lack of diabetes. Treatment for people with developed diabetes contributes to 1 in 4 US dollars in healthcare for the expense groups studied, and over half of the expense is precisely due to diabetes.

Indirect expenses comprise of the following:

- Rising absenteeism ($3.3 billion)
- Increased productivity for the working population while at work ($26.9 billion)
- Lower productivity ($2.3 billion) for those not in employment
- Inability to function due to disability ($37.5 billion)
- Resources wasted due to early death ($19.9 billion; American Diabetes Association 2018).

13.3.2 Regional Economic Burden: Absolute and Relative Global Costs

North America shows the highest absolute costs in 2015 ($499.90 billion [95% CI 478.53–523.03]) and will continue to do so till 2030 in both the baseline ($702.35 billion [670.55–735.94]) and the target scenario ($685.97 billion [654.12–719.44]). Under the past trend's scenario, East Asia and the Pacific region will become the largest contributor to the global economic burden by 2030 (with $796.11 billion [756.97–881.03]). In contrast, while we predict substantial increases in sub-Saharan Africa, the region will remain the smallest contributor to the global economic burden in all scenarios with $36.42 (95% CI 27.1–50.88) to 52.05 billion (38.32–73.47) in 2030 (Bommer et al. 2018).

13.4 Oxidative Stress and Diabetic Complications

Extreme production of reactive species (RS) shows oxidative pressure, which advances pathological conditions in the biological systems. Under normal physiological surroundings, balance exists between the cellular antioxidant defense mechanisms and RS activity, thus retaining the intracellular redox environment. Each change between cellular defense and RS shifts the situation leading to a severe pathological condition (Phaniendra et al. 2015). RS directly attacks different cellular compartments. This may stimulate classical signaling cascades such as cytokines, and protein kinases (Brewer 2011; Nimse and Pal 2015), transcription factors, which leads to inflammatory response activation.

13.4.1 Oxidative-Stress-Induced Pathologies

It is well known that oxidative stress plays a crucial part in the pathogenesis of various acute and chronic diseases (Figure 13.2) (Hassan et al. 2017). Until now, the research and facts have supported the concept of the relation of oxidative stress present in hundreds of clinical conditions (Valko et al. 2005, 2006). Oxidative stress in the kidney has been asserted as the primary cause of diabetic nephroma production (Asadi et al. 2019). Oxidative stress is often involved in the pathophysiology of chronic disease of the kidney (CKD) (Yokozawa et al. 1986).

13.4.2 Oxidative Stress and Diabetic Retinopathy

Enormous studies have demonstrated that ROS plays a vital part in DM issues like diabetic neuropathy, retinopathy, and nephropathy due to changes in the bio-mechanisms involved in microvascular complications (Cecilia et al. 2019).

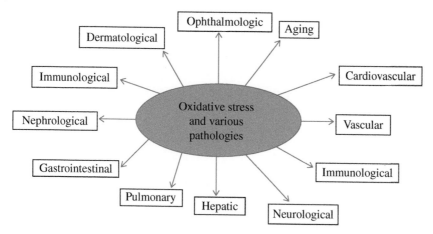

Figure 13.2 Involvement of oxidative stress in various pathologies.

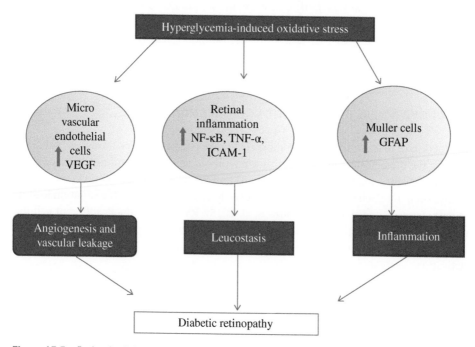

Figure 13.3 Pathophysiology of diabetic retinopathy.

Hyperglycemic conditions promote the stimulation of different pathways, which leads to the development of reactive oxygen species (ROS) by elevated concentrations internally and in the body parts, even at the phase where the antioxidant potential is reached, a condition known as oxidative stress affecting the retinal integrity (Pickering et al. 2018) (Figure 13.3). There are numerous flavonoids that are used in the treatment of diabetic retinopathy (Table 13.1)

Table 13.1 Flavonoids used in the treatment of diabetic retinopathy.

Animal	Model	Treatment	Inference	Outcome	References
Rat	STZ	For 8 weeks, 50–200 mg/kg/day of catechin	Decreased TNF-α, IL-6, IL-1β activation pathway	Anti-inflammation	Wang et al. (2018)
Rat	STZ	For 16 weeks, 100 mg/kg/day of *Morus alba* (mulberry leaves)	Modulation of the polyol pathway Downregulation of caspase-3 and Bax and upregulation of Bcl2	Anti-oxidative, anti-apoptotic, anti-inflammatory	Mahmoud et al. (2017)
Rat	STZ	Reservatrol 5 mg/kg/day, 4 months	Enhanced the degrees of retinas, NF-κB movement with apoptosis rate	Anti-apoptotic and anti-inflammatory	Soufi et al. (2012)
Rat	STZ	Naringenin 50 mg/kg/day, 5 weeks	In the retina of diabetic patients, caspase-3, protein X associated with Bcl-2, B-cell lymphoma 2 (Bcl-2) showed levels in an alleviated manner	Antioxidant anti-diabetic, with antiapoptotic properties	Al-Dosari et al. (2017)
Rat	STZ	Galangin 8 mg/kg BW, 45 days	Galangin results in reduced stimulation of microglial cells, the development of ROS, nuclear factor activation by transcription, and early growth response phosphorylation, and the increased expression of both in vitro and in vivo TNF-α	Antidiabetic and antioxidant activity	Zhang et al. (2019) and Aloud et al. (2017)
Rat	STZ-Nicotinamide	For 45 days, 100 mg/kg of Chyrsin	Increased retinoid binding	Antioxidant	Anitha and Rajadurai (2015)
Rat	STZ	Quercetin 150 mg/kg/day, 20 weeks	Decreases VEGF, MMP-9, MCP-1	Antioxidant, anti-inflammatory	Chen et al. (2017)
Rat	STZ	For 6 weeks, 10–14 mg/kg of Biochanin	Decreases VEGF, IL-1β and TNFα	Anti-angiogenic and anti-inflammation	Mehrabadi et al. (2018)
Rat	STZ	For 12 weeks, 200 mg/kg of Hesperidin	Inhibited degradation of BRB and elevated thickness of the retina, lowered levels of IL-1β, AGE, ICAM-1, TNF-α, VEGF, and glucose in the blood	Anti-inflammatory	Shi et al. (2012)

13.5 Diabetic Cardiomyopathy and Its Pathophysiology

It is characterized by the irregular myocardial function and output in the absence of certain heart disease risk factors in people with diabetes mellitus, like valvular disease, hypertension, and coronary artery disease (Jia et al. 2018). Several mechanisms have been related to the pathophysiology of diabetic cardiomyopathy. Changes in myocardial structure, calcium signaling, and metabolism were identified as early deficits precisely in animal studies and can lead to clinically visible cardiac dysfunction (Boudina and Abel 2010; Jia et al. 2018) (Figure 13.4).

13.5.1 Diabetic Atherogenesis and Cardiomyopathy

Hyperglycemia influences several functions of the diabetic heart; however, the development of reactive oxygen species (ROS) is the underlying factor of adverse tissue remodeling (Kaludercic and Di Lisa 2020). Both initiation of diabetes and the progression of risk-associated symptoms have been linked to ROS and oxidative stress (Giacco and Brownlee 2010). Hence, microvascular complications are associated with exposure to high levels of glucose.

13.5.2 Paleolithic Style Diets in the Prevention of Diabetes and Cardiovascular Diseases

Paleolithic shows the time of Homo genus culture, which begins more than two million years ago since people began cultivating plants (mainly cereal grains) and breeding animals. They acted as hunter-gatherers, consuming wild-animal diets (lean meats, internal organs, with no dairy), with uncultivated plant-sourced diets (mainly apples, non-grains, potatoes, nuts, etc. with no legumes)

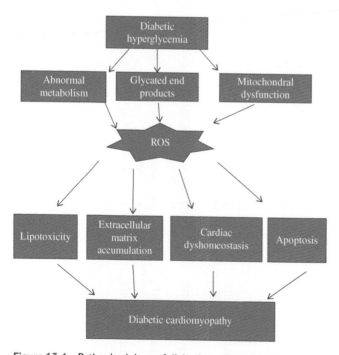

Figure 13.4 Pathophysiology of diabetic cardiomyopathy.

(Klonoff 2009). The Paleolithic diet is an eating pattern that incorporates raw foods from the ecosystem and excludes grains, legumes, and other refined foods. Within the paradigm of the Paleolithic theory, there is a big emphasis on dietary habits, the environmental effects of food decisions, and overall body well-being. The Paleolithic diet encourages ingestion of the following:

- Poultry and meat (with lamb, beef, turkey, chicken, pork [among others])
- Seafood and fish (including salmon, trout, haddock, shrimp, shellfish)
- Eggs
- Vegetables (including carrots, lettuce, onions, spinach, broccoli, tomatoes, peppers)
- Fruits (including bananas, apples, blueberries, pears, avocados, oranges, strawberries)
- Seeds and nuts (including hazelnuts, pumpkin, walnuts, macadamia nuts, almonds, sunflower seeds)
- Fats and oils (including oils of avocado, almond, olive, and coconut)
- Spices including turmeric, garlic, parsley, rosemary (Gupta et al. 2019).

Consuming a Paleolithic-style diet in treatment ($^{1/4}$ 204 intervention group, $^{1/4}$ 202 normal control), a substantial reduction was observed in overall cardiac events and deaths. It was benefited for approximately two years. Twenty-nine of mortality associated with the cardiovascular system was decreased when two servings per week of fish were included in the daily intake (Hristova et al. 2014). In addition to Paleolithic diet, there are various flavonoids that can be used to manage diabetic cardiomyopathy (Table 13.2).

13.6 Diabetic Nephropathy

Diabetic nephropathy is responsible for the failure of the renal system and is across worldwide. The morphologic features involve arteriolar thickening, mesangial extension, interstitial fibrosis, and glomerular hypertrophy. These are all part of microvascular-related complications of diabetes (Testa et al. 2016). Diabetic nephropathy often leads to a gradual decrease in glomerular filtration rate marked by excessive fluid excretion of albumin, glomerular and tubular epithelial hypertrophy, glomerular hyperfiltration, extracellular proteins aggregation, and increased thickness of membrane base (Wang et al. 2019). At a preliminary phase, the first indication is microalbuminuria (appearance of low-level albumin, 30–300 mg/g), accompanying macroalbuminuria (high-level rates, >300 mg/g), progressing to deterioration of renal system and advancement to end-stage renal disease (ESRD) (Dronavalli et al. 2008).

13.6.1 Pathophysiology of Diabetic Nephropathy

Diabetic nephropathy pathogenesis and growth occurs due to associations between metabolic and hemodynamic processes, which are frequently affected in diabetes. The hemodynamic and metabolic irregularities are likely to interfere with each other pathways related to the generation of ROS. Gene regulation and activation of transcription factors are altered due to interactions in the metabolic stimuli with hemodynamic factors. The response of activation including inhibition of different pathways contributes to structural and functional modifications that are clinically expressed as diabetic nephropathy, associated with an increase in albuminuria and reduced renal function (Dronavalli et al. 2008) (Figure 13.5). Numerous studies that have supported the role of flavonoids in diabetic nephropathy are listed in Table 13.3.

Table 13.2 Dietary flavonoid studies done in diabetic animal models.

Animal	Model	Treatment	Result	Effects	References
Mice	STZ	Rutin 60 mg/kg for 12 weeks	Reversed myocardial hypertrophy, with improved extracellular collagen and lipid deposition	Antioxidant, anti-inflammation	Huang et al. (2017)
Rat	STZ	Resveratrol 2.4 mg/kg/day for 8 weeks	Enhances heart efficiency and reduce inflammation of the ventricle with remodeling	Anti-inflammatory	Fiordaliso et al. (2004)
Mice	STZ	Apigenin 100 mg/kg daily for 4 months	Inhibit NF-ÿB translocation and steep-regulate Bax and cleaved-caspase expression 3.	Antioxidant cardioprotective	Liu et al. (2016)
Rat	STZ	*Heracleum persicum* 100–400 mg/kg for 21 days	↓MDA; ↑GSH, CAT and SOD	Antioxidant, anti-inflammatory	Alkan and Celik (2018)
Mice	STZ	Isoquecertin 50–200 mg/kg for 35 days	Reduces the nitrogen content, plasma C-peptides, triglycerides, total cholesterol, and blood urea	Cardioprotective	Wang et al. (2015)
Rat	STZ	Galangin 8 mg/kg for 45 days	The lower level of FFA, cholesterol, PPL, and TG	Antihyperlipidemic	Liu et al. (2019)
Mice	STZ	Scutellarin 24–100 mg/kg/day for 8 weeks	Enhanced nuclear translocation at Nrf2, blocked nuclear translocation at NFKB and improved AKT phosphorylation	Anti-inflammatory antioxidant	Yu et al. (2012)
Rat	STZ	Curcumin100–200 mg/kg daily for 16 weeks	Lower myocardial dysfunction, the stress of oxidation, inflammation and cardiac fibrosis, AGEs accumulation, apoptosis, restoration of phosphorylation of Akt and GSK-3β	Anti-inflammation and antioxidant	Gupta et al. (2015)
Rat	STZ	Genistein 300 mg/kg daily 24 weeks	The administration of genistein to induced animals caused a drop in blood glucose, the amount of expression of proteins, TGF-β1, TNF-α C-reactive protein, and HbA1c	Anti-inflammatory and antioxidant	Chandramohan et al. (2015)
Rat	STZ	Kaempferol 100 mg/kg for 45 days	Glycoprotein concentrations were reduced. It may be due to the formation of the glucose delivery system and even affects the intensity of the insulin binding receptors	Antihyperglycemic	Yu et al. (2017)
Rat	STZ	Gingerol 10 mg/kg for 2 weeks	Decreases BAX, Bcl-2, and caspase-3	Antioxidant and anti-inflammatory	Kashihara et al. (2010)

Note: Downward ↓arrow represents the reduction, and an upward ↑arrow represents an increase.

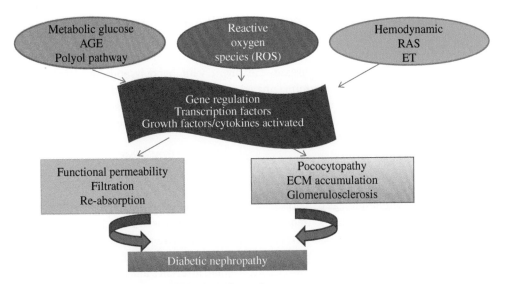

Figure 13.5 Pathophysiology of diabetic nephropathy.

Table 13.3 Results of animal studies done with dietary flavonoids in diabetic nephropathy.

Animal	Model	Treatment	Result	Effect	References
C57BL/6J mice	STZ	Quercetin 10 mg/kg /day for 4 weeks	Diminished polyuria, proteinuria, creatinuria	Antioxidative, antiapoptotic, and renoprotective	Gomes et al. (2015)
Rat	STZ	Kolaviron 100 mg/kg for 6 weeks	Suppresses IL-beta, TNF-α, and IL-1β	Antiapoptotic and antioxidant	Ayepola et al. (2014)
db/db mice	BSO	Cyanidin 10–20 mg/kg for 12 weeks	Reduced renal development of mice α-SMA (α-smooth muscle actin), MMP9 (metalloprotein 9), TGFβ1 (transforming growth factor β 1), fibronectin	Renal protective	Qin et al. (2018)
Rat	STZ	Naringin 20–80 mg/kg for 12 weeks	Restricted oxidative stress by stimulating the antioxidant pathway Nrf2 and by hindering the signaling pathway NF-κB	Anti-inflammation, antioxidant	(Chen et al. (2015)
Rat	STZ	Genistein 25 mg/kg for 8 weeks	Nrf2, HO-1, and NQO1 expression is decreased	Antifibro genic	Jia et al. (2019)
Rat	STZ	Hesperidin 50–150 mg/kg for 10 weeks	Significant rises and regulation of signaling of ARE/Nrf2, synthetase of γ-glutamyl cysteine, p-Nrf2	Anti-inflammatory	Chen et al. (2019)
Rat	STZ	Gingerol 100–400 mg/kg for 6 weeks	Lowe levels of LDL cholesterol, serum glucose, triglycerides, total cholesterol, insulin, phospholipid, and fatty acid	Antioxidant	Li et al. (2012)

13.7   Association Between Diabetes and CNS Disorders

Chronic hyperglycemia causes neurological damage leading to dementia, cognitive dysfunction, and other disorders like Alzheimer's disease. Treatment with hypoglycemia agents prevents neurological-related consequences. Neuroimaging advances have offered further clarity into the physiological and functional effects of diabetes on the CNS (Selvarajah and Tesfaye 2006). It is also associated with different comorbid conditions like fatigue, anxiety, and depression (Mazloom et al. 2013; Butterfield et al. 2014) (Figure 13.6).

13.7.1   Diabetes and Cognitive Impairment

In brain MRI, microvascular damage can present as white-matter hyperintensities (WMHs), cognitive microbes, and lacunar infarcts, frequently known as a disease of cerebral small-vessel disease. WMHs are composition-based defects in the white matter of the cerebral but are associated primarily with perfusion deficits. These are caused due to abnormal structure development of microvascular (modifications of sclerotic in small arterioles and arteries), and activity (impaired control of cerebral blood flow and decreased blood–brain barrier permeability with plasma-fluid leakage). In effect, cerebral microvascular damage is responsible for neuronal cell death, decreased neuronal connectivity, and eventually, brain dysfunction. Dysfunction like dementia may represent diminished cognitive capacity and clinical cognitive disability. In fact, it has been proposed that cerebral microvascular damage leads to depression by affecting the frontal and deep brain structures or their linking mechanisms implicated in the regulation of mood (van Agtmaal et al. 2017; Rensma et al. 2018). Hyperglycemia is responsible for cognitive impairment. It exacerbates BBB breakdown and enhances ROS production, immune response, and Aβ accumulation, contributing eventually to cognitive decline (Uppsala University 2018).

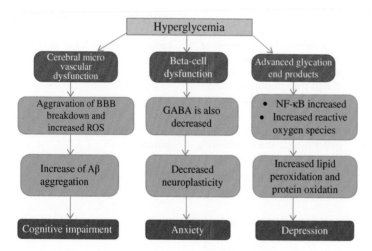

Figure 13.6   Association of diabetes and CNS disorders.

Diabetic rats induced by streptozotocin (STZ) are said to demonstrate deficiencies in cognitive functions, like the output on the Morris water maze (Kamal et al. 2000). Rats diabetes induced by STZ leads to impaired activity of NMDA and glutamate receptors of AMPA (Di Luca et al. 1999) implicated in the learning and memory function. It has been concluded in most animal experiments on diabetes and cognitive function that insulin resistance could lead to a loss of synaptic plasticity and cognitive functions, whereas human research shows cognitive processing could be affected by insulin insensitivity. There is abundant evidence that the neurotransmitter acetylcholine plays a significant role in animal memory control. Also, the neurons with cholinergic involvement in the cortex, hypothalamus, and hippocampus in Alzheimer's disease patients are progressively and exclusively degenerated (Chabot et al. 1997). There are various studies reported supporting the role of flavonoids in the management of diabetes-induced CNS complications in animal models (Table 13.4).

13.7.2 Diabetes-Induced Anxiety and Depression

Anxiety is associated with a human being's emotional aspect and is inherent in nature. It typically strengthens and trains people to face future risks and obstacles, but their chronic and debilitating presence precipitates medical problems recognized as "anxiety disorders." Anxiety was also related to impaired glycemic regulation perceived in diabetic patients. In a survey-based report, it shows that the prevalence of generalized anxiety disorders and subsyndromal anxiety was increased in diabetes relative to those reported in the general population (40% of patients with diabetes have increased levels of stress symptoms). A study showed that clinically relevant anxiety is 20% higher among Americans with diabetes after age regulation, drinking, education, jobs, physical exercise, body mass index (BMI), and socioeconomic status relative to Americans without diabetes. However, GAD and phobia levels are substantially higher in diabetic populations compared with group samples (Thakur et al. 2019).

As the beta cells decline in the amount and depart through the islets as in type 1 diabetes, then GABA is also reduced and hence the beta cells get shielding from GABA. It can degrade and even destroy the remaining beta cells as inflammatory molecules increases in strength (Bickett and Tapp 2016).

Diabetes and depression are two main bidirectional-related infectious illnesses and both propagate like outbreaks in nearly every country across the globe. Co-occurrence in the same case with these two pathologies has significant adverse impacts on the standard of living and reduces the lifespan (Song et al. 2017). There is still compelling evidence increase in the incidence of depression in prediabetic patients and undiagnosed people with diabetes, and a significant rise in diabetic patients diagnosed recently relative to normal adults with glucose metabolism (Bădescu et al. 2016). Previous findings have indicated that about 30% of diabetic patients experience symptoms of depression, which are extremely severe. MDD and diabetes mellitus are associated with elevated stress of oxidation, immune system activity, reduced level of brain monoamine, and impaired synaptic plasticity (Bampi et al. 2020).

Table 13.4 Results of animal models treated with dietary flavonoids in diabetic neuropathy.

Animal	Model	Treatment	Result	Effect	References
Rat	STZ	Curcumin 15–60 mg/kg for 4 weeks	Inhibitory impact on production of TNF-α, IL-1β, and IL-8	Anti-inflammatory	Kulkarni and Dhir (2010)
Rat	STZ	Baicalein 30 mg/kg/day for 4 weeks	↓Oxidative-nitrosative stress and p38 MAPK	↑Nerve conductive velocity	Stavniichuk et al. (2011)
Rat	STZ	Chrysin 30–100 mg/kg for 26 days	↑CAT, SOD, GSH/↓MDA	↑Learning and memory function	Li et al. (2014)
Mice	STZ	Diosmin 50–100 mg/kg for 4 weeks	↓Oxidative stress enzyme activity	↓Glucose level and body weight ↑Nerve function	Jain et al. (2014)
Rat	STZ	Epigallocatechin-gallate (EGCG) 20–40 mg/kg for 7 weeks	↓TBARS and NO ↑SOD	↓Hyperalgesia	Baluchnejadmojara d and Roghani (2012)
Rat	STZ	Hesperidin 25–100 mg/kg, p.o for 4 weeks	↓Free radical generation and proinflammatory cytokines	↓Hyperglycemia and hyperlipidemia ↑Nerve function	Visnagri et al. (2014)
Mice	STZ	Kaempferol 100 mg/kg for 45 days	↓Lipid peroxidation	↓Glucose level	Al-Numair et al. (2015)
Rat	STZ	Luteolin 50–100 mg/kg for 8 weeks	↓Oxidative stress and ChE activity	↓Neuronal injury ↑Cognitive performance	Liu et al. (2013) and Oh (2016)
Rat	STZ	Naringenin 20–100 mg/kg for 8 weeks	↑SOD, CAT, GPx	↓Glucose level ↑NGF, IGF	Hasanein and Fazeli (2014)
Rat	STZ	Proanthocyanidin 250 mg/kg for 24 weeks	↑SOD ↓AGE and MDA	↓Glucose level ↑Nerve conductive velocity	Cui et al. (2008)
Rat	STZ	Puerarin 4–100 nM for 7 days	↓Pain sensitivity	↓Pain sensitivity	Liu et al. (2014)
Rat	STZ	Quercetin 10–40 mg/kg for 8 weeks	Hyperglycemic inhibition and regulation of cytokines of inflammation and stress of oxidative-nitrosative	Neuroprotective	Kandhare et al. (2012)
Rat	STZ	Rutin 5–50 mg/kg for 2 weeks	↑Nrf-2	↓Glucose level ↑Nerve function	Tian et al. (2016)

Note: Downward ↓arrow represents the reduction, and an upward ↑arrow represents an increase.

13.8 Role of Physical Exercise in the Management of Diabetes and Related Disorders

Physical exercise is one of the foundations in the treatment of diabetes mellitus alongside nutrition and treatment since the previous 100 years back (Sigal et al. 2004). Diabetes mellitus, a continuous metabolic illness, is described by an expansion in the blood-glucose level coming about because of a relative insulin insufficiency or insulin opposition or both. As a result, it can prompt glycation of tissues, which continues with metabolic impacts and ends with organ damage. The study focusses throughout the years, detailed that the overall pervasiveness of diabetes mellitus seems, by all accounts, to be expanding alarmingly. It is assessed that 5.4% of all out populace would be influenced by the infection continuously by 2025 as starting reports demonstrated 4.0% in the year 1995. In this way, appropriate administration is ought to be done so as to treat diabetes mellitus (Peirce 1999). Possible mechanisms of exercise include psychological factors, such as increased self-efficacy, a sense of command, distraction, and changes in self-concept, as well as physiological factors such as increased central norepinephrine transmission, changes in the hypothalamic adrenocortical system (Droste et al. 2003), serotonin synthesis and metabolism (Dishman et al. 1997), and endorphins. Regular PA may improve psychological well-being, health-related QOL, and depression in individuals with type 2 diabetes, among whom depression is more common than in the general population (Egede and Zheng 2003).

13.8.1 Types of Exercise and Physical Activity

Aerobic exercise involves repetitive and persistent movement of large muscles (Physical Activity Guidelines Advisory Committee 2008). Activities such as walking, cycling, jogging, and swimming rely primarily on aerobic energy-producing systems. Resistance (strength) training includes exercises with free weights, weight machines, bodyweight, or elastic resistance bands. Flexibility exercises develop a range of motion around joints (Herriott et al. 2004). Balanced exercises benefit posture and prevent falls (Morrison et al. 2010). Activities like tai chi and yoga combine flexibility, balance, and resistance activities.

13.8.2 Benefits of Exercise and Physical Activity

13.8.2.1 Benefits of Aerobic Exercise

Aerobic exercise is the activity that improves oxygen utilization and builds the working of the cardiovascular and respiratory frameworks. Oxygen-consuming activity is a significant helpful methodology for T2DM as it effectively affects physiological boundaries and diminishes the metabolic hazard factors in insulin opposition diabetes mellitus. A few investigations have demonstrated the beneficial outcomes of oxygen-consuming activity dependent on various forces on the improvement of T2DM. Oxygen-consuming activities include swimming, cycling, treadmill, strolling, paddling, running, and bouncing rope (Yamanouchi et al. 1995).

Aerobic exercise leads to increments in mitochondrial thickness, insulin affectability, oxidative chemicals, consistency and reactivity of veins, lung work, resistant capacity, and heart yield (Garber et al. 2011a, b). Moderate to high volumes of high-impact action is related to significantly lower cardiovascular and by and large mortality dangers in both 1 and type 2 diabetes (Sluik et al. 2012). In type 1 diabetes, oxygen-consuming preparation increases cardiorespiratory wellness, diminishes insulin opposition, and improves lipid levels and endothelial capacity (Chimen et al. 2012). In people with type 2 diabetes, normal preparation decreases A1C, triglycerides, pulse, and insulin opposition (Snowling and Hopkins, 2006). On the other hand, high-force span preparing (HIIT) advances the fast improvement of skeletal muscle oxidative limit, insulin affectability, and glycemic control in grown-ups with type 2 diabetes (Little et al. 2011; Jelleyman et al. 2015) and can be performed without crumbling in glycemic control in type 1 diabetes (Tonoli et al. 2012; Dube et al. 2013).

13.8.2.2 Benefits of Resistance Exercise

Resistance exercise induces reasonable glucose control and less insulin obstruction among T2DM. Resistance practices are practices that must be performed against the obstruction. Instances of opposition practices incorporate weight lifting. In contrast to oxygen-consuming activity, obstruction practices are depended on the hardware. High and moderate powers of obstruction practice run between 50 and 75% of 1-repetition most extreme (1-RM) (Boulé et al. 2003). Various investigations have recorded the expected impacts of high-impact preparation have been advantageous in the remedial routine in T2DM patients. Like the oxygen-consuming activity, resistance exercises are helpful devices in the management of T2DM. Obstruction preparing has been accounted to upgrade insulin affectability, day by day vitality use, and personal satisfaction (Poehlman et al. 2000). Besides, obstruction preparing has the potential for expanding muscle quality, lean body, and bone mineral thickness, which could upgrade practical status and glycemic control and aid the anticipation of sarcopenia and osteoporosis (Hurley and Roth 2000; Hunter et al. 2004).

Diabetes is associated with transient risk issues for low muscular strength (Nishitani et al. 2011) and accelerated decline in muscle strength and suitable standing (Anton et al. 2013). The health edges of resistance coaching for all adults embrace enhancements in muscle mass, body composition, strength, physical performance, psychological state, bone mineral density, hormone sensitivity, pressure, lipid profiles, and vas health (Garber et al. 2011a, b). The impact of resistance exercise on glycemic management in one polygenic disorder is unclear (Tonoli et al. 2012). However, resistance exercise will assist in minimizing the risk of exercise-induced hypoglycemia in one polygenic disorder (Yardley et al. 2013). Once resistance and cardiopulmonary exercise are undertaken in one exercise session, playing resistance exercise first leads to less hypoglycemia than once the cardiopulmonary exercise is performed first (Yardley et al. 2012). Resistance exercises for people with kind of polygenic disorder embrace enhancements in glycemic management, hormone resistance, fat mass, pressure, strength, and lean body mass (Gordon et al. 2009).

13.9 Impact of Probiotics in the Management of T2DM

Probiotics are defined as living microorganisms in food and dietary supplements that, upon ingestion in sufficient amounts, can improve the health of the host beyond their inherent basic nutritional content (FAO/WHO 2001). Recently, emerging knowledge suggested that gut microbiota might have a crucial role in the progression and development of T2DM. It had been according that once the microbiome balance is shifted in favor of the unhealthy ones, the amount of metabolic toxin can increase and probably trigger a chronic, inferior inflammation (Zhang and Zhang 2013). Lactobacilli and bifidobacteria are the two most common types of probiotics (Panwar et al. 2013). Probiotics works dynamically by altering the composition of the gut microbiome, thereby maintaining the microbe balance. Some probiotics purport to extend enteral motility, improve enteral barrier performance, stimulate an immune reaction, and modulate inflammatory organic phenomenon within the gut (Senok et al. 2005). Proof from clinical trials suggests that probiotics have a helpful impact on managing canal diseases comparable to irritable internal organ syndrome (Guandalini et al. 2000), looseness of the bowels (McFarland and Dublin 2008), and non-gastrointestinal diseases comparable to allergic diseases (Kalliomäki et al. 2001) and viscus infections in girls (Hilton et al. 1995).

Probiotics have also been reported to reduce blood glucose levels and enhance insulin resistance in rats and humans with diabetes (Yadav et al. 2007; Khalili et al. 2019). Despite the significance of GDM and its effects on maternal and neonatal outcomes, few studies have assessed the effect of probiotics on improving glucose intolerance and insulin resistance, as well as the results of GDM-complicated pregnancies.

13.9.1 Mechanisms by Which Probiotics Boost Glucose Homeostasis

The probiotics-induced improvement in the gut microbiomes in T2DM patients have been linked by some researchers (Larsen et al. 2010; Everard and Cani 2014). It is suggested that the over-growth of certain gram-negative bacteria enhances the risk of T2DM through inflammation path-ways. For example, excessive gram-negative bacterial fragment lipopolysaccharide (LPS) may lead to a leakage of the gut barrier and, as a result, chronic systemic inflammation (Cani et al. 2008; Noble et al. 2017). The gut microbiota may also influence glucose metabolism by modulating the glucagon-like peptide-1 (GLP-1), one of the enteroendocrine peptides produced by L-cell in the gut. The secretion of GLP-1 is associated with a reduction in gastric emptying time and food intake, and an increase in insulin secretion (Tolhurst et al. 2012; Cani et al. 2013). The role of probiotics in improving glycemic control has been investigated in several randomized controlled trials (RCTs). While some trials found that probiotics could lower blood sugar and decrease insulin resistance, the evidence is inconsistent. Previous systematic reviews and meta-analyses have concluded an overall beneficial effect of probiotics in patients with T2DM. However, the literature searches in these systematic reviews do not seem to be comprehensive and the trials included all had a short treatment duration and follow-up period.

13.10 Discussion

Diabetes and the complications of diabetes are particularly common, requiring extra attention to seeking the most appropriate medications. Nature has provided various medications for treating a variety of diseases that involve diabetes since ancient times. Additionally, organic compounds from natural sources have acted as leading components for the creation of novel chemical products that are being transformed into medicines. Plants are an abundant source of complex chemical compounds that are categorized under different phytochemical groups. Flavonoid has historically become one of the most successful sources of phytochemicals with many bioactivities. Studies have demonstrated that various compounds from flavonoid subclasses possess the ability to cure diabetes and control its complications. Discovering its use with various flavonoids and identifying the molecular pathways in diabetic problems for their antidiabetic function and effect can help to establish a stronger treatment plan.

Oxidative stress, commonly observed in diabetic patients, causes the overproduction of highly reactive oxygen species (ROS) and nitrogen species (RNS) from the mitochondrial damage. The unabated overproduction of ROS and RNS can cause damage to the cell membrane and cellular molecules such as proteins, lipids, and DNA. The disturbance in the redox homeostasis not only results in modification of the signaling mechanisms in host cells but also produces detrimental changes in the cell function pathways and production of inflammatory cytokines, consequently resulting in multiple pathological conditions in diabetic patients (Hussain et al. 2016; Oliveira et al. 2018; Kirtonia et al. 2020). Flavonoids and other antioxidants/anti-inflammation diets can play an important role in scavenging the ROS. Thus, the modulation or alleviation of oxidative stress along with lowering of glucose levels in diabetic patients with flavonoids and other hypoglycemic agents and antioxidant phytotherapy, as well as by lifestyle modifications represent a potential strategy in the prevention of diabetes and diabetes-induced complications.

13.11 Concluding Remarks

Exogenous intake of natural bioactive antioxidants can help to maintain the physiological status of cellular antioxidants and consequently prevent the pathogenesis caused by diabetes-induced oxidative stress and excessive production of free radicals. Dietary flavonoids can scavenge free radicals and prevention of cell membrane injury and DNA damage. The clinical and nonclinical studies, as well as some in vivo investigations, provide ample evidence that the polyphenolic compounds present in fruits and vegetables have protective actions to fight diabetic complications. Further clinical studies are needed to establish the long-term safety, efficacy, and dose schedules of flavonoids to prevent and manage diabetic complications. The well-designed, randomized, placebo-controlled, double-blind, and multicenter trials with different bioactive flavonoids will build a stronger foundation for future therapeutic approaches in treating T2DM and its complications.

Conflict of Interest

The authors declare no conflict of interest

References

van Agtmaal, M.J., Houben, A.J., Pouwer, F. et al. (2017). Association of microvascular dysfunction with late-life depression: a systematic review and meta-analysis. *JAMA Psychiatry* 74 (7): 729–739.

Al-Dosari, D.I., Ahmed, M.M., Al-Rejaie, S.S. et al. (2017). Flavonoid naringenin attenuates oxidative stress, apoptosis and improves neurotrophic effects in the diabetic rat retina. *Nutrients* 9 (10): 1161.

Alkan, E.E. and Celik, I. (2018). The therapeutics effects and toxic risk of *Heracleum persicum* Desf. extract on streptozotocin-induced diabetic rats. *Toxicology Reports* 5: 919–926.

Al-Numair, K.S., Chandramohan, G., Veeramani, C. et al. (2015). Ameliorative effect of kaempferol, a flavonoid, on oxidative stress in streptozotocin-induced diabetic rats. *Redox Report* 20 (5): 198–209.

Aloud, A.A., Veeramani, C., Govindasamy, C. et al. (2017). Galangin, a dietary flavonoid, improves antioxidant status and reduces hyperglycemia-mediated oxidative stress in streptozotocin-induced diabetic rats. *Redox Report* 22 (6): 290–300.

American Diabetes Association (2018). Economic costs of diabetes in the US in 2017. *Diabetes Care* 41 (5): 917–928.

Anitha, T. and Rajadurai, M. (2015). Evaluation of biochemical profile of chrysin in streptozotocin-nictonimaide induced diabetic rats. *International Journal of Pharma Bio Sciences* 6 (1): 905–912.

Anton, S.D., Karabetian, C., Naugle, K., and Buford, T.W. (2013). Obesity and diabetes as accelerators of functional decline: can lifestyle interventions maintain functional status in high risk older adults? *Experimental Gerontology* 48 (9): 888–897.

Asadi, S., Goodarzi, M.T., Karimi, J. et al. (2019). Does curcumin or metformin attenuate oxidative stress and diabetic nephropathy in rats? *Journal of Nephropathology* 8 (1): 1–9.

Ayepola, O.R., Cerf, M.E., Brooks, N.L. et al. (2014). Kolaviron, a biflavonoid complex of Garcinia kola seeds modulates apoptosis by suppressing oxidative stress and inflammation in diabetes-induced nephrotoxic rats. *Phytomedicine* 21 (14): 1785–1793.

Bădescu, S.V., Tătaru, C., Kobylinska, L. et al. (2016). The association between diabetes mellitus and depression. *Journal of Medicine and Life* 9 (2): 120.

Bagwe-Parab, S., Kaur, G., Buttar, H.S., and Tuli, H.S. (2019). Absorption, metabolism, and disposition of flavonoids and their role in the prevention of distinctive cancer types. In: *Current Aspects of Flavonoids: Their Role in Cancer Treatment*, 125–137. Singapore: Springer.

Baluchnejadmojarad, T. and Roghani, M. (2012). Chronic oral epigallocatechin-gallate alleviates streptozotocin-induced diabetic neuropathic hyperalgesia in rat: involvement of oxidative stress. *Iranian Journal of Pharmaceutical Research: IJPR* 11 (4): 1243.

Bampi, S.R., Casaril, A.M., Domingues, M. et al. (2020). Depression-like behavior, hyperglycemia, oxidative stress, and neuroinflammation presented in diabetic mice are reversed by the administration of 1-methyl-3-(phenylselanyl)-1H-indole. *Journal of Psychiatric Research* 120: 91–102.

Bickett, A. and Tapp, H. (2016). Anxiety and diabetes: innovative approaches to management in primary care. *Experimental Biology and Medicine* 241 (15): 1724–1731.

Bommer, C., Sagalova, V., Heesemann, E. et al. (2018). Global economic burden of diabetes in adults: projections from 2015 to 2030. *Diabetes Care* 41 (5): 963–970.

Boudina, S. and Abel, E.D. (2010). Diabetic cardiomyopathy, causes and effects. *Reviews in Endocrine and Metabolic Disorders* 11 (1): 31–39.

Boulé, N.G., Kenny, G.P., Haddad, E. et al. (2003). Meta-analysis of the effect of structured exercise training on cardiorespiratory fitness in Type 2 diabetes mellitus. *Diabetologia* 46 (8): 1071–1081.

Brewer, M.S. (2011). Natural antioxidants: Sources, compounds, mechanisms of action, and potential applications. *Comprehensive Reviews in Food Science and Food Safety* 10 (4): 221–247.

Butterfield, D.A., Di Domenico, F., and Barone, E. (2014). Elevated risk of type 2 diabetes for development of Alzheimer disease: a key role for oxidative stress in brain. *Biochimica et Biophysica Acta (BBA)—Molecular Basis of Disease* 1842 (9): 1693–1706.

Cani, P.D., Bibiloni, R., Knauf, C. et al. (2008). Changes in gut microbiota control metabolic endotoxemia-induced inflammation in high-fat diet-induced obesity and diabetes in mice. *Diabetes* 57 (6): 1470–1481.

Cani, P.D., Everard, A., and Duparc, T. (2013). Gut microbiota, enteroendocrine functions and metabolism. *Current Opinion in Pharmacology* 13 (6): 935–940.

Cecilia, O.M., José Alberto, C.G., José, N.P. et al. (2019). Oxidative stress as the main target in diabetic retinopathy pathophysiology. *Journal of Diabetes Research* 2019 (5): 1–21.

Chabot, C., Massicotte, G., Milot, M. et al. (1997). Impaired modulation of AMPA receptors by calcium-dependent processes in streptozotocin-induced diabetic rats. *Brain Research* 768 (1–2): 249–256.

Chandramohan, G., Al-Numair, K.S., Alsaif, M.A. et al. (2015). Antidiabetic effect of kaempferol a flavonoid compound, on streptozotocin-induced diabetic rats with special reference to glycoprotein components. *Progress in Nutrition* 17 (1): 50–57.

Chebil, L., Humeau, C., Falcimaigne, A. et al. (2006). Enzymatic acylation of flavonoids. *Process Biochemistry* 41 (11): 2237–2251.

Chen, F., Zhang, N., Ma, X. et al. (2015). Naringin alleviates diabetic kidney disease through inhibiting oxidative stress and inflammatory reaction. *PLoS One* 10 (11): e0143868.

Chen, B., He, T., Xing, Y. et al. (2017). Effects of quercetin on the expression of MCP-1, MMP-9 and VEGF in rats with diabetic retinopathy. *Experimental and Therapeutic Medicine* 14 (6): 6022–6026.

Chen, Y.J., Kong, L., Tang, Z.Z. et al. (2019). Hesperetin ameliorates diabetic nephropathy in rats by activating Nrf2/ARE/glyoxalase 1 pathway. *Biomedicine and Pharmacotherapy* 111: 1166–1175.

Chimen, M., Kennedy, A., Nirantharakumar, K. et al. (2012). What are the health benefits of physical activity in type 1 diabetes mellitus? A literature review. *Diabetologia* 55 (3): 542–551.

Cho, N., Shaw, J.E., Karuranga, S. et al. (2018). IDF diabetes atlas: global estimates of diabetes prevalence for 2017 and projections for 2045. *Diabetes Research and Clinical Practice* 138: 271–281.

Cook, N.C. and Samman, S. (1996). Flavonoids – chemistry, metabolism, cardioprotective effects, and dietary sources. *The Journal of Nutritional Biochemistry* 7 (2): 66–76.

Cui, X.P., Li, B.Y., Gao, H.Q. et al. (2008). Effects of grape seed proanthocyanidin extracts on peripheral nerves in streptozocin-induced diabetic rats. *Journal of Nutritional Science and Vitaminology* 54 (4): 321–328.

Di Luca, M., Ruts, L., Gardoni, F. et al. (1999). NMDA receptor subunits are modified transcriptionally and post-translationally in the brain of streptozotocin-diabetic rats. *Diabetologia* 42 (6): 693–701.

Dishman, R.K., Renner, K.J., Reigle, T.G. et al. (1997). Activity wheel running reduces escape latency and alters brain monoamine levels after footshock. *Brain Research Bulletin* 42 (5): 399–406.

Dronavalli, S., Duka, I., and Bakris, G.L. (2008). The pathogenesis of diabetic nephropathy. *Nature Clinical Practice Endocrinology and Metabolism* 4 (8): 444–452.

Droste, S.K., Gesing, A., Ulbricht, S. et al. (2003). Effects of long-term voluntary exercise on the mouse hypothalamic–pituitaryadrenocortical axis. *Endocrinology* 144 (7): 3012–3023.

Dube, M.C., Lavoie, C., and Weisnagel, S.J. (2013). Glucose or intermittent high-intensity exercise in glargine/glulisine users with T1DM. *Medicine and Science in Sports and Exercise* 45 (1): 3–7.

Egede, L.E. and Zheng, D. (2003). Independent factors associated with major depressive disorder in a national sample of individuals with diabetes. *Diabetes Care* 26 (1): 104–111.

Everard, A. and Cani, P.D. (2014). Gut microbiota and GLP-1. *Reviews in Endocrine and Metabolic Disorders* 15 (3): 189–196.

FAO/WHO (2001). *Report of a Joint FAO/WHO Expert Consultation on Evaluation of Health and Nutritional Properties of Probiotics in Food Including Powder Milk with Live Lactic Acid Bacteria.* London, ON: World Health Organization and Food and Agriculture Organization of the United Nations.

Fiordaliso, F., Bianchi, R., Staszewsky, L. et al. (2004). Antioxidant treatment attenuates hyperglycemia-induced cardiomyocyte death in rats. *Journal of Molecular and Cellular Cardiology* 37 (5): 959–968.

Garber, C.E., Blissmer, B., Deschenes, M.R. et al. (2011a). Quantity and quality of exercise for developing and maintaining cardiorespiratory, musculoskeletal, and neuromotor fitness in apparently healthy adults: guidance for prescribing exercise. *Medicine and Science in Sports and Exercise* 43 (7): 1334–1359.

Garber, C.E., Blissmer, B., Deschenes, M.R. et al. (2011b). American College of Sports Medicine position stand. Quantity and quality of exercise for developing and maintaining cardiorespiratory, musculoskeletal, and neuromotor fitness in apparently healthy adults: guidance for prescribing exercise. *Medicine and Science in Sports and Exercise* 43 (7): 1334.

Giacco, F. and Brownlee, M. (2010). Oxidative stress and diabetic complications. *Circulation Research* 107 (9): 1058–1070.

Gomes, I.B.S., Porto, M.L., Santos, M.C.L.F.S. et al. (2015). The protective effects of oral lowdose quercetin on diabetic nephropathy in hypercholesterolemic mice. *Frontiers in Physiology* 6: 247.

Gordon, B.A., Benson, A.C., Bird, S.R., and Fraser, S.F. (2009). Resistance training improves metabolic health in type 2 diabetes: a systematic review. *Diabetes Research and Clinical Practice* 83 (2): 157–175.

Guandalini, S., Pensabene, L., Zikri, M.A. et al. (2000). Lactobacillus GG administered in oral rehydration solution to children with acute diarrhea: a multicenter European trial. *Journal of Pediatric Gastroenterology and Nutrition* 30 (1): 54–60.

Gupta, S.K., Dongare, S., Mathur, R. et al. (2015). Genistein ameliorates cardiac inflammation and oxidative stress in streptozotocin-induced diabetic cardiomyopathy in rats. *Molecular and Cellular Biochemistry* 408 (1–2): 63–72.

Gupta, L., Khandelwal, D., Lal, P.R. et al. (2019). Palaeolithic diet in diabesity and endocrinopathies – a vegan's perspective. *European Endocrinology* 15 (2): 77.

Hasanein, P. and Fazeli, F. (2014). Role of naringenin in protection against diabetic hyperalgesia and tactile allodynia in male Wistar rats. *Journal of Physiology and Biochemistry* 70 (4): 997–1006.

Hassan, W., Noreen, H., Rehman, S. et al. (2017). Oxidative stress and antioxidant potential of one hundred medicinal plants. *Current Topics in Medicinal Chemistry* 17 (12): 1336–1370.

Hayat, M., Abbas, M., Munir, F. et al. (2017). Potential of plant flavonoids in pharmaceutics and nutraceutics. *Journal of Biomolecules and Biochemistry* 1 (1): 12–17.

Herriott, M.T., Colberg, S.R., Parson, H.K. et al. (2004). Effects of 8 weeks of flexibility and resistance training in older adults with type 2 diabetes. *Diabetes Care* 27 (12): 2988–2989.

Hilton, E., Rindos, P., and Isenberg, H.D. (1995). Lactobacillus GG vaginal suppositories and vaginitis. *Journal of Clinical Microbiology* 33 (5): 1433.

Hristova, K., Shiue, I., Pella, D. et al. (2014). Prevention strategies for cardiovascular diseases and diabetes mellitus in developing countries: world conference of clinical nutrition 2013. *Nutrition* 30 (9): 1085.

Huang, R., Shi, Z., Chen, L. et al. (2017). Rutin alleviates diabetic cardiomyopathy and improves cardiac function in diabetic ApoEknockout mice. *European Journal of Pharmacology* 814: 151–160.

Hunter, G.R., McCarthy, J.P., and Bamman, M.M. (2004). Effects of resistance training on older adults. *Sports Medicine* 34 (5): 329–348.

Hurley, B.F. and Roth, S.M. (2000). Strength training in the elderly. *Sports Medicine* 30 (4): 249–268.

Hussain, T., Tan, B., Yin, Y. et al. (2016). Oxidative stress and inflammation: what polyphenols can do for us? *Oxidative Medicine and Cellular Longevity* 2016: 1–9.

Jain, D., Bansal, M.K., Dalvi, R. et al. (2014). Protective effect of diosmin against diabetic neuropathy in experimental rats. *Journal of Integrative Medicine* 12 (1): 35–41.

Jelleyman, C., Yates, T., O'Donovan, G. et al. (2015). The effects of high-intensity interval training on glucose regulation and insulin resistance: a meta-analysis. *Obesity Reviews* 16 (11): 942–961.

Jia, G., Hill, M.A., and Sowers, J.R. (2018). Diabetic cardiomyopathy: an update of mechanisms contributing to this clinical entity. *Circulation Research* 122 (4): 624–638.

Jia, Q., Yang, R., Liu, X.F. et al. (2019). Genistein attenuates renal fibrosis in streptozotocin-induced diabetic rats. *Molecular Medicine Reports* 19 (1): 423–431.

Kalliomäki, M., Salminen, S., Arvilommi, H. et al. (2001). Probiotics in primary prevention of atopic disease: a randomised placebo-controlled trial. *The Lancet* 357 (9262): 1076–1079.

Kaludercic, N. and Di Lisa, F. (2020). Mitochondrial ROS formation in the pathogenesis of diabetic cardiomyopathy. *Frontiers in Cardiovascular Medicine* 7: 12.

Kamal, A., Biessels, G.J., Duis, S.E.J. et al. (2000). Learning and hippocampal synaptic plasticity in streptozotocin-diabetic rats: interaction of diabetes and ageing. *Diabetologia* 43 (4): 500–506.

Kandhare, A.D., Raygude, K.S., Kumar, V.S. et al. (2012). Ameliorative effects quercetin against impaired motor nerve function, inflammatory mediators and apoptosis in neonatal streptozotocin-induced diabetic neuropathy in rats. *Biomedicine and Aging Pathology* 2 (4): 173–186.

Kashihara, N., Haruna, Y., Kondeti, V. et al. (2010). Oxidative stress in diabetic nephropathy. *Current Medicinal Chemistry* 17 (34): 4256–4269.

Khalili, L., Alipour, B., Jafarabadi, M.A. et al. (2019). Probiotic assisted weight management as a main factor for glycemic control in patients with type 2 diabetes: a randomized controlled trial. *Diabetology and Metabolic Syndrome* 11 (1): 5.

Kirtonia, A., Sethi, G., and Garg, M. (2020). The multifaceted role of reactive oxygen species in tumorigenesis. *Cellular and Molecular Life Sciences* 77 (22): 1–25.

Klonoff, D.C. (2009). The beneficial effects of a paleolithic diet on type 2 diabetes and other risk factors for cardiovascular disease. *Journal of Diabetes Science and Technology* 3 (6): 1229–1232.

Kulkarni, S.K. and Dhir, A. (2010). An overview of curcumin in neurological disorders. *Indian Journal of Pharmaceutical Sciences* 72 (2): 149.

Kulkarni, Y.A. and Garud, M.S. (2015). Effect of *Bauhinia variegata* Linn. (Caesalpiniaceae) extract in streptozotocin induced type I diabetic rats. *Oriental Pharmacy and Experimental Medicine* 15 (3): 191–198.

Larsen, N., Vogensen, F.K., Van Den Berg, F.W. et al. (2010). Gut microbiota in human adults with type 2 diabetes differs from non-diabetic adults. *PloS One* 5 (2): e9085.

Li, Y., Tran, V.H., Duke, C.C. et al. (2012). Preventive and protective properties of *Zingiber officinale* (ginger) in diabetes mellitus, diabetic complications, and associated lipid and other metabolic disorders: a brief review. *Evidence-based Complementary and Alternative Medicine* 2012 (11): 516870.

Li, R., Zang, A., Zhang, L. et al. (2014). Chrysin ameliorates diabetes-associated cognitive deficits in Wistar rats. *Neurological Sciences* 35 (10): 1527–1532.

Little, J.P., Gillen, J.B., Percival, M.E. et al. (2011). Low-volume high-intensity interval training reduces hyperglycemia and increases muscle mitochondrial capacity in patients with type 2 diabetes. *Journal of Applied Physiology* 111 (6): 1554–1560.

Liu, Y., Tian, X., Gou, L. et al. (2013). Luteolin attenuates diabetes-associated cognitive decline in rats. *Brain Research Bulletin* 94: 23–29.

Liu, M., Liao, K., Yu, C. et al. (2014). Puerarin alleviates neuropathic pain by inhibiting neuroinflammation in spinal cord. *Mediators of Inflammation* 2014 (8): 485927.

Liu, H., Yang, Z., Deng, W. et al. (2016). GW27-e0367 Apigenin attenuates the cardiac remodeling in experimental diabetic cardiomyopathy. *Journal of the American College of Cardiology* 68 (16 Supplement): C14.

Liu, Y., Wang, J., Zhang, X. et al. (2019). Scutellarin exerts hypoglycemic and renal protective effects in db/db mice via the Nrf2/HO-1 signaling pathway. *Oxidative Medicine and Cellular Longevity* 2019: 1354345.

Mahmoud, A.M., El-Twab, S.M.A., and Abdel-Reheim, E.S. (2017). Consumption of polyphenolrich Morus alba leaves extract attenuates early diabetic retinopathy: the underlying mechanism. *European Journal of Nutrition* 56 (4): 1671–1684.

Mazloom, Z., Ekramzadeh, M., and Hejazi, N. (2013). Efficacy of supplementary vitamins C and E on anxiety, depression and stress in type 2 diabetic patients: a randomized, single-blind, placebo-controlled trial. *Pakistan Journal of Biological Sciences* 16 (22): 1597–1600.

McFarland, L.V. and Dublin, S. (2008). Meta-analysis of probiotics for the treatment of irritable bowel syndrome. *World Journal of Gastroenterology: WJG* 14 (17): 2650.

Mehrabadi, M.E., Salemi, Z., Babaie, S. et al. (2018). Effect of biochanin A on retina levels of vascular endothelial growth factor, tumor necrosis factor-alpha and interleukin-1beta in rats with streptozotocin-induced diabetes. *Canadian Journal of Diabetes* 42 (6): 639–644.

Morrison, S., Colberg, S.R., Mariano, M. et al. (2010). Balance training reduces falls risk in older individuals with type 2 diabetes. *Diabetes Care* 33 (4): 748–750.

Moucheraud, C., Lenz, C., Latkovic, M. et al. (2019). Cholinergic system during the progression of Alzheimer's disease: therapeutic implications. *Expert Review of Neurotherapeutics* 8 (11): 1703–1718.

Nimse, S.B. and Pal, D. (2015). Free radicals, natural antioxidants, and their reaction mechanisms. *Pharmacognosy Reviews* 5: 27986–28006.

Nishitani, M., Shimada, K., Sunayama, S. et al. (2011). Impact of diabetes on muscle mass, muscle strength, and exercise tolerance in patients after coronary artery bypass grafting. *Journal of Cardiology* 58 (2): 173–180.

Noble, E.E., Hsu, T.M., and Kanoski, S.E. (2017). Gut to brain dysbiosis: mechanisms linking western diet consumption, the microbiome, and cognitive impairment. *Frontiers in Behavioral Neuroscience* 11: 9.

Oh, Y.S. (2016). Bioactive compounds and their neuroprotective effects in diabetic complications. *Nutrients* 8 (8): 472.

Oliveira, J.S.S.D., Santos, G.D.S., Moraes, J.A. et al. (2018). Reactive oxygen species generation mediated by NADPH oxidase and PI3K/Akt pathways contribute to invasion of Streptococcus agalactiae in human endothelial cells. *Memórias do Instituto Oswaldo Cruz* 113 (6): e140421.

Panwar, H., Rashmi, H.M., Batish, V.K., and Grover, S. (2013). Probiotics as potential biotherapeutics in the management of type 2 diabetes – prospects and perspectives. *Diabetes/Metabolism Research and Reviews* 29 (2): 103–112.

Peirce, N.S. (1999). Diabetes and exercise. *British Journal of Sports Medicine* 33 (3): 161–172.

Phaniendra, A., Jestadi, D.B., and Periyasamy, L. (2015). Free radicals: properties, sources, targets, and their implication in various diseases. *Indian Journal Clinical Biochemicals* 30 (1): 11–26.

Physical Activity Guidelines Advisory Committee (2008). *Physical Activity Guidelines Advisory Committee Report*. Washington, DC: US Department of Health and Human Services. Google Scholar.

Pickering, R.J., Rosado, C.J., Sharma, A. et al. (2018). Recent novel approaches to limit oxidative stress and inflammation in diabetic complications. *Clinical and Translational Immunology* 7 (4): e1016.

Poehlman, E.T., Dvorak, R.V., DeNino, W.F. et al. (2000). Effects of resistance training and endurance training on insulin sensitivity in nonobese, young women: a controlled randomized trial. *The Journal of Clinical Endocrinology and Metabolism* 85 (7): 2463–2468.

Qin, Y., Zhai, Q., Li, Y. et al. (2018). Cyanidin-3-*O*-glucoside ameliorates diabetic nephropathy through regulation of glutathione pool. *Biomedicine and Pharmacotherapy* 103: 1223–1230.

Rensma, S.P., van Sloten, T.T., Launer, L.J. et al. (2018). Cerebral small vessel disease and risk of incident stroke, dementia and depression, and all-cause mortality: a systematic review and meta-analysis. *Neuroscience and Biobehavioral Reviews* 90: 164–173.

Selvarajah, D. and Tesfaye, S. (2006). Central nervous system involvement in diabetes mellitus. *Current Diabetes Reports* 6 (6): 431–438.

Senok, A.C., Ismaeel, A.Y., and Botta, G.A. (2005). Probiotics: facts and myths. *Clinical Microbiology and Infection* 11 (12): 958–966.

Shi, X., Liao, S., Mi, H. et al. (2012). Hesperidin prevents retinal and plasma abnormalities in streptozotocin-induced diabetic rats. *Molecules* 17 (11): 12868–12881.

Sigal, R.J., Kenny, G.P., Wasserman, D.H., and Castaneda-Sceppa, C. (2004). Physical activity/exercise and type 2 diabetes. *Diabetes Care* 27 (10): 2518–2539.

Sluik, D., Buijsse, B., Muckelbauer, R. et al. (2012). Physical activity and mortality in individuals with diabetes mellitus: a prospective study and meta-analysis. *Archives of Internal Medicine* 172 (17): 1285–1295.

Snowling, N.J. and Hopkins, W.G. (2006). Effects of different modes of exercise training on glucose control and risk factors for complications in type 2 diabetic patients: a meta-analysis. *Diabetes Care* 29 (11): 2518–2527.

Song, J., Whitcomb, D.J., and Kim, B.C. (2017). The role of melatonin in the onset and progression of type 3 diabetes. *Molecular Brain* 10 (1): 35.

Soufi, F.G., Mohammad-nejad, D., and Ahmadieh, H. (2012). Resveratrol improves diabetic retinopathy possibly through oxidative stress – nuclear factor κb – apoptosis pathway. *Pharmacological Reports* 64 (6): 1505–1514.

Stavniichuk, R., Drel, V.R., Shevalye, H. et al. (2011). Baicalein alleviates diabetic peripheral neuropathy through inhibition of oxidative–nitrosative stress and p38 MAPK activation. *Experimental Neurology* 230 (1): 106–113.

Testa, R., Bonfigli, A.R., Genovese, S. et al. (2016). The possible role of flavonoids in the prevention of diabetic complications. *Nutrients* 8 (5): 310.

Thakur, A.K., Tyagi, S., and Shekhar, N. (2019). Comorbid brain disorders associated with diabetes: therapeutic potentials of prebiotics, probiotics and herbal drugs. *Translational Medicine Communications* 4 (1): 12.

Tian, R., Yang, W., Xue, Q. et al. (2016). Rutin ameliorates diabetic neuropathy by lowering plasma glucose and decreasing oxidative stress via Nrf2 signaling pathway in rats. *European Journal of Pharmacology* 771: 84–92.

Tolhurst, G., Heffron, H., Lam, Y.S. et al. (2012). Short-chain fatty acids stimulate glucagon-like peptide-1 secretion via the G-protein-coupled receptor FFAR2. *Diabetes* 61 (2): 364–371.

Tonoli, C., Heyman, E., Roelands, B. et al. (2012). Effects of different types of acute and chronic (training) exercise on glycaemic control in type 1 diabetes mellitus. *Sports Medicine* 42 (12): 1059–1080.

Tsuchiya, H. (2010). Structure-dependent membrane interaction of flavonoids associated with their bioactivity. *Food Chemistry* 120 (4): 1089–1096.

Uppsala University (2018). *The Relevance of GABA for Diabetes*. ScienceDaily.

Valko, M., Morris, H., and Cronin, M.T.D. (2005). Metals, toxicity and oxidative stress. *Current Medicinal Chemistry* 12: 1161–1209.

Valko, M., Rhodes, C.J., Moncol, J. et al. (2006). Free radicals, metals and antioxidants in oxidative stress-induced cancer. Chemico--Biological. *Chemico-Biological Interactions* 160: 1–40.

Visnagri, A., Kandhare, A.D., Chakravarty, S. et al. (2014). Hesperidin, a flavanoglycone attenuates experimental diabetic neuropathy via modulation of cellular and biochemical marker to improve nerve functions. *Pharmaceutical Biology* 52 (7): 814–828.

Wang, T., Li, X., Zhou, B. et al. (2015). Anti-diabetic activity in type 2 diabetic mice and α-glucosidase inhibitory, antioxidant and anti-inflammatory potential of chemically profiled pear peel and pulp extracts (*Pyrus* spp.). *Journal of Functional Foods* 13: 276–288.

Wang, W., Zhang, Y., Jin, W. et al. (2018). Catechin weakens diabetic retinopathy by inhibiting the expression of NF-κB signaling pathway-mediated inflammatory factors. *Annals of Clinical and Laboratory Science* 48 (5): 594–600.

Wang, L.P., Gao, Y.Z., Song, B. et al. (2019). MicroRNAs in the progress of diabetic nephropathy: a systematic review and meta-analysis. *Evidence-Based Complementary and Alternative Medicine* 2019 (12): 3513179.

Yadav, H., Jain, S., and Sinha, P.R. (2007). Antidiabetic effect of probiotic dahi containing Lactobacillus acidophilus and Lactobacillus case in high fructose fed rats. *Nutrition* 23 (1): 62–68.

Yamanouchi, K., Shinozaki, T., Chikada, K. et al. (1995). Daily walking combined with diet therapy is a useful means for obese NIDDM patients not only to reduce body weight but also to improve insulin sensitivity. *Diabetes Care* 18 (6): 775–778.

Yardley, J.E., Kenny, G.P., Perkins, B.A. et al. (2012). Effects of performing resistance exercise before versus after aerobic exercise on glycemia in type 1 diabetes. *Diabetes Care* 35 (4): 669–675.

Yardley, J.E., Kenny, G.P., Perkins, B.A. et al. (2013). Resistance versus aerobic exercise: acute effects on glycemia in type 1 diabetes. *Diabetes Care* 36 (3): 537–542.

Yokozawa, T., Zheng, P.D., Oura, H. et al. (1986). Animal model of adenine induced chronic renal failure in rats. *Nephron* 44: 230–234.

Yu, W., Wu, J., Cai, F. et al. (2012). Curcumin alleviates diabetic cardiomyopathy in experimental diabetic rats. *PloS Oone* 7 (12): e52013.

Yu, L.Y., Shi, W.L., and Xin-Gui, G. (2017). Cardio-protective role of gingerol along with prominent anti-diabetic cardiomyopathy action in a streptozotocin-induced diabetes mellitus rat model. *Cell Journal (Yakhteh)* 19 (3): 469.

Zhang, Y. and Zhang, H. (2013). Microbiota associated with type 2 diabetes and its related complications. *Food Science and Human Wellness* 2 (3–4): 167–172.

Zhang, T., Mei, X., Ouyang, H. et al. (2019). Natural flavonoid galangin alleviates microglia-trigged blood–retinal barrier dysfunction during the development of diabetic retinopathy. *The Journal of Nutritional Biochemistry* 65: 1–1.

Index